Steroids and the Nervous System

Steroids and the Nervous System

Editor: Cristin Roth

AMERICAN
MEDICAL PUBLISHERS
www.americanmedicalpublishers.com

AMERICAN
MEDICAL PUBLISHERS
www.americanmedicalpublishers.com

Cataloging-in-Publication Data

Steroids and the nervous system / edited by Cristin Roth.
p. cm.
Includes bibliographical references and index.
ISBN 979-8-88740-474-5
1. Steroid drugs. 2. Neurohormones. 3. Steroid hormones. 4. Neurohormones--Physiological effect.
5. Steroid hormones--Physiological effect. 6. Steroids. 7. Nervous system. I. Roth, Cristin.
RM297.S74 S74 2023
615.36--dc23

American Medical Publishers,
41 Flatbush Avenue,
1st Floor, New York,
NY 11217, USA

ISBN 979-8-88740-474-5 (Hardback)

Contents

Preface

A biologically active organic compound with four rings arranged in a specific molecular configuration is termed as a steroid. Steroid hormones are essential for cell life and they affect the neuroendocrine and behavioral functions in humans. Steroids perform two main biological functions. The first function is that they form an essential part of cell membranes which alters the membrane fluidity. The second function is signal transduction or cell signaling that facilitates cellular response. During early development, steroids regulate the activity and plasticity of neurons and the glial cells. They continue to exert trophic and protective effects on the adult nervous system. Steroids are synthesized by the gonads and adrenal glands, and are transmitted to the brain, spinal cord and the peripheral nerves through the bloodstream. Neurosteroids such as pregnenolone, progesterone, dehydroepiandrosterone and sulfate esters are produced within the nervous system. This book unravels the recent studies related to the importance of steroids in the nervous system. The topics covered herein are of utmost significance and bound to provide incredible insights to the readers. Through this book, we attempt to further enlighten the readers about the new concepts in this field of study.

This book is the end result of constructive efforts and intensive research done by experts in this field. The aim of this book is to enlighten the readers with recent information in this area of research. The information provided in this profound book would serve as a valuable reference to students and researchers in this field.

At the end, I would like to thank all the authors for devoting their precious time and providing their valuable contribution to this book. I would also like to express my gratitude to my fellow colleagues who encouraged me throughout the process.

Editor

Analysis of Clinical Characteristics and Poor Prognostic Predictors in Patients with an Initial Diagnosis of Autoimmune Encephalitis

Xiaowei Qiu[1,2†], Haiqing Zhang[3†], Dongxu Li[1,2], Jing Wang[4], Zhigang Jiang[5], Yuanzhong Zhou[5], Ping Xu[1], Jun Zhang[1], Zhanhui Feng[6], Changyin Yu[1,2] and Zucai Xu[1,2*]*

[1] Department of Neurology, Affiliated Hospital of Zunyi Medical University, Guizhou, China, [2] Key Laboratory of Brain Science, Zunyi Medical University, Guizhou, China, [3] Department of Neurology, The First Affiliated Hospital of Chongqing Medical University, Chongqing, China, [4] Department of Preventive Health Care, Affiliated Hospital of Zunyi Medical University, Guizhou, China, [5] School of Public Health, Zunyi Medical University, Guizhou, China, [6] Department of Neurology, Affiliated Hospital of Guizhou Medical University, Guizhou, China

***Correspondence:**
Changyin Yu
yuchangyin68@163.com
Zucai Xu
docxzc@126.com

†These authors have contributed equally to this work

Purpose: We aimed to retrospectively analyze the clinical features, laboratory and imaging results, and predictors of poor prognosis for patients with an initial diagnosis of autoimmune encephalitis (AE) at the Affiliated Hospital of Zunyi Medical University.

Methods: Fifty patients with an initial diagnosis of AE who were admitted to our hospital from May 2014 to May 2018 were enrolled retrospectively. Clinical characteristics and experimental test data, including the neutrophil-to-lymphocyte ratio (NLR), were collected from medical records within 24 h of admission. Independent prognostic factors were determined by multivariate logistic regression analysis. A good or poor prognosis for patients was defined based on the modified Rankin Scale (mRS). The correlation between the immunotherapy latency and prognostic mRS score was determined using the Spearman rank correlation test.

Results: Univariate analysis indicated that increased NLR ($P = 0.001$), decreased lymphocyte counts ($P = 0.001$), low serum albumin ($P = 0.017$), consciousness disorders ($P = 0.001$), epileptic seizures ($P = 0.007$), extrapyramidal symptoms ($P = 0.042$), abnormal electroencephalogram (EEG) findings ($P = 0.001$), abnormal brain magnetic resonance imaging (MRI) findings ($P = 0.003$), and pulmonary infection complications ($P = 0.000$) were associated with the poor prognosis of AE. Multivariate logistic regression analysis showed that NLR (odds ratio [OR] 2.169, 95% confidence interval [CI] 1.029–4.570; $P < 0.05$) was an independent risk factor for predicting the poor prognosis of AE. NLR > 4.45 was suggested as the cut-off threshold for predicting the adverse outcomes of AE. In addition, we revealed that there was a positive correlation between immunotherapy latency and mRS score ($r_s = 0.535$, $P < 0.05$).

Conclusions: NLR may have predictive value for the poor outcomes of AE. Early initiation of immunotherapy is associated with a good prognosis.

Keywords: autoimmune encephalitis, predictor, neutrophil-to-lymphocyte ratio, immunotherapy, modified Rankin Scale, prognosis

INTRODUCTION

Autoimmune encephalitis (AE) is a severe inflammatory disorder of the brain that is mediated by autoimmune mechanisms and characterized by prominent neuropsychiatric symptoms. AE, which is thought to be associated with antibodies against neuronal cell-surface proteins, ion channels, or receptors (1), accounts for about 20% of all adult encephalitis cases (2). Typical clinical manifestations include epileptic seizures, psychiatric and behavioral disorders, decreased levels of consciousness, memory and cognitive impairment, extrapyramidal symptoms, and central hypoventilation (3, 4). Since the discovery of anti-N-methyl-D-aspartate receptor (anti-NMDAR) antibodies by Dalmau et al. (5), more than a dozen new types of autoantibodies have been identified (6). Anti-NMDAR encephalitis is the most common type of AE, followed by anti-leucine-rich glioma-inactivated 1 (anti-LGI1) encephalitis (7) and anti-γ-aminobutyric acid B receptor (anti-$GABA_BR$) encephalitis. Other types of antibodies include anti-contactin-associated protein-like 2 (anti-CASPR2) antibody and anti-α-amino-3-hydroxy-5-methyl-4-isoxazole propionate receptor (anti-AMPAR) antibody. The presence of corresponding autoantibodies contributes to diagnosis; however, because existing criteria for AE rely on antibody testing and the response to immunotherapy, delays in diagnosis, and missed diagnosis of antibody-negative patients can occur (8). A clinical approach to the diagnosis of AE was put forward jointly by international experts, providing a basis for the early diagnosis of this disease (8). In addition, AE is a severe neurological disorder that is characterized by complicated clinical manifestations and frequent complications. Some cases are associated with tumors. Immunotherapy, intensive care unit (ICU) support, and multidisciplinary treatments can be combined to mitigate the disease (9). At present, the efficacy of immunotherapy and factors that affect patients' poor prognosis have not been determined. Thus, research on the prognostic factors of AE has great clinical and social significance.

AE is recognized as a chronic autoimmune disease characterized by the presence of antigen-specific antibodies in serum and cerebrospinal fluid (CSF) resulting from dysfunction of the immune system regulation and persistent inflammation (10). The neutrophil-to-lymphocyte ratio (NLR) is a commonly used and very significant systemic inflammation biomarker. NLR is calculated as the absolute count of neutrophils divided by the absolute count of lymphocytes (11). Moreover, NLR has been suggested as a marker for the general immune response to various stress stimuli. Prior studies have shown that increased NLR is a prognostic marker in patients with various cancers, including pancreatic cancer, lung cancer, gastric cancer, hepatocellular carcinoma, prostate cancer, and malignant mesothelioma (12–16). In addition, several reports have demonstrated that altered NLR has prognostic value in diabetes mellitus, hypertension, acute myocardial infarction, cerebrovascular disease, peripheral arterial disease, and chronic kidney disease (17–20). Recent studies have also shown that an abnormal NLR level is associated with some autoimmune diseases (21, 22). However, to our knowledge, the relationship between NLR and AE has not been studied so far. Therefore, in this study, we evaluated the association between NLR and prognosis in AE patients and whether NLR is an independent risk factor for predicting the poor prognosis of AE.

METHODS

Research Subjects

This retrospective study complied with the recommendations of the Ethics Committee of Affiliated Hospital of Zunyi Medical University. The protocol was approved by the Ethics Committee of Affiliated Hospital of Zunyi Medical University. All patients or their relatives were informed of the study and signed written informed consent in accordance with the Declaration of Helsinki. We reviewed all the medical records of patients with an initial diagnosis of AE admitted to the Department of Neurology, Affiliated Hospital of Zunyi Medical University, from May 2014 to May 2018. We reassessed the diagnosis basis and followed up with patients by telephone every 3 months after discharge. The inclusion criteria were based on the clinical diagnostic criteria for AE suggested by Mittal and Graus in 2016. Patients were categorized as "definite," "probable," or "possible" according to the adapted criteria (8). The diagnostic criteria for the "definite" group were the detection of antibodies against neuronal membrane or synaptic proteins in CSF and/or serum. Autoantibody-negative but "probable" AE did not meet the diagnostic criteria of the "definite" group but fulfilled all four other criteria supporting AE. Correspondingly, the following exclusion criteria were considered: other acute neurological diseases found during follow-up; not meeting the clinical diagnostic criteria for AE; loss to follow-up; other autoimmune diseases; and incomplete clinical data.

Data Collection

The following basic clinical data were collected: age at onset, sex, clinical manifestations, interval from onset to admission, immunotherapy latency (the time interval from onset to the initiation of immunotherapy), prodromal symptoms, pulmonary infection complications, treatment methods, and hospital stay. In addition, cranial magnetic resonance imaging (MRI) findings, electroencephalogram (EEG) data, laboratory tests, CSF examination (pressure, white blood cell [WBC] counts, and protein, glucose and chloride levels), and autoantibody tests of serum and CSF were reviewed from medical records and electronic databases. The laboratory tests included the following: WBC counts, neutrophil counts, lymphocyte counts, platelet counts, NLR, and the levels of hemoglobin, sodium (Na), potassium (K), chlorine (Cl), calcium (Ca), and albumin. These experimental examinations were recorded within 24 h of admission. NLR was defined as a simple ratio between the absolute neutrophil count and the absolute lymphocyte count. Laboratory tests except NLR were divided into low, normal, and high values based on reference intervals.

Based on previous reports on AE (3), the main symptoms were divided into the following categories: consciousness disorders; epileptic seizures; mental and psychiatric and behavior disorders; and extrapyramidal symptoms. The inflammatory CSF needed to meet at least 2 of the following criteria: an increase in

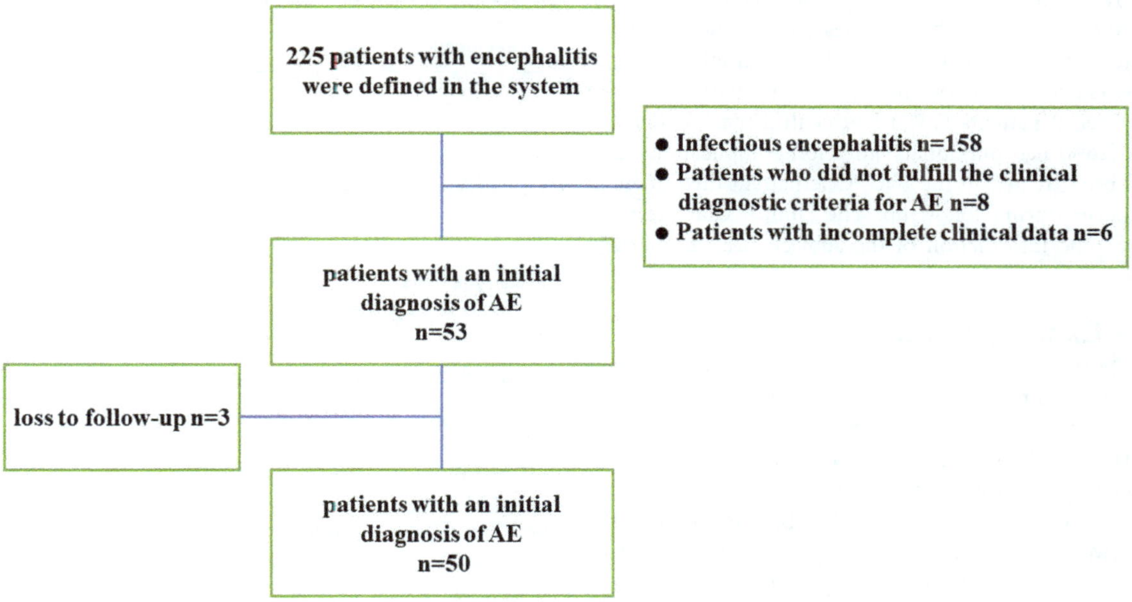

FIGURE 1 | Study flowchart. AE, autoimmune encephalitis.

the number of CSF cells ($\geq$5 leukocytes/mm^3), an increase in the rate of immunoglobulin G (IgG) synthesis, or the appearance of CSF-specific oligoclonal bands. Supportive cranial MRI included T2-weighted fluid-attenuated inversion recovery (FLAIR) hyperintensity on one or both sides of the mesial temporal lobes, multiple inflammatory lesions, or demyelination involving gray and white matter. Supportive EEG included abnormal slow-wave activity and epileptiform discharges (8). Patient serum and CSF samples were simultaneously obtained and sent to Beijing Kindstar Global Company for testing.

Disease Prognosis Evaluation

The modified Rankin Scale (mRS) was used to evaluate neurological function at the time of admission, at discharge from the hospital, and during the follow-up period. The mRS score includes 6 categories (23, 24): if patients had a full recovery (mRS 0 point); if patients had no significant functional impairment and were able to complete all daily duties and activity despite some symptoms (mRS 1 point); if patients had mild-moderate disability and were unable to complete all previous activities but could independently take care of their own affairs (mRS 2–3 points); if patients had severe disability and required others to take care of them (mRS 4 points); if patients had severe disability and required intensive care (mRS 5 points); and death (mRS 6 points). According to the mRS during the follow-up period, we divided all patients into two groups: patients with an mRS score of 0–1 were defined as "good prognosis"; patients with an mRS score of 2–6 were defined as "poor prognosis."

Statistical Analysis

All statistical analyses were performed using SPSS statistical software (version 22.0). Measurement data were presented in the form of "mean $\pm$ standard deviation" and/or "median (range)," whereas count data were presented as number (percentage). Univariate analysis was performed to compare the differences between the two groups. Independent Student's *t*-test was used for normally distributed variables, while the Mann-Whitney test was used for non-normally distributed variables. Categorical variables were compared using the chi-squared test. Logistic regression analysis was performed to determine the independent predictors of poor prognosis. The correlation between the immunotherapy latency and prognostic mRS score was determined using the Spearman rank correlation test. The optimal cutoff value for the NLR to serve as a prognostic marker for AE was determined from receiver operating curve (ROC) analysis. *P*-values < 0.05 (two-sided) were considered statistically significant.

RESULTS

Patient Profile

The search of the electronic database resulted in 225 potential encephalitis cases. A total of 50 patients with AE were included in the study (**Figure 1** provides the flowchart of patient selection). Nine cases with positive antibodies were considered "definite AE," including 7 patients positive for anti-NMDAR antibody, 1 patient positive for anti-GABA$_B$R antibody, and 1 patient positive for anti-AMPAR antibody. Sixteen cases negative for antibodies were considered "probable AE," and 25 cases were categorized as "possible AE." All patients showed acute or subacute onset, and 33 (66%) exhibited prodromal symptoms such as headache and other clinical symptoms of non-specific upper respiratory tract infection symptoms. The average time from onset to admission was 10 days. Thirty-nine patients (78%)

were initially misdiagnosed with viral encephalitis, psychosis, cerebrovascular disease, or other diseases. Among these patients, 2 had lung tumors, 1 had thymoma, and 1 had multiple myeloma. During the entire course of the disease, 19 patients (38%) developed fever, 9 patients (18%) had central hypoventilation, 13 patients (26%) had pulmonary infection complications, and 4 (8%) had been treated in the ICU. One patient died of small cell lung cancer during follow-up. The clinical characteristics and demographic information of the subjects are summarized in **Table 1**.

Auxiliary Examinations

The brain MRI, EEG, and CSF results of all patients were available. EEG findings were abnormal in 33 patients (66%), including 10 patients with epileptiform discharges (such as spike waves, sharp waves, spike slow wave complex, or sharp slow wave complex), 22 patients with unilateral or bilateral non-specific slow waves, and 1 patient with δ brushes. Brain MRI findings showed that the lesions were located in the frontal lobes, temporal lobes, parietal lobes, occipital lobes, insular lobes, hippocampus, basal ganglia, thalamus, cerebellum, cortex, and white matter. Twenty-one patients (42%) had specific T2-signal hyperintensities. These affected brain regions mainly included the medial temporal lobes, frontal and parietal lobes, and/or subcortical regions. Non-specific changes/demyelinating lesions were present in 13 patients (26%), whereas 16 patients had no abnormalities (32%). CSF findings revealed that 21 patients (42%) displayed pleocytosis, and 29 patients (58%) had high concentrations of total protein.

Treatment and Outcome

Twenty (40%) patients received immunotherapy, including eight patients with methylprednisolone (intravenous infusion, 1 g/day; 5 days); two patients with immunoglobulin (intravenous infusions, 0.4 g/kg; 5 days); nine patients with a combination treatment of IVIg and intravenous methylprednisolone; and one patient with a combination therapy of plasma exchange, IVIg, and intravenous methylprednisolone. None of our patients received second-line therapy (rituximab, cyclophosphamide, or other) due to medical insurance restrictions or drug side effects. The median follow-up time was 11 months (8–27 months). At the end of the follow-up period, 33 patients (66%) attained a good prognosis, whereas 17 patients (34%) had poor prognosis. Among all patients, 33 patients (66%) had mRS scores of 0 or 1. Meanwhile, 8 patients (16%) had mRS scores of 2, and 4 patients (8%) had mRS scores of 3. Additionally, 2 patients (4%) reached 4 points, and 2 patients (4%) received 5 points. Unfortunately, 1 patient (2%) died by the end of the study (mRS 6). Three patients relapsed during follow-up. Two patients with anti-NMDAR encephalitis also achieved a good prognosis without immunotherapy.

Predictors of Prognosis

Univariate analysis indicated that there were significant differences between the good and poor outcome groups in laboratory values, including the NLR ($P = 0.001$), lymphocyte counts ($P = 0.001$), and albumin ($P = 0.017$). We found that the median NLR was significantly higher in the poor prognosis group than in the good prognosis group. In addition, consciousness disorders ($P = 0.001$), epileptic seizures ($P = 0.007$), extrapyramidal symptoms ($P = 0.042$), abnormal EEG findings ($P = 0.001$), abnormal MRI findings ($P = 0.003$), and pulmonary infection complications ($P = 0.000$) were associated with worse prognosis of AE (**Table 2**).

All factors with a *P*-value < 0.20 in **Table 2** were included in a multivariate logistic regression model. Multivariate logistic regression analysis showed that NLR (odds ratio [OR] 2.169, 95% confidence interval [CI] 1.029–4.570; $P < 0.05$) was an independent risk factor associated with poor prognosis of AE (**Table 3**). ROC analysis of NLR to predict poor prognosis of AE showed that the area under the curve was 0.866 (95% CI, 0.759–0.974; $P < 0.001$). Based on the ROC curve, the optimal cutoff value was 4.45 (sensitivity, 0.824; specificity, 0.879; shown in **Table 4** and **Figure 2**).

TABLE 1 | Characteristics of the study population ($n = 50$).

Characteristics	Patients (%)
Sex (male/female)	31/19
Age mean, range (years)	39,14–74
Prodromal symptoms	33 (66%)
Interval between onset and Hospitalization mean, range (days)	10,1–60
Fever	19 (38%)
Initial symptoms	
Consciousness disorders	8 (16%)
Epileptic seizures	16 (32%)
Psychiatric and behavior disorders	19 (38%)
Extrapyramidal symptoms	3 (6%)
Other	4 (8%)
Consciousness disorders	25 (50%)
Epileptic seizures	25 (50%)
Psychiatric and behavior disorders	34 (68%)
Extrapyramidal symptoms	17 (34%)
Speech disturbances	5 (10%)
Memory deficits	7 (14%)
Autonomic dysfunction	1 (2%)
Mechanical ventilation	9 (18%)
Abnormal EEG results	33 (66%)
Abnormal brain MRI results	21 (42%)
Increased CSF pressure	9 (18%)
Increased CSF protein	29 (58%)
Increased CSF WBC counts	21 (42%)
Neutrophil count (10^9 /L) (median IQR)	5.30 (3.73–8.20)
Lymphocyte count (10^9 /L) (median IQR)	1.66 (1.14–2.03)
NLR (median IQR)	3.72 (2.16–5.56)
Pulmonary infection complications	13 (26%)
Tumor	4 (8%)
Immunotherapy	20 (40%)
Average hospital stay, range (days)	22.5, 5–99

IQR, interquartile range; EEG, electroencephalogram; MRI, magnetic resonance imaging; CSF, cerebral spinal fluid; NLR, neutrophil-to-lymphocyte ratio.

TABLE 2 | Univariate analysis of prognostic factors associated with AE.

Variables	Good prognosis ($n = 33$)	Poor prognosis ($n = 17$)	P-value
Age (years), (mean ± SD)	39.06 ± 17.74	38.06 ± 19.33	0.855
Sex			
Male	19 (57.6%)	12 (70.6%)	0.369
Female	14 (42.4%)	5 (29.4%)	
Duration from onset to admission			
≤2 wk	26 (78.8%)	13 (76.5%)	0.851
>2 wk	7 (21.2%)	4 (23.5%)	
Fever			
≤ 37.5°C	21 (63.6%)	10 (58.8%)	0.740
>37.5°C	12 (36.4%)	7 (41.2%)	
Consciousness disorders			
Yes	11 (33.3%)	14 (82.4%)	**0.001**
No	22 (66.7%)	3 (17.6%)	
Epileptic seizures			
Yes	12 (36.4%)	13 (76.5%)	**0.007**
No	21 (63.6%)	4 (23.5%)	
Psychiatric and behavior disorders			
Yes	22 (66.7%)	12 (70.6%)	0.778
No	11 (33.3%)	5 (29.4%)	
Extrapyramidal symptoms			
Yes	8 (24.2%)	9 (52.9%)	**0.042**
No	25 (75.8%)	8 (47.1%)	
Brain MRI results			
Abnormal	9 (27.3%)	12 (70.6%)	**0.003**
Normal	24 (72.7%)	5 (29.4%)	
EEG results			
Abnormal	17 (48.5%)	16 (94.1%)	**0.001**
Normal	16 (51.5%)	1 (5.9%)	
CSF pressure, mmH$_2$O			
≥230	5 (15.2%)	4 (23.5%)	0.465
<230	28 (84.8%)	13 (76.5%)	
CSF WBC count			
Normal	19 (57.6%)	10 (58.8%)	0.933
High	14 (42.4%)	7 (41.2%)	
CSF protein level, mg/L			
≤400	13 (39.4%)	8 (47.1%)	0.603
>400	20 (60.6%)	9 (52.9%)	
CSF glucose level			
Low	1 (3.0%)	1 (5.9%)	0.655
Normal	27 (81.8%)	12 (70.6%)	
High	5 (15.2%)	4 (23.5%)	
CSF chloride level			
Low	1 (3.0%)	1 (5.9%)	0.830
Normal	29 (87.9%)	15 (88.2%)	
High	3 (9.1%)	1 (5.9%)	
Blood potassium level			
Low	5 (15.2%)	5 (29.4%)	0.232
Normal	28 (84.8%)	12 (70.6%)	
Blood sodium level			
Low	6 (18.2%)	5 (29.4%)	0.221
Normal	27 (81.8%)	11 (64.7%)	
High	0 (0.0%)	1 (5.9%)	
Blood chlorine level			
Low	2 (6.1%)	2 (11.8%)	0.277
Normal	31 (93.9%)	14 (82.4%)	
High	0 (0%)	1 (5.9%)	
Blood calcium level			
Low	12 (36.4%)	8 (47.1%)	0.465
Normal	21 (63.6%)	9 (52.9%)	
Albumin			
Low	18 (54.5%)	15 (88.2%)	**0.017**
Normal	15 (45.5%)	3 (11.8%)	
WBC count			
Normal	26 (78.8%)	12 (70.6%)	0.520
High	7 (21.2%)	5 (29.4%)	
Neutrophil count			
Normal	24 (72.7%)	9 (52.9%)	0.162
High	9 (27.3%)	8 (47.1%)	
Lymphocyte count			
Low	2 (6.1%)	8 (47.1%)	**0.001**
Normal	31 (93.9%)	9 (52.9%)	
Hemoglobin			
Low	10 (30.3%)	7 (41.2%)	0.603
Normal	22 (66.7%)	10 (58.8%)	
High	1 (3.0%)	0 (0%)	
Platelet count			
Low	1 (3%)	2 (11.8%)	0.203
Normal	22 (66.7%)	13 (76.5%)	
High	10 (30.3%)	2 (11.8%)	
NLR (median IQR)	2.92 (1.87–4.01)	5.60(4.56–11.49)	**0.001**
Mechanical ventilation			
Yes	4 (12.1%)	5 (29.4%)	0.236
No	29 (87.9%)	12 (70.6%)	
Pulmonary infection complications			
Yes	3 (9.1%)	10 (58.8%)	**0.000**
No	30 (90.9%)	7 (41.2%)	

AE, autoimmune encephalitis; SD, standard deviation; IQR, interquartile range; EEG, electroencephalogram; MRI, magnetic resonance imaging; CSF, cerebral spinal fluid; WBC, white blood cell; NLR, neutrophil-to-lymphocyte ratio. Reference interval: CSF WBC count: 0–5 × 10^6/L; CSF protein level, 200–400 mg/L; CSF glucose level, 2.5–4.4 mmol/L; CSF chloride level, 120–130 mmol/L; blood potassium level, 3.5–5.3 mmol/L; blood sodium level, 137–147 mmol/L; blood chlorine level, 99–110 mmol/L; blood calcium level, 2.20–2.65 mmol/L; albumin, 40–55 g/L; WBC count, 3.5–10 × 10^9/L; neutrophil count, 1.8–6.3 × 10^9/L; lymphocyte count, 1.1–3.2 × 10^9/L; hemoglobin, 115–150 g/L; platelet count, 101–320 × 10^9/L. P values < 0.05 are considered statistically significant.

The Spearman rank correlation test was performed to analyze the correlation between the immunotherapy latency and prognostic mRS scores of 20 patients who received

TABLE 3 | Multivariate analysis of factors associated with a poor prognosis.

Variables	OR	95% CI	*P*-value
Consciousness disorders	11.995	0.173–833.456	0.251
Epileptic seizures	1.003	0.31–32.757	0.999
Extrapyramidal symptoms	10.157	0.529–195.094	0.124
EEG results	18.206	0.209–1586.043	0.203
Brain MRI results	1.189	0.53–26.628	0.913
Pulmonary infection complications	1.071	0.029–40.049	0.970
Albumin	1.792	0.100–32.115	0.692
Neutrophil count	0.089	0.002–3.640	0.201
Lymphocyte count	6.918	0.059–812.704	0.426
NLR	2.169	1.029–4.570	0.042

OR, odds ratio; CI, confidence interval; EEG, electroencephalogram; MRI, magnetic resonance imaging; NLR, neutrophil-to-lymphocyte ratio.

TABLE 4 | Receiver operating characteristic curve-related statistical indicators.

Prediction	AUC	95% CI	*P*
NLR	0.866	0.759–0.974	<0.001

NLR, neutrophil-to-lymphocyte ratio; AUC, area under the curve; CI, confidence interval.

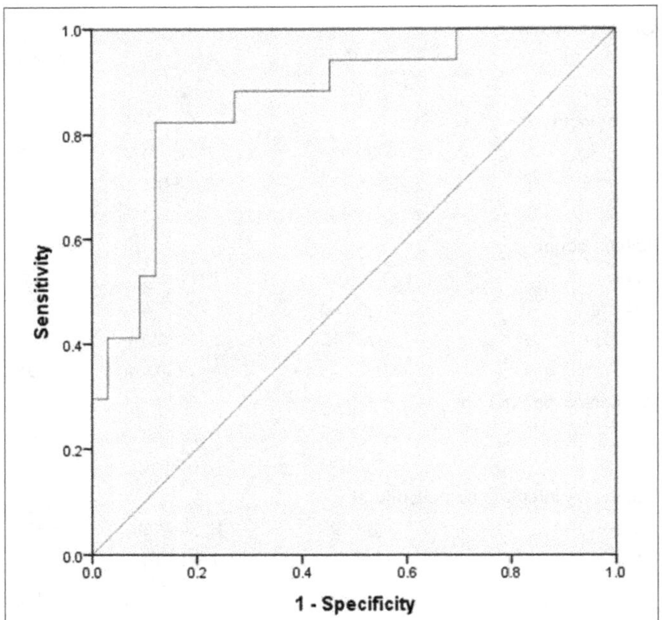

FIGURE 2 | ROC curve of the predictive value of NLR for poor prognosis of AE.

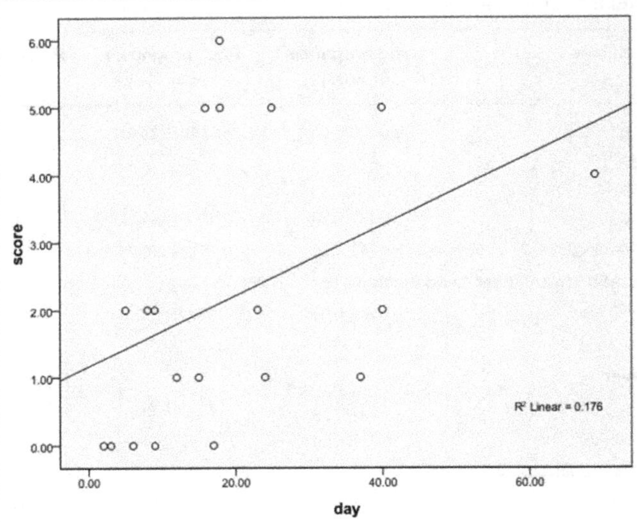

FIGURE 3 | The correlation between the immunotherapy latency and the prognostic mRS scores of 20 patients who received immunotherapy.

immunotherapy. There was a positive correlation between the immunotherapy latency and mRS score ($r_s = 0.535$, $P < 0.05$; **Figure 3**).

DISCUSSION

In this study, we retrospectively analyzed patients with an initial diagnosis of AE. We focused on clinical features, laboratory and imaging examinations, and EEG findings; moreover, we evaluated which factors are related to a poor prognosis. This study revealed that an increase in NLR was an independent risk factor for predicting the poor prognosis of AE. Prior to our study, the role of NLR in AE had not been examined, and this study presented a novel finding to predict the poor prognosis of AE.

AE is an increasingly recognized immune-mediated brain disease (10). This disease includes a heterogeneous group of encephalitic syndromes, which is divided into the following categories: new-type AE associated with antibodies to neural surface antigens and classic paraneoplastic limbic encephalitis (LE) associated with onconeural antibodies against intracellular antigens (25). It is reported that cases with surface antigen antibodies present a different immune reaction than that of cases with intracellular antigen antibodies. T cells are thought to play a cytotoxic role in cases with intracellular antigen antibodies (26), whereas antibody and/or complement-mediated mechanisms are considered to be responsible for neurodegeneration in encephalitis with surface antigen antibodies (10). Chronic inflammation, which is triggered by the overproduction of autoantibodies, inflammatory cytokine release, and deposition of the immune complex, plays an important role in the disease development process of AE (25). Abnormal immune regulation and persistent inflammation are critical pathological manifestations in the disease development process of AE.

NLR has been suggested as an indicator of systemic inflammation (11, 27). Compared with independent neutrophils, lymphocytes, and total white blood cell counts, NLR is less affected by various physiological and pathological conditions. NLR is an inexpensive, easily measurable, and widely available blood test affected by both innate immune response (mediated by neutrophils) and adaptive immune response (mediated by lymphocytes) (20). Changes in NLR may reflect the shifting balance between inflammatory activity and immune activity

(28). Inflammation is a response to acute or chronic tissue damage caused by infection, ischemic injury, physical injury, and other types of trauma. When these conditions occur, the immune system will lead neutrophils, lymphocytes and other inflammatory cells to accumulate in the site of damage (14). Under inflammatory conditions, neutrophil and lymphocyte counts present temporary changes. High levels of neutrophil infiltration may result from cytotoxicity in response to changes in the balance of pro-inflammatory and anti-inflammatory cytokines (29). The reason why NLR can predict prognosis may be summarized in two aspects: neutrophils are associated with a much quicker response, while lymphocytes are involved with more adaptive, chronic responses of the immune system (30). In the process of inflammation and immunity, neutrophils can destroy tissue directly by producing the enzyme myeloperoxidase and free radicals, and regulating the activity of other cell types (31). Moreover, some treatments such as immunotherapy can cause changes in NLR. Therefore, the routine blood results in our study were recorded within 24 h of admission to avoid interference from immunotherapy.

As an indicator of systemic inflammation, NLR has been frequently used to predict outcomes in many diseases. Prior studies have shown that altered NLR is related to decreased overall survival (OS) in various cancers. For example, Ma et al. detected that NLR is a significant predictor for recurrence in stage III melanoma patients (32). Shimada et al. suggested a high preoperative NLR as a biomarker to identify patients with a poor prognosis after resection for primary gastric cancer (33). Azab et al. found that NLR level >3.3 is an independent significant predictor of mortality in patients with breast cancer (34). Some studies have also reported that increased NLR is associated with higher rates of mortality in patients with acute heart failure or acute coronary syndrome (31, 35). In addition, a high NLR is also associated with a risk of death in critically ill patients, including patients with severe sepsis or septic shock (27, 36). Kim et al. demonstrated that NLR is a stronger independent predictor of postoperative acute kidney injury (AKI) (37). Another retrospective study of prognostic factors in patients with acute respiratory distress syndrome (ARDS) suggested that a high NLR (>14) independently predicts a poor prognosis in patients with ARDS (38). Based on recent studies, NLR is increased in patients with autoimmune diseases. In a previous study on the relationship between NLR and systemic lupus erythematosus (SLE), a high NLR was independently associated with SLE (39). In a meta-analysis on the relationship between hematological indices and autoimmune rheumatic diseases (ARDs), including ankylosing spondylitis (AS), Behçet's disease (BD), and rheumatoid arthritis (RA), NLR was recommended as a diagnostic biomarker for ARDs (22). Our study results extended previous reports on the prognostic role of NLR.

In fact, in clinical work, antibody-positive AEs are the minority, while most AEs are probable AEs or possible AEs. Several previous studies on prognostic factors of AE also evaluated different AEs, including "definite" and "probable" AE cases, in the same study (2, 40). In our study, among patients who received antibody testing, the proportion of patients with a definite diagnosis of AE (36%) was in the range reported in the literature (2, 40, 41). AE can appear as several different syndromes, classically presenting with decreased levels of consciousness (symptoms progress over a period of days or weeks) that eventually develops into coma (42). Extrapyramidal symptoms, such as dystonic seizures, chorea, or abnormal posture of the limbs, occur with anti-NMDAR encephalitis. In adults with anti-NMDAR encephalitis, facial, and limb writhing movements may be most notable in the comatose phases of the disease (43). In our data, 71% (5/7) of patients with anti-NMDAR encephalitis developed extrapyramidal symptoms. Seizures are common in AE and may occur at any stage of the disease, and studies have revealed that status epilepticus can predict a poor outcome for encephalitis (44, 45). Several studies on the death factors of encephalitis in the ICU have shown that status epilepticus, central hypoventilation, and complications (such as multiple organ dysfunction or severe pulmonary infection) are predictors of poor prognosis of encephalitis (44, 46, 47). However, in our study, consciousness disorders, epileptic seizures, extrapyramidal symptoms, and pulmonary infection complications were associated with adverse outcomes but were not independent predictors of poor prognosis. This result may be attributed to the following reason. With the development of diagnostic techniques and the availability of effective treatments, the predictors of poor prognosis may change. For example, a retrospective study of anti-NMDAR encephalitis also found that disturbance of consciousness, central hypoventilation, and complications are not independent predictors of poor prognosis (48). Another French study reported that status epilepticus in patients with anti-NMDA receptor encephalitis is unrelated to poor prognosis (49). Our results were essentially consistent with the results of previous related studies.

Serum albumin has been suggested as a prognostic factor in various diseases, including Guillain-Barre syndrome (GBS) (50). Jang et al. reported that low albumin levels are a significant indicator of AE prognosis (51). In our study, low albumin was associated with poor prognosis in univariate analysis but not in multivariate logistic regression analysis. This result may be because albumin levels in patients with low albumin have been improved during hospitalization without affecting patients' prognosis.

In most cases of AE, brain MRI shows normal or only non-specific inflammation changes (52). Some abnormal cases may present with increased signal on T2-weighted images, especially in the medial temporal lobe. In our study, abnormal MRI findings were associated with poor prognosis of AE in univariate analysis. The reason for this finding may be related to the anatomy and physiological functions of the involved brain regions. Frontal and temporal lobe lesions can easily lead to psychiatric symptoms and secondary epilepsy seizures; parietal lobe lesions are susceptible to sensory disturbances, and basal ganglia lesions are prone to causing extrapyramidal symptoms or paralysis, among other nervous system sequelae. EEG often exhibits focal or diffuse slow-wave activity associated with one or more epileptic foci in all types of AE. In addition to what may be called an "extreme triangle brush" pattern in patients with anti-NMDAR encephalitis, there are no characteristic EEG abnormalities for other forms of AE (53). However, in the acute phase of encephalitis, aggravation of slow-wave activity is often accompanied by disturbance of consciousness, indicating that the injury is severe. Some studies have reported that EEG can predict prognosis in autoimmune or infective encephalitis, and normal EEG is a predictor of good prognosis (54). In our study, abnormal EEG was associated with poor prognosis of AE in univariate analysis. This study demonstrated that inflammatory changes in CSF are not related to prognosis. Although some patients with AE have moderately increased CSF lymphocytes, a lack of increase in cell numbers does not rule out this diagnosis (52). Most patients with AE have detectable neuronal autoantibodies in the CSF even if the CSF test is normal (8).

Immunotherapy for AE includes first-line therapy (steroids, IVIg, plasma exchange, or all) and second-line therapy (rituximab, cyclophosphamide, or other). Steroids are always the first option. Two weeks or more should be allowed for first-line therapies to work. If the patient remains very ill after first-line treatments, second-line therapy is typically administered (43). In the present study, early initiation of immunotherapy was associated with a good prognosis. Correspondingly, previous studies suggested that early immunotherapy improves the outcome of AE. A multi-institutional observational study of the prognosis of 577 patients with anti-NMDAR encephalitis showed a correlation between early immunotherapy and good prognosis, and it took more than 18 months for patients to recover (55). Another study suggested that patients who received immunotherapy within 40 days of onset had a better outcome than those who started immunotherapy after 40 days of onset (56). Our results were consistent with those of previous studies. Notably, not all patients with AE will respond to immunotherapy, but this does not mean that patients with AE cannot achieve a good outcome without immunotherapy. For example, in our study, two patients with anti-NMDAR encephalitis also achieved a good prognosis without immunotherapy. Therefore, considering the response to immunotherapy as a part of the diagnostic criteria of AE is not unreasonable. The speed of recovery, degree of residual deficit, and frequency of relapse differ greatly in different types of AE (8).

There is no known laboratory marker that predicts the poor prognosis of AE. Our study is the first to investigate the prognostic value of NLR in patients with AE. NLR has the advantage of low economic cost, no damage, and convenience. However, our study has several limitations. First, the present study was a retrospective design, thus, controlling for confounding factors was difficult. Prospective validation of NLR is required. Second, this study was conducted in a single institution, and the sample size of this study was small. Third, other inflammatory biomarkers, such as C-reactive protein (CRP), were not investigated, and the relationship between NLR and other inflammatory biomarkers could not be evaluated. Finally, there is still no consensus on the cutoff values to define the levels of NLR. The optimal cutoff value found in our study was 4.45, which is different from the values used in prior studies. The difference in cutoff points may be due to differences in the study population.

In conclusion, our study found that NLR may have predictive value for the poor outcomes of AE. Prospective validation of NLR is required. In addition, we revealed that early initiation of immunotherapy was associated with a good prognosis.

ETHICS STATEMENT

This study was carried out in accordance with the recommendations of the ethical guidelines of the Declaration of Helsinki with written informed consent from all subjects. All subjects gave written informed consent in accordance with the Declaration of Helsinki.

AUTHOR CONTRIBUTIONS

XQ, HZ, CY, and ZX contributed to the conception and design of the work. XQ, HZ, and DL contributed to the acquisition, analysis, and interpretation of the data. HZ, DL, JW, PX, and JZ prepared figures and tables. XQ and HZ contributed to drafting the manuscript. XQ, ZJ, YZ, and CY contributed to statistical analysis. XQ, HZ, ZF, and ZX discussed the results. XQ and ZX revised the manuscript. XQ and HZ contributed equally and share first authorship.

FUNDING

This study was supported by grants from the National Natural Science Foundation of China (No: 81660227 and 81560224), the Guizhou Provincial Science and Technology Foundation (No: [2015] 7471), and the Zunyi City Science and Technology Foundation (No: [2018] 64).

ACKNOWLEDGMENTS

The authors are sincerely grateful for the support of the Department of Neurology, Affiliated Hospital of Zunyi Medical University. In addition, we thank all of the subjects who participated in this study.

REFERENCES

1. Lancaster E, Dalmau J. Neuronal autoantigens–pathogenesis, associated disorders and antibody testing. *Nat Rev.* (2012) 8:380–90. doi: 10.1038/nrneurol.2012.99
2. Harutyunyan G, Hauer L, Dunser MW, Moser T, Pikija S, Leitinger M, et al. Risk factors for intensive care unit admission in patients with autoimmune encephalitis. *Front Immunol.* (2017) 8:835. doi: 10.3389/fimmu.2017.00835
3. Lim M, Hacohen Y, Vincent A. Autoimmune encephalopathies. *Pediatr Clin N Am.* (2015) 62:667–85. doi: 10.1016/j.pcl.2015.03.011
4. Granerod J, Ambrose HE, Davies NW, Clewley JP, Walsh AL, Morgan D, et al. Causes of encephalitis and differences in their clinical presentations in England: a multicentre, population-based prospective study. *Lancet.* (2010) 10:835–44. doi: 10.1016/S1473-3099(10)70222-X
5. Dalmau J, Tuzun E, Wu HY, Masjuan J, Rossi JE, Voloschin A, et al. Paraneoplastic anti-N-methyl-D-aspartate receptor encephalitis associated

with ovarian teratoma. *Ann Neurol.* (2007) 61:25–36. doi: 10.1002/ana.21050

6. Graus F, Dalmau J. CNS autoimmunity: new findings and pending issues. *Lancet.* (2012) 11:17–9. doi: 10.1016/S1474-4422(11)70280-0
7. van Sonderen A, Petit-Pedrol M, Dalmau J, Titulaer MJ. The value of LGI1, Caspr2 and voltage-gated potassium channel antibodies in encephalitis. *Nat Rev Neurol.* (2017) 13:290–301. doi: 10.1038/nrneurol.2017.43
8. Graus F, Titulaer MJ, Balu R, Benseler S, Bien CG, Cellucci T, et al. A clinical approach to diagnosis of autoimmune encephalitis. *Lancet Neurol.* (2016) 15:391–404. doi: 10.1016/S1474-4422(15)00401-9
9. Mittal MK, Rabinstein AA, Hocker SE, Pittock SJ, Wijdicks EF, McKeon A. Autoimmune encephalitis in the ICU: analysis of phenotypes, serologic findings, and outcomes. *Neurocritic Care.* (2016) 24:240–50. doi: 10.1007/s12028-015-0196-8
10. Bien CG, Vincent A, Barnett MH, Becker AJ, Blumcke I, Graus F, et al. Immunopathology of autoantibody-associated encephalitides: clues for pathogenesis. *Brain J Neurol.* (2012) 135:1622–38. doi: 10.1093/brain/aws082
11. Zahorec R. Ratio of neutrophil to lymphocyte counts-rapid and simple parameter of systemic inflammation and stress in critically ill. *Bratislavske Lekarske Listy.* (2001) 102:5–14.
12. Xiao Y, Xie Z, Shao Z, Chen W, Xie H, Qin G, et al. Neutrophil and lymphocyte counts at diagnosis are associated with overall survival of pancreatic cancer: a retrospective cohort study. *Medicine.* (2016) 95:e5024. doi: 10.1097/MD.0000000000005024
13. Feng F, Sun L, Zheng G, Liu S, Liu Z, Xu G, et al. Low lymphocyte-to-white blood cell ratio and high monocyte-to-white blood cell ratio predict poor prognosis in gastric cancer. *Oncotarget.* (2017) 8:5281–91. doi: 10.18632/oncotarget.14136
14. Wang L, Liang D, Xu X, Jin J, Li S, Tian G, et al. The prognostic value of neutrophil to lymphocyte and platelet to lymphocyte ratios for patients with lung cancer. *Oncol Lett.* (2017) 14:6449–56. doi: 10.3892/ol.2017.7047
15. Okamura Y, Sugiura T, Ito T, Yamamoto Y, Ashida R, Mori K, et al. Neutrophil to lymphocyte ratio as an indicator of the malignant behaviour of hepatocellular carcinoma. *Br J Surg.* (2016) 103:891–8. doi: 10.1002/bjs.10123
16. Tural Onur S, Sokucu SN, Dalar L, Iliaz S, Kara K, Buyukkale S, et al. Are neutrophil/lymphocyte ratio and platelet/lymphocyte ratio reliable parameters as prognostic indicators in malignant mesothelioma? *Ther Clin Risk Manage.* (2016) 12:651–6. doi: 10.2147/TCRM.S104077
17. Meng LB, Yu ZM, Guo P, Wang QQ, Qi RM, Shan MJ, et al. Neutrophils and neutrophil-lymphocyte ratio: Inflammatory markers associated with intimal-media thickness of atherosclerosis. *Thrombosis Res.* (2018) 170:45–52. doi: 10.1016/j.thromres.2018.08.002
18. Demirkol S, Balta S, Unlu M, Arslan Z, Cakar M, Kucuk U, et al. Neutrophils/lymphocytes ratio in patients with cardiac syndrome X and its association with carotid intima-media thickness. *Clin Appl Thrombosis/Hemostasis.* (2014) 20:250–5. doi: 10.1177/1076029612467227
19. Pichler M, Hutterer GC, Stoeckigt C, Chromecki TF, Stojakovic T, Golbeck S, et al. Validation of the pre-treatment neutrophil-lymphocyte ratio as a prognostic factor in a large European cohort of renal cell carcinoma patients. *Br J Cancer.* (2013) 108:901–7. doi: 10.1038/bjc.2013.28
20. Sawant AC, Adhikari P, Narra SR, Srivatsa SS, Mills PK, Srivatsa SS. Neutrophil to lymphocyte ratio predicts short- and long-term mortality following revascularization therapy for ST elevation myocardial infarction. *Cardiol J.* (2014) 21:500–8. doi: 10.5603/CJ.a2013.0148
21. Hu ZD, Sun Y, Guo J, Huang YL, Qin BD, Gao Q, et al. Red blood cell distribution width and neutrophil/lymphocyte ratio are positively correlated with disease activity in primary Sjogren's syndrome. *Clin Biochem.* (2014) 47:287–90. doi: 10.1016/j.clinbiochem.2014.08.022
22. Hao X, Li D, Wu D, Zhang N. The relationship between hematological indices and autoimmune rheumatic diseases (ARDs), a meta-analysis. *Sci Rep.* (2017) 7:10833. doi: 10.1038/s41598-017-11398-4
23. van Swieten JC, Koudstaal PJ, Visser MC, Schouten HJ, van Gijn J. Interobserver agreement for the assessment of handicap in stroke patients. *Stroke.* (1988) 19:604–7. doi: 10.1161/01.STR.19.5.604
24. Lim JA, Lee ST, Jung KH, Kim S, Shin JW, Moon J, et al. Anti-N-methyl-d-aspartate receptor encephalitis in Korea: clinical features, treatment, and outcome. *J Clin Neurol.* (2014) 10:157–61. doi: 10.3988/jcn.2014.10.2.157
25. Dalmau J, Rosenfeld MR. Autoimmune encephalitis update. *Neuro-oncology.* (2014) 16:771–8. doi: 10.1093/neuonc/nou030
26. Graus F, Saiz A, Dalmau J. Antibodies and neuronal autoimmune disorders of the CNS. *J Neurol.* (2010) 257:509–17. doi: 10.1007/s00415-009-5431-9
27. Salciccioli JD, Marshall DC, Pimentel MA, Santos MD, Pollard T, Celi LA, et al. The association between the neutrophil-to-lymphocyte ratio and mortality in critical illness: an observational cohort study. *Critic Care.* (2015) 19:13. doi: 10.1186/s13054-014-0731-6
28. Yang HJ, Guo Z, Yang YT, Jiang JH, Qi YP, Li JJ, et al. Blood neutrophil-lymphocyte ratio predicts survival after hepatectomy for hepatocellular carcinoma: a propensity score-based analysis. *World J Gastroenterol.* (2016) 22:5088–95. doi: 10.3748/wjg.v22.i21.5088
29. Summers C, Singh NR, White JF, Mackenzie IM, Johnston A, Solanki C, et al. Pulmonary retention of primed neutrophils: a novel protective host response, which is impaired in the acute respiratory distress syndrome. *Thorax.* (2014) 69:623–9. doi: 10.1136/thoraxjnl-2013-204742
30. Dunn GP, Okada H. Principles of immunology and its nuances in the central nervous system. *Neuro-oncology.* (2015) 17(Suppl 7):vii3–vii8. doi: 10.1093/neuonc/nov175
31. Benites-Zapata VA, Hernandez AV, Nagarajan V, Cauthen CA, Starling RC, Tang WH. Usefulness of neutrophil-to-lymphocyte ratio in risk stratification of patients with advanced heart failure. *Am J Cardiol.* (2015) 115:57–61. doi: 10.1016/j.amjcard.2014.10.008
32. Ma J, Kuzman J, Ray A, Lawson BO, Khong B, Xuan S, et al. Neutrophil-to-lymphocyte Ratio (NLR) as a predictor for recurrence in patients with stage III melanoma. *Sci Rep.* (2018) 8:4044. doi: 10.1038/s41598-018-22425-3
33. Shimada H, Takiguchi N, Kainuma O, Soda H, Ikeda A, Cho A, et al. High preoperative neutrophil-lymphocyte ratio predicts poor survival in patients with gastric cancer. *Gastric Cancer.* (2010) 13:170–6. doi: 10.1007/s10120-010-0554-3
34. Azab B, Bhatt VR, Phookan J, Murukutla S, Kohn N, Terjanian T, et al. Usefulness of the neutrophil-to-lymphocyte ratio in predicting short- and long-term mortality in breast cancer patients. *Ann Surg Oncol.* (2012) 19:217–24. doi: 10.1245/s10434-011-1814-0
35. Acet H, Ertas F, Bilik MZ, Akil MA, Ozyurtlu F, Aydin M, et al. The relationship between neutrophil to lymphocyte ratio, platelet to lymphocyte ratio and thrombolysis in myocardial infarction risk score in patients with ST elevation acute myocardial infarction before primary coronary intervention. *Adv Int Cardiol.* (2015) 11:126–35. doi: 10.5114/pwki.2015.52286
36. Riche F, Gayat E, Barthelemy R, Le Dorze M, Mateo J, Payen D. Reversal of neutrophil-to-lymphocyte count ratio in early versus late death from septic shock. *Critic Care.* (2015) 19:439. doi: 10.1186/s13054-015-1144-x
37. Kim WH, Park JY, Ok SH, Shin IW, Sohn JT. Association between the neutrophil/lymphocyte ratio and acute kidney injury after cardiovascular surgery: a retrospective observational study. *Medicine.* (2015) 94:e1867. doi: 10.1097/MD.0000000000001867
38. Wang Y, Ju M, Chen C, Yang D, Hou D, Tang X, et al. Neutrophil-to-lymphocyte ratio as a prognostic marker in acute respiratory distress syndrome patients: a retrospective study. *J Thoracic Dis.* (2018) 10:273–82. doi: 10.21037/jtd.2017.12.131
39. Li L, Xia Y, Chen C, Cheng P, Peng C. Neutrophil-lymphocyte ratio in systemic lupus erythematosus disease: a retrospective study. *Int J Clin Exp Med.* (2015) 8:11026–31.
40. Harutyunyan G, Hauer L, Dunser MW, Karamyan A, Moser T, Pikija S, et al. Autoimmune encephalitis at the neurological intensive care unit: etiologies, reasons for admission and survival. *Neurocritic Care.* (2017) 27:82–9. doi: 10.1007/s12028-016-0370-7
41. Hacohen Y, Wright S, Waters P, Agrawal S, Carr L, Cross H, et al. Paediatric autoimmune encephalopathies: clinical features, laboratory investigations and outcomes in patients with or without antibodies to known central nervous system autoantigens. *J Neurol Neurosurg Psychiatry.* (2013) 84:748–55. doi: 10.1136/jnnp-2012-303807
42. Hoftberger R, Titulaer MJ, Sabater L, Dome B, Rozsas A, Hegedus B, et al. Encephalitis and GABAB receptor antibodies: novel findings in a new case series of 20 patients. *Neurology.* (2013) 81:1500–6. doi: 10.1212/WNL.0b013e3182a9585f
43. Lancaster E. The diagnosis and treatment of autoimmune encephalitis. *J Clin Neurol.* (2016) 12:1–13. doi: 10.3988/jcn.2016.12.1.1

44. Thakur KT, Motta M, Asemota AO, Kirsch HL, Benavides DR, Schneider EB, et al. Predictors of outcome in acute encephalitis. *Neurology.* (2013) 81:793–800. doi: 10.1212/WNL.0b013e3182a2cc6d
45. Kalita J, Mani VE, Bhoi SK, Misra UK. Spectrum and outcome of acute infectious encephalitis/encephalopathy in an intensive care unit from India. *QJM.* (2017) 110:141–8. doi: 10.1093/qjmed/hcw132
46. Venkatesan A. Epidemiology and outcomes of acute encephalitis. *Curr Opin Neurol.* (2015) 28:277–82. doi: 10.1097/WCO.0000000000000199
47. Chi X, Wang W, Huang C, Wu M, Zhang L, Li J, et al. Risk factors for mortality in patients with anti-NMDA receptor encephalitis. *Acta Neurol Scand.* (2017) 136:298–304. doi: 10.1111/ane.12723
48. Wang W, Li JM, Hu FY, Wang R, Hong Z, He L, et al. Anti-NMDA receptor encephalitis: clinical characteristics, predictors of outcome and the knowledge gap in southwest China. *Eur J Neurol.* (2016) 23:621–9. doi: 10.1111/ene.12911
49. de Montmollin E, Demeret S, Brule N, Conrad M, Dailler F, Lerolle N, et al. Anti-N-Methyl-d-aspartate receptor encephalitis in adult patients requiring intensive care. *Am J Respir Critic Care Med.* (2017) 195:491–9. doi: 10.1164/rccm.201603-0507OC
50. Fokkink WR, Walgaard C, Kuitwaard K, Tio-Gillen AP, van Doorn PA, Jacobs BC. Association of albumin levels with outcome in intravenous immunoglobulin-treated guillain-barre syndrome. *JAMA Neurol.* (2017) 74:189–96. doi: 10.1001/jamaneurol.2016.4480
51. Jang Y, Lee ST, Kim TJ, Jun JS, Moon J, Jung KH, et al. High albumin level is a predictor of favorable response to immunotherapy in autoimmune encephalitis. *Sci Rep.* (2018) 8:1012. doi: 10.1038/s41598-018-19490-z
52. Dalmau J, Graus F. Antibody-mediated encephalitis. *N Engl J Med.* (2018) 378:840–51. doi: 10.1056/NEJMra1708712
53. Schmitt SE, Pargeon K, Frechette ES, Hirsch LJ, Dalmau J, Friedman D. Extreme delta brush: a unique EEG pattern in adults with anti-NMDA receptor encephalitis. *Neurology.* (2012) 79:1094–100. doi: 10.1212/WNL.0b013e3182698cd8
54. Sutter R, Kaplan PW, Cervenka MC, Thakur KT, Asemota AO, Venkatesan A, et al. Electroencephalography for diagnosis and prognosis of acute encephalitis. *Clin Neurophysiol.* (2015) 126:1524–31. doi: 10.1016/j.clinph.2014.11.006
55. Titulaer MJ, McCracken L, Gabilondo I, Armangué T, Glaser C, Iizuka T, et al. Treatment and prognostic factors for long-term outcome in patients with anti-NMDA receptor encephalitis: an observational cohort study. *Lancet Neurol.* (2013) 12:157–65. doi: 10.1016/S1474-4422(12)70310-1
56. Irani SR, Bera K, Waters P, Zuliani L, Maxwell S, Zandi MS, et al. N-methyl-D-aspartate antibody encephalitis: temporal progression of clinical and paraclinical observations in a predominantly non-paraneoplastic disorder of both sexes. *Brain.* (2010) 133:1655–67. doi: 10.1093/brain/awq113

2

Epidemiology of Antibody-Positive Autoimmune Encephalitis in Southwest China: A Multicenter Study

Yixue Gu[1†], Min Zhong[2†], Liang He[3†], Wei Li[4], Yuanyuan Huang[5], Jing Liu[6], Yangmei Chen[3] and Zheng Xiao[1]*

[1] Department of Neurology, First Affiliated Hospital of Chongqing Medical University, Chongqing, China, [2] Department of Neurology, Children's Hospital of Chongqing Medical University, Chongqing, China, [3] Department of Neurology, The Second Affiliated Hospital of Chongqing Medical University, Chongqing, China, [4] Department of Neurology, Daping Hospital & Research Institute of Surgery, The Army Military Medical University, Chongqing, China, [5] Department of Neurology, Southwest Hospital, The Third Military Medical University (Army Medical University), Chongqing, China, [6] Department of Neurology, Chongqing Three Gorges Central Hospital, Chongqing, China

***Correspondence:**
Zheng Xiao
xiaozhenghf@126.com

† These authors have contributed equally to this work

In recent years, as an increasing number of neuronal autoantibodies have been detected and used for clinical diagnosis, clinicians have become more aware of autoimmune encephalitis, causing its reported incidence to trend upward over several years. To date, however, there has been no large-scale epidemiological survey of autoimmune encephalitis in adults and children, and its epidemiological characteristics remain unclear. Six main types of antibodies are detected and used to diagnose autoimmune encephalitis in Chongqing, Southwestern China: anti-NMDA receptor antibody, anti-$GABA_B$ receptor antibody, anti-LGI1 antibody, anti-CASPR2 antibody, anti-AMPA1 receptor antibody, and anti-AMPA2 receptor antibody. From January 2012 to February 2018, 189 patients at six general hospitals in Chongqing were diagnosed with autoimmune encephalitis and were positive for neuronal autoantibodies. In this report, the epidemic situation and the antibody distribution among these patients are analyzed and described in detail. The differences in disease severity among different ages and between the sexes are evaluated, and the correlation between antibody titer and disease severity is also assessed.

Keywords: autoimmune encephalitis, epidemiology, age, sex, neuronal autoantibodies

INTRODUCTION

Encephalitis has high incidence and mortality rates worldwide (1), with a reported mortality rate of 8–18.45% (2–4). The term autoimmune encephalitis (AE) refers in general to a large group of diseases caused by an antigen-antibody reaction by the immune system to the central nervous system (5). The main clinical characteristics of AE are acute or subacute seizures of epilepsy, cognitive impairment, and mental symptoms. The disease spectrum of AE has been expanding since the first case of teratoma-related anti-N-methyl-D-aspartate (NMDA) receptor encephalitis was reported in 2007 (6). With the continuous progress and implementation of detection methods, a growing number of cases of AE with positivity for different autoantibodies have been diagnosed and reported. As an important cause of encephalitis, autoimmunity is receiving increasing attention from medical staff.

Investigations have shown that AE affects the quality of life of those affected and imposes a serious economic burden on both patients and society (7). Because the clinical manifestations of AE are very complex, the condition is difficult to diagnose, although early intervention is important for improving the prognosis of these patients (8). Neuronal autoantibodies are key for the diagnosis of AE, and changes in antibody titer are closely related to the clinical course (9). Neuronal autoantibodies identify subtypes of AE and help clinicians detect cases with atypical clinical manifestations. Therefore, antibody measurement is a critical step in the diagnosis of AE (5).

To date, there have been few epidemiological investigations of AE, and there are currently no data from large-scale epidemiological investigations. Thus, the epidemiological characteristics of the condition are still unclear. Six main types of antibodies are detected and used for the diagnosis of AE in Chongqing, Southwestern China: anti-NMDA receptor (NMDAR) antibody, anti-gamma-aminobutyric acid-B receptor ($GABA_BR$) antibody, anti-leucine-rich glioma-inactivated 1 (LGI1) antibody, anti-contactin-associated protein-like 2 (CASPR2) antibody, anti-α-amino-3-hydroxy-5-methyl-4-isoxazolepropionic acid 1 (AMPA1) receptor antibody, and anti-α-amino-3-hydroxy-5-methyl-4-isoxazolepropionic acid 2 (AMPA2) receptor antibody. In this study, the epidemiological characteristics of 189 patients with AE and antibody positivity were analyzed according to the diagnostic criteria of AE (5). The findings will provide clinicians with an improved understanding of the epidemiological characteristics of AE and contribute to speeding the diagnostic process and improving patient prognosis.

METHODS

Study Population

Data were collected from six large general hospitals in Chongqing, Southwestern China. From January 2012 to February 2018, 189 patients with AE were diagnosed with antibody positivity. The patients' medical records, laboratory results, cost information, and prognoses were reviewed and registered by a neurologist.

Inclusion Criteria

According to the AE diagnostic criteria published in *The Lancet Neurology* (5), the following four criteria were used, along with positivity for neuron surface antibodies: (1) subacute onset (rapid progression over <3 months); working memory deficits, epilepsy, or psychiatric symptoms related to the limbic system; (2) bilateral brain abnormalities highly restricted to the medial temporal lobe on T2-weighted fluid-attenuation inversion recovery MRI; (3) at least one of the following: 1) an increase in the number of cerebrospinal fluid (CSF) cells (white blood cell count exceeding $5/mm^3$) 2) EEG indicating epilepsy or slow-wave activity in the medial temporal lobe; and (4) reasonable exclusion of other diseases.

Exclusion Criteria

The exclusion criteria for the study were as follows: (1) no lumbar puncture CSF examination performed or incomplete clinical data from the period of hospitalization; (2) central nervous system infection caused by specific intracranial pathogens; (3) thyroid disease, a recent history of thyroid hormone replacement, or a lack of test results on thyroid function and antibodies; (4) an immunosuppressed state (including long-term immunosuppressive therapy due to chemotherapy, organ transplantation, or cancer); and (5) loss to follow-up.

This study was approved by the ethics committees of the six participating hospitals. All patients or their families were informed of the study and gave signed consent to allow the use of their medical records for the study.

Antibody Detection Methods

Six hospitals sent CSF and serum to the same laboratory, which began to detect AE-related antibodies in June 2011. Six types of antibodies were detected: anti-NMDAR antibody, anti-$GABA_BR$ antibody, anti-LGI1 antibody, anti-CASPR2 antibody, anti-AMPA1 receptor antibody, and anti-AMPA2 receptor antibody. The laboratory used indirect immunofluorescence (IIF) assays for antibody detection. A cell-based assay (CBA) with high specificity and sensitivity was used to analyze the CSF and serum of each patient. The initial dilution titers of CSF and serum were 1:1 and 1:10, respectively. Serum antibody titers were considered weakly positive at 1:10, positive at 1:32 to 1:100, and strongly positive at 1:320. The titers of CSF antibodies were considered weakly positive at 1:1, positive at 1:3.2 to 1:10, and strongly positive at 1:32 or above.

Statistical Analysis

The classification variables are described as percentages, and the characteristics of each subgroup are represented by the median. The chi-squared test or Fisher's exact test was used to compare differences among the subsets of classification variables. An independent-sample t-test was employed to compare differences among subgroups of continuous variables. The Wilcoxon signed-rank test was applied to compare differences among subgroups of hierarchical data. Spearman correlation analysis was used to analyze correlations among classified variables. SPSS 25.0 software was utilized to analyze and sort the data, with $P < 0.05$ indicating a significant difference.

RESULTS

Baseline Demography and Incidence Trends

From January 2012 to 2018, 189 patients with AE and neuronal autoantibody positivity were diagnosed at six large general hospitals in Southwestern China. Samples from 457 patients with suspected AE were analyzed for antibodies, with a positivity rate of 41.36%. Five patients died, giving a mortality rate of 2.65%. In terms of prognosis, the Glasgow Outcome Scale (GOS) was used for evaluation. Those discharged with a score of >4 had a good prognosis, those discharged with a score of 2–3 had a poor prognosis, and those with a score of 1 died.

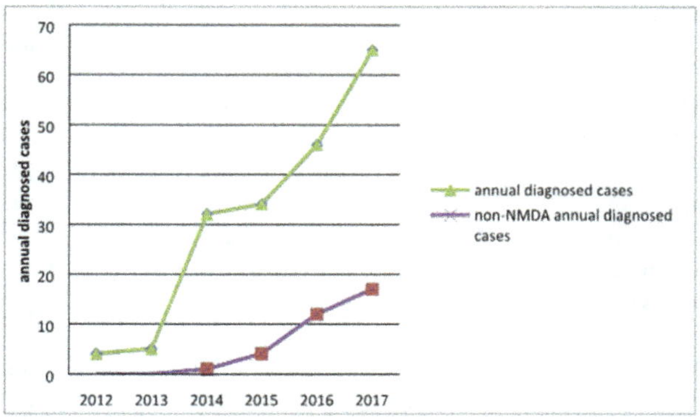

FIGURE 1 | Trends in the numbers of annual diagnosed cases of AE and non-NMDAR encephalitis.

The prognosis was good in 161 cases (85.19%). There were 41 cases (21.69%) in spring, 42 cases (22.22%) in summer, 59 cases (31.22%) in autumn, and 44 cases (24.87%) in winter. The median hospitalization time was 21 days, and the median hospitalization expenses were 4623.35 USD.

Among the 189 patients, females (116, 61.38%) outnumbered males (73, 38.62%) by a statistically significant margin ($\chi^2 = 9.783$, $P = 0.002$). The youngest patient was 1 year and 6 months old, and the oldest was 70 years old; the median age was 16 years. Among all patients, 99 (52.38%) were under 18 years old, 58 (30.69%) were 18–44 years old, 26 (7.72%) were 45–59 years old, and 6 (3.17%) were aged 60 years or older. The vast majority (83.07%) of patients were children and young adults ($\chi^2 = 213.556$, $P = 0.000$).

Of the 189 patients, 4 were diagnosed in 2012, accounting for 2.12% of all patients; 5 in 2013, accounting for 2.65%; and 32 in 2014, accounting for 16.93%; there were 34 cases (17.99%) in 2015 and 46 (24.34%) in 2016. In 2017, there were 65 cases, accounting for 34.39%. Three cases were confirmed in January and February 2018. The annual number of confirmed cases trended upward, as shown in **Figure 1**. With the development of diagnostic methods, an increasing number of autoimmune antibodies are used in clinical diagnosis. Using non-NMDAR antibodies, 1 case was diagnosed in 2014, 5 in 2015, 12 in 2016, 17 in 2017, and 2 in 2018, as shown in **Figure 1**.

Antibody Distribution

Among the 189 patients, 153 (80.95%) were positive for anti-NMDAR antibody, 14 (7.41%) for anti-GABA$_B$R antibody, 9 (4.76%) for anti-LGI1 antibody, 5 (2.65%) for anti-CASPR2 antibody, 3 (1.59%) for both anti-NMDAR and anti-GABA$_B$R antibodies, 3 (1.59%) for both anti-LGI1 and anti-CASPR2 antibodies, 1 (0.53%) for both anti-NMDAR and anti-CASPR2 antibodies, and 1 (0.53%) for both anti-AMPA2 receptor and anti-CASPR2 antibodies. Most of the patients were positive for anti-NMDAR antibody ($\chi^2 = 72.429$, $P = 0.000$).

Regarding the 153 patients with anti-NMDAR antibody positivity, 146 (95.42%) were CSF positive, and 123 (80.39%) were seropositive. The titer for the antibody is shown in **Table 1**.

TABLE 1 | Details of antibody titers in the CSF and serum of one antibody-positive patient.

		Negative	Weakly positive	Positive	Strongly positive
NMDAR	CSF	7	6	112	28
	Serum	30	17	98	8
GABA$_B$R	CSF	1	2	7	4
	Serum	1	4	7	2
LGI1	CSF	3	2	4	0
	Serum	1	1	7	0
CASPR2	CSF	4	0	1	0
	Serum	1	4	0	0

CSF testing was more sensitive than serum testing ($\chi^2 = 16.264$, $P = 0.000$), and the antibody titers were higher in the CSF than in the serum ($\chi^2 = 16.264$, $P = 0.000$). Among the 14 patients with anti-GABA$_B$R antibody positivity, 13 (92.86%) were CSF positive, and 13 (92.86%) were seropositive. There was no difference in the positivity rate or titer of anti-GABA$_B$R antibody between CSF and serum. Among the 9 LGI1-positive patients, 6 (66.67%) were CSF positive, and 8 (88.89%) were seropositive. The positive rate of serum was higher than that of CSF, but the difference was not significant. Among the 5 CASPR2-positive patients, 1 (20.00%) was CSF positive, and 4 (80%) were seropositive. Although the number of samples was small, the anti-CASPR2 positivity rate of serum was significantly higher than that of CSF.

Concurrent positivity for two types of antibodies was found in 8 patients. Further details on double-positive cases are shown in **Table 2**. Among the patients with LGI1 + CASPR2 positivity, 1 was strongly positive for CASPR2 in the CSF, whereas the antibody titers in the other patients were weakly positive or positive. In addition, only one of the five patients with anti-CASPR2 antibody positivity was CSF positive. All five patients with anti-CASPR2 antibody positivity were also positive for other antibodies, and only one of the five patients was CSF positive for anti-CASPR2 antibody. Presumably, the rate of CSF positivity for anti-CASPR2 antibody is low among AE patients in general.

Analysis of Factors Correlated With Disease Severity

Differences in Disease Severity Between the Sexes

We found that there were differences between males and females with regard to comorbid tumors and prognosis (**Table 3**). Male patients had tumors in 6 cases (8.22%), and female patients had tumors in 5 cases (4.31%). In the past, it was believed that women were more likely than men to have tumors as a comorbidity with AE, especially given the strong relationship between teratoma and anti-NMDAR encephalitis. However, in our study, male AE patients were more likely than females to have tumors, and 1/2 of males with tumors had GABA$_B$R-positive pulmonary tumors. Fifty-six male patients (76.71%) had a good prognosis, and 105 female patients (92.92%) had a good prognosis; thus, more women than men had a good prognosis, and the difference was significant ($\chi^2 = 6.766$, $P = 0.009$). Among the patients who died, 3 were (4.11%) male and 2 (1.72%) female. Although the

TABLE 2 | Details of antibody titers in the CSF and serum of patients who were positive for two antibody types concurrently.

Antibodies	Cases	Antibody titer
NMDAR + $GABA_BR$	Case 1	CSF NMDAR: weakly positive $GABA_BR$: positive Serum $GABA_BR$: positive
	Case 2	CSF NMDAR: positive $GABA_BR$: positive Serum NMDAR: positive $GABA_BR$: positive
	Case 3	CSF NMDAR: positive $GABA_BR$: positive Serum NMDAR: positive $GABA_BR$: positive
LGI1+ CASPR2	Case 1	CSF LGI1: positive CASPR2: strongly positive Serum Negative
	Case 2	CSF Negative Serum LGI1: weakly positive CASPR2: positive
	Case 3	CSF Negative Serum LGI1: weakly positive CASPR2: positive
NMDAR + CASPR2	Case 1	CSF NMDAR: positive Serum NMDAR: weakly positive CASPR2: weakly positive
AMPA2 receptor + CASPR2	Case 1	CSF AMPA2 receptor: positive Serum AMPA2 receptor: weakly positive CASPR2: weakly positive

TABLE 3 | Details regarding disease severity indicators in males and females.

	Male	Female
ICU (no.)	25	41
Ventilator use (no.)	9	9
Tumor (no.)	6	5
Surgery (no.)	1	2
Median hospitalization days	21	23
Median hospitalization costs (USD)	4622.27	5005.11
Prognosis		
GOS ≥4	56	105
2–3	14	9
1	3	2

mortality rate of males was higher than that of females, there was no significant difference ($\chi^2 = 0.990$, $P = 0.376$). Moreover, despite being more susceptible than males to AE, females had a better prognosis.

Differences in Disease Severity Among Different Age Groups

We found that there were differences in antibody distribution, combined tumors, ICU occupancy, and ventilator use between adults and children (**Table 4**). There were 34 AE cases with non-NMDAR antibody positivity (37.78%) in adults and 2 cases (2.02%) in children. Therefore, non-NMDAR antibody-positive encephalitis was more common among adults than children ($\chi^2 = 38.272$, $P = 0.000$). There were 11 adult patients and no child patients with cancer; accordingly, adults were more likely than children to have tumors ($\chi^2 = 12.848$, $P = 0.000$). Additionally, a greater number of adults (56, accounting for 62.22% of all adults) than children (fewer than 10, accounting for 10.10% of all children) were admitted to the ICU. This difference was statistically significant ($\chi^2 = 65.253$, $P = 0.000$). Among adults, 13 used ventilators, accounting for 14.44% of all adults; among

TABLE 4 | Details regarding disease severity indicators in different age groups.

	Adult	Children
ICU (no.)	56	10
Ventilator use (no.)	13	5
Tumor (no.)	11	0
Surgery (no.)	3	0
Median hospitalization days	22	22
Median hospitalization costs (USD)	5005.11	4623.35
Prognosis		
GOS ≥4	80	81
2–3	8	15
1	2	3

children, 5 used ventilators, accounting for 5.05% of all children. Overall, adult patients used ventilators at a higher rate than children did ($\chi^2 = 4.828$, $P = 0.028$).

Relationship Between Antibody Titer and Disease Severity

Because the antibody status of the double-positive patients was complex, those 8 out of 189 patients were excluded from this subgroup analysis. Among the 181 patients with single antibody positivity (**Table 5**), correlation analysis showed that the antibody titer in the CSF was positively correlated with ICU admission (rs = 0.234, $P = 0.002$), with ventilator use (rs = 0.254, $P = 0.001$), and with the presence of tumors (rs = 0.200, $P = 0.007$). There was also a positive correlation between CSF antibody titers and prognosis, but it was not significant ($P = 0.135$). In addition, our analysis found that the serum antibody titer was negatively correlated with ICU admission (rs = −0.329, $P = 0.000$). Conversely, there was no significant correlation between the serum antibody titer and other indicators, such as ventilator use and prognosis.

DISCUSSION

Since Dalmau et al. (10) proposed the condition of anti-NMDAR encephalitis, an increasing number of AE-related autoantibodies have been detected and used for clinical diagnosis. To date, however, there has been no large-scale epidemiological survey of AE in adults and children, and its epidemiological characteristics remain unclear. In 2016, *The Lancet Neurology* published diagnostic criteria for AE, emphasizing the diagnostic significance of AE-related autoantibodies (5). The epidemiological characteristics of 189 patients with AE and autoimmune antibody positivity in the CSF or serum were retrospectively analyzed in this study.

The most commonly detected synaptic receptor antibodies in Southwestern China are the anti-NMDAR, anti-AMPA1 receptor, anti-AMPA2 receptor, anti-$GABA_BR$, anti-LGI1-related, and anti-CASPR2-related antibodies. In the present study, 457 patients with suspected or confirmed AE were examined for serum and CSF antibodies. The positivity rate for antibodies was 41.36%. In a study by Lai et al. (11), 35.78% of patients with AE were positive for antibodies.

TABLE 5 | Details regarding disease severity indicators in relation to different antibody titers in the CSF and serum.

	CSF				Serum			
	Negative	Weakly positive	Positive	Strongly positive	Negative	Weakly positive	Positive	Strongly positive
ICU (no.)	4	5	29	19	21	16	19	5
Ventilator use (no.)	0	1	7	9	6	2	6	2
Tumor (no.)	0	0	5	5	3	0	6	1
Surgery (no.)	0	0	1	2	1	0	1	1
Median hospitalization days	14	19.5	22	30	21	20	23	24.5
Median hospitalization costs (USD)	2439.89	5041.56	4676.74	6391.01	4802.69	4919.42	4700.65	4535.96
Prognosis								
GOS ≥4	13	9	107	24	28	22	95	8
2–3	2	1	14	6	5	2	15	1
1	0	0	3	2	2	1	3	1

The rate of good prognosis was 85.19%, and the mortality rate was 2.65%. This finding is consistent with previous studies, indicating that the overall prognosis of AE is good. One study of 571 patients with anti-NMDAR encephalitis by Kayser et al. (12) reported that 83% of the patients recovered completely or partially. However, in a study by Yeshokumar et al. (13), the mortality rate was 12%; the rate of good prognosis was only 53%, and the rate of poor prognosis was 34%. The differences in the results of that study and of ours may be due to differences in prognosis prediction. The previous study scored prognosis using the modified Rankin scale (mRS), whereas we used the GOS. Moderately disabled patients were classified in our study as having a good prognosis, while the study by Yeshokumar et al. classified such patients as having a poor prognosis. Some scholars have found that among all cases of encephalitis, AE has an especially poor prognosis, with 56% of AE patients dying or having severe disabilities (2, 3). The reason why patient prognosis in previous studies differs so greatly from that in the present study may be that the prognosis of AE associated with tumors is worse than that of non-tumor-related AE. As our study did not involve paraneoplastic AE, the overall prognosis was good.

In terms of the time distribution of AE, there is no previous literature specifying the incidence by season. This study found that autumn (September-November) was the most common season, accounting for 31.22% of all cases, although there was no significant difference among seasons.

With regard to sex distribution, women (61.38%) were significantly more likely than men (38.62%) to have AE. This sex distribution is consistent with previously reported statistics for AE (13). Some possible mechanisms are that estrogen enhances humoral immunity (14) and that mutation of X chromosome-linked genes leads to differential expression of pathogenic genes, leading to the occurrence of autoimmune diseases (15, 16).

In our analysis of age distribution, we observed that the majority of patients were under 45 years old (83.07%). This result is consistent with reported data on other autoimmune diseases in children and young adults. In a study by Titulaer et al. (17), 577 patients had antibody-confirmed anti-NMDAR encephalitis, 95% of whom were under 45 years old, and 37% of whom were children. However, the effect of age on autoimmune diseases is unclear. Some studies suggest that the connection may be related to changes in hormone levels after middle age and that the decrease in estrogen in females weakens the immune response (14).

From 2012 to present, the number of confirmed cases of AE has increased annually, which may be related to increasing awareness of AE among clinicians. In 2007, Dalmau et al. (10) first reported anti-NMDAR encephalitis and found that it was closely related to teratoma. In 2009, Lai et al. (11) reported anti-AMPA receptor encephalitis for the first time, presenting 10 cases associated with type 1 and type 2 glutamate receptors. In 2010, Lancaster et al. (18) first reported and described $GABA_BR$ encephalitis and found that it may be associated with small cell lung cancer. In the same year, Lai et al. (19) first reported anti-LGI1 antibody-related encephalitis and anti-CASPR2 antibody-related encephalitis associated with voltage-gated potassium channels in *The Lancet Neurology*. Since then, a variety of neuronal autoantibodies have been reported. According to the results of our study, the number of confirmed cases of non-NMDAR encephalitis is also increasing yearly, which may be related to the expansion of the known neuronal autoantibody spectrum and the gradual adoption of antibody detection.

In this study, 189 patients were diagnosed with AE and were antibody positive. The majority were positive for anti-NMDAR antibody (80.95%), followed by anti-$GABA_BR$ (7.41%), LGI1-related (4.76%), CASPR2-related (2.65%), NMDAR+$GABA_BR$ (1.59%), LGI1+CASPR2 (1.59%), NMDAR+CASPR2 (0.53%), and AMPA2 receptor+CASPR2 antibodies (0.53%). The distribution of antibodies in this study is fundamentally consistent with that of previous studies. In a study by McCracken (20), 78.82% of patients were positive for antibodies against NMDAR, followed by $GABA_BR$ (4.71%), LGI1 (4.71%), CASPR2 (2.35%), and others (9.41%). In addition, Guan et al. (21) found 12.9% of 4,106 encephalitis patients to be positive for anti-NMDAR antibody, 12.8% for anti-LGI1 antibody, 5.6% for anti-$GABA_BR$ antibody, 1.3% for anti-CASPR2 antibody, and 0.6% for anti-AMPA receptor antibody.

The present study found that CSF detection was 15.03% more sensitive than serum detection for patients with anti-NMDAR encephalitis and that the antibody titer in the CSF was higher than that in the serum ($P = 0.000$), which was consistent with previous studies. For example, Gresa-Arribas et al. (9) found that in NMDAR encephalitis, CSF was a more sensitive sample type than blood for detecting anti-NMDAR antibodies. By comparing matched serum and CSF samples, Titulaer et al. (17) also found that the detection sensitivity of CSF was ∼15% higher than that of serum for anti-NMDAR encephalitis. However, there was no difference in sensitivity or antibody titer between serum and CSF in other types of antibody-positive AE.

In addition, although the number of CASPR2 antibody-positive patients was small, only 5 cases were CSF positive, and simultaneous detection of CASPR2 and other antibodies in the CSF was found for only one of the five patients. Thus, the positivity rate for CASPR2 in the CSF appears to be low. Bien et al. (22) found that 5 (33.33%) of 15 patients with CASPR2 receptor encephalitis were positive for anti-CASPR2 antibody in the CSF. The sensitivity of the CSF in the previous study was higher than that observed in the present study.

When we analyzed factors related to disease severity, we found that, despite significantly outnumbering male patients, female patients had a better prognosis. In a study by Harutyunyan (23), 16 (59.26%) of 27 AE patients admitted to the ICU were male whereas 11 (40.74%) were female, suggesting that males have more severe disease than females. Additionally, Murphy et al. (24) reported that when BXSB mice developed spontaneous lupus syndrome as an autoimmune disease, males tended to exhibit more severe clinical symptoms than females; the average survival time of male mice was also significantly shorter than that of female mice. Subramanian et al. (25) found that the Toll-like receptor 7 (TRL7) gene, which is related to immunogenesis and development, was heterotopic from the X chromosome to the Y chromosome and was overexpressed, which may explain the autoimmune symptoms in male mice.

The present study found that adult patients with AE are more likely than children to suffer from non-NMDAR encephalitis and to have tumors. Previous studies have shown that anti-AMPA receptor encephalitis may be associated with thymoma, small cell lung cancer, and breast cancer (19, 26, 27); anti-$GABA_BR$ encephalitis was also associated with small cell lung cancer in another report (18). These reports were consistent with the three cases of $GABA_BR$ encephalitis with lung tumors found in this study. Anti-LGI1 antibody-related encephalitis and anti-CASPR2 antibody-related encephalitis may also be associated with thymoma (19, 28). In general, adults are more likely to have non-NMDAR encephalitis because they have a higher incidence of tumors than children have (29).

In our analysis of the relationship between antibody titers and disease severity, we found that antibody titers in the CSF were positively correlated with ICU admission, ventilator use, and tumors, which reflect the severity of the disease. Gresa-Arribas et al. (9) have also indicated that antibody titers are higher in severe and teratoma patients. In addition, there was no direct correlation between CSF antibody titers and prognosis in our study, whereas Gresa-Arribas et al. (9) reported that the CSF and serum titers of patients with a poor prognosis were higher than those of patients with a good prognosis. Regardless, Broadley et al. (30) believe that the relationship between CSF titer and prognosis is not exact.

Our study has the following limitations. First, the sample size of the present study was insufficient. Nonetheless, as the number of cases is small for certain low-incidence types of AE, such as anti-CASPR2 antibody-related encephalitis, it is difficult to carry out a statistical analysis. Second, many more autoimmune antibodies are currently tested than the six antibodies mentioned in this paper. However, from 2012 to 2018, the main antibodies detected in Southwestern China were the six described herein. Therefore, we evaluated only these six antibodies. Additional antibodies could be assessed in follow-up studies.

CONCLUSION

AE is an inflammatory disorder of the brain that has very complex clinical manifestations and is difficult to diagnose. In recent years, the number of confirmed cases of AE has been increasing annually. Early intervention is very important to improve the prognosis of patients. Neuronal autoantibodies are often a key diagnostic basis in the diagnosis of AE. In our study, 41.36% of patients with suspected AE tested positive for antibodies, and their overall prognosis was good. Women outnumbered men in our sample. There were slightly more children than adults, and children and young adults accounted for the vast majority. Anti-NMDAR encephalitis accounted for the majority of cases; for this type, the sensitivity of antibody detection was higher in the CSF than in the serum, and the antibody titer was also higher in CSF than in serum. It is worth mentioning that the positivity rate for the anti-CASPR2 antibody was higher in serum than in CSF in anti-CASPR2-positive encephalitis cases, with or without concurrent positivity for other antibodies. Analysis of the factors related to the severity of the disease showed that the prognosis of women was better than that of men, that adults were more likely than children to suffer from non-NMDAR encephalitis, and that adults were more likely than children to have tumors. CSF antibody titers were positively correlated with ICU admission, ventilator use, and tumor complications, which may reflect the severity of the disease. However, there was no direct correlation between CSF antibody titers and prognosis. Understanding the epidemiological characteristics of AE can help increase the speed of diagnosis and improve the prognosis of AE patients.

AUTHOR CONTRIBUTIONS

All authors listed have made a substantial, direct and intellectual contribution to the work, and approved it for publication.

FUNDING

This study was supported by the National Natural Science Foundation of China (grant numbers 81071040, 81471320), and Natural Science Foundation of Chongqing, China (cstc2016jcyjA0337; cstc2018jscx-msybX0121). None of the institution or individual influence the study design, the collection, analysis and interpretation of data, the writing of the report or the decision to submit the manuscript for publication.

REFERENCES

1. Venkatesan A, Tunkel AR, Bloch KC, Lauring AS, Sejvar J, Bitnun A, et al. Case definitions, diagnostic algorithms, and priorities in encephalitis: consensus statement of the international encephalitis consortium. *Clin Infect Dis.* (2013) 57:1114–28. doi: 10.1093/cid/cit458
2. Granerod J, Ambrose HE, Davies NW, Clewley JP, Walsh AL, Morgan D, et al. Causes of encephalitis and differences in their clinical presentations in England: a multicentre, population-based prospective study. *Lancet Infect Dis.* (2010) 10:835–44. doi: 10.1016/S1473-3099(10)70222-X
3. Mailles A, Stahl JP. Steering Committee and Investigators Group. Infectious encephalitis in france in 2007: a national prospective study. *Clin Infect Dis.* (2009) 49:1838–47. doi: 10.1086/648419
4. Thakur KT, Motta M, Asemota AO, Kirsch HL, Benavides DR, Schneider EB, et al. Predictors of outcome in acute encephalitis. *Neurology.* (2013) 81:793–800. doi: 10.1212/WNL.0b013e3182a2cc5d
5. Graus F, Titulaer MJ, Balu R, Benseler S, Bien CG, Cellucci T, et al. A clinical approach to diagnosis of autoimmune encephalitis. *Lancet Neurol.* (2016) 15:391–404. doi: 10.1016/S1474-4422(15)00401-9
6. Sansing LH, Tüzün E, Ko MW, Baccon J, Lynch DR, Dalmau J. A patient with encephalitis associated with NMDA receptor antibodies. *Nat Clin Pract Neurol.* (2007) 3:291–6. doi: 10.1038/ncpneuro0493
7. Cohen J, Sotoca J, Gandhi S, Yeshokumar AK, Gordon-Lipkin E, Geocadin RG, et al. Autoimmune encephalitis: a costly condition. *Neurology.* (2019) 92:e964–72. doi: 10.1212/WNL.0000000000006990
8. Vollmer TL, McCarthy M. Autoimmune encephalitis: a more treatable tragedy if diagnosed early. *Neurology.* (2016) 86:1655–6. doi: 10.1212/WNL.0000000000002641
9. Gresa-Arribas N, Titulaer MJ, Torrents A, Aguilar E, McCracken L, Leypoldt FLancet, et al. Antibody titres at diagnosis and during follow-up of anti-NMDA receptor encephalitis: a retrospective study. *Lancet Neurol.* (2014) 13:167–77. doi: 10.1016/S1474-4422(13)70282-5
10. Dalmau J, Tüzün E, Wu HY, Masjuan J, Rossi JE, Voloschin A, et al. Paraneoplastic anti-N-methyl-D-aspartate receptor encephalitis associated with ovarian teratoma. *Ann Neurol.* (2007) 61:25–36. doi: 10.1002/ana.21050
11. Lai M, Hughes EG, Peng X, Zhou L, Gleichman AJ, Shu H, et al. AMPA receptor antibodies in limbic encephalitis alter synaptic receptor location. *Ann Neurol.* (2009) 65:424–34. doi: 10.1002/ana.21589
12. Kayser MS, Titulaer MJ, Gresa-Arribas N, Dalmau J. Frequency and characteristics of isolated psychiatric episodes in anti-N-methyl-d-aspartate receptor encephalitis. *JAMA Neurol.* (2013) 70:1133–9. doi: 10.1001/jamaneurol.2013.3216
13. Yeshokumar AK, Gordon-Lipkin E, Arenivas A, Cohen J, Venkatesan A, Saylor D, et al. Neurobehavioral outcomes in autoimmune encephalitis. *J Neuroimmunol.* (2017) 312:8–14. doi: 10.1016/j.jneuroim.2017.08.010
14. Cutolo M, Sulli A, Straub RH. Estrogen metabolism and autoimmunity. *Autoimmun Rev.* (2012) 11:A460–4. doi: 10.1016/j.autrev.2011.11.014
15. Selmi C. The X in sex: how autoimmune diseases revolve around sex chromosomes. *Best Pract Res Clin Rheumatol.* (2008) 22:913–22. doi: 10.1016/j.berh.2008.09.002
16. Voskuhl RR, Sawalha AH, Itoh Y. Sex chromosome contributions to sex differences in multiple sclerosis susceptibility and progression. *Mult Scler.* (2018) 24:22–31. doi: 10.1177/1352458517737394
17. Titulaer MJ, McCracken L, Gabilondo I, Armangué T, Glaser C, Iizuka T, et al. Treatment and prognostic factors for long-term outcome in patients with anti-NMDA receptor encephalitis: an observational cohort study. *Lancet Neurol.* (2013) 12:157–65. doi: 10.1016/S1474-4422(12)70310-1
18. Lancaster E, Lai M, Peng X, Hughes E, Constantinescu R, Raizer J, et al. Antibodies to the GABA(B) receptor in limbic encephalitis with seizures: case series and characterisation of the antigen. *Lancet Neurol.* (2010) 9:67–76. doi: 10.1016/S1474-4422(09)70324-2
19. Lai M, Huijbers MG, Lancaster E, Graus F, Bataller L, Balice-Gordon R, et al. Investigation of LGI1 as the antigen in limbic encephalitis previously attributed to potassium channels: a case series. *Lancet Neurol.* (2010) 9:776–85. doi: 10.1016/S1474-4422(10)70137-X
20. McCracken L, Zhang J, Greene M, Crivaro A, Gonzalez J, Kamoun M, et al. Improving the antibody-based evaluation of autoimmune encephalitis. *Neurol Neuroimmunol Neuroinflamm.* (2017) 4:e404. doi: 10.1212/NXI.0000000000000404
21. Guan HZ, Ren HT, Cui LY. Autoimmune encephalitis: an expanding frontier of neuroimmunology. *Chin Med J.* (2016) 129:1122–7. doi: 10.4103/0366-6999.180514
22. Bien CG, Mirzadjanova Z, Baumgartner C, Onugoren MD, Grunwald T, Holtkamp M, et al. Anti-contactin-associated protein-2 encephalitis: relevance of antibody titres, presentation and outcome. *Eur J Neurol.* (2017) 24:175–86. doi: 10.1111/ene.13180
23. Harutyunyan G, Hauer L, Dünser MW, Karamyan A, Moser T, Pikija S, et al. Autoimmune encephalitis at the neurological intensive care unit: etiologies, reasons for admission and survival. *Neurocrit Care.* (2017) 27:82–9. doi: 10.1007/s12028-016-0370-7
24. Murphy ED, Roths JB. A Y chromosome associated factor in strain BXSB producing accelerated autoimmunity and lymphoproliferation. *Arthritis Rheum.* (1979) 22:1188–94. doi: 10.1002/art.1780221105
25. Subramanian S, Tus K, Li QZ, Wang A, Tian XH, Zhou J, et al. A Tlr7 translocation accelerates systemic autoimmunity in murine lupus. *Proc Natl Acad Sci USA.* (2006) 103:9970–5. doi: 10.1073/pnas.0603912103
26. Joubert B, Kerschen P, Zekeridou A, Desestret V, Rogemond V, Chaffois MO, et al. Clinical spectrum of encephalitis associated with antibodies against the α-amino-3-hydroxy-5-methyl-4-isoxazolepropionic acid receptor: case series and review of the literature. *JAMA Neurol.* (2015) 72:1163–9. doi: 10.1001/jamaneurol.2015.1715
27. Spatola M, Dalmau J. Seizures and risk of epilepsy in autoimmune and other inflammatory encephalitis. *Curr Opin Neurol.* (2017) 30:345–53. doi: 10.1097/WCO.0000000000000449
28. Irani SR, Alexander S, Waters P, Kleopa KA, Pettingill P, Zuliani L, et al. Antibodies to Kv1 potassium channel-complex proteins leucine-rich, glioma inactivated 1 protein and contactin-associated protein-2 in limbic encephalitis, Morvan's syndrome and acquired neuromyotonia. *Brain.* (2010) 133:2734–48. doi: 10.1093/brain/awq213
29. Engels EA. Epidemiology of thymoma and associated malignancies. *J Thorac Oncol.* (2010) 5(10 Suppl. 4):S260–5. doi: 10.1097/JTO.0b013e3181f1f62d
30. Broadley J, Seneviratne U, Beech P, Buzzard K, Butzkueven H, O'Brien T, et al. Prognosticating autoimmune encephalitis: a systematic review. *J Autoimmun.* (2019) 96:24–34. doi: 10.1016/j.jaut.2018.10.014

3

Sex Steroids, Adult Neurogenesis and Inflammation in CNS Homeostasis, Degeneration and Repair

*Tracy A. Larson**

Department of Biology, University of Virginia, Charlottesville, VA, United States

Correspondence:
Tracy A. Larson
larson.tracy@virginia.edu

Sex steroidal hormones coordinate the development and maintenance of tissue architecture in many organs, including the central nervous systems (CNS). Within the CNS, sex steroids regulate the morphology, physiology, and behavior of a wide variety of neural cells including, but not limited to, neurons, glia, endothelial cells, and immune cells. Sex steroids spatially and temporally control distinct molecular networks, that, in turn modulate neural activity, synaptic plasticity, growth factor expression and function, nutrient exchange, cellular proliferation, and apoptosis. Over the last several decades, it has become increasingly evident that sex steroids, often in conjunction with neuroinflammation, have profound impact on the occurrence and severity of neuropsychiatric and neurodegenerative disorders. Here, I review the foundational discoveries that established the regulatory role of sex steroids in the CNS and highlight recent advances toward elucidating the complex interaction between sex steroids, neuroinflammation, and CNS regeneration through adult neurogenesis. The majority of recent work has focused on neuroinflammatory responses following acute physical damage, chronic degeneration, or pharmacological insult. Few studies directly assess the role of immune cells in regulating adult neurogenesis under healthy, homeostatic conditions. As such, I also introduce tractable, non-traditional models for examining the role of neuroimmune cells in natural neuronal turnover, seasonal plasticity of neural circuits, and extreme CNS regeneration.

Keywords: apoptosis, astrocyte, microglia, neural homeostasis, neural plasticity, neurodegenerative, neurogenesis, steroidal hormone

INTRODUCTION

Sex steroids coordinate the development and maintenance of male and female reproductive systems, and a multitude of other organ systems, including the digestive, metabolic, skeletal, immune, and nervous systems. Sex steroids are robust regulators of many diseases that, unsurprisingly, occur in organ systems in which steroidal hormones regulate development and homeostasis. Steroidal hormones influence morphology, physiology, and ultimately behavior from the cellular level to the organismal level through a variety of effectors, or classes of sex steroids, their specific receptor types, and several intracellular signaling pathways. In this manner, sex steroids spatially and temporally coordinate vast molecular networks. These networks regulate processes including, but not limited to, cellular proliferation, differentiation, motility, survival, and apoptosis. Specifically within the central nervous system (CNS) sex steroids directly regulate neural activity, nitric oxide signaling, and growth factor expression, among others (1). Through these and other direct processes, sex steroids also secondarily affect the birth and survival of neuronal, glial, and endothelial cells.

Within the context of immune function, sex steroids exert effects on and are one of many effectors of inflammatory cells and immune responses within the CNS. It has become increasingly evident over the last 30 years that the prevalence and severity of neuropsychiatric and neurodegenerative diseases with a neuroinflammatory component are linked to genetic sex [i.e., male versus female (2, 3)]. For example, women are more frequently diagnosed with atypical depression, depression with anxiety, and more severe progression of Alzheimer's Disease than men [reviewed in Ref. (3)]. As such, recent efforts have focused on understanding the implications of estrogen interactions with the neuroimmune system, primarily in the context of neurodegenerative disease and the possible use of estrogens and inhibitors of estrogen signaling as therapeutics. However, there is mounting evidence that the two other classes of sex steroids, androgens and progestogens, also modulate immune responses. Moreover, all of the sex steroids along with the classically described inflammatory cells have emerged as critical players in maintaining cell and tissue integrity under homeostatic and non-pathological conditions. Thus, understanding the role of all sex steroids, in all sexes, and under non-pathological conditions is paramount for unraveling the complex interactions between the hormonal, specifically sex steroidal, and immune systems, and for ultimately developing therapeutics for maintaining and restoring proper cognitive function.

In this review, I aim to present a comprehensive and integrative view of the independent, antagonistic, and synergistic impacts of sex steroids, the neuroinflammatory system, and neural stem cells (NSCs) for neural homeostasis, neuroprotection, and repair following neural insult. After providing a brief overview on sex steroid biosynthesis and intracellular signaling mechanisms, I discuss the steroidal hormone regulation of neural activity and synaptic plasticity, growth factor expression and responses, and apoptosis. With the intent to bridge three vast and recently converging areas of focus in neuroscience, I first lay a framework by describing the impacts of sex steroids on various neural and inflammatory cell types, including NSCs, neural endothelial cells, microglia, astrocytes, and leukocytes, among others. I then discuss the most recent findings at the intersections of sex steroids, neuroinflammation, and postnatal neurogenesis. I finally present several new models that have great potential to provide novel insights into inflammatory regulation of homeostasis, natural plasticity of neurogenesis, and extreme functional repair and recovery following neural damage and degeneration.

SEX STEROID BIOSYNTHESIS AND SIGNALING MECHANISMS

Two major classes of sex steroids, androgens and estrogens, were classically delineated as male- and female-specific hormones as a result of their respective pronounced synthesis in the testes and ovaries and their generalized roles in promoting secondary masculinizing and feminizing effects. Yet, the discovery of extra-gonadal biosynthesis of estrogens from androgens in adipose tissue in 1947 (4) and the birth of the "organizational hypothesis" in 1959 from work that demonstrated testosterone feminizes the CNS of the guinea pig [(5) and reviewed in Ref. (6)] revolutionized the thought and study of sex steroid function. Subsequently, estrogens and androgens have been discovered to be synthesized and exert regulatory effects in multiple organ systems in both males and females.

The three major types of endogenous estrogens are estrone (E_1), 17β-estradiol (E_2), and estriol (E_3), with E_2 being the most prevalent and potent form of circulating estrogen. The primary mode of E_2 biosynthesis occurs *via* the precursor, estrone, which itself is synthesized from androstenedione produced in the theca internal cells of the ovaries in females (**Figure 1**). The enzyme 5α-reductase, also called aromatase, converts androstenedione to E_1, which itself can be converted into E_2 by 17β-hydroxysteroid dehydrogenase (17β-HSD). In both males and females, 17β-HSD can also convert androstenedione into testosterone, which can be converted into E_2 by aromatase [reviewed in Ref. (7)]. After the discovery of extra-gonadal biosynthesis of E_2 in adipocytes, evidence of E_2 biosynthesis has been observed in astrocytes, neurons, and ependymal cells of the brain, osteoblasts, fibroblasts, adrenocortical cells, parietal cells of the intestines, smooth arterial muscle cells, and splenic T cells [reviewed in Ref. (8)].

The androgens testosterone (T) and androstenedione are synthesized primarily by the Leydig cells of the testes (in males) and the zona reticular and zona fasciculate of the adrenal cortex in males and females (**Figure 1**). Circulating plasma T and androstenedione can be converted to dihydrotestosterone (DHT), a potent androgen receptor ligand, by the enzyme 5α-reductase in target tissues. Likewise, dehydroepiandrosterone (DHEA), also known as androstenolone, is produced in both males and females in the adrenals [reviewed in Ref. (7)]. Circulating DHEA can be converted into both DHT and estrogens in peripheral tissues and itself can bind the different estrogen receptors with varying affinities [for more see Ref. (9)]. As mentioned, T and androstenedione can also be converted to E_2 by aromatase in both males and females.

A third class of sex steroids, progestins, includes progesterone, which is synthesized from pregnenolone in the corpus luteum of the ovaries and in the adrenal cortex (**Figure 1**). Progesterone can be converted by 7α-hydroxyprogesterone into androstenedione, which, again, is a precursor of T and E_1 [reviewed in Ref. (7)]. Extra-gonadal and extra-adrenal production of progesterones has also been observed in the pineal, thalamus, cerebellum, and tectum among other areas of the CNS (10).

At peripheral target sites, all steroid hormones bind nuclear and transmembrane receptors to drive complex, yet precisely tuned cell-type specific signaling responses. Briefly, the estrogens E_1, E_2, and E_3 diffuse across the lipid membrane and bind cytoplasmic estrogen receptors alpha (ERα) and beta [ERβ; for more on affinities, see Ref. (11)]. Ligand-bound ERα and ERβ dimerize, rapidly translocate to the nucleus, and directly regulate transcription of over 3,600 mammalian genes (12). Estrogens can also bind the G-protein-coupled receptors GPER (primarily expressed in adipocytes and intestinal cells), GPER1 (neural and adrenocortical cells), and GPER30 [endothelial cells; reviewed in Ref.

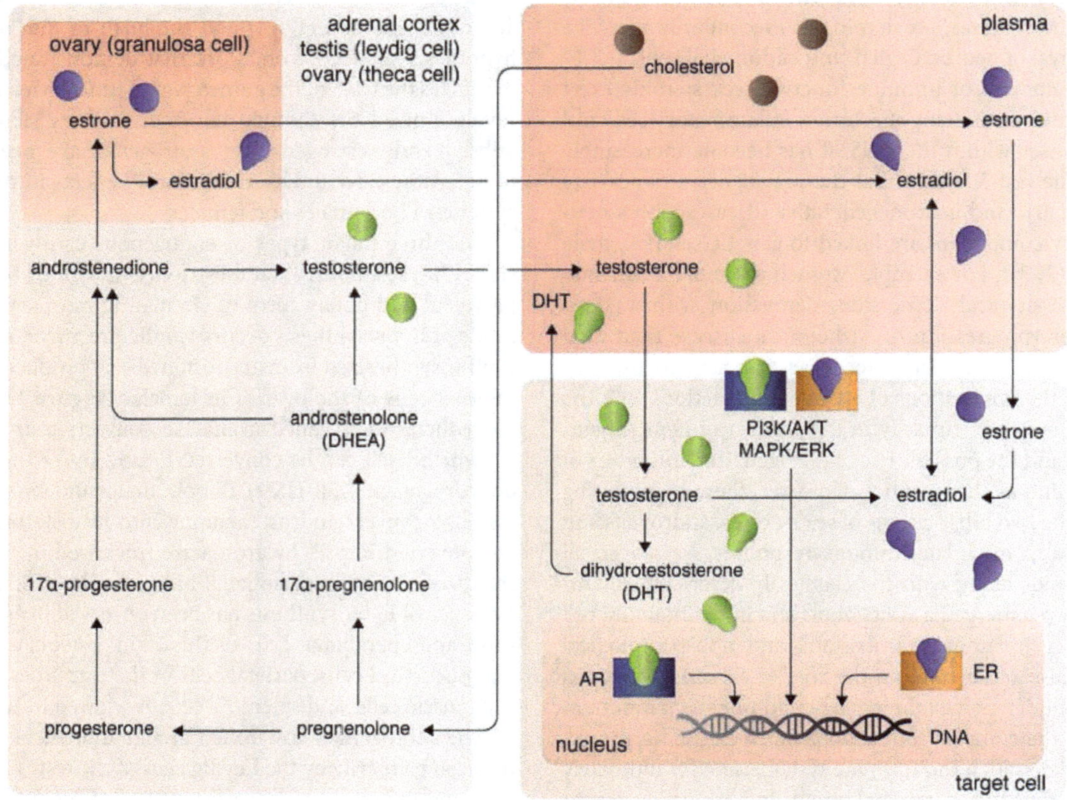

FIGURE 1 | Biosynthesis and localization of sex steroids, with a focus on estrogens and androgens.

(13)]. Estrogen-activation of the GPERs (and likely membrane-associated ERs, as well) initiates PI3K/AKT and MAPK/ERK signaling pathways (13), that in turn coordinate the transcription and translation of whole gene families that regulate cellular processes including, but not limited, to cellular differentiation, proliferation, survival, and apoptosis (14). Similarly, androgens and progesterones exert their functional effects on transcription and translation through intracellular canonical genomic signaling and the non-genomic signaling cascades PI3K/AKT and MAPK/ERK (15, 16). Differential androgen signaling depends on cytoplasmic- versus membrane-targeted isoforms of the androgen receptor gene (16). By contrast progesterone receptors, like estrogen receptors, are encoded by distinct genes and include the intracellular receptors PR-A and PR-B and the membrane progesterone receptor isoforms alpha (mPRα), beta (mPRβ), and gamma (mPRγ) (17). Further, contributing to the complexity of sex steroid receptor signaling mechanisms, unbound estrogen and androgen receptors can bypass activation by their cognate ligands and functionally bind to transcription response elements, albeit with much lower affinity (16).

OVERVIEW OF SEX STEROID FUNCTIONS WITHIN THE CNS

Through their various metabolites, receptors, receptor isoforms, and intracellular signaling mechanisms, sex steroids regulate vast molecular networks to spatially and temporally coordinate a multitude of processes related to cellular proliferation, motility, differentiation, and survival. Within the CNS, sex steroid signaling directly regulates neural activity, growth factor expression, endothelial cell and NSC proliferation, survival, and apoptosis (15, 18).

Neural Activity and Synaptic Plasticity

During development sex steroids, especially estrogens, play a pivotal role in arborization, synaptogenesis, and circuit formation (19). For example, the structural, connective, and physiological differences between the male and female brain are a result of gonadal steroid action during development. Regardless of genetically determined sex, morphological, and physiological masculinization of the brain occurs with exposure to E_2 but not DHT during a restricted developmental window [reviewed in Ref. (6)]. Feminization of the brain and behavior results from a lack of early steroidal hormone exposure (6). One mechanism through which E_2 affects the development of neural connections is through the modulation of glutamatergic synapse formation. For example, in the developing hippocampus, E_2 bound ERα stimulates expression of vesicular glutamate transporter 1 and the post-synaptic NMDA receptor, which in turn increases glutamatergic synapse formation of hippocampal neurons (20). For more information on these and other mechanisms driving sexual differentiation of the brain see Ref. (6).

Sex steroids also critically regulate neural activity and synaptic plasticity to influence circuit structure and activity in the adult CNS (**Figure 2**). In hippocampal CA1 pyramidal neurons of adult female rats, E_2 increases NMDA and AMPA receptor activity, which in turn increase neuronal sensitivity to NMDA (21). This E_2-mediated enhancement in NMDA sensitivity drives increased dendritic spine density of the pyramidal neurons (21). The influence of progesterone in modulation of dendritic spine formation and neural activity is, however, less clear and complicated by age and prior steroidal hormone exposure. For example, Edwards et al. found that progesterone enhances evoked responses from CA1 field recordings of adult female hippocampal slices (22), whereas Ito et al. observed no effect of progesterone on long-term potentiation in CA1 slices from 4-week-old rats (23). Moreover, progesterone and E_2 treatment together diminishes the enhanced glutamate-mediated release of intracellular calcium that each hormone has when administered independently (24).

Aside from canonical genomic signaling at the nucleus, sex steroids can rapidly modulate synaptic transmission through changes in spine density and neuron sensitivity within the synaptic process itself. For instance, T and DHT positively regulate spine formation through extranuclear ARs localized within dendritic spines and activation of local MAPK/ERK signaling (25). Local activation of MAPK/ERK drives rapid cytoskeletal and proteomic changes necessary for spinogenesis and plasticity (discussed further below). Similarly, ERα localizes not only within post-synaptic CA1 spines (26) but also pre-synaptic CA3 terminals, where it rapidly promotes long-term depression and spine formation through MAPK signaling (27).

Growth Factor Regulation

Over 40 years ago, sex steroids, specifically estrogens, were hypothesized to act in conjunction with neurotrophins to induce classic growth factor responses including increased cellular proliferation, differentiation, and survival (28). Subsequently, interactions between sex steroids and neurotrophins have been identified as critical regulators of sex-associated differences in body mass, cardiac function, bone mineral density; hepatic regeneration; tumor formation, and growth; and neural cell function and plasticity [reviewed in Ref. (29)]. Specifically within the CNS, sex steroid receptors co-localize with growth factor receptors including the insulin growth factor (IGF1) receptor IGFR, the low-affinity nerve growth factor receptor p75NTR, and the tropomyosin receptor kinase (trk) family—trkA (nerve growth factor; NGF), trkB (brain-derived neurotrophic factor and neurotrophin 4; BDNF and NT-4), trkC (NT-3). Co-localization occurs within, but is not limited to, the developing mammalian forebrain (30), cerebellum (31), and cortex [*in vitro* (32)], and the telencephalic nucleus HVC [proper name (33)] of the avian song production circuit (**Figure 3**) among other regions functionally related to the song system (34, 35). Such co-localization of steroidal hormone receptors and neurotrophic receptors drives neurotrophic-dependent processes through one or more of several mechanisms including: (1) convergence on the PI3K/AKT and MAPK/ERK signaling pathways to increase transcription and translation of gene families related to well-characterized neurotrophic processes, (2) autonomous enhancement in expression of neurotrophins and their cognate receptors, and (3) a cascade effect driving non-autonomous expression of neurotrophins.

Sex steroids and growth factors synergistically interact through convergence on the PI3K/AKT and MAPK/ERK signaling pathways to directly and indirectly modulate activity of downstream signaling cascades, transcription factors, and translation machinery. For example, PI3K activation by ligand-bound sex steroid receptors and/or growth factor receptors results in phosphorylation of AKT, which ultimately increases CREB-mediated transcription and ribosomal S6 kinase translation *via* mTOR activation (36). Likewise, both PI3K and MAPK activation increase

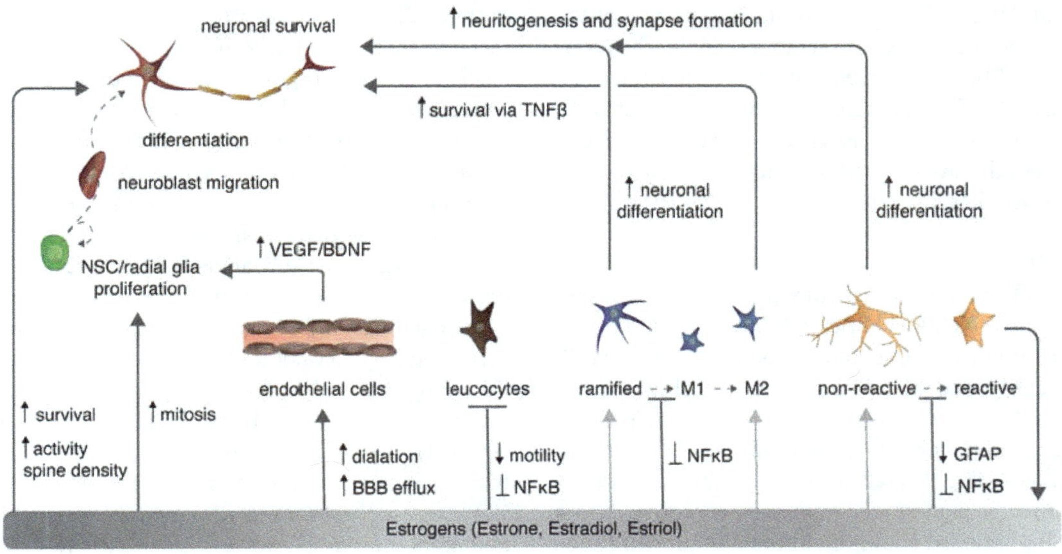

FIGURE 2 | The effects of estrogen on various cell types in the central nervous system. Light gray arrows indicate that estrogens have an effect on neurons via the given cell type to which the arrow points.

phosphorylation of GS3Kβ, inhibiting GS3Kβ's pro-apoptotic effects (37). As eluded to above, convergence on the PI3K and MAPK cascades can occur not only within the neuronal soma but also in pre- and post-synapses to drive rapid local responses to sex steroids and growth factors. Within the nucleus, E_2 directly regulates transcription through ER activity at estrogen response elements located in the promotor region of several growth factors—VEGF, transforming growth factor alpha (TGF-α), BDNF, NT-4, and NGF [reviewed in Ref. (2)]. Alternatively, within the dendritic spines, sex steroids can bind extranuclear ERs and ARs to enhance local BDNF translation *via* activation of PI3K/AKT and MAPK/ERK (25, 38). This in turn supports cytoskeletal rearrangement of dendritic spines and ultimately long-term potentiation by upregulating: the structural proteins growth-associated protein 43 and microtubule-associated protein 2 [reviewed in Ref. (19)]; the phosphorylation of the actin cleaving protein coffilin (39); and synthesis of essential synaptic proteins such as PSD-95 (40). In this manner, sex steroids and neurotrophins, specifically BDNF, rapidly modulate dendritic spine formation and stabilization to facilitate synaptic and circuit plasticity. At the pre-synaptic terminal, E_2 also increases retrograde transport of BDNF through a trkB-dependent mechanism in olfactory bulb neurons (41), possibly supporting antagonistic neurotrophic signaling, neuronal competition, and circuit plasticity (42).

Sex steroids can also drive autonomous and non-autonomous up regulation of both self and different neurotrophins and their cognate receptors. To highlight one example of many, in songbirds, testosterone, and specifically its E_2 metabolite, upregulates the expression of VEGF and the VEGF receptor-R2 in endothelial cells within the highly neurogenic nucleus HVC (**Figure 3**). VEGF in turn induces expansion of the local microvasculature through a sex steroid-independent increase in endothelial cell mitosis (43). Within 1 week of testosterone treatment not only new and mature endothelial cells, but also neurons and astroglia within HVC, upregulate synthesis of BDNF (43). BDNF is both required for and promotes the addition of adult-born projection neurons into HVC (43, 44), thus facilitating growth of the song control circuit and increased quality of singing behavior [reviewed in Ref. (45)]. This example not only demonstrates the neurotrophic cascade effect of sex steroids acting in concert with growth factors, but also introduces effects on vasculature and NSCs that sex steroids have often in conjunction with activation of growth factor signaling.

Vasculature

Sex steroids modulate cerebrovasculature function through several mechanisms, of which I will briefly discuss three [for more, see Ref. (46, 47)]: angiogenesis and endothelial cell survival, vascular contractility, and blood–brain barrier (BBB) permeability (**Figure 2**). Angiogenesis requires proliferation, migration, alignment, and differentiation of endothelial cells. Sex steroids, specifically estrogens, regulate all of these processes. Estradiol directly and indirectly increases the expression of growth factors including VEGF (discussed above) and fibroblast growth factor 2 (FGF2) that in turn increase the proliferation of endothelial cells (48). Estrogens also stimulate endothelial cell adhesion and migration through FGF-mediated increases in expression of surface integrins (49) and the formation of capillary-like structures with an internal lumen *in vitro* (50). Conversely, progesterone suppresses endothelial cell proliferation through nuclear progesterone receptor-mediated arrest of endothelial cells in the G1 phase (51).

Sex steroids also modulate cerebrovascular contractility. Chronic exposure to estrogens decreases vasculature tone and increases nitric oxide-dependent dilation in both males and females (52, 53). Estrogens promote vasodilation through both transcriptional increases in vasodilators including prostacyclin, endothelial nitric oxide synthase (eNOS), among others [reviewed in Ref. (46)], and posttranscriptional mechanisms. For example, E_2 not only enhances eNOS protein and mRNA expression through nuclear ERα (54, 55), but also eNOS activation through PI3K/AKT-mediated phosphorylation of eNOS at serine 1177 (56, 57). Together, increased production and activation of eNOS promotes nitric oxide production and, consequently, endothelium relaxation.

The BBB is a specialized cerebrovascular structure composed of endothelial cells encased in a basement membrane. The BBB is supported by astrocytic feet, pericytes, and local neurons that collectively form the neurovascular unit [NVU; reviewed in Ref. (47)]. The NVU regulates the influx and efflux of ions, molecules, and cells across the BBB to maintain homeostasis (47). Unique from other endothelial cells, the endothelial cells of the BBB are connected with tight junctions and adherin junctions that restrict the paracellular permeability of the BBB (47). By controlling the flow of ions, the BBB creates a high trans-endothelial electrical resistance, which decreases the ability of polar molecules to penetrate the BBB (58). Transport of substances across the BBB is limited to the passive diffusion of low molecular weight lipophilic molecules, polar nutrients including glucose and amino acids *via* solute carriers, and receptor- and adsorptive-mediated transcytosis of specific high molecular weight molecules such as insulin (59).

Sex steroids modulate the permeability of the BBB by enhancing nutrient and efflux transporter expression. Specifically, estrogens increase endothelial expression of glucose transporter 1, which facilitates 2-deoxy-D-glucose uptake into the BBB endothelial cells and transcytosis (60). Estrogens also modulate efflux transporter expression. Efflux transporters, predominately the adenosine triphosphate (ATP) binding cassette (ABC) transporters, prevent many lipophilic molecules from entering the brain and thus limit exposure to potentially harmful molecules (47). The activity of the ABC transporter sub family G member 2 (ABCG2)—alternatively known as the breast cancer related protein—is controlled by estrogens *via* ERβ (61). In endothelial cells, ligand-bound ERβ reduces phosphorylation of AKT, which subsequently reduces the expression and activity of ABCG2 through ubiquitination and proteosomal degradation (61). The decreased expression of ABCG2 results in not only decreased efflux of harmful molecules out of the brain, including amyloid-β protein (62), but also increased transcytosis of molecules such as tyrosine kinase inhibitors and xenobiotics (e.g., pharmaceuticals).

Although untested to my knowledge, the ability of sex steroids to alter BBB permeability through changes in growth factor expression and non-genomic PI3K/AKT signaling seems likely.

The growth factor VEGF increases tight junction permeability *via* VEGFR2-mediated phosphorylation and decreases in the expression of a critical regulatory protein of paracellular permeability, occludin (63). Given the previously discussed E_2-mediated increases in VEGF expression in endothelial cells, E_2 likely increases permeability of the BBB *via* VEGF-mediated decreases in occludin expression. Likewise, protein kinase C, an upstream regulator of PI3K/AKT signaling also reduces the expression of another tight junction protein claudin-5 (64). Thus, activation of PKC and PI3K/AKT signaling *via* ligand-bound sex steroid receptors may also decrease claudin-5 expression to increase permeability across the BBB.

Estrogens also repress inflammatory-mediated increases in leukocyte diapedesis, or transmigration, across the BBB. Secreted inflammatory factors including nuclear factor kappa-light-chain-enhancer of activated B cells (NFκB) and interleukin-1 beta (IL1β) increase transcriptional activation of cellular adhesion molecules (CAMs). CAMs mediate leukocyte–endothelial cell interactions are necessary for diapedesis and infiltration of leukocytes into the CNS. E_2 attenuates the release IL1β by astrocytes, activation of NFκB, and expression of ICAM1 (64), thus decreasing the permeability of the BBB to leukocytes. In this manner, E_2 is thought to mitigate inflammation following stroke or traumatic brain injury.

Oligodendrocytes

Oligodendrocytes are type of neuroglia that support and maintain the integrity of axons in the CNS. During early development oligodendrocyte precursors arise from neuroepithelial cells in the ventral ventricular zone (VZ) of the embryonic spinal cord and then migrate to and populate the VZs of the brain (65). As the last cell type to populate the CNS, oligodendrocyte precursor cells (OPCs) migrate into the gray and white matter of the entire embryonic CNS. The migration of OPCs is guided by growth factors including platelet-derived growth factor and FGF, netrins, semaphorins, and the chemokine CXCL1 [reviewed in Ref. (66)]. After migration, OPCs differentiate into other two types of oligodendrocytes: (1) myelin forming oligodendrocytes, which ensheath axons with an approximately 1 μm think myelin sheet and (2) non myelin forming oligodendrocytes, also known as perineuronal or satellite oligodendrocytes, which might play a role in the demyelination of nude neurons [reviewed in Ref. (67)]. Oligodendrocytes not only provide trophic support with production and secretion of glial cell line-derived neurotrophic factor, BDNF, and IGF1, but also electrically insulate axons, promote clustering of sodium channels at nodes of Ranvier, and promote microtubule stability in the axon (66).

Interestingly, myelination of axons by oligodendrocytes is tightly controlled by the neuron rather than a preprogrammed developmental clock within the oligodendrocytes themselves. The primary cue for oligodendrocyte ensheathment of axons is electrical activity of neurons. Electrically active neurons downregulate the polysialylated neural cell adhesion molecule (PSA-NCAM), allowing NCAM–NCAM adhesion required for oligodendrocyte–neuron interactions. Neuron firing also causes release of adenosine and ATP during the action potential. Adenosine and ATP promotes OPC differentiation and stimulation of astrocytes, which in turn secrete leukemia inhibitory factor to induce oligodendrocyte myelination (66). After associating with and receiving signals to ensheath by neurons, oligodendrocytes upregulate transport of myelin proteins transcripts, including proteolipid protein (PLP) and myelin basic protein (MBP), to the wrapping processes. PLP and MBP facilitate ensheathment by assisting with membrane trafficking and vertically coupling the multiple layers of membrane of the sheath, respectively (66).

Oligodendrocytes express both nuclear and non-nuclear ERs and PRs, and as such are directly modulated by sex steroids. During development estradiol promotes myelination in the neonatal rat brain, giving rise to higher numbers of oligodendrocytes in female-derived oligodendrocyte cultures than male-derived cultures (68) and possibly contributing to the well-documented higher incidence of neurological autoimmune diseases in females. More specifically, E_2, but not progesterone or testosterone, delays the exit of OPCs from the cell cycle, thereby increasing OPC proliferation (68). E_2 also enhances sheath formation through genomic ER signaling at an estrogen response element for MBP (68, 69) and resulting increases of MBP expression (70). Likewise, progesterone also enhances the formation of MBP and PLP positive membrane sheets through the progesterone receptor, although the precise signaling mechanism is still unknown (68, 71). Progesterone, as well as E_2, also facilitate remyelination following pathological demyelination in the CNS (72, 73). Given the high incidence of autoimmune disorders like multiple sclerosis (MS) in women, demyelination and subsequent remyelination unsurprisingly involves complex interactions between the immune system and steroidal hormones, and as such, will be discussed further below.

Postnatal Neurogenesis

Contrary to popular belief, new neurons are generated in the CNS from NSCs and neural progenitor cells (NPCs) throughout the entirety of vertebrates' lives. Pioneering studies in mammals and songbirds in the 1960s and 1980s provided the first evidence that new neurons arise in the adult brain (74) and that adult-born neurons functionally integrate into pre-existing neural circuits and acquire mature neuronal phenotypes (75). Since the discovery of adult neurogenesis several hypotheses regarding the function of adult-born neurons and neuronal turnover have been proposed. The replacement of older neurons by adult-born neurons has been proposed to enable the learning of new memories (76–78), the maintenance older memories (79, 80), the replacement of over-excited neurons (80), or the replacement of neurons weakened by DNA damage or loss of trophic support (81). Many studies have tested these and other hypotheses, however, no studies have conclusively supported or eliminated any of these possible functions of neuronal turnover (78, 81). Here, I will limit discussion to the complex, yet fine-tuned processes of adult neurogenesis, as broadly defined to include proliferation of NSCs, migration of neuroblasts, and the incorporation and survival of adult-born neurons in functional neural circuits. I will briefly introduce studies that highlight the modulation of adult neurogenesis by sex steroids, as the topic has been extensively reviewed in the past. Although many extrinsic and intrinsic factors such as non-steroidal hormones (e.g., glucocorticoids), morphogens (e.g., Shh, Wnt, BMP), neurotrophins, and neural activity also coordinate the processes of adult neurogenesis, in this review I will primarily focus on the role of the neuroinflammatory cells as a major regulator (below). For exhaustive discussion of these and a broad range of other adult neurogenesis related topics including functional importance, consider consulting Ref. (82).

Niches and Proliferation

Adult neurogenesis occurs across all investigated vertebrates (and some invertebrates) with varying spatial localization: addition of adult-born neurons is limited primarily to the olfactory bulb and the hippocampus of mammals, but occurs broadly across the telencephalon of birds, and the telencephalon, diencephalon, optic tectum, cerebellum, and hindbrain of fish [**Figure 3** (83)]. True stem cells are defined by two critical characteristics: (1) the ability to self-renew through proliferation and (2) the ability to give rise to multiple cell types through differentiation of progeny. The NSCs of the adult vertebrate brain are self renewing and thought to be multipotent, giving rise to neurons, astrocytes, and oligodendrocytes. Two major models have been proposed to describe the identity of NSC. Briefly, one model posits that non radial glial cells characterized by their expression of sex determining region Y-box 2 (Sox2) are the putative multipotent NSCs, whereas the other model suggests that radial glial cells expressing glial fibrillary acidic protein (GFAP) give rise to adult-born neurons and glia [reviewed in Ref. (84, 85)]. Given that both models are supported by experimental evidence (84, 85) and are not necessarily mutually exclusive, diversity in putative NSCs might represent the spatiotemporal diversity of adult neurogenesis not only across species, but also between neurogenic brain regions within a given species. Alternatively, true stem cells in the adult brain might not exist as a single cell, but rather might represent a whole population of unipotent NPCs, which independently give rise to either neurons, astroglia, or oligodendrocytes.

The dynamic lineages of progeny derived from NSCs, including both lineage-non-restricted NPCs and lineage-restricted NPCs like OPCs, further complicate the identity of putative NSCs in the adult vertebrate brain. For example, in the mammalian brain there are two major neurogenic regions: the ventricular–subventricular zone (V–SVZ) of the lateral ventricles and the subgranular zone (SGZ) of the dentate gyrus (DG). The NSCs of the V–SVZ are GFAP positive radial glia-like B cells. B cells are generally quiescent but can be activated by various signaling factors from other cells in the neurogenic niche and transform into GFAP negative transit-amplifying C cells [for mechanisms see Ref. (85)]. Type C NPCs actively proliferate giving rise to doublecortin (DCX) expressing type A neuroblasts that ultimately populate the olfactory bulb [reviewed in Ref. (84, 86)]. Likewise, the NSCs of the SGZ include type I GFAP expressing radial glial-like cells, which give rise to GFAP negative type II NPCs. The type II NPCs are further divided into two subpopulations: (1) type IIa, which express Mashl and Sox2 and are highly prolific and (2) type IIb, which express Proxl, NeuroD1, and DCX for early commitment to the neuroblast fate [reviewed in Ref. (84, 86)]. Type IIb neuroblasts ultimately incorporate into the local network in the granular cell layer of the DG.

The conservation of NSCs/NPCs lineage relationships across neurogenic niches within mammals and more generally across vertebrates, suggests a common evolutionary origin for the development of NSC/NPC pools in the adult vertebrate brain. For example, the adult avian brain contains proliferative type B cells in the VZ of the telencephalon that give rise to type A migrating neuroblasts (87). NSCs of the adult zebrafish telencephalon exists as type I GFAP positive cells that are quiescent until transforming into type II GFAP positive radial glial cells. Interestingly, the slowly proliferative type II cells can give rise to both new type I cells through Notch signaling and highly proliferative type III GFAP negative neuroblasts [reviewed in Ref. (88)]. These transit-amplifying type III neuroblasts can continue to proliferate, but can also begin fate specification by turning on PSA-NCAM and the pro-neural gene ascl1 (88). The NSCs/NPCs of the neurogenic niches in the zebrafish cerebellum and optic tectum express the classic NPC marker Sox2 and PCNA, but not GFAP (88).

Although it is generally accepted that adult neurogenesis continuously occurs across all non-human vertebrate lifespans [albeit to a lesser extent with age (89, 90)], the degree to which NSC/NPC proliferation occurs across the human lifespan has become a matter of recent intense debate. In 1998 NPCs in the human brain were first identified in postmortem hippocampal tissue of cancer patients who previously received an injection of the thymidine analog bromodeoxyuridine (91)—a commonly used reagent for labeling mitotic cells. BrdU-labeled cells were identified in the granule cell layer, the SGZ, and the hilus of the DG (91). Given that the average age of the patients examined in this study was 64.4 ± 2.9 years, the authors concluded that adult neurogenesis occurs throughout life in the human DG (91). In 2013 Spalding et al. birth dated hippocampal neurons in humans exposed to nuclear-bomb-test-derived 14C and calculated that around 700 new neurons are generated in the hippocampus per day with a turnover rate of 1.75% annually in nearly one-third of the population of hippocampal neurons (92). Again, the authors concluded that although the majority of hippocampal neurons do not turnover (thus the average age of hippocampal neurons increases with the age of the individual), turnover does indeed continue throughout the entire human lifespan (92). Moreover, in April of 2018 neurogenesis was found to persist in postmortem adult hippocampi of otherwise healthy humans ranging in age from 14 to 79 years (93). The degree to which hippocampal neurogenesis occurs subsequent to the first year of life, however, has recently been challenged. Using postmortem and postoperative samples of human hippocampi, Sorrells et al. reported in March of 2018 that proliferation in the DG peaks at 14 gestational weeks and decreases rapidly by 22 gestational weeks (94). By 7 years of age, nestin, vimentin, or GFAP positive cells with NSC/NPC morphology were not detectable in the SGZ or hilus of the DG, suggesting that the proliferative progenitor pool is near completely, if not entirely, depleted by 7 years of age (94). The apparent contradictions across studies regarding the degree to which adult neurogenesis occurs throughout the human lifespan likely arises from the large diversity in the manner through which the human samples were obtained. Given the difficulty in obtaining human samples in general and the near impossibility of controlling for the plethora of factors that alter adult neurogenesis in these human studies participants, the issue of degree to which NSC/

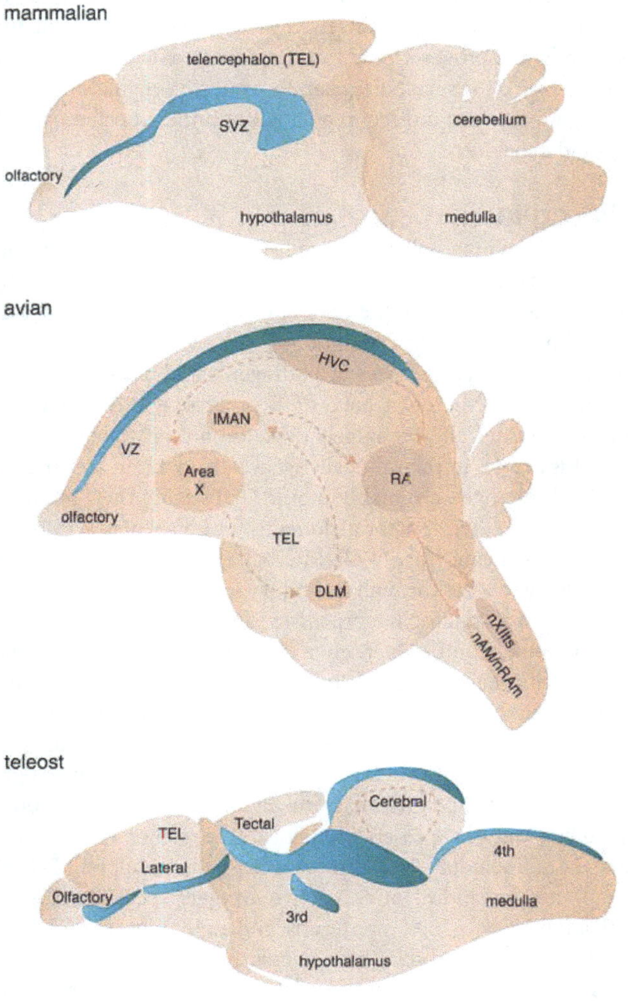

FIGURE 3 | Neurogenic niches in mammals, songbirds, and teleost fishes. Niches are colored blue. Dashed arrows in the avian brain represent the anterior forebrain pathway responsible for song learning, whereas solid arrows in the avian schematic represent the song motor pathway of songbirds. Both pathways are simplified for clarity.

NPC proliferation occurs in humans will likely continue to be debated for some time.

Migration

Generally, migration of neuroblasts occurs between one and fourteen days following birth by means of one of three modes—radial, tangential, or undirected wandering migration. In the mammalian CNS, neuroblasts originating from precursors in the SGZ translocate by means of radial migration into layer CA1 of the hippocampus, although typically after tangentially migrating independent of radial glia cells along the local vasculature (95). Alternatively, neuroblasts from the V-SVZ tangentially migrate to the olfactory bulb along chains of PSA-NCAM positive cells forming the rostral migratory stream (96). These PSA-NCAM positive chains consist of a network of differentiated neurons, astrocytes, and tanycytes (97). Migration of neuroblasts along the rostral migratory stream into the olfactory bulb occurs at a rate of nearly 120 µm/h [*in vitro* (98)] and as such generally occurs over 2 days and 2 weeks (99). In the mammalian brain (and other vertebrate brains too), radial glia, microvasculature, and the cells of the PSA-NCAM chains provide trophic support for the migrating neuroblasts through a multitude of factors including, but not limited to, IGF1 and BDNF (95, 100).

In songbirds, a small fraction of the neuroblasts originating from the lateral ventricles migrate mediolaterally along the fibers of radial glia projecting through the telencephalon (101, 102). However, not all neurogenic regions of the avian brain contain radial fibers (102). Rather, neuroblasts translocating to the olfactory bulb migrate tangentially on chains of PSA-NCAM in the avian telencephalon (74). Neuroblasts destined for HVC wander from the VZ without apparent directionality to and within HVC (103).

Integration and Survival

Newly generated neuroblasts undergo fairly dramatic attrition before successful incorporation into their respective neural circuits: generally around 50% of neuroblast die via programmed cell death across all neurogenic regions of all vertebrate brains investigated. The "selection process" on neuroblasts is tightly regulated by a plethora of factors, including sex steroids, neurotrophins, and inflammatory cytokines, among many others [for mechanisms see Ref. (82)]. In the DG nearly half of adult-born neurons die within 2 weeks of birth. The neuroblasts that survive the initial culling begin neurite outgrowth with dendrites extending into the molecular layer of the DG and axon extension into the hilus of the DG. By 2 weeks, nascent neurons in the DG begin spinogenesis and the axons begin forming functional connections on CA3 pyramidal neurons in the hilus. By 28 days, adult-born neurons of the DG become fully mature and indistinguishable in morphology, physiology, and behavior from pre-existing mature CA1 neurons [reviewed in Ref. (104)].

After 2–14 days, neuroblast arising from the V–SVZ exit the rostral migratory stream and migrate radially into the olfactory bulb, but not before nearly half of neuroblasts undergo apoptosis (99). Between 15 and 30 days, the persisting olfactory bulb neuroblasts differentiate into one of two types of local interneurons. The vast majority, around 95%, differentiate into GABAergic granule cells, whereas the remaining 5% differentiate into periglomerular neurons expressing either GABA, or dopamine, or both (99).

As is true with the other populations of new neurons in the mammalian brain, nearly 50% of all cells born from NSCs/NPCs undergo apoptosis during migration to their final destination in the avian brain as well (105). The majority of investigations characterizing the fate of neuroblasts in the avian brain originate from studies in the song control circuit, although recently studies have also examined adult neurogenesis in the avain hippocampus (106). Within the song control circuit nascent HVC projection neurons begin to express neuronal markers and form synapses on targets up to 4 mm away in the robust nucleus of archopallium (RA) as early as 2 weeks of age (105). By 28 days to 8 months, most new HVC neurons that survive the initial stages of culling form synapses onto RA neurons (105, 107). These new HVC to RA projection neurons persist for months (108) to years (109, 110), depending on their time of birth and the presence of sex steroids [reviewed in Ref. (81)].

Sex Steroidal Modulation

Sex steroids have complex roles in regulating adult neurogenesis, as broadly defined. Both E_2 and progesterone treatment independently increase mitosis of NSCs/NPCs [**Figure 2** (111, 112)]. However, as is the case with modulation of dendritic spine density (above), progesterone and E_2 reduce the effect of each steroidal hormone when administered together (112). Several studies have shown that natural seasonal plasticity of androgens and castration with supplementation of exogenous androgens enhance the survival of new neurons in both mammals and birds [reviewed in Ref. (3, 81)]. More specifically, the androgen metabolite DHT consistently promotes new neuron survival, whereas the metabolite E_2 has mixed effects, depending on the mammalian species examined, the sex of the animal, and timing and duration of E_2 exposure [reviewed in Ref. (3)]. Alternatively, in HVC of both male and female birds, both DHT and E_2 act independently and synergistically to enhance addition and survival of new neurons (113, 114). Sex steroids exert these pro-neurogenic effects by promoting increased DNA synthesis, transcription, and growth factor signaling and processes [for more see Ref. (3, 15, 81)].

Apoptosis

As discussed throughout, sex steroids generally promote the survival of new and mature neurons. Estrogens, however, have also been proposed to potentiate excitotoxic neuronal death, especially following pathological damage (2). This working hypothesis is supported by the increased sensitivity and excitability of neurons exposed to E_2 *via* estrogen-mediated increases in NMDA and AMPA receptor activity (discussed above). Increased firing of neurons, specifically through NMDA signaling in turn rapidly increases E_2 synthesis (115), and thus can drive a feed-forward cycle that could result in excitotoxic cell death. In this context, estrogens facilitate seizure activity in both animal models and humans (116, 117) through the initiation of an NMDA–E_2 positive-feedback loop (118). Clearly, there exists a fine balance between the beneficial and harmful effects of sex steroids in the maintenance of homeostasis and on neuron survival. And so, careful analysis of the spatiotemporal expression of sex steroids across the sexes and the effects of interactions between the classes of sex steroids on cell proliferation, behavior, and survival is critical for garnering a more thorough understanding of the basic biology and potential restorative value of sex steroids.

SEX STEROID ACTION ON NEUROINFLAMMATORY CELLS

Sex steroids play a pivotal role in the development and function of the immune system through both rapid and long-term mechanisms. Besides regulating the proliferation, migration, and differentiation of immune cells, sex steroids are generally neuroprotective under inflammatory conditions. The anti-inflammatory potential of sex steroids, specifically estrogens, originates from observations that the drop in steroidal hormones associated with menopause increases the incidence of neuroinflammatory associated neuropathologies [reviewed in Ref. (119)]. Subsequently, estrogens, and progesterones to a more limited degree, have been demonstrated to exert their generally protective regulatory action through direct and indirect regulation of immune cell morphology and behavior.

Microglia

Microglia are macrophage-like cells that originate from myeloid precursors during early development and migrate to and take up permanent residence in the developing CNS (120). The primary role of microglia is to continuously survey the microenvironment, remove cell debris and pathogens, and activate reactive inflammation. Microglia have both protective and destructive impacts in the CNS that largely depend on their state of activation (**Figure 4**). In the un-challenged, healthy brain "resting" or ramified microglia are highly motile (121) using their branches for surveilling their territorial domains for excess neural cells and synapses to phagocytose (122). Microglia remain in the resting or non-activated state through inhibitory signals from the neurons on which the microglial processes directly reside (123). The loss of connection between microglia and neurons, for example during neuronal death, accelerates the activation and response of microglia (123). With neural damage or loss of homeostasis, microglia become polarized to one of two states: M1 and M2 [mechanisms reviewed in Ref. (124)]. Inflammatory M1 microglia induce classical, and often harmful, cytotoxic responses through enhanced antigen presentation and the release of cytotoxic mediators, including NO, tumor necrosis factor alpha (TNFα), IL-1β, prostaglandin, and reactive oxygen species following activation by cytokines, interferons, and endotoxins [reviewed in Ref. (125)]. M1 microglia can molecularly switch to M2 microglia [reviewed in Ref. (124)], which phagocytose dying neurons and promote neurite outgrowth, oligodendrocyte fate specification, and angiogenesis following neuronal death (126–128). The switching between cell types and the balance between protective and restrictive outcomes depends on regulatory molecules in the local environment, including sex steroids, among many others [reviewed in Ref. (124, 125, 129)].

Administration of sex steroids before or after insult generally reduces infarct volume following middle cerebral artery occlusion [MCAO; reviewed in Ref. (129)], with evidence that this neuroprotective effect of sex steroids is mediated in part through microglia. For example, administration of E_2 and progesterone reduces the attraction of microglia (and leukocytes) to the MCAO-induced penumbra in both male and female rats (130). Moreover, the typically observed pro-inflammatory cytokines CCL2, CCL5, and IL-6 are lower in the penumbra following E_2 and progesterone treatment, suggesting that activation of local microglia is also suppressed by E_2 and progesterone (130).

Likewise, E_2 disrupts microglia activation following stimulation with lipopolysaccharide (LPS)—a lipoglycan endotoxin isolated from the outer membrane of Gram-negative bacteria and commonly used to mimic CNS infection and induce microglia activation (131). Typically, LPS activates the innate immune receptor toll-like 4 [TLR4 (132)] to induce microglia activation *via* MAPK phosphorylation and NFκB nuclear translocation (133,

134). In turn, microglia stimulated by LPS increase expression of pro-inflammatory cytokines (e.g., TNFα), cyclooxygenase-2), and NOS (135). E_2 activation of microglial ERα, but not ERβ, inhibits the LPS-induced translocation of NFκB family proteins to the nucleus and, consequently, reduces NFκB-dependent transcriptional activity and the resultant inflammatory response [**Figure 2** and **4** (136)]. Further supporting a role for E_2–ERα in microglia reactivity, exogenous systemic supplementation of E_2 prevents LPS-induced microglial activation and expression of neuroinflammatory mediators, specifically, metalloproteinase 9, and complement C3 receptor in mice (137). However, this impact of exogenous E_2 on microglia reactivity is lost in ERα-null mice (137).

The effects of steroidal hormones, however, might not be universal across the sexes: in cultured microglia isolated from neonatal hippocampus of male and female rats, E_2 administration following LPS stimulation of the *ex vivo* microglia attenuates IL-1β mRNA upregulation in male but not female microglia (138). The anti- and pro-inflammatory impact of E_2 on male and female neonatal microglia, respectively, indicates that E_2 drives differential microglia responses in males and females during development likely contributes to sexual differentiation of the CNS (139) and that the differential impact of E_2 across the sexes have effects beyond development. Given the above evidence that E_2 plays pro-neuroprotective and anti-inflammatory roles in the adult female CNS, additional studies directly testing the role of E_2 and the other sex steroids to determine when the switch between E_2-dependent pro- and anti-inflammatory effects occurs in females are necessary.

Astroglia

Astroglia, a sub-type of macroglial cells, comprise nine biochemically and developmentally distinct forms including radial, fibrous, protoplasmic, among others (140). As discussed above, radial astroglia (more commonly referred to simply as radial glia) are organized in planes perpendicular to the ventricle with one of their two projections extended toward the ventricle and the other deep into the gray matter. As such, radial glia structurally and trophically support migrating neuroblasts and, in doing so, play an extensive role in neural development and adult neurogenesis (**Figure 2** and **4**). Fibrous astroglia reside along white matter tracts and exhibit long unbranched fiber-like process, whereas protoplasmic astroglia are found throughout gray matter and are characterized by many fine branching processes uniformly distributed around the soma in the classic stellate pattern. Both fibrous and protoplasmic astrocytes establish highly organized territorial domains with their processes, one of which, the "end foot" contacts an intraparenchymal blood vessel whereas the other processes extend into and survey the surrounding microenvironment. In this manner, all astrocytes bi-directionally connect nutrient sources (e.g., cerebrospinal fluid and blood) to nearby glia, neuropil, and synapses, allowing for dynamic responses to microenvironmental changes [reviewed in Ref. (141)].

Under healthy physiological conditions, astrocytes maintain homeostasis and play key specialized roles in the CNS [reviewed in Ref. (142)]. For example, astrocytes not only facilitate high frequency neuronal firing through buffering of local pH (143), uptake of interstitial K+ (144) and glutamate recycling (145), but also modulate neural activity and the propagation of action potentials through the release of glutamate, GABA and calcium, among other "gliotransmitters" (141, 146). Astrocytes also supply energy and nutrients to cells of the CNS through several mechanisms, including, but not limited to: (1) rapid vasodilation during neural activity to increase the availability of oxygen and glucose (147), (2) storage and release of glycogen [reviewed in Ref. (148)], and (3) production, secretion, and distribution of cholesterols that cannot cross the BBB (149). And finally, under normal physiological conditions, non-reactive astrocytes, like ramified microglia, regulate the formation and pruning of synapses (150, 151).

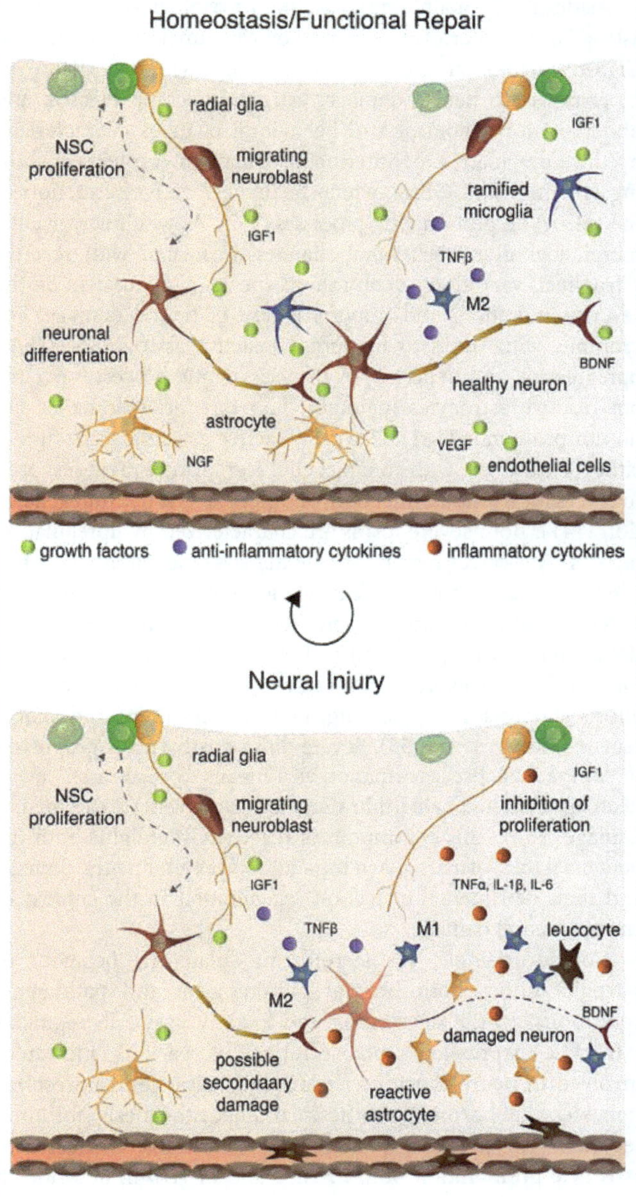

FIGURE 4 | Cellular interactions in homeostatic, injury-induced, and reparative conditions.

Aside from maintaining stable physiological conditions, astroglia also perform immunological functions similar to CNS-resident microglia and macrophages (**Figure 2** and **4**). In response to neural damage, astroglia become reactive and undergo morphological and behavioral changes characterized by the upregulation of intermediate filament proteins including vimentin and GFAP, which facilitate reactive retraction of the astrocytic perisynaptic processes (152). As with microglia, the morphological and behavioral changes associated with reactive astrogliosis vary along a continuous spectrum dependent on the severity and the spatiotemporal extent of neural damage. For example, with "mild to moderate" reactive astrogliosis, GFAP upregulation and hypertrophy of perisynaptic processes occurs, but reactive astrocytes maintain their territorial domains and do not proliferate (141). "Severe" reactive astrogliosis occurs as either "diffuse" or "with compact glial scar formation" in response to severe focal lesions, infection, or other chronic neurodegeneration (141). Both severe forms are characterized by upregulation of GFAP, processes hypertrophy, extensive intermingling of territorial domains, cytokine release and leukocyte, microglia, and T-cell recruitment, astrocytic proliferation, and reorganization of tissue architecture [reviewed in Ref. (141, 153)]. Moreover, the increased GFAP expression by astrocytes during reactive astrogliosis suppresses neurite outgrowth *in vitro* (154) and axonal regeneration *in vivo* (155). Severe diffuse astrogliosis progresses to compact glial scar formation as a means to cordon off severe necrosis and leukocyte infiltration and to prevent further neural damage (156). This continuum of reactivity highlights both the beneficial roles of astroglia in the acute stages after neural damage and their detrimental effects on regeneration in the context of chronic neural damage.

Not surprisingly, sex steroids modulate the behavior of astroglia under both normal physiological and pathogenic conditions. In the developing and healthy brain, E_2 regulates astrocytic expression and secretion of various molecules involved in neurotransmitter transport, mitochondria respiration, steroidal hormone synthesis, and neuritogenesis [for more see Ref. (157)]. Under pathological conditions, E_2 decreases astrocyte proliferation both *in vitro* and *in vivo* in addition to reducing cytokine secretion and glial scar formation (158–160). The modulation of the astrogliotic response by E_2 begins at the morphological activation of astrocytes: E_2 decreases the expression of GFAP and vimentin after injury-induced neuronal loss, ultimately preventing reactive astrogliosis [**Figure 2** (159, 161)]. Interestingly, E_2 stimulates GFAP expression in olfactory bulb astrocytes (162) and increases astrocytic proliferation in white matter (163), suggesting regional and astrocyte-type differences in response to sex steroids and possibly even impacts on neuroprotection.

Generally, sex steroids suppress astrocytic secretion of pro-inflammatory molecules and the subsequent recruitment of additional inflammatory cells. For instance, as with microglial activation, E_2 prevents LPS stimulated translocation of NFκB to the nucleus and production of TNFα, NO, IL-1β, and IL-6 in astrocytes (164–166). As mentioned above, E_2 suppression of NFκB in astrocytes also results in decreased astrocytic expression of ICAM1 (64), a CAMs that mediates leukocyte–endothelial cell interactions necessary for transmigration of leukocytes across the BBB into the CNS. In this manner, E_2 synthesis and secretion by astrocytes may decrease the permeability of the BBB to leukocytes and contribute to the mitigation of inflammation and glial scaring following neural damage.

Neuronal injury within the mammalian and avian CNS routinely enhances the expression and activity of aromatase (167, 168), which, consequently, permits increases in local estrogen synthesis and confers neuroprotection [**Figure 2** (169)]. Important to understanding mechanisms of injury-induced aromatase activity, upregulation of aromatase occurs in and around the lesion site regardless of the whether or not the affected brain region produces aromatase under normal physiological conditions (170, 171). In fact, this upregulation of aromatase occurs specifically within the locally activated astrocytes. These astrocytes in turn synthesize and secrete estradiol to decrease local neuronal apoptosis (169), as well as likely inducing nearby proliferation of NSCs and migration of neuroblasts to the region of damage [(discussed above and below (172)].

Macrophages, Neutrophils, Monocytes, Dendritic Cells (DCs), and Lymphocytes

In addition to microglia and macroglia, sex steroids modulate inflammation through other inflammatory cells as well. CNS-resident macrophages, neutrophils, non-proliferative monocytes, antigen presenting myeloid cells (i.e., DCs), and lymphocytes (i.e., T-, B-, and natural killer cells) continuously surveil the CNS, rapidly infiltrate sites of injury to clear dead cells and pathogens, recruit additional inflammatory cells for tissue repair, and in some contexts, provide protection from similar future insults. Generally, macrophages, monocytes, and neutrophils minimize inflammation through the phagocytosis of dead cells and debris and the release of cytokines and chemokines to recruit additional leukocytes (e.g., monocytes, neutrophils, etc.) to the CNS and site of injury [reviewed in Ref. (173)]. Another phagocyte, the DC, serves as a sentinel by sensing the local environment through continuous and regular endocytosis. Depending on the environmental signals perceived, DCs dictate the type of inflammatory response initiated through differential secretion of cytokines, some of which promote the differentiation of activated T cells, reviewed in Ref. (174). Differentiated T cells can in turn secrete cytokines, stimulate the activation other cell types (e.g., DCs, macrophages, B cells, etc.), and initiate cytotoxic "killer" functions (174). Together, the degree of collaboration of different inflammatory cell types promotes a unique step-wise program and cytokine profile dictating the impact of the inflammatory response. Although initially beneficial, extensive or overreactive activation and recruitment of leukocytes, DCs, and lymphocytes can push the inflammatory response beyond beneficial toward detrimental in terms of neuroprotection and repair (175).

The majority of evidence supporting a role for sex steroids in regulating these other inflammatory cells originates with male-female differences in insult-responsive cell numbers, with a few exceptions [reviewed in Ref. (173)]. For instance, resident macrophages have higher TLR expression and phagocytic activity in females than males, which possibly contributes to the greater response efficiency and survival of females during sepsis (176).

Likewise, plasmic neutrophil counts correlate with systemic estrogen levels (177). Although vastly understudied, the mechanistic role of estrogens in regulating leukocytes, lymphocytes, and DCs is becoming more evident. In addition to decreasing NκFB nuclear translocation and TNFα, IL-1β, and IL-6 expression in microglia and astrocytes, E_2 regulates macrophages and monocytes stimulated with LPS or other neural trauma through these same mechanisms [**Figure 2** (178, 179)]. Neutrophils decrease IL-1β and IL-6 secretion following injury to the carotid arteries when exposed to E_2 (180). Estrogens also regulate the motility of monocytes and neutrophils: E_2 not only decreases transcytosis of leukocytes across the BBB through changes in BBB permeability (discussed above), but also modulates leukocyte migration through direct action on the leukocytes themselves. Specifically, E_2 decreases CXCR2, a chemokine receptor that mediates monocyte and neutrophil adhesion and chemotaxis, following cytokine stimulation or injury (180–182). As such, E_2 suppression of leukocyte migration across the BBB and within the CNS may restrict recruitment of inflammatory cells and, in turn severe inflammatory responses to promote sex steroid dependent neuroprotection.

Estrogens also regulate myeloid cell and lymphocyte differentiation and function, and thus DCs and T cells are involved in mediating the neuroprotective effects of estrogens. For instance, estrogen signaling *via* ERα is necessary for DC differentiation and modulates the acquisition of DC effector functions (183). The estrogen estriol (E_3) promotes immune self-tolerance functions of DCs through increased expression of anti-inflammatory cytokines IL-10 and TGF-β and decreased expression of pro-inflammatory cytokines IL-12 and IL-6 (183). Likewise, E_2 promotes the development and function of regulatory T cells, which participate in the maintenance of self-tolerance and, when aberrant, autoimmune disorders through upregulation of the transcriptional factor FoxP3 within T cells (184). Together these data provide the beginnings of a mechanistic understanding for the well-known female sex bias in the development of neurological autoimmune disorders and psychiatric disease [for more, see Ref. (185)]. Future efforts examining the influence of steroidal hormones on myeloid cell and lymphocyte physiology and impacts are undoubtably justified.

INTEGRATION OF SEX STEROIDS, NEUROGENESIS, AND NEUROINFLAMMATION

The first conclusive evidence that inflammation impacts adult neurogenesis came in 2003 from a study showing that a 4-week infusion of LPS into the hippocampus decreased NSC proliferation (186). The same year another study demonstrated that systemic inflammation induced through intraperitoneal injection of LPS similarly decreased NSC proliferation (187). Moreover, the LPS-mediated impairment of adult neurogenesis was ameliorated by the administration of inhibitors of microglia activation, minocycline and indomethacin, suggesting microglia were likely regulating NSC behavior (186, 187). Given the 4-week time course of LPS infusion, the observed decrease in NSC proliferation could have resulted from increased NSC apoptosis (122) and reduction of neuroblast incorporation into circuits (188). Yet, subsequent studies have confirmed that LPS promotes a neuroinflammatory response, including depression of NSC proliferation, through direct stimulation of astrocytes and microglia in addition to indirect recruitment of leukocytes, specifically monocytes and neutrophils (189, 190).

Recent studies highlight the dynamic role of inflammatory cells, their interactions, and their responses in modulating adult neurogenesis and the regenerative capabilities of the CNS. Most of such efforts have focused on neuroinflammatory responses to physical damage, such as ischemia and traumatic brain injury, or pharmacological insult, including treatment with LPS or pro-inflammatory cytokines and chemokines. Currently, few studies have directly assessed the role of immune cells in regulating adult neurogenesis, as broadly defined here to include NSC proliferation, neuroblast migration, and nascent neuronal differentiation and survival, under healthy, homeostatic conditions. Below, I briefly discuss advances in understanding the damage-induced inflammatory response on NSC and their nascent progeny after first highlighting the few studies that have addressed the impact of non-reactive and alternatively activated (i.e., M2) microglia on neurogenesis.

Regulation of Adult Neurogenesis by Microglia

Ramified, unchallenged microglia play a pivotal role in homeostasis not only in the parenchyma (above) but also in the neurogenic niches of the CNS. Ramified microglia instruct neuronal differentiation of neuroblasts through the secretion of a still unknown factor [**Figures 2** and **4**; (191)] and facilitates clearance by phagocytosis of the ~50% of neuroblasts that do not differentiate and functionally incorporate into circuits (122). Likewise, alternatively activated M2 microglia promote pro-neurogenic effects through the release of anti-inflammatory cytokines including IL-4, IL-10, and TGFβ; tpysinogen, a precursor of the enzyme trypsin; and growth factor such as IGF1 and BDNF [**Figures 2** and **4**; reviewed in Ref. (124)]. For instance, chronic elevation of microglial TGFβ enhances the survival of proliferative NSC and the differentiation of progeny into the neuronal (as opposed to glial) lineage (192). Likewise, microglia stimulated with IL-4 or IL-10 enhance NPC proliferation, perhaps through the upregulation of IGF1 production following anti-inflammatory cytokine stimulation (193, 194).

Reactive M1 microglia also have immediate beneficial impacts on recovery from neural insult, as they facilitate the initial clearance of debris. Typically, however, in the context of neurogenic repair following clearance of injury- or pathogen-induced neuronal death, M1 microglia have detrimental effects on neurogenesis (**Figure 4**). M1 microglia secretion of pro-inflammatory cytokines, including TNFα, IL-1β, IL-6, and INF-γ (195), directly impair NSC proliferation, suggesting that the NSCs themselves are capable of detecting and responding to certain cytokines. Besides modulating NSC proliferation, these cytokines impair other processes of adult neurogenesis (as broadly defined) from the migration and differentiation of neuroblasts to final incorporation and survival of new neurons. For instance, IL-1β not only decreases NSC proliferation but also impairs the survival of neuroblasts and hinders neuronal differentiation (196). Although not tested directly as an output of microglia, administration of TNFα, a secreted factor of M1 microglia, promotes the apoptosis of NSC (197) and increases the proportion of daughter cells that differentiate into the astrocytic as opposed to neuronal lineage (198). Likewise, IL-6 reduces NPC proliferation through promotion of progenitor differentiation, albeit into neurons (199).

The differential beneficial and detrimental impacts of microglia underscore the need to further characterize microglial behaviors in healthy and neurodegenerative conditions, and to elucidate mechanisms driving molecular and behavioral switches between states of microglial activation. Additional, carefully controlled studies will also be important for deciphering upstream and downstream regulatory mechanisms of cytokines, growth factors, and other signaling factors: research efforts should be made to disentangle the beneficial versus detrimental impacts of microglia on themselves, other inflammatory cells (astrocytes, leukocytes, DCs, T cells), and CNS-resident cells (endothelial cells of the parenchymal vasculature and BBB, neurons).

Astroglia, Aromatase, and Adult Neurogenesis

As mentioned above, astroglia can synthesize and secrete E_2. In songbirds, the number of newly generated cells positively correlates with the number of precursor radial glial cell processes expressing aromatase (200). Likewise, the degree of neurogenesis also correlates positively with the number of aromatase expressing non-precursor astrocytes, and this correlation is abolished with ovariectomy and administration of aromatase inhibitors (172, 201). Non-precursor astrocytes also actively regulate the differentiation and survival of newly generated neurons (**Figures 2** and **4**). For instance, astrocytic expression of ephrin-B2 induces neuronal differentiation *via* EphB4 receptors on NSCs and subsequent activation of Wnt signaling (202). Moreover, astrocytes facilitate dendritic spine maturation and synapse formation of adult-born neurons through vesicular release of D-serine, a co-agonist (along with glycine) of the NMDA receptor expressed by new neurons (203). However, very few studies have directly tested roles for activated, immunogenic astroglia in regulating NSC proliferation, neuroblast migration and differentiation, or neuronal incorporation and survival. Given the similarities in activation responses between microglia and astroglia, one could easily deduce that if astroglia directly regulate NSCs, then the initial astrogliotic response following injury would likely promote neurogenesis, whereas chronic astrogliosis likely hinders NSC proliferation and new neuron differentiation and survival.

Regulation of Myelination Through Sex Steroid Impacts on Immune Cells

Sex steroids also enhance the myelination of new neurons and the remyelination of mature neurons following pathological demyelination. As discussed above, under non-pathological conditions sex steroids directly promote the proliferation of OPCs, differentiation of new oligodendrocytes and stimulate oligodendrocyte activities including sheath synthesis and wrapping of axons. The impact of sex steroids on oligodendrocyte behavior also occurs indirectly through immune cell-mediated interactions. For example, the CNS autoimmune disorder MS is more prevalent in women than men. Moreover, the characteristic relapsing and progressive sclerotic plaques and demyelination of MS can be alleviated by treatment with sex steroidal hormones (204). In a murine model of MS administration of the copper chelator cuprizone induces toxic demyelination, which is lessened in severity by treatment with progesterone (73). Likewise, treatment with E_2 following cuprizone administration also ameliorates demyelination and promotes myelin repair (163). Progesterone and E_2 both independently induce IGF1 expression in astrocytes, which in turn promotes the proliferation of OPCs and the differentiation of progeny into myelinating oligodendrocytes (163, 205). The beneficial impact of estrogens is, at least in part, mediated through ERα-dependent signaling in reactive astroglia. Treatment of experimental autoimmune encephalomyelitis (EAE) mice, another model for MS, with the selective ERα agonist PLP peptide 139–151 (PPT), decreases the production of TNFα, interferon-γ, and IL-6 in addition to decreasing the recruitment of macrophages and T cells and EAE-associated demyelination (206–208). Conditional gene deletions of ERα in astroglia, but not neurons, reversed the effect of PPT treatment on macrophage and T cell recruitment and prevented estrogen-mediated attenuation of gliosis and axonal degeneration in EAE mice (208). The ERβ agonist WAY-202041 has minimal reported effects on EAE-induced cytokine production (206). Interestingly, however, ERβ, but not ERα, is expressed in microglia. Treatment of EAE mice with the selective ERβ agonist LY3201 promotes microglia to retain their ramified morphology and, as such, reduces microglia NFκB activation and iNOS expression (209).

Microglia and astroglia, in addition to other immune cell types, facilitate not only debris removal following demyelination, axonal damage, and neuronal death, but also neurogenesis, gliogenesis, nascent cell fate specification, arbor and synapse maturation, and nude axonal ensheathment. Although sex steroids clearly modulate the behavior and impact of immune cells, gaps in our understanding of the complex interactions between immune cells, neural cells, and sex hormones still exist. Thus, directly testing the relative impact of reactive astrogliosis and activated microglia on adult neurogenesis and gliogenesis will be essential for understanding not only the unique roles of micro- and macroglia during regeneration but also the manner through which astrocytic and microglial responses integrate into the larger orchestra of neuroinflammation.

FUTURE DIRECTIONS: EMERGING MODELS OF NEUROINFLAMMATION AND REGENERATION

The role of inflammation in neurocognitive disorders and employment of sex steroidal and anti-inflammatory therapeutics has been discussed extensively in past reviews. So instead, here, I limit the discussion to emerging models of neuroinflammation and regeneration. For more information on the role of inflammation in relatively well-characterized psychiatric and neurodegenerative disorders and classes of therapeutics see **Table 1**.

Neurological Diseases With Recently Discovered Immune Component

The reemergence of fetal microcephaly as a result of maternal Zika viral infection has recently leapt onto the main stage as a neurodevelopmental disorder with an underlying neuroimmune component. This is not to suggest that Zika virus (ZIKV) is the only neurological disease with developing evidence for an inflammatory component, but it certainly of recent piqued interest, and thus, I will briefly discuss ZIKV-induced microcephaly here. Following the detection of ZIKV in the fetal brain (220) and establishment of a causal relationship between ZIKV infection and microcephaly (221) in 2016, ZIKV was discovered to infect NPCs and attenuate their growth (222). Specifically within radial glia progenitor cells, ZIKV reduces proliferation and promotes premature differentiation through ZIKV protein NS2A destabilization of the adherens junction complex, and as a result, mis-scaffolding of the radial processes (223). Two other ZIKV proteins, NS4A and NS4B, cooperatively inhibit AKT and mTOR signaling in NSCs, leading to decreased proliferation and increased autophogy of the NSC (224). ZIKV also infects microglia of human fetal brain, rendering the microglia reactive. ZIKV-infected microglia secrete high levels of pro-inflammatory factors TNF-α, IL-1β, IL-6, among several others (225), which likely further decreases embryonic neurogenesis through mechanisms discussed above. Cleary, additional studies determining the mechanisms of ZIKV's negative impact on neurogenesis and neuroinflammation are warranted and these mechanisms will certainly be taken into consideration during the development of therapeutics and vaccines. Given that ZIKV infects both stem cells and microglia consequently decreasing neurogenesis, it will be important to evaluate potential long-term consequences of infection in the adult brain. Postfetal infection with ZIKV will most certainly negatively impact the maintenance of neural homeostasis through aberrations in NSC and neuroinflammatory cell behavior. Thus, it seems likely that postfetal infection with ZIKV could result in the manifestation of neuropsychiatric and neurodegenerative disorders associated with disruptions in neurogenesis and chronic neural inflammation (see **Table 1**).

Non-Traditional Model With High Natural Neuronal Turnover and Plasticity

Songbirds provide a powerful model for understanding the mechanisms, including those of the neurcimmune system, that regulate natural neuronal turnover during periods of homeostatic stability and robust plasticity. Avian song learning and production are regulated by discrete, well-characterized and intertwined circuits—the anterior forebrain pathway and song production pathway, respectively (**Figure 3**). The song production pathway includes the highly neurogenic nucleus HVC and its target nucleus, the robust nucleus of the archopallium (RA). In temporal resident and migratory (226) birds (most often the males), both HVC and RA undergo dramatic sex steroid dependent physiological and morphological changes between environmental seasons [reviewed in Ref. (227)]. Early each breeding season (spring) HVC and RA nearly double in volume. The increase in HVC volume results largely from the addition of over 50,000 new neurons to a pre-breeding season neuronal population of around 100,000 [numbers from Gambel's white-crowned sparrows (*Zonotrichia leucophrys gambelii*) (228, 229) and vary across species (226)]. Alternatively, the growth of RA volume results from increases in neuron size and spacing, but not number (228, 229). Both HVC and RA demonstrate evidence of increased neural activity during the breeding season (230, 231), which has been proposed to be one function of the seasonal uptick in addition of new HVC neurons (81). The seasonal growth of the song production pathway nuclei is concomitantly linked to increased rate and quality of singing behavior (232), which is used most typically by male birds for territory maintenance and mate attraction. As seasonally plastic songbirds transition into the non breeding season (fall), plasmic levels of sex steroids decrease and the song production pathway regresses (89, 233, 234). Regression of HVC occurs very rapidly, with the caspase-mediated apoptosis of 50,000 neurons (a mixture of new and old neurons) occurring between one and four days following transition into non-breeding conditions (89, 235). As soon as one day following transition, song rate and quality also decreases dramatically (89).

Importantly, yet unsurprisingly given the evidence above, systemic inflammation negatively impacts hormonal responses and behavior in songbirds. Subcutaneous injection of LPS in the songbird Gambel's white-crowned sparrow prompts a rapid increase in plasma corticosterone levels, suppresses luteinizing hormone (a trigger of gonad growth and production of sex steroids), and impairs total activity encompassing decreases in food and water intake, singing, and territorial aggression (236). These observations in conjunction with the known upregulation of aromatase expression by astroglia in the zebra finch telencephalon following

TABLE 1 | Neurological disorders with known inflammatory component and therapeutics.

Psychiatric disorders	
Depression	(119, 210)
Schizophrenia	(119)
Autism	(211, 212)
Neurodegernative disorders	
Multiple sclerosis	(119, 213)
Amyotrophic lateral sclerosis	(119)
Parkinson's disease	(119, 214, 215)
Alzheimer's disease	(15, 119)
Traumatic injury	
Cerebral ischemia	(119, 216)
Aging	(3, 210)
Therapeutics	
Selective estrogen receptor modulators	(15, 217)
Blood–brain barrier	(1, 46, 47)
Macrophage delivery	(218)
Mesenchymal stem cells	(216, 219)
Neural stem cells	(216, 219)

injury (171, 201) firmly establish that inflammation impacts the avian CNS and likely plays a role in neural homeostasis and seasonal plasticity of the song circuits.

Interestingly, the seasonal regression of HVC through caspase-mediated apoptosis is necessary for reactive proliferation of neural stem/progenitor cells in the nearby VZ and subsequent HVC neuronal addition (89, 235, 237). Given the likely role of phagocytic cells in the clearance of dying HVC neurons, microglia, and astrocytes may confer the signal of neuronal death in HVC to the VZ neural stem/progenitor cells. If so, the potential for understanding the functions and mechanisms of microglia and astrocytes during natural death or turnover of neurons and the functional incorporation of new long-range projection neurons [as opposed to interneurons or locally projecting adult-born neurons in mammals (81, 104)] is unparalleled. However, to date, any functional mechanistic connections between sex steroid dependent neural plasticity, natural reactive neurogenesis, and neuroinflammatory involvement remains to be directly tested.

Songbirds also provide a tractable model for investigating the interactions between neurogenesis, neuroinflammation, and sex steroid levels, both elevated and basal in both males and females. Although all passerine songbirds have the neural circuits controlling song learning and production, not all songbirds are seasonally plastic. For example, zebra finches are highly social opportunistic breeders, and as such, do not have photoperiod-dependent seasonality of either systemic testosterone levels or HVC neuronal addition. Yet, even in non-seasonally plastic species of songbirds, new neurons do continuously enter and incorporate within HVC, replacing older HVC to RA projection neurons (110). Thus, comparative studies across species or manipulative studies in both seasonal and opportunistic species could provide mechanistic insight into the neuroimmune modulatory effects of sex steroids across the sexes and under varying reproductive states.

Non-Traditional Model With High Regenerative Capacity

Teleost fishes have the most widespread and pronounced adult neurogenesis of any vertebrate examined, with 12–16 proliferative zone distributed across telencephalon, diencephalon, optic tectum, cerebellum, and hindbrain of fish [**Figure 3**; (83)]. Teleosts have indeterminate growth (i.e., continue to grow throughout life), and adult neurogenesis has been proposed to function not only in corresponding growth of the CNS but also in replacing naturally dying neurons [reviewed in Ref. (81, 238)]. The mechanisms of adult neurogenesis in teleost fish are characteristic of those in mammals and birds, with a few exceptions—for more on localization of proliferative zones and mechanisms, see Ref. (238).

Across all vertebrates traumatic brain injury is characterized by apoptosis of neurons, glia, and endothelial cells, inflammation, proliferation of micro- and macroglial cells, and increased neural stem/progenitor cell proliferation. Depending on the severity of the lesion, the secondary effects can include a penumbra of degeneration, inflammation, and breakdown of the BBB, all of which further complicate regenerative abilities and functional recovery of behavior. After traumatic brain injury, bony fishes have the remarkable ability to not only upregulate the proliferation of NSCs and migration of neuroblasts, but to functionally incorporate new neurons that survive long term and to near completely restore tissue architecture at the site of the lesion [reviewed in Ref. (239)]. The first evidence of such brain regeneration in fish came from optic tectum lesion experiments in juvenile carp (*Carassium carassium*), in which the size of the remaining progenitor zone correlated with the degree of tissue restoration (240). Reactive proliferation also occurs in the cerebellum of weakly electric fish (*Apteronotus leptorhynchus*) as soon as one day following apoptosis-mediated clearance of cells at the lesion site (241, 242). Apoptosis rather than necrosis at the lesion promotes a "clean" type of cell death, which has been proposed to contribute to the remarkable regenerative ability of fishes (241). Likewise, zebrafish exhibit reactive progenitor cell proliferation, neuroblast migration, nascent neuronal incorporation, and restoration of tissue architecture following stab lesions through the olfactory bulb and into the telencephalon (243).

Many factors regulate teleost reactive neurogenesis [reviewed in Ref. (239)], including inflammation. Traumatic injury to the zebrafish telencephalon stimulates the activation of microglia, infiltration of leukocytes, and the secretion of pro-inflammatory cytokines TNFα, IL-1β, and IL-8 (244). Upregulation of cysteinyl leukotriene receptor 1 expression in the NPC niche is also induced by traumatic brain injury as wells as cerebroventricular microinjection of the immunogenic zymosan A BioParticles (244). Moreover, administration of leukotriene C4, a ligand for CysLT1, enhances NPC proliferation without physical injury, suggesting cysteinyl leukotriene signaling is an essential regulator of the inflammatory-mediated neurogenic response in zebrafish (244). The chemokine receptor CXCR5 is expressed within and is a critical regulatory signal for the proliferation of the radial neural progenitors of the zebrafish telencephalon following stab lesion (245).

The profound regenerative ability of the fish CNS begs the question, "why is regeneration relatively limited in the mammalian brain?" Comparative studies uncovering the conserved and evolutionarily distinct molecular mechanisms that govern regenerative neurogenesis will inform not only neuroimmune and regenerative biology generally but also neurological disease etiology, and treatments that enhance NSC activity and successful neuroblast incorporation and survival.

CONCLUDING REMARKS

Although still not extensively examined, there clearly exist important links between sex steroids, neuroinflammatory responses, and adult neurogenesis. In this review, I have provided convincing evidence that sex steroids independently influence the processes and mechanisms of adult neurogenesis and neuroimmune responses. Moreover, sex steroids are secreted as an effector of the inflammatory response, and so likely influence immune cell-mediated homeostatic neurogenesis and neural repair. Integration of the sub-fields of sex steroids, neuroinflammation, and neurogenesis will embolden a better understanding of basic biology of NSCs and neuroimmune function, as well as the etiology of neural disorders—those with established and emerging evidence of a neuroimmune component. Ultimately, future studies exploiting the intersection of sex steroids, inflammation, and neurogenesis will spur the development of novel therapeutic strategies for the treatment of neuropsychiatric and neurodegenerative disorders. The future of neuroinflammation and adult neurogenesis research will no doubt be complicated, but will also certainly be exciting and rewarding!

AUTHOR CONTRIBUTIONS

The author confirms being the sole contributor of this work and approved it for publication.

ACKNOWLEDGMENTS

Supported by Pratt and UVa startup funds to TL. The author thanks Sandy R. Larson for extensive discussions, guidance, and editorial comments and David M. Parichy for editorial comments.

REFERENCES

1. Pelligrino DA, Galea E. Estrogen and cerebrovascular physiology and pathophysiology. *Jpn J Pharmacol* (2001) 86:137–58. doi:10.1254/jjp.86.137
2. Strom JO, Theodorsson A, Theodorsson E. Mechanisms of estrogens' dose-dependent neuroprotective and neurodamaging effects in experimental models of cerebral ischemia. *Int J Mol Sci* (2011) 12:1533–62. doi:10.3390/ijms12031533
3. Mahmoud R, Wainwright SR, Galea LA. Sex hormones and adult hippocampal neurogenesis: regulation, implications, and potential mechanisms. *Front Neuroendocrinol* (2016) 41:129–52. doi:10.1016/j.yfrne.2016.03.002
4. Hemsell DL, Grodin JM, Brenner PF, Siiteri PK, MacDonald PC. Plasma precursors of estrogen. II. Correlation of the extent of conversion of plasma androstenedione to estrone with age. *J Clin Endocrinol Metab* (1974) 38:476–9. doi:10.1210/jcem-38-3-476
5. Phoenix CH, Goy RW, Gerall AA, Young WC. Organizing action of prenatally administered testosterone propionate on the tissues mediating mating behavior in the female guinea pig. *Endocrinology* (1959) 65:369–82. doi:10.1210/endo-65-3-369
6. McCarthy MM. Estradiol and the developing brain. *Physiol Rev* (2008) 88:91–124. doi:10.1152/physrev.00010.2007
7. Payne AH, Hales DB. Overview of steroidogenic enzymes in the pathway from cholesterol to active steroid hormones. *Endocr Rev* (2004) 25:947–70. doi:10.1210/er.2003-0030
8. Barakat R, Oakley O, Kim H, Jin J, Ko CJ. Extra-gonadal sites of estrogen biosynthesis and function. *BMB Rep* (2016) 49:488–96. doi:10.5483/BMBRep.2016.49.9.141
9. Webb SJ, Geoghegan TE, Prough RA, Michael Miller KK. The biological actions of dehydroepiandrosterone involves multiple receptors. *Drug Metab Rev* (2006) 38:89–116. doi:10.1080/03602530600569877
10. Hanukoglu I, Karavolas HJ, Goy RW. Progesterone metabolism in the pineal, brain stem, thalamus and corpus callosum of the female rat. *Brain Res* (1977) 125:313–24. doi:10.1016/0006-8993(77)90624-2
11. Blair RM, Fang H, Branham WS, Hass BS, Dial SL, Moland CL, et al. The estrogen receptor relative binding affinities of 188 natural and xenochemicals: structural diversity of ligands. *Toxicol Sci* (2000) 54:138–53. doi:10.1093/toxsci/54.1.138
12. Carroll JS, Meyer CA, Song J, Li W, Geistlinger TR, Eeckhoute J, et al. Genome-wide analysis of estrogen receptor binding sites. *Nat Genet* (2006) 38:1289–97. doi:10.1038/ng1901
13. Prossnitz ER, Arterburn JB, Sklar LA. GPR30: a G protein-coupled receptor for estrogen. *Mol Cell Endocrinol* (2007) 265-266:138–42. doi:10.1016/j.mce.2006.12.010
14. Singh M. Ovarian hormones elicit phosphorylation of Akt and extracellular-signal regulated kinase in explants of the cerebral cortex. *Endocrine* (2001) 14:407–15. doi:10.1385/ENDO:14:3:407
15. Brinton RD, Thompson RF, Foy MR, Baudry M, Wang J, Finch CE, et al. Progesterone receptors: form and function in brain. *Front Neuroendocrinol* (2008) 29:313–39. doi:10.1016/j.yfrne.2008.02.001
16. Leung JK, Sadar MD. Non-genomic actions of the androgen receptor in prostate cancer. *Front Endocrinol* (2017) 8:2. doi:10.3389/fendo.2017.00002
17. Thomas P, Pang Y. Protective actions of progesterone in the cardiovascular system: potential role of membrane progesterone receptors (mPRs) in mediating rapid effects. *Steroids* (2013) 78:583–8. doi:10.1016/j.steroids.2013.01.003
18. Suzuki S, Brown CM, Wise PM. Neuroprotective effects of estrogens following ischemic stroke. *Front Neuroendocrinol* (2009) 30:201–11. doi:10.1016/j.yfrne.2009.04.007
19. Toran-Allerand CD, Singh M, Setalo G Jr. Novel mechanisms of estrogen action in the brain: new players in an old story. *Front Neuroendocrinol* (1999) 20:97–121. doi:10.1006/frne.1999.0177
20. Jelks KB, Wylie R, Floyd CL, McAllister AK, Wise P. Estradiol targets synaptic proteins to induce glutamatergic synapse formation in cultured hippocampal neurons: critical role of estrogen receptor-alpha. *J Neurosci* (2007) 27:6903–13. doi:10.1523/JNEUROSCI.0909-07.2007
21. Woolley CS, Weiland NG, McEwen BS, Schwartzkroin PA. Estradiol increases the sensitivity of hippocampal CA1 pyramidal cells to NMDA receptor-mediated synaptic input: correlation with dendritic spine density. *J Neurosci* (1997) 17:1848–59. doi:10.1523/JNEUROSCI.17-05-01848.1997
22. Edwards HE, Epps T, Carlen PL, MacLusky NJ. Progestin receptors mediate progesterone suppression of epileptiform activity in tetanized hippocampal slices in vitro. *Neuroscience* (2000) 101:895–906. doi:10.1016/S0306-4522(00)00439-5
23. Ito K, Skinkle KL, Hicks TP. Age-dependent, steroid-specific effects of oestrogen on long-term potentiation in rat hippocampal slices. *J Physiol* (1999) 515(Pt 1):209–20. doi:10.1111/j.1469-7793.1999.209ad.x
24. Nilsen J, Brinton RD. Impact of progestins on estrogen-induced neuroprotection: synergy by progesterone and 19-norprogesterone and antagonism by medroxyprogesterone acetate. *Endocrinology* (2002) 143:205–12. doi:10.1210/endo.143.1.8582
25. Hatanaka Y, Hojo Y, Mukai H, Murakami G, Komatsuzaki Y, Kim J, et al. Rapid increase of spines by dihydrotestosterone and testosterone in hippocampal neurons: dependence on synaptic androgen receptor and kinase networks. *Brain Res* (2015) 1621:121–32. doi:10.1016/j.brainres.2014.12.011
26. Adams MM, Fink SE, Shah RA, Janssen WG, Hayashi S, Milner TA, et al. Estrogen and aging affect the subcellular distribution of estrogen receptor-alpha in the hippocampus of female rats. *J Neurosci* (2002) 22:3608–14.
27. Mukai H, Tsurugizawa T, Murakami G, Kominami S, Ishii H, Ogiue-Ikeda M, et al. Rapid modulation of long-term depression and spinogenesis via synaptic estrogen receptors in hippocampal principal neurons. *J Neurochem* (2007) 100:950–67. doi:10.1111/j.1471-4159.2006.04264.x
28. Sirbasku DA. Hormone-responsive growth in vivo of a tissue culture cell line established from the MT-W9A rat mammary tumor. *Cancer Res* (1978) 38:1154–65.
29. Sohrabji F. Estrogen-IGF-1 interactions in neuroprotection: ischemic stroke as a case study. *Front Neuroendocrinol* (2015) 36:1–14. doi:10.1016/j.yfrne.2014.05.003
30. Miranda RC, Sohrabji F, Toran-Allerand CD. Neuronal colocalization of mRNAs for neurotrophins and their receptors in the developing central nervous system suggests a potential for autocrine interactions. *Proc Natl Acad Sci U S A* (1993) 90:6439–43. doi:10.1073/pnas.90.14.6439
31. Haghir H, Rezaee AA, Nomani H, Sankian M, Kheradmand H, Hami J. Sexual dimorphism in expression of insulin and insulin-like growth factor-I receptors in developing rat cerebellum. *Cell Mol Neurobiol* (2013) 33:369–77. doi:10.1007/s10571-012-9903-6
32. Toran-Allerand CD. Mechanisms of estrogen action during neural development: mediation by interactions with the neurotrophins and their receptors? *J Steroid Biochem Mol Biol* (1996) 56:169–78. doi:10.1016/0960-0760(95)00234-0

33. Reiner A, Perkel DJ, Mello CV, Jarvis ED. Songbirds and the revised avian brain nomenclature. *Ann N Y Acad Sci* (2004) 1016:77–108. doi:10.1196/annals.1298.013
34. Wade J. TrkB-like immunoreactivity in the song system of developing zebra finches. *J Chem Neuroanat* (2000) 19:33–9. doi:10.1016/S0891-0618(00)00051-X
35. Wissman AM, Brenowitz EA. The role of neurotrophins in the seasonal-like growth of the avian song control system. *J Neurosci* (2009) 29:6461–71. doi:10.1523/JNEUROSCI.0638-09.2009
36. Altamirano F, Oyarce C, Silva P, Estrada M. Testosterone activates mTOR/S6K1 pathway through intracellular calcium and ERK in cardiomyocytes. *FASEB J* (2008) 22:742.4.
37. Sanchez JF, Sniderhan LF, Williamson AL, Fan S, Chakraborty-Sett S, Maggirwar SB. Glycogen synthase kinase 3beta-mediated apoptosis of primary cortical astrocytes involves inhibition of nuclear factor kappaB signaling. *Mol Cell Biol* (2003) 23:4649–62. doi:10.1128/MCB.23.13.4649-4662.2003
38. Mannella P, Brinton RD. Estrogen receptor protein interaction with phosphatidylinositol 3-kinase leads to activation of phosphorylated Akt and extracellular signal-regulated kinase 1/2 in the same population of cortical neurons: a unified mechanism of estrogen action. *J Neurosci* (2006) 26:9439–47. doi:10.1523/JNEUROSCI.1443-06.2006
39. Kramar EA, Chen LY, Brandon NJ, Rex CS, Liu F, Gall CM, et al. Cytoskeletal changes underlie estrogen's acute effects on synaptic transmission and plasticity. *J Neurosci* (2009) 29:12982–93. doi:10.1523/JNEUROSCI.3059-09.2009
40. Srivastava DP, Waters EM, Mermelstein PG, Kramar EA, Shors TJ, Liu F. Rapid estrogen signaling in the brain: implications for the fine-tuning of neuronal circuitry. *J Neurosci* (2011) 31:16056–63. doi:10.1523/JNEUROSCI.4097-11.2011
41. Jezierski MK, Sohrabji F. Estrogen enhances retrograde transport of brain-derived neurotrophic factor in the rodent forebrain. *Endocrinology* (2003) 144:5022–9. doi:10.1210/en.2003-0724
42. Deppmann CD, Mihalas S, Sharma N, Lonze BE, Niebur E, Ginty DD. A model for neuronal competition during development. *Science* (2008) 320:369–73. doi:10.1126/science.1152677
43. Louissaint A Jr, Rao S, Leventhal C, Goldman SA. Coordinated interaction of neurogenesis and angiogenesis in the adult songbird brain. *Neuron* (2002) 34:945–60. doi:10.1016/S0896-6273(02)00722-5
44. Rasika S, Alvarez-Buylla A, Nottebohm F. BDNF mediates the effects of testosterone on the survival of new neurons in an adult brain. *Neuron* (1999) 22:53–62. doi:10.1016/S0896-6273(00)80678-9
45. Brenowitz EA. Testosterone and brain-derived neurotrophic factor interactions in the avian song control system. *Neuroscience* (2013) 239:115–23. doi:10.1016/j.neuroscience.2012.09.023
46. Duckles SP, Krause DN. Cerebrovascular effects of oestrogen: multiplicity of action. *Clin Exp Pharmacol Physiol* (2007) 34:801–8. doi:10.1111/j.1440-1681.2007.04683.x
47. Witt KA, Sandoval KE. Steroids and the blood-brain barrier: therapeutic implications. *Adv Pharmacol* (2014) 71:361–90. doi:10.1016/bs.apha.2014.06.018
48. Garmy-Susini B, Delmas E, Gourdy P, Zhou M, Bossard C, Bugler B, et al. Role of fibroblast growth factor-2 isoforms in the effect of estradiol on endothelial cell migration and proliferation. *Circ Res* (2004) 94:1301–9. doi:10.1161/01.RES.0000127719.13255.81
49. Klein S, Giancotti FG, Presta M, Albelda SM, Buck CA, Rifkin DB. Basic fibroblast growth factor modulates integrin expression in microvascular endothelial cells. *Mol Biol Cell* (1993) 4:973–82. doi:10.1091/mbc.4.10.973
50. Arnaoutova I, Kleinman HK. In vitro angiogenesis: endothelial cell tube formation on gelled basement membrane extract. *Nat Protoc* (2010) 5:628–35. doi:10.1038/nprot.2010.6
51. Vazquez F, Rodriguez-Manzaneque JC, Lydon JP, Edwards DP, O'Malley BW, Iruela-Arispe ML. Progesterone regulates proliferation of endothelial cells. *J Biol Chem* (1999) 274:2185–92. doi:10.1074/jbc.274.4.2185
52. Geary GG, Krause DN, Duckles SP. Estrogen reduces myogenic tone through a nitric oxide-dependent mechanism in rat cerebral arteries. *Am J Physiol* (1998) 275:H292–300.
53. Geary GG, Krause DN, Duckles SP. Gonadal hormones affect diameter of male rat cerebral arteries through endothelium-dependent mechanisms. *Am J Physiol Heart Circ Physiol* (2000) 279:H610–8. doi:10.1152/ajpheart.2000.279.2.H610
54. McNeill AM, Kim N, Duckles SP, Krause DN, Kontos HA. Chronic estrogen treatment increases levels of endothelial nitric oxide synthase protein in rat cerebral microvessels. *Stroke* (1999) 30:2186–90. doi:10.1161/01.STR.30.10.2186
55. Geary GG, McNeill AM, Ospina JA, Krause DN, Korach KS, Duckles SP. Selected contribution: cerebrovascular nos and cyclooxygenase are unaffected by estrogen in mice lacking estrogen receptor-alpha. *J Appl Physiol (1985)* (2001) 91:2391–9; discussion 2389–90. doi:10.1152/jappl.2001.91.5.2391
56. Haynes MP, Sinha D, Russell KS, Collinge M, Fulton D, Morales-Ruiz M, et al. Membrane estrogen receptor engagement activates endothelial nitric oxide synthase via the PI3-kinase-Akt pathway in human endothelial cells. *Circ Res* (2000) 87:677–82. doi:10.1161/01.RES.87.8.677
57. Stirone C, Boroujerdi A, Duckles SP, Krause DN. Estrogen receptor activation of phosphoinositide-3 kinase, akt, and nitric oxide signaling in cerebral blood vessels: rapid and long-term effects. *Mol Pharmacol* (2005) 67:105–13. doi:10.1124/mol.104.004465
58. Butt AM, Jones HC, Abbott NJ. Electrical resistance across the blood-brain barrier in anaesthetized rats: a developmental study. *J Physiol* (1990) 429:47–62. doi:10.1113/jphysiol.1990.sp018243
59. Abbott NJ, Patabendige AA, Dolman DE, Yusof SR, Begley DJ. Structure and function of the blood-brain barrier. *Neurobiol Dis* (2010) 37:13–25. doi:10.1016/j.nbd.2009.07.030
60. Shi J, Simpkins JW. 17 beta-estradiol modulation of glucose transporter 1 expression in blood-brain barrier. *Am J Physiol* (1997) 272:E1016–22.
61. Hartz AM, Madole EK, Miller DS, Bauer B. Estrogen receptor beta signaling through phosphatase and tensin homolog/phosphoinositide 3-kinase/Akt/glycogen synthase kinase 3 down-regulates blood-brain barrier breast cancer resistance protein. *J Pharmacol Exp Ther* (2010) 334:467–76. doi:10.1124/jpet.110.168930
62. Do TM, Noel-Hudson MS, Ribes S, Besengez C, Smirnova M, Cisternino S, et al. ABCG2- and ABCG4-mediated efflux of amyloid-beta peptide 1-40 at the mouse blood-brain barrier. *J Alzheimers Dis* (2012) 30:155–66. doi:10.3233/JAD-2012-112189
63. Harhaj NS, Felinski EA, Wolpert EB, Sundstrom JM, Gardner TW, Antonetti DA. VEGF activation of protein kinase C stimulates occludin phosphorylation and contributes to endothelial permeability. *Invest Ophthalmol Vis Sci* (2006) 47:5106–15. doi:10.1167/iovs.06-0322
64. Galea E, Santizo R, Feinstein DL, Adamsom P, Greenwood J, Koenig HM, et al. Estrogen inhibits NF kappa B-dependent inflammation in brain endothelium without interfering with I kappa B degradation. *Neuroreport* (2002) 13:1469–72. doi:10.1097/00001756-200208070-00024
65. Richardson WD, Kessaris N, Pringle N. Oligodendrocyte wars. *Nat Rev Neurosci* (2006) 7:11–8. doi:10.1038/nrn1826
66. Bradl M, Lassmann H. Oligodendrocytes: biology and pathology. *Acta Neuropathol* (2010) 119:37–53. doi:10.1007/s00401-009-0601-5
67. Kipp M, Hochstrasser T, Schmitz C, Beyer C. Female sex steroids and glia cells: impact on multiple sclerosis lesion formation and fine tuning of the local neurodegenerative cellular network. *Neurosci Biobehav Rev* (2016) 67:125–36. doi:10.1016/j.neubiorev.2015.11.016
68. Marin-Husstege M, Muggironi M, Raban D, Skoff RP, Casaccia-Bonnefil P. Oligodendrocyte progenitor proliferation and maturation is differentially regulated by male and female sex steroid hormones. *Dev Neurosci* (2004) 26:245–54. doi:10.1159/000082141
69. Bourdeau V, Deschenes J, Metivier R, Nagai Y, Nguyen D, Bretschneider N, et al. Genome-wide identification of high-affinity estrogen response elements in human and mouse. *Mol Endocrinol* (2004) 18:1411–27. doi:10.1210/me.2003-0441
70. Jung-Testas I, Renoir M, Bugnard H, Greene GL, Baulieu EE. Demonstration of steroid hormone receptors and steroid action in primary cultures of rat glial cells. *J Steroid Biochem Mol Biol* (1992) 41:621–31. doi:10.1016/0960-0760(92)90394-X
71. Kashani IRP, Hedayatpour AP, Pasbakhsh PP, Kafami LP, Khallaghi BM, Malek FM. Progesterone enhanced remyelination in the mouse corpus callosum after cuprizone induced demyelination. *Iran J Med Sci* (2015) 40:507–14.
72. Kipp M, Beyer C. Impact of sex steroids on neuroinflammatory processes and experimental multiple sclerosis. *Front Neuroendocrinol* (2009) 30:188–200. doi:10.1016/j.yfrne.2009.04.004

73. El-Etr M, Rame M, Boucher C, Ghoumari AM, Kumar N, Liere P, et al. Progesterone and nestorone promote myelin regeneration in chronic demyelinating lesions of corpus callosum and cerebral cortex. *Glia* (2015) 63: 104–17. doi:10.1002/glia.22736
74. Altman J, Das GD. Autoradiographic and histological evidence of postnatal hippocampal neurogenesis in rats. *J Comp Neurol* (1965) 124:319–35. doi:10.1002/cne.901240303
75. Paton JA, Nottebohm FN. Neurons generated in the adult brain are recruited into functional circuits. *Science* (1984) 225:1046–8. doi:10.1126/science.6474166
76. Nottebohm F. From bird song to neurogenesis. *Sci Am* (1989) 260:74–9. doi:10.1038/scientificamerican0289-74
77. Kempermann G. Why new neurons? Possible functions for adult hippocampal neurogenesis. *J Neurosci* (2002) 22:635–8.
78. Deng W, Aimone JB, Gage FH. New neurons and new memories: how does adult hippocampal neurogenesis affect learning and memory? *Nat Rev Neurosci* (2010) 11:339–50. doi:10.1038/nrn2822
79. Barnea A, Pravosudov V. Birds as a model to study adult neurogenesis: bridging evolutionary, comparative and neuroethological approaches. *Eur J Neurosci* (2011) 34:884–907. doi:10.1111/j.1460-9568.2011.07851.x
80. Wilbrecht L, Kirn JR. Neuron addition and loss in the song system: regulation and function. *Ann N Y Acad Sci* (2004) 1016:659–83. doi:10.1196/annals.1298.024
81. Brenowitz EA, Larson TA. Neurogenesis in the adult avian song-control system. *Cold Spring Harb Perspect Biol* (2015) 7. doi:10.1101/cshperspect.a019000
82. Cold Spring Harbor. *Neurogenesis*. New York: Cold Spring Harbor Laboratory Press (2015).
83. Kaslin J, Ganz J, Brand M. Proliferation, neurogenesis and regeneration in the non-mammalian vertebrate brain. *Philos Trans R Soc Lond B Biol Sci* (2008) 363:101–22. doi:10.1098/rstb.2006.2015
84. Alvarez-Buylla A, Garcia-Verdugo JM, Tramontin AD. A unified hypothesis on the lineage of neural stem cells. *Nat Rev Neurosci* (2001) 2:287–93. doi:10.1038/35067582
85. Ming GL, Song H. Adult neurogenesis in the mammalian brain: significant answers and significant questions. *Neuron* (2011) 70:687–702. doi:10.1016/j.neuron.2011.05.001
86. Tobin MK, Bonds JA, Minshall RD, Pelligrino DA, Testai FD, Lazarov O. Neurogenesis and inflammation after ischemic stroke: what is known and where we go from here. *J Cereb Blood Flow Metab* (2014) 34:1573–84. doi:10.1038/jcbfm.2014.130
87. Alvarez-Buylla A, Garcia-Verdugo JM, Mateo AS, Merchant-Larios H. Primary neural precursors and intermitotic nuclear migration in the ventricular zone of adult canaries. *J Neurosci* (1998) 18:1020–37. doi:10.1523/JNEUROSCI.18-03-01020.1998
88. Schmidt R, Strahle U, Scholpp S. Neurogenesis in zebrafish – from embryo to adult. *Neural Dev* (2013) 8:3. doi:10.1186/1749-8104-8-3
89. Larson TA, Thatra NM, Lee BH, Brenowitz EA. Reactive neurogenesis in response to naturally occurring apoptosis in an adult brain. *J Neurosci* (2014) 34:13066–76. doi:10.1523/JNEUROSCI.3316-13.2014
90. Apple DM, Solano-Fonseca R, Kokovay E. Neurogenesis in the aging brain. *Biochem Pharmacol* (2017) 141:77–85 doi:10.1016/j.bcp.2017.06.116
91. Eriksson PS, Perfilieva E, Bjork-Eriksson T, Alborn AM, Nordborg C, Peterson DA, et al. Neurogenesis in the adult human hippocampus. *Nat Med* (1998) 4:1313–7. doi:10.1038/3305
92. Spalding KL, Bergmann O, Alkass K, Bernard S, Salehpour M, Huttner HB, et al. Dynamics of hippocampal neurogenesis in adult humans. *Cell* (2013) 153:1219–27. doi:10.1016/j.cell.2013.05.002
93. Boldrini M, Fulmore CA, Tartt AN, Simeon LR, Pavlova I, Poposka V, et al. Human hippocampal neurogenesis persists throughout aging. *Cell Stem Cell* (2018) 22:589–99.e5. doi:10.1016/j.stem.2018.03.015
94. Sorrells SF, Paredes MF, Cebrian-Silla A, Sandoval K, Qi D, Kelley KW, et al. Human hippocampal neurogenesis drops sharply in children to undetectable levels in adults. *Nature* (2018) 555:377–81. doi:10.1038/nature25975
95. Sun GJ, Zhou Y, Stadel RP, Moss J, Yong JH, Ito S, et al. Tangential migration of neuronal precursors of glutamatergic neurons in the adult mammalian brain. *Proc Natl Acad Sci U S A* (2015) 112:9484–9. doi:10.1073/pnas.1508545112
96. Doetsch F, Alvarez-Buylla A. Network of tangential pathways for neuronal migration in adult mammalian brain. *Proc Natl Acad Sci U S A* (1996) 93:14895–900. doi:10.1073/pnas.93.25.14895
97. Rousselot P, Nottebohm F. Expression of polysialylated N-CAM in the central nervous system of adult canaries and its possible relation to function. *J Comp Neurol* (1995) 356:629–40. doi:10.1002/cne.903560411
98. Wichterle H, Garcia-Verdugo JM, Alvarez-Buylla A. Direct evidence for homotypic, glia-independent neuronal migration. *Neuron* (1997) 18:779–91. doi:10.1016/S0896-6273(00)80317-7
99. Petreanu L, Alvarez-Buylla A. Maturation and death of adult-born olfactory bulb granule neurons: role of olfaction. *J Neurosci* (2002) 22:6106–13. doi:10.1523/JNEUROSCI.22-14-06106.2002
100. Jiang J, McMurtry J, Niedzwiecki D, Goldman SA. Insulin-like growth factor-1 is a radial cell-associated neurotrophin that promotes neuronal recruitment from the adult songbird edpendyma/subependyma. *J Neurobiol* (1998) 36:1–15. doi:10.1002/(SICI)1097-4695(199807)36:1<1::AID-NEU1>3.0.CO;2-6
101. Alvarez-Buylla A, Nottebohm F. Migration of young neurons in adult avian brain. *Nature* (1988) 335:353–4. doi:10.1038/335353a0
102. Alvarez-Buylla A, Theelen M, Nottebohm F. Mapping of radial glia and of a new cell type in adult canary brain. *J Neurosci* (1988) 8:2707–12. doi:10.1523/JNEUROSCI.08-08-02707.1988
103. Vellema M, van der Linden A, Gahr M. Area-specific migration and recruitment of new neurons in the adult songbird brain. *J Comp Neurol* (2010) 518:1442–59. doi:10.1002/cne.22281
104. Kempermann G, Song H, Gage FH. Neurogenesis in the adult hippocampus. *Cold Spring Harb Perspect Biol* (2015) 7:a018812. doi:10.1101/cshperspect.a018812
105. Kirn JR, Fishman Y, Sasportas K, Alvarez-Buylla A, Nottebohm F. Fate of new neurons in adult canary high vocal center during the first 30 days after their formation. *J Comp Neurol* (1999) 411:487–94. doi:10.1002/(SICI)1096-9861(19990830)411:3<487::AID-CNE10>3.0.CO;2-M
106. Sherry DF, Hoshooley JS. Seasonal hippocampal plasticity in food-storing birds. *Philos Trans R Soc Lond B Biol Sci* (2010) 365:933–43. doi:10.1098/rstb.2009.0220
107. Scott BB, Lois C. Developmental origin and identity of song system neurons born during vocal learning in songbirds. *J Comp Neurol* (2007) 502:202–14. doi:10.1002/cne.21296
108. Kirn JR, Alvarez-Buylla A, Nottebohm F. Production and survival of projection neurons in a forebrain vocal center of adult male canaries. *J Neurosci* (1991) 11:1756–62. doi:10.1523/JNEUROSCI.11-06-01756.1991
109. Barnea A, Nottebohm F. Seasonal recruitment of hippocampal neurons in adult free-ranging black-capped chickadees. *Proc Natl Acad Sci U S A* (1994) 91:11217–21. doi:10.1073/pnas.91.23.11217
110. Walton C, Pariser E, Nottebohm F. The zebra finch paradox: song is little changed, but number of neurons doubles. *J Neurosci* (2012) 32:761–74. doi:10.1523/JNEUROSCI.3434-11.2012
111. Tanapat P, Hastings NB, Gould E. Ovarian steroids influence cell proliferation in the dentate gyrus of the adult female rat in a dose- and time-dependent manner. *J Comp Neurol* (2005) 481:252–65. doi:10.1002/cne.20385
112. Wang JM, Johnston PB, Ball BG, Brinton RD. The neurosteroid allopregnanolone promotes proliferation of rodent and human neural progenitor cells and regulates cell-cycle gene and protein expression. *J Neurosci* (2005) 25:4706–18. doi:10.1523/JNEUROSCI.4520-04.2005
113. Rasika S, Nottebohm F, Alvarez-Buylla A. Testosterone increases the recruitment and/or survival of new high vocal center neurons in adult female canaries. *Proc Natl Acad Sci U S A* (1994) 91:7854–8. doi:10.1073/pnas.91.17.7854
114. Brenowitz EA, Lent K. Act locally and think globally: intracerebral testosterone implants induce seasonal-like growth of adult avian song control circuits. *Proc Natl Acad Sci U S A* (2002) 99:12421–6. doi:10.1073/pnas.192308799
115. Hojo Y, Hattori TA, Enami T, Furukawa A, Suzuki K, Ishii HT, et al. Adult male rat hippocampus synthesizes estradiol from pregnenolone by cytochromes P45017alpha and P450 aromatase localized in neurons. *Proc Natl Acad Sci U S A* (2004) 101:865–70. doi:10.1073/pnas.2630225100
116. Backstrom T. Epileptic seizures in women related to plasma estrogen and progesterone during the menstrual cycle. *Acta Neurol Scand* (1976) 54:321–47. doi:10.1111/j.1600-0404.1976.tb04363.x
117. Beraudi A, Bruno V, Battaglia G, Biagioni F, Rampello L, Nicoletti F, et al. Pharmacological activation of mGlu2/3 metabotropic glutamate receptors

protects retinal neurons against anoxic damage in the goldfish *Carassius auratus*. *Exp Eye Res* (2007) 84:544–52. doi:10.1016/j.exer.2006.11.008

118. Sato SM, Woolley CS. Acute inhibition of neurosteroid estrogen synthesis suppresses status epilepticus in an animal model. *Elife* (2016) 5. doi:10.7554/eLife.19109
119. Pozzi S, Benedusi V, Maggi A, Vegeto E. Estrogen action in neuroprotection and brain inflammation. *Ann N Y Acad Sci* (2006) 1089:302–23. doi:10.1196/annals.1386.035
120. Ginhoux F, Greter M, Leboeuf M, Nandi S, See P, Gokhan S, et al. Fate mapping analysis reveals that adult microglia derive from primitive macrophages. *Science* (2010) 330:841–5. doi:10.1126/science.1194637
121. Nimmerjahn A, Kirchhoff F, Helmchen F. Resting microglial cells are highly dynamic surveillants of brain parenchyma in vivo. *Science* (2005) 308:1314–8. doi:10.1126/science.1110647
122. Sierra A, Encinas JM, Deudero JJP, Chancey JH, Enikolopov G, Overstreet-Wadiche LS, et al. Microglia shape adult hippocampal neurogenesis through apoptosis-coupled phagocytosis. *Cell Stem Cell* (2010) 7:483–95. doi:10.1016/j.stem.2010.08.014
123. Hoek RM, Ruuls SR, Murphy CA, Wright GJ, Goddard R, Zurawski SM, et al. Down-regulation of the macrophage lineage through interaction with OX2 (CD200). *Science* (2000) 290:1768–71. doi:10.1126/science.290.5497.1768
124. Sierra A, Beccari S, Diaz-Aparicio I, Encinas JM, Comeau S, Tremblay ME. Surveillance, phagocytosis, and inflammation: how never-resting microglia influence adult hippocampal neurogenesis. *Neural Plast* (2014) 2014:610343. doi:10.1155/2014/610343
125. Prinz M, Priller J. Microglia and brain macrophages in the molecular age: from origin to neuropsychiatric disease. *Nat Rev Neurosci* (2014) 15:300–12. doi:10.1038/nrn3722
126. Hu X, Li P, Guo Y, Wang H, Leak RK, Chen S, et al. Microglia/macrophage polarization dynamics reveal novel mechanism of injury expansion after focal cerebral ischemia. *Stroke* (2012) 43:3063–70. doi:10.1161/STROKEAHA.112.659656
127. Miron VE, Boyd A, Zhao JW, Yuen TJ, Ruckh JM, Shadrach JL, et al. M2 microglia and macrophages drive oligodendrocyte differentiation during CNS remyelination. *Nat Neurosci* (2013) 16:1211–8. doi:10.1038/nn.3469
128. Wang G, Zhang J, Hu X, Zhang L, Mao L, Jiang X, et al. Microglia/macrophage polarization dynamics in white matter after traumatic brain injury. *J Cereb Blood Flow Metab* (2013) 33:1864–74. doi:10.1038/jcbfm.2013.146
129. Habib P, Beyer C. Regulation of brain microglia by female gonadal steroids. *J Steroid Biochem Mol Biol* (2015) 146:3–14. doi:10.1016/j.jsbmb.2014.02.018
130. Dang J, Mitkari B, Kipp M, Beyer C. Gonadal steroids prevent cell damage and stimulate behavioral recovery after transient middle cerebral artery occlusion in male and female rats. *Brain Behav Immun* (2011) 25:715–26. doi:10.1016/j.bbi.2011.01.013
131. Buttini M, Limonta S, Boddeke HW. Peripheral administration of lipopolysaccharide induces activation of microglial cells in rat brain. *Neurochem Int* (1996) 29:25–35. doi:10.1016/0197-0186(95)00141-7
132. Shimazu R, Akashi S, Ogata H, Nagai Y, Fukudome K, Miyake K, et al. MD-2, a molecule that confers lipopolysaccharide responsiveness on toll-like receptor 4. *J Exp Med* (1999) 189:1777–82. doi:10.1084/jem.189.11.1777
133. Heese K, Fiebich BL, Bauer J, Otten U. NF-kappaB modulates lipopolysaccharide-induced microglial nerve growth factor expression. *Glia* (1998) 22:401–7. doi:10.1002/(SICI)1098-1136(199804)22:4<401::AID-GLIA9>3.0.CO;2-5
134. Santa-Cecilia FV, Socias B, Ouidja MO, Sepulveda-Diaz JE, Acuna L, Silva RL, et al. Doxycycline suppresses microglial activation by inhibiting the p38 MAPK and NF-kB signaling pathways. *Neurotox Res* (2016) 29:447–59. doi:10.1007/s12640-015-9592-2
135. Choi HB, Khoo C, Ryu JK, van Breemen E, Kim SU, McLarnon JG. Inhibition of lipopolysaccharide-induced cyclooxygenase-2, tumor necrosis factor-alpha and [Ca2+]i responses in human microglia by the peripheral benzodiazepine receptor ligand PK11195. *J Neurochem* (2002) 83:546–55. doi:10.1046/j.1471-4159.2002.01122.x
136. Ghisletti S, Meda C, Maggi A, Vegeto E. 17beta-estradiol inhibits inflammatory gene expression by controlling NF-kappaB intracellular localization. *Mol Cell Biol* (2005) 25:2957–68. doi:10.1128/MCB.25.8.2957-2968.2005
137. Vegeto E, Bonincontro C, Pollio G, Sala A, Viappiani S, Nardi F, et al. Estrogen prevents the lipopolysaccharide-induced inflammatory response in microglia. *J Neurosci* (2001) 21:1809–18. doi:10.1523/JNEUROSCI.21-06-01809.2001
138. Loram LC, Sholar PW, Taylor FR, Wiesler JL, Babb JA, Strand KA, et al. Sex and estradiol influence glial pro-inflammatory responses to lipopolysaccharide in rats. *Psychoneuroendocrinology* (2012) 37:1688–99. doi:10.1016/j.psyneuen.2012.02.018
139. VanRyzin JW, Pickett LA, McCarthy MM. Microglia: driving critical periods and sexual differentiation of the brain. *Dev Neurobiol* (2017). doi:10.1002/dneu.22569
140. Emsley JG, Macklis JD. Astroglial heterogeneity closely reflects the neuronal-defined anatomy of the adult murine CNS. *Neuron Glia Biol* (2006) 2:175–86. doi:10.1017/S1740925X06000202
141. Sofroniew MV, Vinters HV. Astrocytes: biology and pathology. *Acta Neuropathol* (2010) 119:7–35. doi:10.1007/s00401-009-0619-8
142. Lundgaard I, Osorio MJ, Kress BT, Sanggaard S, Nedergaard M. White matter astrocytes in health and disease. *Neuroscience* (2014) 276:161–73. doi:10.1016/j.neuroscience.2013.10.050
143. Chesler M, Kaila K. Modulation of pH by neuronal activity. *Trends Neurosci* (1992) 15:396–402. doi:10.1016/0166-2236(92)90191-A
144. Walz W. Role of astrocytes in the clearance of excess extracellular potassium. *Neurochem Int* (2000) 36:291–300. doi:10.1016/S0197-0186(99)00137-0
145. Oliet SH, Piet R, Poulain DA. Control of glutamate clearance and synaptic efficacy by glial coverage of neurons. *Science* (2001) 292:923–6. doi:10.1126/science.1059162
146. Sasaki T, Matsuki N, Ikegaya Y. Action-potential modulation during axonal conduction. *Science* (2011) 331:599–601. doi:10.1126/science.1197598
147. Takano T, Tian GF, Peng W, Lou N, Libionka W, Han X, et al. Astrocyte-mediated control of cerebral blood flow. *Nat Neurosci* (2006) 9:260–7. doi:10.1038/nn1623
148. Belanger M, Allaman I, Magistretti PJ. Brain energy metabolism: focus on astrocyte-neuron metabolic cooperation. *Cell Metab* (2011) 14:724–38. doi:10.1016/j.cmet.2011.08.016
149. Dietschy JM, Turley SD. Thematic review series: brain lipids. Cholesterol metabolism in the central nervous system during early development and in the mature animal. *J Lipid Res* (2004) 45:1375–97. doi:10.1194/jlr.R400004-JLR200
150. Ullian EM, Sapperstein SK, Christopherson KS, Barres BA. Control of synapse number by glia. *Science* (2001) 291:657–61. doi:10.1126/science.291.5504.657
151. Chung WS, Clarke LE, Wang GX, Stafford BK, Sher A, Chakraborty C, et al. Astrocytes mediate synapse elimination through MEGF10 and MERTK pathways. *Nature* (2013) 504:394–400. doi:10.1038/nature12776
152. Lepekhin EA, Eliasson C, Berthold CH, Berezin V, Bock E, Pekny M. Intermediate filaments regulate astrocyte motility. *J Neurochem* (2001) 79:617–25. doi:10.1046/j.1471-4159.2001.00595.x
153. Ubogu EE, Cossoy MB, Ransohoff RM. The expression and function of chemokines involved in CNS inflammation. *Trends Pharmacol Sci* (2006) 27:48–55. doi:10.1016/j.tips.2005.11.002
154. Menet V, Gimenez YRM, Sandillon F, Privat A. GFAP null astrocytes are a favorable substrate for neuronal survival and neurite growth. *Glia* (2000) 31:267–72. doi:10.1002/1098-1136(200009)31:3<267::AID-GLIA80>3.0.CO;2-N
155. Cho KS, Yang L, Lu B, Feng Ma H, Huang X, Pekny M, et al. Re-establishing the regenerative potential of central nervous system axons in postnatal mice. *J Cell Sci* (2005) 118:863–72. doi:10.1242/jcs.01658
156. Voskuhl RR, Peterson RS, Song B, Ao Y, Morales LB, Tiwari-Woodruff S, et al. Reactive astrocytes form scar-like perivascular barriers to leukocytes during adaptive immune inflammation of the CNS. *J Neurosci* (2009) 29:11511–22. doi:10.1523/JNEUROSCI.1514-09.2009
157. Azcoitia I, Santos-Galindo M, Arevalo MA, Garcia-Segura LM. Role of astroglia in the neuroplastic and neuroprotective actions of estradiol. *Eur J Neurosci* (2010) 32:1995–2002. doi:10.1111/j.1460-9568.2010.07516.x
158. Zhang L, Li B, Zhao W, Chang YH, Ma W, Dragan M, et al. Sex-related differences in MAPKs activation in rat astrocytes: effects of estrogen on cell death. *Brain Res Mol Brain Res* (2002) 103:1–11. doi:10.1016/S0169-328X(02)00379-0
159. Ciriza I, Carrero P, Azcoitia I, Lundeen SG, Garcia-Segura LM. Selective estrogen receptor modulators protect hippocampal neurons from kainic

acid excitotoxicity: differences with the effect of estradiol. *J Neurobiol* (2004) 61:209–21. doi:10.1002/neu.20043

160. Barreto G, Santos-Galindo M, Diz-Chaves Y, Pernia O, Carrero P, Azcoitia I, et al. Selective estrogen receptor modulators decrease reactive astrogliosis in the injured brain: effects of aging and prolonged depletion of ovarian hormones. *Endocrinology* (2009) 150:5010–5. doi:10.1210/en.2009-0352
161. Garcia-Estrada J, Del Rio JA, Luquin S, Soriano E, Garcia-Segura LM. Gonadal hormones down-regulate reactive gliosis and astrocyte proliferation after a penetrating brain injury. *Brain Res* (1993) 628:271–8. doi:10.1016/0006-8993(93)90964-O
162. Lewis DK, Johnson AB, Stohlgren S, Harms A, Sohrabji F. Effects of estrogen receptor agonists on regulation of the inflammatory response in astrocytes from young adult and middle-aged female rats. *J Neuroimmunol* (2008) 195:47–59. doi:10.1016/j.jneuroim.2008.01.006
163. Acs P, Kipp M, Norkute A, Johann S, Clarner T, Braun A, et al. 17beta-estradiol and progesterone prevent cuprizone provoked demyelination of corpus callosum in male mice. *Glia* (2009) 57:807–14. doi:10.1002/glia.20806
164. Dodel RC, Du Y, Bales KR, Gao F, Paul SM. Sodium salicylate and 17beta-estradiol attenuate nuclear transcription factor NF-kappaB translocation in cultured rat astroglial cultures following exposure to amyloid A beta(1-40) and lipopolysaccharides. *J Neurochem* (1999) 73:1453–60. doi:10.1046/j.1471-4159.1999.0731453.x
165. Kipp M, Karakaya S, Johann S, Kampmann E, Mey J, Beyer C. Oestrogen and progesterone reduce lipopolysaccharide-induced expression of tumour necrosis factor-alpha and interleukin-18 in midbrain astrocytes. *J Neuroendocrinol* (2007) 19:819–22. doi:10.1111/j.1365-2826.2007.01588.x
166. Cerciat M, Unkila M, Garcia-Segura LM, Arevalo MA. Selective estrogen receptor modulators decrease the production of interleukin-6 and interferon-gamma-inducible protein-10 by astrocytes exposed to inflammatory challenge in vitro. *Glia* (2010) 58:93–102. doi:10.1002/glia.20904
167. Schlinger BA, Amur-Umarjee S, Shen P, Campagnoni AT, Arnold AP. Neuronal and non-neuronal aromatase in primary cultures of developing zebra finch telencephalon. *J Neurosci* (1994) 14:7541–52. doi:10.1523/JNEUROSCI.14-12-07541.1994
168. Garcia-Segura LM, Wozniak A, Azcoitia I, Rodriguez JR, Hutchison RE, Hutchison JB. Aromatase expression by astrocytes after brain injury: implications for local estrogen formation in brain repair. *Neuroscience* (1999) 89:567–78. doi:10.1016/S0306-4522(98)00340-6
169. Saldanha CJ, Rohmann KN, Coomaralingam L, Wynne RD. Estrogen provision by reactive glia decreases apoptosis in the zebra finch (*Taeniopygia guttata*). *J Neurobiol* (2005) 64:192–201. doi:10.1002/neu.20147
170. Peterson RS, Saldanha CJ, Schlinger BA. Rapid upregulation of aromatase mRNA and protein following neural injury in the zebra finch (*Taeniopygia guttata*). *J Neuroendocrinol* (2001) 13:317–23. doi:10.1046/j.1365-2826.2001.00647.x
171. Duncan KA, Saldanha CJ. Neuroinflammation induces glial aromatase expression in the uninjured songbird brain. *J Neuroinflammation* (2011) 8:81. doi:10.1186/1742-2094-8-81
172. Peterson RS, Fernando G, Day L, Allen TA, Chapleau JD, Menjivar J, et al. Aromatase expression and cell proliferation following injury of the adult zebra finch hippocampus. *Dev Neurobiol* (2007) 67:1867–78. doi:10.1002/dneu.20548
173. Ritzel RM, Capozzi LA, McCullough LD. Sex, stroke, and inflammation: the potential for estrogen-mediated immunoprotection in stroke. *Horm Behav* (2013) 63:238–53. doi:10.1016/j.yhbeh.2012.04.007
174. D'Agostino PM, Gottfried-Blackmore A, Anandasabapathy N, Bulloch K. Brain dendritic cells: biology and pathology. *Acta Neuropathol* (2012) 124:599–614. doi:10.1007/s00401-012-1018-0
175. Akopov SE, Simonian NA, Grigorian GS. Dynamics of polymorphonuclear leukocyte accumulation in acute cerebral infarction and their correlation with brain tissue damage. *Stroke* (1996) 27:1739–43. doi:10.1161/01.STR.27.10.1739
176. Scotland RS, Stables MJ, Madalli S, Watson P, Gilroy DW. Sex differences in resident immune cell phenotype underlie more efficient acute inflammatory responses in female mice. *Blood* (2011) 118:5918–27. doi:10.1182/blood-2011-03-340281
177. Bain BJ, England JM. Variations in leucocyte count during menstrual cycle. *Br Med J* (1975) 2:473–5. doi:10.1136/bmj.2.5969.473
178. Kramer PR, Kramer SF, Guan G. 17 beta-estradiol regulates cytokine release through modulation of CD16 expression in monocytes and monocyte-derived macrophages. *Arthritis Rheum* (2004) 50:1967–75. doi:10.1002/art.20309
179. Murphy AJ, Guyre PM, Pioli PA. Estradiol suppresses NF-kappa B activation through coordinated regulation of let-7a and miR-125b in primary human macrophages. *J Immunol* (2010) 184:5029–37. doi:10.4049/jimmunol.0903463
180. Miller AP, Feng W, Xing D, Weathington NM, Blalock JE, Chen YF, et al. Estrogen modulates inflammatory mediator expression and neutrophil chemotaxis in injured arteries. *Circulation* (2004) 110:1664–9. doi:10.1161/01.CIR.0000142050.19488.C7
181. Lei ZB, Fu XJ, Lu ZT, Wang BC, Liu XL, You NZ. Effect of estradiol on chemokine receptor CXCR2 expression in rats: implications for atherosclerosis. *Acta Pharmacol Sin* (2003) 24:670–4.
182. Geraldes P, Gagnon S, Hadjadj S, Merhi Y, Sirois MG, Cloutier I, et al. Estradiol blocks the induction of CD40 and CD40L expression on endothelial cells and prevents neutrophil adhesion: an ERalpha-mediated pathway. *Cardiovasc Res* (2006) 71:566–73. doi:10.1016/j.cardiores.2006.05.015
183. Douin-Echinard V, Laffont S, Seillet C, Delpy L, Krust A, Chambon P, et al. Estrogen receptor alpha, but not beta, is required for optimal dendritic cell differentiation and [corrected] CD40-induced cytokine production. *J Immunol* (2008) 180:3661–9. doi:10.4049/jimmunol.180.6.3661
184. Polanczyk MJ, Carson BD, Subramanian S, Afentoulis M, Vandenbark AA, Ziegler SF, et al. Cutting edge: estrogen drives expansion of the CD4+CD25+ regulatory T cell compartment. *J Immunol* (2004) 173:2227–30. doi:10.4049/jimmunol.173.4.2227
185. Kayser MS, Dalmau J. The emerging link between autoimmune disorders and neuropsychiatric disease. *J Neuropsychiatry Clin Neurosci* (2011) 23:90–7. doi:10.1176/appi.neuropsych.23.1.90
186. Ekdahl CT, Claasen JH, Bonde S, Kokaia Z, Lindvall O. Inflammation is detrimental for neurogenesis in adult brain. *Proc Natl Acad Sci U S A* (2003) 100:13632–7. doi:10.1073/pnas.2234031100
187. Monje ML, Toda H, Palmer TD. Inflammatory blockade restores adult hippocampal neurogenesis. *Science* (2003) 302:1760–5. doi:10.1126/science.1088417
188. Belarbi K, Arellano C, Ferguson R, Jopson T, Rosi S. Chronic neuroinflammation impacts the recruitment of adult-born neurons into behaviorally relevant hippocampal networks. *Brain Behav Immun* (2012) 26:18–23. doi:10.1016/j.bbi.2011.07.225
189. Ji KA, Yang MS, Jeong HK, Min KJ, Kang SH, Jou I, et al. Resident microglia die and infiltrated neutrophils and monocytes become major inflammatory cells in lipopolysaccharide-injected brain. *Glia* (2007) 55:1577–88. doi:10.1002/glia.20571
190. Johann S, Kampmann E, Denecke B, Arnold S, Kipp M, Mey J, et al. Expression of enzymes involved in the prostanoid metabolism by cortical astrocytes after LPS-induced inflammation. *J Mol Neurosci* (2008) 34:177–85. doi:10.1007/s12031-007-9028-4
191. Walton NM, Sutter BM, Laywell ED, Levkoff LH, Kearns SM, Marshall GP II, et al. Microglia instruct subventricular zone neurogenesis. *Glia* (2006) 54:815–25. doi:10.1002/glia.20419
192. Battista D, Ferrari CC, Gage FH, Pitossi FJ. Neurogenic niche modulation by activated microglia: transforming growth factor beta increases neurogenesis in the adult dentate gyrus. *Eur J Neurosci* (2006) 23:83–93. doi:10.1111/j.1460-9568.2005.04539.x
193. Butovsky O, Ziv Y, Schwartz A, Landa G, Talpalar AE, Pluchino S, et al. Microglia activated by IL-4 or IFN-gamma differentially induce neurogenesis and oligodendrogenesis from adult stem/progenitor cells. *Mol Cell Neurosci* (2006) 31:149–60. doi:10.1016/j.mcn.2005.10.006
194. Annenkov A. The insulin-like growth factor (IGF) receptor type 1 (IGF1R) as an essential component of the signalling network regulating neurogenesis. *Mol Neurobiol* (2009) 40:195–215. doi:10.1007/s12035-009-8081-0
195. Vallieres L, Campbell IL, Gage FH, Sawchenko PE. Reduced hippocampal neurogenesis in adult transgenic mice with chronic astrocytic production of interleukin-6. *J Neurosci* (2002) 22:486–92. doi:10.1523/JNEUROSCI.22-02-00486.2002
196. Wu MD, Hein AM, Moravan MJ, Shaftel SS, Olschowka JA, O'Banion MK. Adult murine hippocampal neurogenesis is inhibited by sustained IL-1beta and not rescued by voluntary running. *Brain Behav Immun* (2012) 26:292–300. doi:10.1016/j.bbi.2011.09.012

197. Seguin JA, Brennan J, Mangano E, Hayley S. Proinflammatory cytokines differentially influence adult hippocampal cell proliferation depending upon the route and chronicity of administration. *Neuropsychiatr Dis Treat* (2009) 5:5–14.
198. Johansson S, Price J, Modo M. Effect of inflammatory cytokines on major histocompatibility complex expression and differentiation of human neural stem/progenitor cells. *Stem Cells* (2008) 26:2444–54. doi:10.1634/stemcells.2008-0116
199. Ben-Hur T, Ben-Menachem O, Furer V, Einstein O, Mizrachi-Kol R, Grigoriadis N. Effects of proinflammatory cytokines on the growth, fate, and motility of multipotential neural precursor cells. *Mol Cell Neurosci* (2003) 24:623–31. doi:10.1016/S1044-7431(03)00218-5
200. Peterson RS, Lee DW, Fernando G, Schlinger BA. Radial glia express aromatase in the injured zebra finch brain. *J Comp Neurol* (2004) 475:261–9. doi:10.1002/cne.20157
201. Lee DW, Fernando G, Peterson RS, Allen TA, Schlinger BA. Estrogen mediation of injury-induced cell birth in neuroproliferative regions of the adult zebra finch brain. *Dev Neurobiol* (2007) 67:1107–17. doi:10.1002/dneu.20564
202. Ashton RS, Conway A, Pangarkar C, Bergen J, Lim KI, Shah P, et al. Astrocytes regulate adult hippocampal neurogenesis through ephrin-B signaling. *Nat Neurosci* (2012) 15:1399–406. doi:10.1038/nn.3212
203. Sultan S, Li L, Moss J, Petrelli F, Casse F, Gebara E, et al. Synaptic integration of adult-born hippocampal neurons is locally controlled by astrocytes. *Neuron* (2015) 88:957–72. doi:10.1016/j.neuron.2015.10.037
204. Gold SM, Voskuhl RR. Estrogen treatment in multiple sclerosis. *J Neurol Sci* (2009) 286:99–103. doi:10.1016/j.jns.2009.05.028
205. Chesik D, De Keyser J. Progesterone and dexamethasone differentially regulate the IGF-system in glial cells. *Neurosci Lett* (2010) 468:178–82. doi:10.1016/j.neulet.2009.10.051
206. Elloso MM, Phiel K, Henderson RA, Harris HA, Adelman SJ. Suppression of experimental autoimmune encephalomyelitis using estrogen receptor-selective ligands. *J Endocrinol* (2005) 185:243–52. doi:10.1677/joe.1.06063
207. Morales LB, Loo KK, Liu HB, Peterson C, Tiwari-Woodruff S, Voskuhl RR. Treatment with an estrogen receptor alpha ligand is neuroprotective in experimental autoimmune encephalomyelitis. *J Neurosci* (2006) 26:6823–33. doi:10.1523/JNEUROSCI.0453-06.2006
208. Spence RD, Hamby ME, Umeda E, Itoh N, Du S, Wisdom AJ, et al. Neuroprotection mediated through estrogen receptor-alpha in astrocytes. *Proc Natl Acad Sci U S A* (2011) 108:8867–72. doi:10.1073/pnas.1103833108
209. Wu WF, Tan XJ, Dai YB, Krishnan V, Warner M, Gustafsson JA. Targeting estrogen receptor beta in microglia and T cells to treat experimental autoimmune encephalomyelitis. *Proc Natl Acad Sci U S A* (2013) 110:3543–8. doi:10.1073/pnas.1300313110
210. Kohman RA, Rhodes JS. Neurogenesis, inflammation and behavior. *Brain Behav Immun* (2013) 27:22–32. doi:10.1016/j.bbi.2012.09.003
211. Frick LR, Williams K, Pittenger C. Microglial dysregulation in psychiatric disease. *Clin Dev Immunol* (2013) 2013:608654. doi:10.1155/2013/608654
212. McCarthy MM, Wright CL. Convergence of sex differences and the neuroimmune system in autism spectrum disorder. *Biol Psychiatry* (2017) 81:402–10. doi:10.1016/j.biopsych.2016.10.004
213. Vegeto E, Benedusi V, Maggi A. Estrogen anti-inflammatory activity in brain: a therapeutic opportunity for menopause and neurodegenerative diseases. *Front Neuroendocrinol* (2008) 29:507–19. doi:10.1016/j.yfrne.2008.04.001
214. Mori K, Kaneko YS, Nakashima A, Nagasaki H, Nagatsu T, Nagatsu I, et al. Subventricular zone under the neuroinflammatory stress and Parkinson's disease. *Cell Mol Neurobiol* (2012) 32:777–85. doi:10.1007/s10571-011-9783-1
215. Morale MC, Serra PA, L'Episcopo F, Tirolo C, Caniglia S, Testa N, et al. Estrogen, neuroinflammation and neuroprotection in Parkinson's disease: glia dictates resistance versus vulnerability to neurodegeneration. *Neuroscience* (2006) 138:869–78. doi:10.1016/j.neuroscience.2005.07.060
216. Xu W, Zheng J, Gao L, Li T, Zhang J, Shao A. Neuroprotective effects of stem cells in ischemic stroke. *Stem Cells Int* (2017) 2017:4653936. doi:10.1155/2017/4653936
217. Arevalo MA, Diz-Chaves Y, Santos-Galindo M, Bellini MJ, Garcia-Segura LM. Selective oestrogen receptor modulators decrease the inflammatory response of glial cells. *J Neuroendocrinol* (2012) 24:183–90. doi:10.1111/j.1365-2826.2011.02156.x
218. Tong HI, Kang W, Davy PM, Shi Y, Sun S, Allsopp RC, et al. Monocyte trafficking, engraftment, and delivery of nanoparticles and an exogenous gene into the acutely inflamed brain tissue – evaluations on monocyte-based delivery system for the central nervous system. *PLoS One* (2016) 11:e0154022. doi:10.1371/journal.pone.0154022
219. Russo I, Barlati S, Bosetti F. Effects of neuroinflammation on the regenerative capacity of brain stem cells. *J Neurochem* (2011) 116:947–56. doi:10.1111/j.1471-4159.2010.07168.x
220. Mlakar J, Korva M, Tul N, Popovic M, Poljsak-Prijatelj M, Mraz J, et al. Zika virus associated with microcephaly. *N Engl J Med* (2016) 374:951–8. doi:10.1056/NEJMoa1600651
221. Rasmussen SA, Jamieson DJ, Honein MA, Petersen LR. Zika virus and birth defects – reviewing the evidence for causality. *N Engl J Med* (2016) 374:1981–7. doi:10.1056/NEJMsr1604338
222. Tang H, Hammack C, Ogden SC, Wen Z, Qian X, Li Y, et al. Zika virus infects human cortical neural progenitors and attenuates their growth. *Cell Stem Cell* (2016) 18:587–90. doi:10.1016/j.stem.2016.02.016
223. Yoon KJ, Song G, Qian X, Pan J, Xu D, Rho HS, et al. Zika-virus-encoded NS2A disrupts mammalian cortical neurogenesis by degrading adherens junction proteins. *Cell Stem Cell* (2017) 21:349–58.e6. doi:10.1016/j.stem.2017.07.014
224. Liang Q, Luo Z, Zeng J, Chen W, Foo SS, Lee SA, et al. Zika virus NS4A and NS4B proteins deregulate Akt-mTOR signaling in human fetal neural stem cells to inhibit neurogenesis and induce autophagy. *Cell Stem Cell* (2016) 19:663–71. doi:10.1016/j.stem.2016.07.019
225. Lum FM, Low DK, Fan Y, Tan JJ, Lee B, Chan JK, et al. Zika Virus Infects Human Fetal Brain Microglia and Induces Inflammation. *Clin Infect Dis* (2017) 64(7):914–20. doi:10.1093/cid/ciw878
226. Tramontin AD, Brenowitz EA. Seasonal plasticity in the adult brain. *Trends Neurosci* (2000) 23:251–8. doi:10.1016/S0166-2236(00)01558-7
227. Brenowitz EA, Beecher MD. Song learning in birds: diversity and plasticity, opportunities and challenges. *Trends Neurosci* (2005) 28:127–32. doi:10.1016/j.tins.2005.01.004
228. Smith GT, Brenowitz EA, Wingfield JC. Roles of photoperiod and testosterone in seasonal plasticity of the avian song control system. *J Neurobiol* (1997) 32:426–42. doi:10.1002/(SICI)1097-4695(199704)32:4<426::AID-NEU6>3.0.CO;2-8
229. Tramontin AD, Hartman VN, Brenowitz EA. Breeding conditions induce rapid and sequential growth in adult avian song control circuits: a model of seasonal plasticity in the brain. *J Neurosci* (2000) 20:854–61. doi:10.1523/JNEUROSCI.20-02-00854.2000
230. Wennstrom KL, Reeves BJ, Brenowitz EA. Testosterone treatment increases the metabolic capacity of adult avian song control nuclei. *J Neurobiol* (2001) 48:256–64. doi:10.1002/neu.1055
231. Meitzen J, Weaver AL, Brenowitz EA, Perkel DJ. Plastic and stable electrophysiological properties of adult avian forebrain song-control neurons across changing breeding conditions. *J Neurosci* (2009) 29:6558–67. doi:10.1523/JNEUROSCI.5571-08.2009
232. Meitzen J, Thompson CK, Choi H, Perkel DJ, Brenowitz EA. Time course of changes in Gambel's white-crowned sparrow song behavior following transitions in breeding condition. *Horm Behav* (2009) 55:217–27. doi:10.1016/j.yhbeh.2008.10.006
233. Kirn J, O'Loughlin B, Kasparian S, Nottebohm F. Cell death and neuronal recruitment in the high vocal center of adult male canaries are temporally related to changes in song. *Proc Natl Acad Sci U S A* (1994) 91:7844–8. doi:10.1073/pnas.91.17.7844
234. Thompson CK, Bentley GE, Brenowitz EA. Rapid seasonal-like regression of the adult avian song control system. *Proc Natl Acad Sci U S A* (2007) 104:15520–5. doi:10.1073/pnas.0707239104
235. Thompson CK, Brenowitz EA. Caspase inhibitor infusion protects an avian song control circuit from seasonal-like neurodegeneration. *J Neurosci* (2008) 28:7130–6. doi:10.1523/JNEUROSCI.0663-08.2008
236. Owen-Ashley NT, Turner M, Hahn TP, Wingfield JC. Hormonal, behavioral, and thermoregulatory responses to bacterial lipopolysaccharide in captive and free-living white-crowned sparrows (*Zonotrichia* leucophrys gambelii). *Horm Behav* (2006) 49:15–29. doi:10.1016/j.yhbeh.2005.04.009
237. Thompson CK, Brenowitz EA. Neurogenesis in an adult avian song nucleus is reduced by decreasing caspase-mediated apoptosis. *J Neurosci* (2009) 29:4586–91. doi:10.1523/JNEUROSCI.5423-08.2009
238. Ganz J, Brand M. Adult neurogenesis in fish. *Cold Spring Harb Perspect Biol* (2016) 8. doi:10.1101/cshperspect.a019018
239. Kizil C, Kaslin J, Kroehne V, Brand M. Adult neurogenesis and brain regeneration in zebrafish. *Dev Neurobiol* (2012) 72:429–61. doi:10.1002/dneu.20918

240. Kirsche W, Kirsche K. [Experimental studies on the problem of regeneration and function of the tectum opticum of *Carassium carassium* L]. *Z Mikrosk Anat Forsch* (1961) 67:140–82.
241. Zupanc GK, Kompass KS, Horschke I, Ott R, Schwarz H. Apoptosis after injuries in the cerebellum of adult teleost fish. *Exp Neurol* (1998) 152:221–30. doi:10.1006/exnr.1998.6853
242. Zupanc GK, Ott R. Cell proliferation after lesions in the cerebellum of adult teleost fish: time course, origin, and type of new cells produced. *Exp Neurol* (1999) 160:78–87. doi:10.1006/exnr.1999.7182
243. Kroehne V, Freudenreich D, Hans S, Kaslin J, Brand M. Regeneration of the adult zebrafish brain from neurogenic radial glia-type progenitors. *Development* (2011) 138:4831–41. doi:10.1242/dev.072587
244. Kyritsis N, Kizil C, Zocher S, Kroehne V, Kaslin J, Freudenreich D, et al. Acute inflammation initiates the regenerative response in the adult zebrafish brain. *Science* (2012) 338:1353–6. doi:10.1126/science.1228773
245. Kizil C, Dudczig S, Kyritsis N, Machate A, Blaesche J, Kroehne V, et al. The chemokine receptor cxcr5 regulates the regenerative neurogenesis response in the adult zebrafish brain. *Neural Dev* (2012) 7:27. doi:10.1186/1749-8104-7-27

4

Brain-Derived Steroids, Behavior and Endocrine Conflicts Across Life History Stages in Birds

John C. Wingfield[1], Douglas W. Wacker[2], George E. Bentley[3] and Kazuyoshi Tsutsui[4]*

[1] Department of Neurobiology Physiology and Behavior, University of California, Davis, Davis, CA, United States, [2] Division of Biological Sciences, School of STEM, University of Washington Bothell, Bothell, WA, United States, [3] Department of Integrative Biology, Helen Wills Neuroscience Institute, University of California, Berkeley, Berkeley, CA, United States, [4] Department of Biology, Waseda University, Shinjuku, Japan

***Correspondence:**
John C. Wingfield
jcwingfield@ucdavis.edu

Biological steroids were traditionally thought to be synthesized exclusively by the adrenal glands and gonads. Recent decades have seen the discovery of neurosteroid production that acts locally within the central nervous system to affect physiology and behavior. These actions include, for example, regulation of aggressive behavior, such as territoriality, and locomotor movement associated with migration. Important questions then arose as to how and why neurosteroid production evolved and why similar steroids of peripheral origin do not always fulfill these central roles? Investigations of free-living vertebrates suggest that synthesis and action of bioactive steroids within the brain may have evolved to regulate expression of specific behavior in different life history stages. Synthesis and secretion of these hormones from peripheral glands is broadcast throughout the organism *via* the blood stream. While widespread, general actions of steroids released into the blood might be relevant for regulation of morphological, physiological, and behavioral traits in one life history stage, such hormonal release may not be appropriate in other stages. Specific and localized production of bioactive steroids in the brain, but not released into the periphery, could be a way to avoid such conflicts. Two examples are highlighted. First, we compare the control of territorial aggression of songbirds in the breeding season under the influence of gonadal steroids with autumnal (non-breeding) territoriality regulated by sex steroid production in the brain either from circulating precursors such as dehydroepiandrosterone or local central production of sex steroids *de novo* from cholesterol. Second, we outline the production of 7α-hydroxypregnenolone within the brain that appears to affect locomotor behavior in several contexts. Local production of these steroids in the brain may provide specific regulation of behavioral traits throughout the year and independently of life history stage.

Keywords: territorial aggression, life history stages, aromatase, dehydropepiandrosterone, 7α-hydroxypregnenolone, locomotor activity, neurosteroid

INTRODUCTION

The life cycles of animals consist of life history stages such as breeding, migration, molt, and non-breeding expressed at appropriate times of year and with specific durations matched to seasonal change [e.g., Ref. (1, 2)]. Each stage has a unique suite of sub-stages in which animals exhibit morphological, physiological, and behavioral adaptations to changing environmental and social conditions.

Some traits may be expressed across multiple life history stages. However, the neuroendocrine and peripheral endocrine regulation of those traits in one stage might be different in another stage. Examples include the regulation of territorial aggression across breeding and non-breeding seasons (3–5), the control of locomotor activity in seasonal migration and facultative movements to avoid perturbations of the environment [e.g., Ref. (6–8)].

There is growing evidence that the neuroendocrine and endocrine cascades involved in regulation of morphology, physiology, and behavior across different life history stages can be altered at many different levels [e.g., Ref. (9); **Figure 1**]. Localized regulatory mechanisms in one life history stage allow trait modulation without the effects associated with signals that act throughout the organism such as hormones secreted into the bloodstream acting on multiple tissues. Thus, conflict between the need for the expression of a particular trait that can be regulated by a particular hormone and the inappropriate co-regulation of other physiological or behavioral responses to that hormone at the wrong season can be avoided. These regulatory processes can be organized into three major categories [see **Figure 1** (10, 11)]:

1. Secretion—cascades of hormone secretion [e.g., the hypothalamo-pituitary-gonad (HPG) axis, **Figure 2**] in which hormones are broadcast throughout the organism's bloodstream and have as many potential targets as cells or tissues that possess receptors for that hormone.
2. Transport—transport systems by which hormones are transported in the blood [e.g., corticosteroid-binding globulins (CBG)], or are selectively taken up by organs and tissues *via* other cellular transport proteins (e.g., the blood–brain barrier).
3. Response—regulated responses of target cells to, and fine-tuned synthesis/availability of, paracrine, neuroendocrine, and endocrine secretions that can facilitate appropriate life history stage changes. These processes may involve alterations to receptor expression within a target cell, actions of metabolizing enzymes that can promote or deactivate a hormone (e.g., steroid metabolizing enzymes in many tissues that regulate local substrate availability for endocrine signaling systems), and a complex system of proteins that can act as enhancers or inhibitors of gene expression. It is possible to take this further downstream to protein synthesis, packaging, and actions, but these are beyond the scope of this paper.

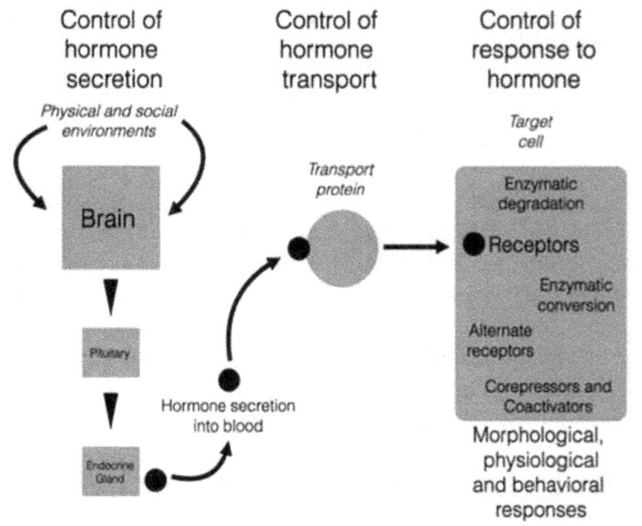

FIGURE 1 | There are three components of the action of hormones that can be regulated in diverse ways. The left-hand part of the figure shows the triggering of neural, neuroendocrine, and endocrine cascades that result in production of a highly specific secreted signal. The central part of the figure shows that after secretion into the blood, many hormones (particularly steroids, thyroid hormones, and some peptides) are transported by carrier proteins. Once the hormonal signal reaches the target cell (e.g., a neuron in the brain), it can act in various ways by binding to membrane or nuclear receptors that trigger extremely complex actions in a cell. Note that all three components are sites of regulation that could change daily or seasonally, or vary among individuals, populations, sex, or in response to unique experience of the environment. It is possible that this scheme is highly conserved across vertebrates and that different species modulate different components and still achieve the same behavioral and physiological end points. See text for more details. From Wingfield (10), courtesy of the American Ornithologist's Union and Wingfield (11), courtesy of Elsevier.

An example of a secretion–transport–response system is the production and action of sex steroids (**Figure 2**), in which the HPG cascade leading to testosterone secretion has multiple levels of possible regulation. Many species of vertebrates have highly specific androgen-binding proteins in the blood, including sex hormone-binding globulin, which is absent in birds, as well as CBG, which binds both glucocorticoids and sex steroids (12–14). The CBG gene has recently been identified in birds (15) and will allow future studies on CBG regulation. Target cell responses can be regulated in various ways, including the transformation of testosterone to estradiol and thus activation of a different array of receptor types [**Figure 2** (16, 17)]. Also, testosterone can be deactivated by 5β-reductase to 5β-dihydrotestosterone that is generally regarded as inert and does not bind to androgen receptors (ARs) [**Figure 2** (18–20)]. Note that peripheral secretion of sex steroids (left-hand side of **Figures 1** and **2**) results in broadcast of hormones to the entire organism through the blood stream, whereas actions at target cells (right-hand part of the **Figures 1** and **2**) allows local adjustment of the responses to a hormone. Steroids produced within the brain also allow paracrine actions at very localized sites without the additional effects on general morphological, physiological, and behavioral responses that occur when the hormone is broadcast through the blood stream [e.g., Ref. (11)]. These flexible points of regulation allow for the fine-tuning of trait expression to meet the specific demands of a stimulus, while keeping the animal within the necessary constraints of its current life history stage.

The secretion–transport–response regulatory model allows for the progressive localization of the effects of blood borne hormones (**Figure 2**; Figure S1 in Supplementary Material). Secretion cascades are generally broadcast to the whole organism whereas transport and especially target cell responses can be tailored to specific situations, environmental change, and life history stage. Environmental cues emanating from changing conditions can have direct effects on the secretion–transport–response system (e.g., temperature-related changes in hormone metabolism) or,

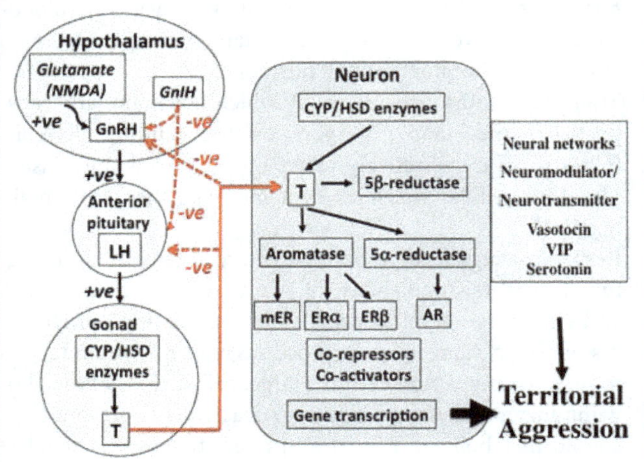

FIGURE 2 | Control mechanisms for territorial aggression in birds in spring. There are three major components to control mechanisms. First, the regulation of hormone secretion from the hypothalamo–pituitary–gonad axis (left part of the figure), transport of hormones such as testosterone in the blood (lines in red), and the mechanisms associated with action of the hormone in the target cell, in this case a neuron in the brain (central part of the figure). The net result is regulation of territorial aggression by neural networks (right-hand part of the figure). This three-part system of control of hormone secretion, transport, and effects on target organs is an important concept because it offers many points of potential regulation. The secretion component on the left summarizes how sensory information, in this case social, in transduced through neurotransmitter, e.g., glutamate (NMDA), and neuroendocrine secretions such as gonadotropin-releasing hormone (GnRH) and gonadotropin-inhibiting hormone (GnIH) into release of gonadotropins luteinizing hormone (LH) and follicle-stimulating hormone (not shown) from the anterior pituitary into the blood. LH travels to the gonad where it acts on cells that express steroidogenic enzymes to stimulate secretion of the sex steroid hormone testosterone (T) that is in turn released into the blood. Local actions of T in the testis include regulation of spermatogenesis, but it is also released into the blood in many avian species during breeding. Among many actions of T are effects on territorial aggression, and negative feedback on neuroendocrine and pituitary secretions (red lines). In birds, T circulates bound weakly to corticosteroid-binding globulin before entering target neurons involved in the expression of territorial aggression (center of figure). Once T has entered a target neuron, it has four potential fates. First, it can bind directly to the androgen receptor (AR), a member of the type 1 genomic receptors that become gene transcription factors once they are bound to T. Second, T can be converted to estradiol (E2) by the enzyme aromatase. E2 can then bind to either estrogen receptor alpha (ERα) or estrogen receptor beta (ERβ) both of which are genomic receptors that regulate gene transcription, but different genes from those regulated by AR. Third, T can be converted to 5α-dihydrotestosterone that also binds to AR and cannot be aromatized thus enhancing the AR gene transcription pathway. Fourth, T can be converted to 5β-dihydrotestosterone that binds to no known receptors and also cannot be aromatized indicating a deactivation shunt. The possibility of a rapid acting membrane receptor (non-genomic) should also be considered. A complex system of co-repressors and co-activators of genomic steroid receptor action are also known. Furthermore, it is now known that many neurons in vertebrate brains express all the enzymes required to synthesize T and E2 *de novo* from cholesterol or from circulating inert steroid hormone precursors such as dehydroepiandrosterone, androstenedione, and progesterone. The end result is regulatory action on neural networks that regulate expression of territorial aggression. Several neurotransmitters and neuromodulators such as arginine vasotocin, vasoactive intestinal peptide (VIP), and serotonin as also involved at this level. Evidence suggests that the basic secretory, transport, and action mechanisms are conserved across vertebrates. However, it is also clear that there are very many points at which the expression of territorial aggression may be affected indicating almost limitless combinations of possible regulatory mechanisms. From Wingfield (10), courtesy of the American Ornithologist's Union and Wingfield (11), courtesy of Elsevier.

more commonly, can be signalized *via* neural perception and transduction [Figure S1 in Supplementary Material, see Ref. (21)]. Mechanisms by which environmental cues can affect transport mechanisms and specific target cell responses remain much less well known. For example, it appears that the testes of zebra finches, *Taenopygia guttata*, can integrate and respond to cues of stress directly, rather than relying on a hormonal cascade initiated by the brain (22, 23), but it is not known exactly why the brain is bypassed in this instance. The evolutionary origins of the endocrine axes have seemingly resulted in a remarkable flexibility of response of different tissues (24).

Neurosteroids in Vertebrate Brains

Sex steroids have multiple peripheral and central actions on physiological traits. Sex steroids are not only produced solely by gonads and adrenal glands, but also by the brain [e.g., Ref. (5, 9, 25–31)]. In seasonally breeding vertebrates, neurally derived sex steroids produced in the non-breeding season do not influence reproductive traits *per se*, as very little sex steroid from this source reaches the blood stream and such neurosteroids are synthesized and act in a paracrine fashion in localized areas of the brain (32). Still, neurosteroids can have numerous effects on behavioral traits such as locomotor activity, aggression, reproduction, body temperature, and blood pressure (9, 29, 33–38). In addition, steroids in specific brain nuclei show seasonal changes in concentration, independently of circulating steroids [e.g., Ref. (39)]. These neurosteroids then act in a variety of brain regions to facilitate appropriate behavior for each life history stage (3, 28, 30, 40, 41).

The seasonal regulation of neurosteroid expression is not restricted to sex steroids. In a study on Japanese newts, *Cynops pyrrhogaster*, concentrations of pregnenolone and progesterone in the brain were higher in animals exposed to long spring-like vs. short winter-like day lengths, whereas experimental manipulation of environmental temperature had no effect (28). The newt brain expresses enzymes that synthesize 7α-hydroxypregnenolone *de novo* from cholesterol, and this neurosteroid activates locomotor activity associated with spring breeding. Moreover, the effect of 7α-hydroxypregnenolone on locomotor activity was blocked by dopamine D2-like receptor antagonists (27).

TWO EXAMPLES OF FLEXIBILITY IN STEROID MECHANISMS OF ACTION

We will focus next on two examples in which local production and paracrine actions of steroids in the brain can have major impacts on control of behavior and potentially avoid evolutionary costs of peripheral endocrine secretions at the wrong time.

Androgen/Estrogen Control of Avian Territorial Aggression Across Life History Stages

Although male territorial aggression was classically thought to be associated with circulating testosterone, work over the last 30 years suggests that the neural sensitivity to sex steroids, and the synthesis and action of both androgens and estrogens can modulate such behavior (32, 38, 42, 43). These are particularly important findings with regards to seasonal animals that express aggression during non-breeding life history stages when high circulating testosterone levels would likely lead to inappropriately timed reproductive behavior. For example, the Pacific Northwest subspecies of the song sparrow (*Melospiza melodia morphna*) shows high levels of aggressive territoriality and circulating testosterone during its breeding life history stage, low levels of testosterone and aggression during the autumnal molt, and high levels of aggression, but very low levels of circulating testosterone during the post-molt, non-breeding period (44). Our three-point secretion–transport–response regulatory model helps to explain how such behavioral expression is achieved across these different life history stages.

Secretion and production of sex steroids that modulate territorial aggression in the song sparrow change seasonally. For example, there is evidence for local production of testosterone and 17β-estradiol in the brain, both *de novo* from cholesterol and from circulating precursors (32, 33, 39). An example of the latter is dehydroepiandrosterone (DHEA), which is released by the adrenal glands, liver, and other peripheral organs, taken up by brain regions, and converted locally to more bioactive steroids (39). Neural steroid production allows for animals to retain actions of sex steroids in regions of the brain relevant to aggression, while avoiding the complication and inappropriate activation of morphology, physiology, and behavior associated with reproduction at the wrong time of year (45). Measurement of circulating DHEA indicates seasonal changes associated with territorial behavior in different life history stages in some species [e.g., Ref. (3, 19)] but not others [e.g., Ref. (46)]. In the song sparrow, circulating DHEA levels are highest during breeding and non-breeding when aggression is highest and lower during the molt, when aggression is also low, suggesting that circulating DHEA acts to promote life history appropriate aggression in this species (39).

The peripheral transport of DHEA and its movement into the brain, especially in birds, is not well characterized. In humans and some other vertebrates, DHEA travels in a hydrophilic sulfated form, DHEAS [e.g., Ref. (47)]. However, in birds, including the song sparrow, DHEA circulates primarily in its non-sulfated form [e.g., Ref. (39)]. Once DHEA arrives at its targets in the brain, it is possible that it has direct effects *via* ERβ, sigma-1, and/or GABAA receptor activation (48–50), though the affinity of DHEA for these receptors can be very low and more work is needed to assess the physiological and behavioral relevance of these possibilities. It is perhaps more likely that DHEA exerts the bulk of its effects on aggression *via* local conversion to testosterone, 5α-dihydrotestosterone, and 17β-estradiol, and subsequent activation of androgen and estrogen receptors.

Although circulating DHEA levels are equally high in breeding and non-breeding song sparrows, its local conversion to testosterone/estrogen in the brain may be more important during the non-breeding life history sub-stage (51). The activity of 3β-hydroxysteroid dehydrogenase/Δ^5-Δ^4-isomerase (3β-HSD), the enzyme that catalyzes transformation of DHEA to androstenedione, is higher during non-breeding vs. breeding in many brain regions that comprise neural networks underlying social behavior (30). Furthermore, DHEA is rapidly metabolized in such brain regions in dominant male song sparrows during aggressive interactions (42). These same interactions do not alter plasma DHEA levels. Evidence suggests that DHEA is eventually converted to 17β-estradiol to facilitate non-breeding aggression in this species.

Fadrozole, an inhibitor of aromatase, the enzyme that catalyzes the transformation of androgens to estrogens, reduces non-breeding, but not breeding aggression in song sparrows (20). That the precursor, DHEA might play a more prominent role in steroid-dependent, non-breeding aggression makes intuitive sense, as elevated circulating testosterone likely provides ample substrate to brain regions modulating aggression during the breeding period. Furthermore, castration of male song sparrows had no effect on territorial aggression in autumn suggesting that gonadal sources of androgen were not essential for expression of territoriality (52). These findings strengthen the hypothesis that circulating steroid hormone precursors such as DHEA and/or local production of sex steroids in the brain are requisite for expression of aggression in the non-breeding season in some species.

Estrogen synthesis can also be modified to facilitate appropriate behavioral responses. Changes in estrogen synthesis can occur in response to immediate environmental or social cues. For example, aromatase can be rapidly inactivated *via* phosphorylation (53), which may help to quickly alter behavior when an immediate context warrants it, though much more work is needed to address the behavioral relevance of these acute changes (16, 54). Estrogen synthesis can also change seasonally, potentially facilitating life history stage appropriate responses. In the male song sparrow, aromatase activity is highest in the ventromedial telencephalon, home to the medial amygdala, during breeding and non-breeding life history stages, when aggression is also at its height (3). The expression of aromatase mRNA also changes seasonally in multiple brain regions associated with the control of social behavior in the male song sparrow (5). Aromatase expression in the ventromedial nucleus of the hypothalamus (VMH), a brain region known to be involved in aggression-seeking behavior in rats (55), is equally high during breeding and non-breeding, when aggression is also highest, suggesting that the VMH may also mediate aggressive responses in birds (5). Aromatase expression in the preoptic area (POA), a brain region long known to be involved in the regulation of reproductive behavior and physiology, is both elevated during breeding and increased by administration of exogenous DHEA in male song sparrows, suggesting that this androgen/estrogen precursor may mediate different effects in different life history stages (56).

Androgen and estrogen receptor sensitivity may also be modulated to promote life history stage appropriate behavior. For example, neural AR mRNA expression changes seasonally in male song sparrows, with higher levels in the POA, the periventricular nucleus of the medial striatum (pvMSt), and paraHVC, a region of the song control system, during breeding (5). Exogenously administered DHEA increases AR expression in many of the same regions, again suggesting a role for this hormone in the seasonal modulation of social behaviors in this species (56). Current evidence suggests that DHEA, its transport to the brain from peripheral tissues, and its local conversion to androgens and estrogens helps promote life history appropriate behaviors, including seasonal aggression, in the male song sparrow. Adjustments of AR and aromatase gene expression have also been associated with aggressive responses to simulated territorial intrusions in dark-eyed juncos, *Junco hyemalis* (43), and differences in estrogen receptor alpha (ERα) expression are associated morph-specific variation in aggressive song in white-throated sparrows, *Zonotrichia albicollis* (57). In juncos, there were no changes in ERα expression, however (58), highlighting the importance of considering species-specific differences when assessing steroid responses relating to avian territorial aggression. Changes in sex steroid receptors in specific areas of the brain appear to be a widespread mechanism by which the sensitivity of neural tissue is regulated [e.g., Ref. (59, 60)].

Potential Roles of Neurosteroids on Animal Movement Including Migration

A second example of how the secretion–transport–response regulatory model approach informs hypotheses about how potential conflicts of steroid control of life history stages in different contexts might be avoided, involves the role of the neurosteroid 7α-hydroxypregnenolone in regulation of locomotor activity. Regular avian migrations (e.g., spring and autumn) have well-established endocrine control mechanisms [e.g., Ref. (7, 61)]. However, control mechanisms associated with specific environmental cues in one migration life history stage may have conflicts of action for the other. For example, spring migration toward a breeding area occurs during increasing day length but decreasing temperature and trophic resources as animals move north. By contrast, autumn migration toward a wintering area occurs during decreasing day length but temperatures tend to be higher as the animals move south and trophic resources are good, even increasing [e.g., Ref. (6)]. It is likely that these cues are differently transduced and integrated across these life history stages, even though the resulting migratory behaviors are similar in appearance. Furthermore, other types of animal movements such as facultative movements in response to local conditions may be different again (8). Nevertheless, common mechanisms may exist at fundamental neural levels across life history stages and facultative contexts, and there is preliminary evidence that the paracrine actions of 7α-hydroxypregnenolone may play a key role.

7α-Hydroxypregnenolone has been shown to affect locomotor behavior in newts, fish, and quail [e.g., Ref. (27, 34, 36, 40)]. Prolactin mediates 7α-hydroxypregnenolone action on spring migration in Japanese newts (62) and during upstream migration in chum salmon, *Oncorhynchus keta*, possibly *via* actions on dopaminergic neurons in the magnocellular preoptic nucleus (63). There are also strong circadian effects on 7α-hydroxypregnenolone that are possibly mediated by melatonin (36, 64), setting the stage for circadian control of locomotor behavior.

To assess the distribution and actions of 7α-hydroxypregnenolone in a migratory songbird, the white-crowned sparrow, *Zonotrichia leucophrys gambelii* (see Presentation S1 in Supplementary Material for methods and details), we collected brains from photostimulated birds that were in the spring migratory life history stage and divided them into regions. Left and right hemispheres were analyzed for differences in 7α-hydroxypregnenolone synthesis and concentrations, respectively. We also collected brains from birds in the non-migratory stage and analyzed 7α-hydroxypregnenolone synthesis separately in the cerebrum, diencephalon, mesencephalon, and cerebellum. There were no significant differences in 7α-hydroxypregnenolone synthesis in any brain region between the "migratory phase" and "non-migratory phase" (**Figure 3**).

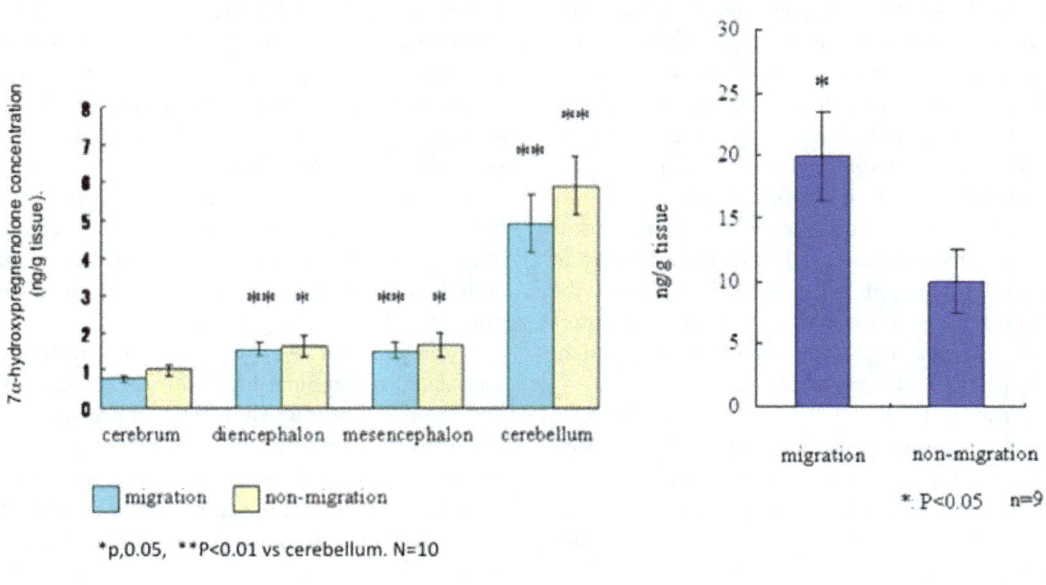

FIGURE 3 | Left panel. Synthesis of 7α-hydroxypregnenolone in different brain regions of the white-crowned sparrow, *Zonotrichia leucophrys gambelii*. Right panel. Whole brain concentrations of 7α-hydroxypregnenolone in white-crowned sparrows, in migratory and non-migratory life history stages.

However, 7α-hydroxypregnenolone synthesis in the cerebellum was higher than those in other brain regions in both males and females and regardless of migratory and non-migratory states (**Figure 3**; Figure S2 in Supplementary Material).

By GC-Ms analysis for 7α-hydroxypregnenolone concentration, we combined different brain regions (cerebrum + diencephalon + mesencephalon + cerebellum) due to the small tissue amounts involved. Results from this analysis suggest that 7α-hydroxypregnenolone concentration during the spring migratory phase is higher than that during the non-migration phase (**Figure 3**, right-hand panel). Note also that white-crowned sparrows in the vernal migratory stage exhibited very high levels of nocturnal migratory restlessness (*Zugunruhe*) compared with photorefractory birds that were molting and not migrating (Figure S3 in Supplementary Material). A higher concentration of 7α-hydroxypregnenolone during the migratory stage may depend on the amount of its precursor pregnenolone. An analysis of P450scc producing pregnenolone may be required in order to fully elucidate the dynamics of 7α-hydroxypregnenolone synthesis during this life history stage.

To determine central behavioral effects of 7α-hydroxypregnenolone infused into the third ventricle of white-crowned sparrows, birds in the molt life history stage were used, i.e., birds not showing migratory behavior (Figure S4 in Supplementary Material). Birds were then video-recorded for 30 min post-infusion, but most of the effects occurred in the first 10 min. 7α-Hydroxypregnenolone significantly inhibited perch-hopping behavior at a dose of 200 ng in 2 μl of vehicle in molting birds, but there was a great deal of variance in the data (top panel of Figure S4 in Supplementary Material). Overall, there was a decrease in perch-hops of approximately 30% compared with activity following saline infusions in the same birds (Figure S4 in Supplementary Material). There was approximately a 90% decrease in some individuals. In a follow-up study, infusion of 7α-hydroxypregnenolone at high and low doses into white-crowned sparrows had no effect on locomotor behavior during the spring migration life history stage (lower panel, Figure S4 in Supplementary Material). These data suggest seasonal and state dependent differences in actions of neurosteroids. Further studies attempting to block the actions of 7α-hydroxypregnenolone in spring and autumn migration will be critical.

PERSPECTIVE

The regulation of morphological, physiological, and behavioral traits specific to life history stages is mediated through endocrine, neuroendocrine, and paracrine secretions. When a specific trait may be expressed in more than one life history stage, the potential for conflict and decreased fitness arises, and the regulation of that trait may differ across those stages. In other words, hormonal regulation appropriate for one life history stage may not be suitable for another. As mentioned earlier, sex steroids of gonadal origin that affect territorial aggression in the breeding season are dependent on the HPG axis and are broadcast throughout an organism *via* the blood stream. In a non-breeding life history stage, such peripheral secretion of sex steroids would also activate morphological, physiological, and behavioral responses that would be inappropriate for that life history stage. Instead, local production of sex steroids in specific areas of the brain regulate territorial aggression during non-breeding, thereby helping to avoid the costs of action of gonadal sources of sex steroids in peripheral tissues.

In other cases, production of neurosteroids in localized, specific, brain regions may regulate behavioral and physiological traits that are expressed throughout the life cycle, and also on facultative bases. The role of 7α-hydroxypregnenolone may fit this scenario, especially in relation to its actions on locomotor activity. Although 7α-hydroxypregnenolone levels in the brain were higher in white-crowned sparrows in migratory vs. non-migratory life history stages (**Figure 3**), the effects of central infusion are difficult to interpret (Figure S4 in Supplementary Material). This may have been because birds were already showing maximum migratory activity, or that other regions of the brain may be important for regulation of migratory behavior. Nonetheless, future investigations will be needed to determine how 7α-hydroxypregnenolone might be important for regulation of migration, and whether this regulation changes across the two migratory life history stages (vernal and autumnal migrations) in the white-crowned sparrow.

Haraguchi et al. (65) have shown that 7α-hydroxyprogesterone can increase locomotor activity following restraint stress in newts, and, along with elevated corticosterone, may regulate behavioral responses to environmental perturbations. The possibility that this neurosteroid is involved in the rapid regulation of facultative movements associated with environmental perturbations during all life history stages is an exciting hypothesis. Facultative movements could occur at any time as part of the corticosteroid-induced emergency life history stage, for example, in response to a storm or increased predator pressure [e.g., Ref. (66, 67)]. Facultative movements would need to cease once suitable alternate habitat is found for the individual to survive the perturbation. 7α-hydroxypregnenolone is one neural paracrine signal that may be involved in both seasonal and facultative behavioral changes. It may also play a role in suppressing activity in molting white-crowned sparrows.

How hormone and neurohormone secretion, transport, and response are integrated to achieve the appropriate morphological, physiological, and behavioral response to life history stage and environmental and social changes requires further integrated studies. Coordination of the biological actions of these newly discovered autocrine and paracrine actions in the brain especially need more investigation in relation to life history stage and other environmental contexts. Understanding each organism's physiological and behavioral requirements across life history stages will allow us to identify the endocrine conflicts each faces as their requirements change. This has the potential to enlighten us as to how novel autocrine and paracrine actions within the brain and other tissues are coordinated and provide insights into the selection pressures that have driven the evolution of these systems.

AUTHOR CONTRIBUTIONS

JW wrote the original review and all other authors contributed equally to edits, addition of relevant references, and conceptual development.

ACKNOWLEDGMENTS

JW is grateful for a series of grant from the National Science Foundation (IBN-9631350 and IBN-0317141), and a subcontract of NIH grant RO1 MH61994-01, Barney Schlinger P.I. U.C.LA. Wingfield also acknowledges the Endowed Chair in Physiology, University of California, Davis. All animal procedures were approved by the University of Washington and University of California, Davis, Institutional Animal Care and Use Committees.

REFERENCES

1. Wingfield JC. Organization of vertebrate annual cycles: implications for control mechanisms. *Philos Trans R Soc Lond B Biol Sci* (2008) 363:425–41. doi:10.1098/rstb.2007.2149
2. Wingfield JC. Comparative endocrinology, environment and global change. *Gen Comp Endocrinol* (2008) 157:207–16. doi:10.1016/j.ygcen.2008.04.017
3. Soma KK, Schlinger BA, Wingfield JC, Saldanha CJ. Brain aromatase, 5 α-reductase, and 5 β-reductase change seasonally in wild male song sparrows: relationship to aggressive and sexual behavior. *J Neurobiol* (2003) 56:209–21. doi:10.1002/neu.10225
4. Wacker DW, Schlinger BA, Wingfield JC. Combined effects of DHEA and fadrozole on aggression and neural VIP immunoreactivity in the non-breeding male song sparrow. *Horm Behav* (2008) 53:287–94. doi:10.1016/j.yhbeh.2007.10.008
5. Wacker DW, Wingfield JC, Davis JE, Meddle SL. Seasonal changes in aromatase and androgen receptor, but not estrogen receptor mRNA expression in the brain of the free-living male song sparrow, *Melospiza melodia morphna*. *J Comp Neurol* (2010) 518:3819–35. doi:10.1002/cne.22426
6. Ramenofsky M, Wingfield JC. Regulation of migration. *Bioscience* (2007) 57:135–43. doi:10.1641/B570208
7. Ramenofsky M, Wingfield JC. Regulation of complex behavioral transitions: migration to breeding. *Anim Behav* (2016) 124:299–306. doi:10.1016/j.anbehav.2016.09.015
8. Wingfield JC, Ramenofsky M. Corticosterone and facultative dispersal in response to unpredictable events. *Ardea* (1997) 85:155–66.
9. Schmidt KL, Pradhan DS, Shah AH, Charlier TD, Chin EH, Soma KK. Neurosteroids, immunosteroids, and the balkanization of endocrinology. *Gen Comp Endocrinol* (2008) 157:266–74. doi:10.1016/j.ygcen.2008.03.025
10. Wingfield JC. Regulatory mechanisms that underlie phenology, behavior, and coping with environmental perturbations: an alternate look at biodiversity. *Auk* (2012) 129:1–7. doi:10.1525/auk.2012.129.1.1
11. Wingfield JC. Ecophysiological studies of hormone-behavior relations in birds: future challenges in a changing world. 3rd ed. In: Pfaff DW, Joëls M, editors. *Hormones, Brain and Behavior*. (Vol. 2), New York: Academic Press (2017). p. 321–45.
12. Charlier TD, Underhill C, Hammond GL, Soma KK. Effects of aggressive encounters on plasma corticosteroid-binding globulin and its ligands in white-crowned sparrows. *Horm Behav* (2009) 56:339–47. doi:10.1016/j.yhbeh.2009.06.012
13. Malisch JL, Breuner CW. Steroid-binding proteins and free steroids in birds. *Mol Cell Endocrinol* (2010) 316:42–52. doi:10.1016/j.mce.2009.09.019
14. Schoech SJ, Romero LM, Moore IT, Bonier F. Constraints, concerns and considerations about the necessity of estimating free glucocorticoid concentrations for field endocrine studies. *Funct Ecol* (2013) 27:1100–6. doi:10.1111/1365-2435.12142
15. Vaschenko G, Das S, Moon K-M, Rogalski JC, Taves MD, Soma KK, et al. Identification of avian corticosteroid-binding globulin (SerpinA6) reveals the molecular basis of evolutionary adaptations in SerpinA6 structure and function as a steroid-binding protein. *J Biol Chem* (2016) 291(21):11300–12. doi:10.1074/jbc.M116.714378
16. Charlier TD, Cornil CA, Ball GF, Balthazart J. Diversity of mechanisms involved in aromatase regulation and estrogen action in the brain. *Biochim Biophys Acta* (2010) 1800(10):1094–105. doi:10.1016/j.bbagen.2009.12.010
17. Balthazart J, Choleris E, Remage-Healey L. Steroids and the brain: 50 years of research, conceptual shifts and the ascent of non-classical and membrane-initiated actions. *Horm Behav* (2018) 99:1–8. doi:10.1016/j.yhbeh.2018.01.002
18. Hutchison JB, Steimer T. Brain 5β-reductase: a correlate of behavioral sensitivity to androgen. *Science* (1981) 213:244–6. doi:10.1126/science.7244635
19. Soma KK, Bindra RK, Gee J, Wingfield J, Schlinger BA. Androgen metabolizing enzymes show region-specific changes across the breeding season in the brain of a wild breeding songbird. *J Neurobiol* (1999) 41:176–88. doi:10.1002/(SICI)1097-4695(19991105)41:2<176::AID-NEU2>3.0.CO;2-2
20. Soma KK, Sullivan K, Wingfield JC. Combined aromatase inhibitor and antiandrogen treatment decreases territorial aggression in a wild songbird during the non-breeding season. *Gen Comp Endocrinol* (1999) 115:442–53. doi:10.1006/gcen.1999.7334
21. Wingfield JC, Mukai M. Endocrine disruption in the context of life cycles: environmental perturbations, global change and the adrenocortical response to stress. *Gen Comp Endocrinol* (2009) 163:92–6. doi:10.1016/j.ygcen.2009.04.030
22. Lynn SE, Perfito N, Guardardo D, Bentley GE. Food, stress, and circulating testosterone: cue integration by the testes, not the brain, in male zebra finches (*Taeniopygia guttata*). *Gen Comp Endocrinol* (2015) 215:1–9. doi:10.1016/j.ygcen.2015.03.010
23. Ernst DK, Lynn SE, Bentley GE. Differential response of GnIH in the brain and gonads following acute stress in a songbird. *Gen Comp Endocrinol* (2016) 227:51–7. doi:10.1016/j.ygcen.2015.05.016
24. Bentley GE, Wilsterman K, Ernst DK, Lynn SE, Dickens MJ, Calisi RM, et al. Neural versus gonadal GnIH: are they independent systems? A mini-review. *Integr Comp Biol* (2017) 57:1194–203. doi:10.1093/icb/icx085
25. Ukena K, Honda Y, Inai Y, Kohchi C, Lea RW, Tsutsui K. Expression and activity of 3β-hydroxysteroid dehydrogenase/delta5-delta4-isomerase in different regions of the avian brain. *Brain Res* (1999) 818:536–42. doi:10.1016/S0006-8993(98)01296-7
26. Matsunaga M, Ukena K, Tsutsui K. Expression and localization of cytochrome P450 17α-hydroxylase/c17,20-lyase in the avian brain. *Brain Res* (2001) 899:112–22. doi:10.1016/S0006-8993(01)02217-X
27. Matsunaga M, Ukena K, Baulieu E-E, Tsutsui K. 7α-hydroxypregnenolone acts as a neuronal activator to stimulate locomotor activity of breeding newts by means of the dopaminergic system. *Proc Natl Acad Sci U S A* (2004) 101:17282–7. doi:10.1073/pnas.0407176101
28. Inai Y, Nagai K, Ukena K, Oishii T, Tsutsui K. Seasonal changes in neurosteroid concentrations in the amphibian brain and environmental factors regulating their changes. *Brain Res* (2003) 959:214–25. doi:10.1016/S0006-8993(02)03745-9
29. Do Rego JL, Seong JY, Burel D, Lepronce J, Luu-The V, Tsutsui K, et al. Neurosteroid biosynthesis: enzymatic pathways and neuroendocrine regulation by neurotransmitters and neuropeptides. *Front Neuroendocrinol* (2009) 30:259–301. doi:10.1016/j.yfrne.2009.05.006
30. Pradhan DS, Newman AE, Wacker DW, Wingfield JC, Schlinger BA, Soma KK. Aggressive interactions rapidly increase androgen synthesis in the brain during the non-breeding season. *Horm Behav* (2010) 57:381–9. doi:10.1016/j.yhbeh.2010.01.008
31. Tsutsui K, Matsanuga M, Miyabara H, Ukena K. Neurosteroid biosynthesis in the quail brain: a review. *J Exp Zool* (2006) 305A:733–42. doi:10.1002/jez.a.302
32. Schlinger BA. Steroids in the avian brain: heterogeneity across space and time. *J Ornithol* (2015) 156(Suppl 1):S419–24. doi:10.1007/s10336-015-1184-7
33. Schlinger BA, Arnold AP. Brain is the major site of estrogen synthesis in a male songbird. *Proc Natl Acad Sci U S A* (1991) 88:4191–4. doi:10.1073/pnas.88.10.4191

34. Tsutsui K, Yamazaki T. Avian neurosteroids. 1. Pregnenolone synthesis in the quail brain. *Brain Res* (1995) 678:1–9. doi:10.1016/0006-8993(95)00116-8
35. Matsunaga M, Ukena K, Tsutsui K. Androgen biosynthesis in the avian brain. *Brain Res* (2002) 948:180–5. doi:10.1016/S0006-8993(02)03147-5
36. Tsutsui K, Inoue K, Miyabara H, Suzuki S, Ogura Y, Haraguchi S. 7α-hydroxypregnenolone mediates melatonin action underlying diurnal locomotor rhythms. *J Neurosci* (2008) 28:2158–67. doi:10.1523/JNEUROSCI.3562-07.2008
37. Schlinger BA, Pradhan DS, Soma KK. 3β-HSD activates DHEA in the songbird brain. *Neurochem Int* (2008) 52:611–20. doi:10.1016/j.neuint.2007.05.003
38. Schlinger BA, Brenowitz EA. Neural and hormonal control of birdsong. In: Pfaff DW, Arnold AP, Etgen AM, Fahrbach SE, Rubin RT, editors. *Hormones, Brain and Behavior*. (Vol. 2), San Diego: Academic Press (2009). p. 897–941.
39. Soma KK, Wingfield JC. Dehydroepiandrosterone in songbird plasma: seasonal regulation and relationship to territorial aggression. *Gen Comp Endocrinol* (2001) 123:144–55. doi:10.1006/gcen.2001.7657
40. Tsutsui K, Ukena K, Usui M, Sakamoto H, Takase M. Novel brain function: biosynthesis and actions of neurosteroids in neurons. *Neurosci Res* (2000) 36:261–73. doi:10.1016/S0168-0102(99)00132-7
41. Koibuchi N, Kimura-Kuroda J, Ikeda Y, Tsutsui K. Cerebellum, a target for hormonal signaling. *Cerebellum* (2008) 7:499–504. doi:10.1007/s12311-008-0015-2
42. Heimovics SA, Prior NH, Ma C, Soma KK. Rapid effects of an aggressive interaction on dehydroepiandrosterone, testosterone and estradiol levels in the male song sparrow brain: a seasonal comparison. *J Neuroendocrinol* (2016) 28:12345. doi:10.1111/jne.12345
43. Rosvall KA, Bergeon-Burns CM, Barske J, Goodson J, Schlinger BA, Sengelaub DR, et al. Neural sensitivity to sex steroids predicts individual differences in aggression: implications for behavioral evolution. *Proc Biol Sci* (2012) 279(1742):3547–55. doi:10.1098/rspb.2012.0442
44. Wingfield JC, Hahn TP. Testosterone and territorial behaviour in sedentary and migratory sparrows. *Anim Behav* (1994) 47(1):77–89. doi:10.1006/anbe.1994.1009
45. Wingfield JC, Lynn SE, Soma KK. Avoiding the 'costs' of testosterone: ecological bases of hormone-behavior interactions. *Brain Behav Evol* (2001) 57(5):239–51. doi:10.1159/000047243
46. Landys MM, Goymann W, Soma KK, Slagsvold T. Year-round territorial aggression is independent of plasma DHEA in the European nuthatch *Sitta europaea*. *Horm Behav* (2013) 63:166–72. doi:10.1016/j.yhbeh.2012.10.002
47. Labrie F, Belanger A, Simard J, Luu-The V, Labrie C. DHEA and peripheral androgen and estrogen formation: intracrinology. *Ann N Y Acad Sci* (1995) 774:16–28. doi:10.1111/j.1749-6632.1995.tb17369.x
48. Chen F, Knecht K, Birzin E, Fisher J, Wilkinson H, Mojena M, et al. Direct agonist/antagonist functions of dehydroepiandrosterone. *Endocrinology* (2005) 146:4568–76. doi:10.1210/en.2005-0368
49. Sousa A, Ticku MK. Interactions of the neurosteroid dehydroepiandrosterone sulfate with the $GABA_A$ receptor complex reveals that it may act via the picrotoxin site. *J Pharmacol Exp Ther* (1997) 282:827–33.
50. Maurice T, Su TP. The pharmacology of sigma-1 receptors. *Pharmacol Ther* (2009) 124:195–206. doi:10.1016/j.pharmthera.2009.07.001
51. Heimovics SA, Trainor BC, Soma KK. Rapid effects of estradiol on aggression in birds and mice: the fast and the furious. *Integr Comp Biol* (2015) 55:281–93. doi:10.1093/icb/icv048
52. Wingfield JC. Regulation of territorial behavior in the sedentary song sparrow, *Melospiza melodia morphna*. *Horm Behav* (1994) 28:1–15. doi:10.1006/hbeh.1994.1001
53. Ubuka T, Haraguchi S, Tobari Y, Narihiro M, Ishikawa K, Hayashi T, et al. Hypothalamic inhibition of socio-sexual behavior by increasing neuroestrogen synthesis. *Nat Commun* (2014) 5:3061. doi:10.1038/ncomms4061
54. Comito D, Pradhan DS, Karleen BJ, Schlinger BA. Region-specific rapid regulation of aromatase activity in zebra finch brain. *J Neurochem* (2016) 136(6):1177–85. doi:10.1111/jnc.13513
55. Falkner AL, Grosenick L, Davidson TJ, Deisseroth K, Lin D. Hypothalamic control of male aggression-seeking behavior. *Nat Neurosci* (2016) 19(4):596–604. doi:10.1038/nn.4264
56. Wacker DW, Khalaj LJ, Jones LJ, Champion TL, Davis JE, Meddle SL, et al. Dehydroepiandrosterone heightens aggression and increases androgen receptor and aromatase mRNA expression in the brain of a male songbird. *J Neuroendocrinol* (2016) 28. doi:10.1111/jne.12443
57. Horton BM, Hudson WH, Ortlund EA, Shirk S, Thomas JW, Young ER, et al. Estrogen receptor α polymorphism in a species with alternative behavioral phenotypes. *Proc Natl Acad Sci U S A* (2014) 111:1443–8. doi:10.1073/pnas.1317165111
58. Bergeon-Burns CM, Rosvall KA, Ketterson ED. Neural steroid sensitivity and aggression: comparing individuals of two songbird sub-species. *J Evol Biol* (2013) 26:820–31. doi:10.1111/jeb.12094
59. Canoine V, Fusani L, Schlinger B, Hau M. Low sex steroids, high steroid receptors: increasing the sensitivity of the nonreproductive brain. *Dev Neurobiol* (2007) 67:57–67. doi:10.1002/dneu.20296
60. Voigt C, Goymann W. Sex-role reversal is reflected in the brain of African black coucals (*Centropus grillii*). *Dev Neurobiol* (2007) 67:1560–73. doi:10.1002/dneu.20528
61. Wingfield JC, Ramenofsky M. Hormone-behavior interrelationships of birds in response to weather. In: Jane Brockmann H, Roper TJ, Naguib M, Mitani JC, Simmons LW, editors. *Advances in the Study of Behavior*. Vol. 43. Burlington: Academic Press (2011). p. 93–188. Elsevier Inc. Academic Press.
62. Haraguchi S, Koyama T, Hasanuma I, Vaudry H, Tsutsui K. Prolactin increases synthesis of 7α-hydroxypregnenolone, a key factor for induction of locomotor activity, in breeding male newts. *Endocrinology* (2010) 151:2211–22. doi:10.1210/en.2009-1229
63. Haraguchi S, Yamamoto Y, Suzuki Y, Chang JH, Koyama T, Sato M, et al. 7α-hydroxypregnenolone, a key neuronal modulator of locomotion, stimulates upstream migration by means of the dopaminergic system in salmon. *Sci Rep* (2015) 5:12546. doi:10.1038/srep12546
64. Tsutsui K, Haraguchi S, Inoue K, Miyabara H, Suzuki S, Ubuka T. Control of circadian activity of birds by the interaction of melatonin with 7a-hydroxypregnenolone, a newly discovered neurosteroid stimulating locomotion. *J Ornithol* (2012) 153(Suppl 1):S235–43. doi:10.1007/s10336-011-0795-x
65. Haraguchi S, Koyama T, Hasunuma I, Okuyama S-I, Ubuka T, Kikuyama S, et al. Acute stress increases the synthesis of 7α-hydroxypregnenolone, a new key steroid stimulating locomotor activity, through corticosterone action in newts. *Endocrinology* (2012) 153:794–805. doi:10.1210/en.2011-1422
66. Wingfield JC. The comparative biology of environmental stress: behavioral endocrinology and variation in ability to cope with novel, changing environments. *Anim Behav* (2013) 85:1127–33. doi:10.1016/j.anbehav.2013.02.018
67. Wingfield JC. Ecological processes and the ecology of stress: the impacts of abiotic environmental factors. *Funct Ecol* (2013) 27:37–44. doi:10.1111/1365-2435.12039

5

Gonadal Hormones and Retinal Disorders

Raffaele Nuzzi[1], Simona Scalabrin[1], Alice Becco[1] and Giancarlo Panzica[2,3]*

[1]Eye Clinic, Department of Surgical Sciences, University of Turin, Turin, Italy, [2]Laboratory of Neuroendocrinology, Department of Neuroscience Rita Levi-Montalcini, University of Torino, Torino, Italy, [3]Neuroscience Institute Cavalieri-Ottolenghi (NICO), Orbassano, Italy

***Correspondence:**
Raffaele Nuzzi
raffaele.nuzzi@unito.it

Aim: Gonadal hormones are essential for reproductive function, but can act on neural and other organ systems, and are probably the cause of the large majority of known sex differences in function and disease. The aim of this review is to provide evidence for this hypothesis in relation to eye disorders and to retinopathies in particular.

Methods: Epidemiological studies and research articles were reviewed.

Results: Analysis of the biological basis for a relationship between eye diseases and hormones showed that estrogen, androgen, and progesterone receptors are present throughout the eye and that these steroids are locally produced in ocular tissues. Sex hormones can have a neuroprotective action on the retina and modulate ocular blood flow. There are differences between the male and the female retina; moreover, sex hormones can influence the development (or not) of certain disorders. For example, exposure to endogenous estrogens, depending on age at menarche and menopause and number of pregnancies, and exposure to exogenous estrogens, as in hormone replacement therapy and use of oral contraceptives, appear to protect against age-related macular degeneration (both drusenoid and neurovascular types), whereas exogenous testosterone therapy is a risk factor for central serous chorioretinopathy. Macular hole is more common among women than men, particularly in postmenopausal women probably owing to the sudden drop in estrogen production in later middle age. Progestin therapy appears to ameliorate the course of retinitis pigmentosa. Diabetic retinopathy, a complication of diabetes, may be more common among men than women.

Conclusion: We observed a correlation between many retinopathies and sex, probably as a result of the protective effect some gonadal hormones may exert against the development of certain disorders. This may have ramifications for the use of hormone therapy in the treatment of eye disease and of retinal disorders in particular.

Keywords: gonadal hormones, estrogens, hormone therapy, eye disorders, retinopathies, optic nerve, age-related macular degeneration, sex-related differences

INTRODUCTION

There is a growing body of evidence for the importance of gonadal hormone action in the function of the reproductive and other systems (1), including bone (2) and cardiovascular system. Sex hormones (androgenic, estrogenic, and progestinic) are produced by both sexes, though the quantity and mode differ by sex and age. Moreover, they are produced, not only by the gonads, but also by other organs (3, 4), including the central nervous system (CNS) in which estrogens are thought to exert a neuroprotective role (5, 6).

Historically, interactions between gonadal hormones and the eye have received scarce attention; however, recent research into sex-related differences has begun to reveal possible links between estrogens and eye diseases, i.e., glaucoma, age-related macular degeneration (AMD), and cataracts. This has carried over into the evaluation of the implications that postmenopausal hormone replacement therapy (HRT) and anti-estrogenic therapy in breast cancer could have for concomitant eye disorders (7).

Since, research in this area is still at its beginning, the available studies are few and often limited in sample size; this does not allow to reach a univocal and definitive answer about the relationship between sex, sex hormones, and ocular pathologies. The purpose of this review is, therefore, to summarize the results currently present in the literature.

BASICS OF BIOLOGY AND EPIDEMIOLOGY OF INTERACTION BETWEEN GONADAL HORMONES AND THE EYE

Presence of Hormone Receptors in the Human Eye

The eye was long considered a "sexually neutral" structure, meaning that it was believed that there were no differences in ocular physiology and pathology between the sexes. Today, however, we know that differences among sexes exist both in the physiology and in the pathology of the eye. In fact, the eye is a target for sex steroid hormones as demonstrated by the large presence of sex steroid hormone receptors (SSHRs). The SSHRs' mRNAs are present everywhere in the eye (8): cornea, lens, iris, ciliary body, retina, lacrimal gland, meibomian gland, conjunctiva [for a complete list of citations see Ref. (9)]. In all these locations, estrogen receptor α (ERα), estrogen receptor β (ERβ), progesterone receptor, and androgen receptor (AR) mRNAs have been detected.

The distribution of SSHRs in the eye varies by sex and age, which partly explains the difference in the epidemiology of certain eye diseases (9). PCR assay, Western blot, and immunohistochemical analysis have demonstrated the presence of ER-α protein in the retina and RPE of young women, but not in postmenopausal women or men (10).

In addition to AR mRNA (8), the AR protein is present in the lachrymal and meibomian glands, the cornea, the bulbar conjunctiva, the lens, and the RPE, together with 5α-reductase (the enzyme converting testosterone into the more powerful dihydrotestosterone, DHT) type 1 and 2 mRNA (8).

Synthesis of Steroids in the Retina

The mammalian retina has the ability of synthetize neurosteroids (pregnenolone, progesterone, dehydroepiandrosterone, desoxycorticosterone, 3 alpha, 5 alpha-tetrahydrodesoxycorticosterone, 3 alpha-hydroxy-5 alpha-dihydro-progesterone, 17-hydroxyprogesterone, and 17-hydroxypregnenolone) from cholesterol, as demonstrated by using retinal explants, thus excluding interferences from circulating steroids (11).

Following studies demonstrated also the presence of steroidogenic enzymes (mRNA and protein) in the retina (12): cytochrome CYP11A1 (CYP450scc) that converts cholesterol in pregnenolone; 3-β-hydroxysteroid dehydrogenase which converts pregnenolone in progesterone; cytochrome CYP17A1 (P450c17) involved in the production of 17-α-hydroxymetabolites; and CYP19A1 (P450 aromatase) which converts testosterone in 17-β-estradiol [(11, 13, 14), **Figure 1**]. Cholesterol, which activates the metabolic cascade leading to the production of E_2, is also produced in the retina: HMG-CoA reductase, the main enzyme for cholesterol synthesis, is present in the RPE, photoreceptors, and Müller cells. Exogenous cholesterol, on the other hand, is derived from high-density and low-density lipoproteins (HDL and LDL, respectively) that bind to specific receptors of the retinal cells (15). The principal limiting steps for estrogen production in the retina are the regulation of CYP450scc and aromatase enzymatic activities (14) (**Figure 1**). The steroidogenic enzymes are found in retinal neurons, glial cells, and photoreceptors in amounts similar to those observed in other part of the CNS (16). Enzymes' concentration is greatest in the internal nuclear layer, which is considered the principal site of retinal steroids' synthesis (14).

Finally, it is important to note that estrogens and androgens are also produced outside the retina (gonads, adrenals) and, through the blood flow, they can reach the eye where, in males, circulating testosterone may be locally metabolized in 17-β-estradiol. Diseases or functional alterations linked to steroid hormones may, therefore, be due to both retinal steroidogenic enzyme failure (short-term effects?), alterations in the gonadal and adrenal hormone supply (long-term effects?), or both conditions.

Differences in Retinal Function between Men and Women

There are marked sex-related differences in ocular anatomy and pathophysiology, particularly for the retina. Studies on mice have identified differences in retinal structure between males and females and found that, as measured by multifocal electroretinography (mfERG), retinal function is better in females of reproductive age than in males and older females (17). Similar mfERG studies on humans found a statistically significant difference in neuroretinal function between men and women below 50 years, but not after this age; in addition, neuroretinal function was lowest in women who received a hysterectomy during reproductive age, with subsequent iatrogenic-induced menopause. These findings suggest that the estrogenic cycle has a beneficial effect on neuroretinal function and that estrogens may have a protective role (18).

Sex-Related Differences in the Prevalence of Eye Disorders

Sex-related differences in eye anatomy and physiology are reflected in disease processes (19). Cataracts, for example, are far more prevalent among women than men: the prevalence of lens opacities in women aged between 65 and 74 years is 24–27%, but only 14–20% in their male counterparts (20–23). Estrogen levels, besides other risk factors, appear to play a role. Numerous studies have shown that HRT is a protective factor in postmenopausal

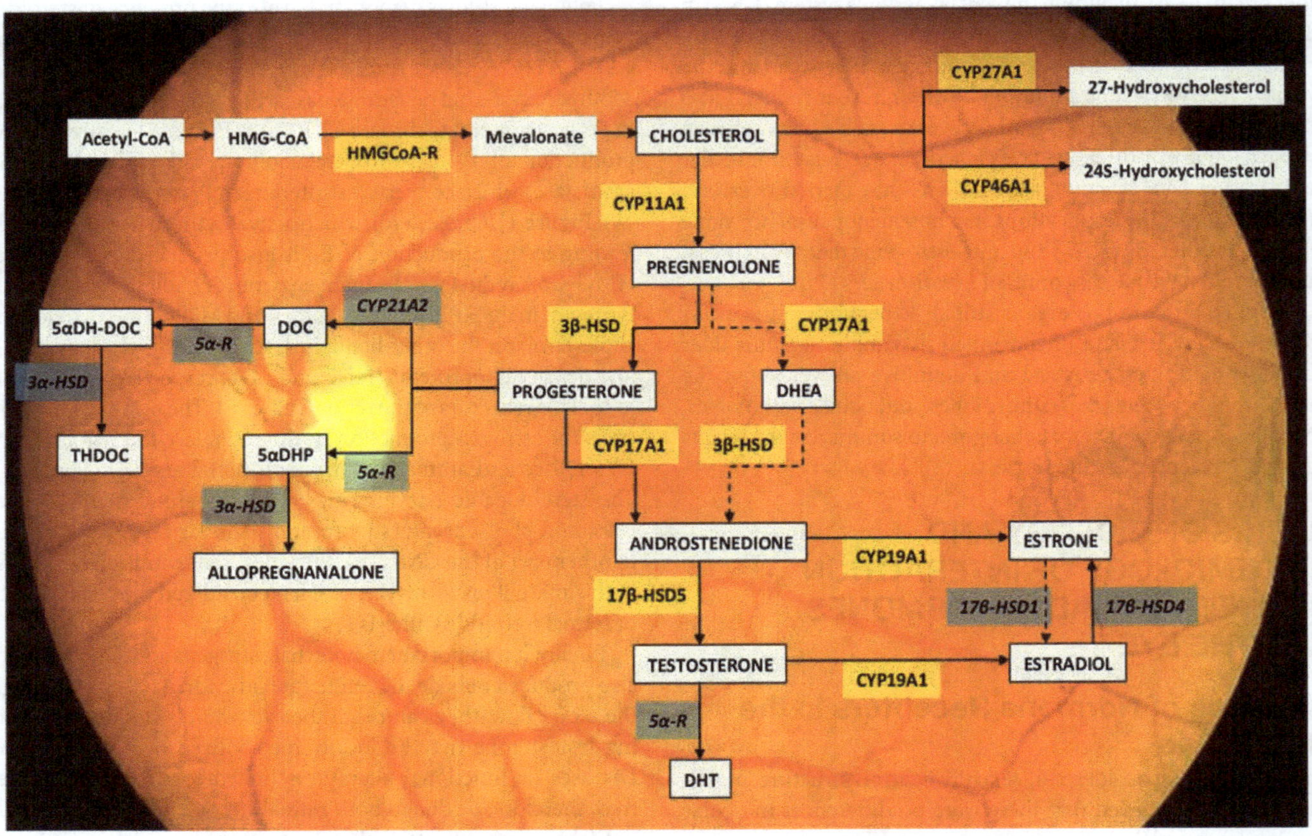

FIGURE 1 | Neurosteroid synthesis in the retina. The drawing report of the metabolic pathway leading to estradiol synthesis within the retina (11, 14). The steroidogenic enzymes already identified for their mRNA, activity or immunolocalization are indicated within yellow boxes. The enzymes still lacking of identification are indicated within the grey boxes. Dotted lines indicate so far unclear enzymatic activities. Abbreviations: 3β-HSD, 3β-hydroxysteroid dehydrogenase; 3α-HSD, 3α-hydroxysteroid dehydrogenase; 5αDH-DOC, 5 alpha-dihydrodeoxycorticosterone; 5αDHP, 5α-dihydroprogesterone; 5α-R, 5α-Reductase; 17β-HSD1, 17β-hydroxysteroid dehydrogenases 1; 17β-HSD4, 17β-hydroxysteroid dehydrogenases 4; 17β-HSD5, 17β-hydroxysteroid dehydrogenases 5; DHEA, dehydroepiandrosterone; DHT, dihydrotestosterone; DOC, deoxycorticosterone; HMG-CoA, hydroxymethylglutaryl-CoA; HMGCoA-R, hydroxymethylglutaryl-CoA reductase.

women and that late menopause or early menarche, both of which augment estrogen exposure, lower the risk of cataracts in advanced age (24–27). The main protective action of estrogens on the lens is probably due to their antioxidant properties (28). With the onset of menopause, the drop in estrogen levels increases the risk of cataracts in older women. Differently, the levels of estrogen converted by aromatase from testosterone in men do not seem to be age dependent, affording men greater protection against the development of cataracts (29). This sex-related difference in eye disorders is not always so distinct. For example, sex is not considered a factor in AMD (30, 31), though some studies have suggested its higher prevalence among women (32, 33). When distinguished by type of AMD, neovascular (34) and drusenoid (32) forms are more prevalent among women. As reported for cataracts, longer exposure to estrogens or HRT confers a lower risk of developing AMD in later age (35, 36), suggesting that this is due to the antioxidant and anti-inflammatory actions of estrogen (37, 38).

Glaucoma is also more frequent in women (39), though this is more likely linked to the longer life expectancy of women and as such is an age-related risk factor (40). Nonetheless, sex-related differences have been associated with different types of glaucoma: a study conducted on an Asian population (39) reported that angle-closure glaucoma is more prevalent among women; other studies reported the same findings for white and black populations (41, 42), but other studies found that, after adjusting for age and population, angle-closure glaucoma is more common among men (40, 43). Sex-related differences in the prevalence of diabetic retinopathy are associated with the difference in the prevalence of diabetes. Though more men than women are affected by type 1 diabetes (44) no study to date has found a significant difference in its prevalence (45, 46). Similarly, no statistically significant sex-related differences in the prevalence of diabetic retinopathy associated with type 2 diabetes have been established, though some studies have suggested that it is more frequent among men (47, 48).

Various other risk factors besides sex alone need to be taken into account (49). For example, in a study on a rural south Indian population, Nirmalan et al. (50) tried to understand if female reproductive factors (age at menarche and menopause, number of pregnancies, etc.) were related with eye diseases. The study found no association with cataracts, open-angle glaucoma, macular degeneration, or myopia; nonetheless, the study presented several limitations, including the fact that the data on reproductive factors were gleaned from self-report questionnaires and that eye disorders were diagnosed in most subjects during the course of the study.

NEUROPROTECTIVE EFFECT OF SEX HORMONES

Preclinical Studies

Several studies have investigated whether estrogens have a neuroprotective role and, if so, through which mechanisms they exert such action. Nixon et al. (51) examined the role of hormones in elevated levels of glutamate, which has a neurotoxic effect. High glutamate concentrations inhibit the cysteine/glutamate transporter, which reduces the production of glutathione, an antioxidant. This decrease leads to the augmented production of reactive oxygen species (52), which, owing to oxidative damage, promote the development of eye diseases, such as AMD (53) and retinitis pigmentosa (54). The experiment was carried out *in vitro* on 661 W cells, i.e., a mouse cone photoreceptor cell line, and demonstrated that E_2 and the non-feminizing estrogen analogs ZYC-26 and ZYC-3 exert a protective action against the damage induced by 5 μM of glutamate. It was also observed that the protective effect of ZYC-26 and ZYC-3 is not exerted *via* the classic estrogen receptors ERα and ERβ, as demonstrated by the persistent protective action despite the use of an estrogen receptor pan-antagonist (ICI182780) and the lack of a protective effect after the use of the two agonists of ERα and ERβ. Based on these results, it was hypothesized that non-feminizing hormones could be used in the treatment of neurodegenerative eye disorders, and thus avert the side effects of prolonged estrogen therapy. Mo et al. (55) investigated intracellular neuroprotective mechanisms in ovariectomized mice, as measured by electroretinography of light-induced apoptosis in retinal cells. Following intravitreal administration of 17β-estradiol, retinal function was preserved due to the reduction of neuronal apoptosis. The involved pathway is PI3k/Akt activation: administration of a PI3K inhibitor (LY294002) increases retinal neuronal apoptosis, while the administration of estrogens leads to the translocation of NF-kB p65 from the cytosol to the nucleus, which is inhibited in the presence of LY294002. These results demonstrated that the protective action of estrogen on the retina is exerted *via* activation of the PI3K/Akt cascade and concludes with the nuclear translocation of NF-kB (55). The mechanism of action reported in this study is not the only one through which sex hormones exert their neuroprotective effect.

Estrogens also have a protective effect on intraretinal synapses. Kaja et al. (56) used a mouse model in which mild retinal ischemia was induced by transient occlusion of the middle cerebral artery. This experimental condition is ideal for examining the earliest stages of retinal damage that precede the development of neurodegenerative processes. Synaptic activity was measured using an immunoreactive technique based on the detection of Vesl-1L7Homer 1c (V-1L), a neuronal cytosolic protein involved in receptor clustering for neurotransmitters and in neuronal development and plasticity. V-1L is also a good marker to evaluate the changes in synaptic connectivity during the early stages of apoptosis of retinal ganglion cells. The study (56) found that retinal ischemia, though mild, can significantly reduce the number of V-1L-positive synapses in the internal plexiform layer of the retina, and increase the number of neuronal apoptotic cells in the ganglion cell layer. Estrogen administration exerts a protective effect by reducing the percentage of cells undergoing apoptosis and by preventing early ischemia-induced changes preceding apoptosis in the synaptic connections.

The neuroprotective action of estrogens appears to be closely linked to their antioxidant activity. Among the studies investigating this property, the early study by Moosmann et al. (57) merits mention as it demonstrated that the antioxidant-neuroprotective action of the hormones is not due to their genomic property, i.e., their ability to influence the transcription of specific genes, but rather because of their chemical properties as hydrophobic phenolic molecules. Estrogens were compared with other phenol molecules: the results showed that the protective effect against glutamate-induced oxidative toxicity in neuronal mouse cells was present in all the compounds studied and that the dose to obtain this effect was also the same. The study also showed that there is no correlation between estrogen strength and its antioxidant properties. The discovery of the dissociation between the hormonal effect and the neuroprotective effect could open the way to the development of new therapies using molecules that possess the same protective properties as estrogens, but without the unwanted effects associated with their activities as sex hormones.

Nakazawa et al. (58) investigated differences in neuroprotective activity between "endogenous" estrogens (produced in ovary) and "exogenous" estrogens (administrated through intravitreal injection) in a mouse model by comparing their neuroprotective effects against retinal ganglion cell (RGC) death following axotomy of the optic nerve, which mimics glaucoma-induced RGC death. To evaluate endogenous estrogen activity, samples of retinal tissue from female mice, ovariectomized or not, served as controls in which RGC density was measured. While ovariectomy had no effect on RGC density, the density was significantly reduced in mice that received ovariectomy and axotomy as compared to those that received only axotomy. These findings underscored the neuroprotective role of endogenous estrogens. In the evaluation of exogenous estrogens, ovariectomized mice administered intravitreal 17β-estradiol had a reduction in RGC death correlated with axotomy. The neuroprotective role of estrogens in this experimental condition indicates the potential for estrogen therapy in persons with etiologically similar eye diseases, such as glaucoma. In the second part of the study, the researchers wanted to identify the mechanism by which the exogenous estrogens exert their neuroprotective action. Immunoblot assay and immunohistochemical analysis showed that following intravitreal administration of E_2, activation of the ERK signal transduction pathway, and c-Fos was augmented, whereas no change in PI3K/Act activation was observed. This finding was then confirmed in an experiment using U1026, an ERK inhibitor. Administration of U0126 before administration of E_2 inhibited the neuroprotective effect of the estrogens (58).

Another molecular mechanism by which estrogens exert their neuroprotective effect involves upregulation of stromal cell-derived factor 1 (SDF-1). SDF-1 protects against retinal ischemia *via* its powerful chemotactic effect that promote tissue repair and the migration of stem cells produced in bone marrow to the site of damage (59). To demonstrate this factor's mechanism of action, transient retinal ischemia was induced by increasing intraocular pressure (IOP) to 110 mm Hg in a mouse model. Following reperfusion, the expected increase in mRNA and SDF-1 was measured *via* real-time PCR and Western blot. To evaluate the role of estrogens, E_2 was administered peripherally before inducing ischemia and SDF-1 was measured. The increased quantity of SDF-1 indicated that also in this condition estrogens play a neuroprotective role in reducing retinal damage (60).

Several studies aimed to determine whether only estrogens exerted neuroprotective action or other sex hormones, such as progesterone possessed similar properties (61). Progesterone was administered by peripheral infusion to one half of a population of male rats that had undergone photostress-induced retinal degeneration. Electroretinography showed no statistically significant differences between the two cohorts. The study findings suggested that progesterone has no protective effects similar to those of estrogens.

Clinical Studies

In addition to preclinical animal studies, also clinical studies have been performed, including a population-based study in postmenopausal Korean women (62) in which the women were administered a questionnaire investigating their gynecological characteristics and whether they were taking estrogens as HRT. The women also received an eye examination, which revealed a higher prevalence of eye diseases, including anterior polar cataracts and other retinal disorders in the women not receiving HRT, suggesting its neuroprotective action.

EFFECT OF SEX HORMONES ON OCULAR BLOOD FLOW

Besides acting directly on retinal neuronal cells, sex hormones can also influence tissue perfusion by modulating retinal and choroid blood flow. A recent review of the literature (63) on sex differences in ocular blood flow sought to determine the possible role of sex hormones. The rationale for the study was derived from the fact that the eye diseases in which reduced blood flow is considered a causal or contributing factor, including AMD (64–66), glaucoma (67, 68), and diabetic retinopathy (69–71) are also those for which a sex-related correlation with prevalence has been found, suggesting that sex hormones may be implicated in the development of these diseases. Estrogens appear to play a protective role probably because of their vasodilatory action in reducing vascular resistance. This finding is shared by several studies that compared blood flow velocity and resistance of the ophthalmic artery and the central retinal artery in pre- and postmenopausal women. Blood flow velocity was higher and vascular resistance indices were lower in the premenopausal women (72), whereas vascular resistance of the central retinal artery was reduced after estrogen administration as compared to placebo (73). Retinal blood flow was higher in women receiving HRT than in those naïve to HRT (74); however, the evidence was not sufficiently strong to recommend HRT in the treatment of these conditions.

While estrogens exert a vasodilatory effect on retinal perfusion, testosterone, like progesterone, has the opposite effect (72). Progesterone exerts a vasoconstrictive effect on ocular blood flow. As demonstrated by color Doppler imaging (75), progesterone increases the resistance of ophthalmic and retinal arteries. In women of reproductive age, progesterone was found to antagonize the vasodilatory effect of estrogen during the menstrual cycle, as measured with the pulsatility index of the central retinal artery (76).

The role of HRT has been extensively studied because of the implications it can have for postmenopausal women with eye diseases. Postmenopausal women receiving HRT or not were compared with regards to blood flow in the inferotemporal retinal artery (ITRA), the peripapillary retina, and the margin of the optic nerve head, as measured using stereometric parameters and electroretinography (73). Blood flow in the ITRA was significantly higher and trophism of the optic nerve head and surrounding area was better in those receiving HRT. The effect of estradiol on retinal perfusion was investigated using ovariectomized mice; in this model E_2 treatment improved retinal perfusion mainly through the increase in blood flow. Both HRT and administration of E_2 exert a protective effect on the retina and the retinal nerve fiber layer by modulating tissue perfusion.

Harris-Yitzhak et al. (77) compared blood flow velocity in the retrobulbar arteries of postmenopausal women receiving HRT or not and young women of reproductive age. Hemodynamic resistance in the ophthalmic artery was lower in the young women and those receiving HRT than in the postmenopausal women not receiving HRT, whereas central retinal artery blood flow was similar for all three groups. Blood flow in the posterior ciliary arteries was better in the young women than in the two groups of postmenopausal women in which blood flow was similar. These findings suggested that HRT may modulate resistance in the ophthalmic artery, whereas its effect on other arteries is less pronounced, since changes in blood perfusion in these areas seem to be related to age.

Other studies have compared the effect of estradiol and testosterone on ocular hemodynamics by measuring the serum levels of the two hormones in pre- and postmenopausal women not receiving HRT, in addition to evaluating *via* color Doppler blood flow velocity and vascular resistance in the ophthalmic and central retinal arteries (72). The findings showed that peak systolic blood flow velocity in the ophthalmic artery correlated with serum estradiol levels, whereas vascular resistance of the central retinal artery decreased with increasing levels of estrogens in both groups of women. Peak systolic blood flow velocity correlated negatively with serum testosterone levels in the premenopausal women, whereas vascular resistance increased with higher testosterone levels. The two hormones were found to exert opposite effects: testosterone seemed to exert an antagonist effect as compared to estrogen.

The action of testosterone on ocular hemodynamics has also been studied in men, in which testosterone levels are naturally higher than in women. Low testosterone levels correlated with hypertension and higher cardiovascular risk (78, 79). There are also population-based differences. In fact, Malan et al. (80) described differences for the cardiometabolic prognosis and intraocular perfusion pressure in two cohorts of black and white men aged between 28 and 68 years. Only in white men there was a positive correlation between free testosterone levels and retinal vessel diameter (except for the central retinal artery in which the vessel diameter was inversely proportional to testosterone levels). The findings suggested a population-based protective effect of testosterone on vascularization and retinal perfusion, probably linked to the vasodilatory effect in the microvasculature.

DISEASES OF THE RETINA, OPTIC NERVE, AND POSSIBLE SEX-RELATED EFFECTS

In this section of the review we tried, for each pathology, to collect the evidence in favor of the correlation with sex hormones and those against (**Table 1**).

Age-Related Macular Degeneration

Evidence for the Protective Effect of Estrogens

Age-related macular degeneration is a progressive multifactorial eye disease that leads to deterioration of vision, loss of spatial and color vision, and adaptation to darkness (81–85). According to the World Health Organization, AMD is the cause of blindness in 10% of cases. Histological hallmarks are degeneration of the RPE, Bruch's membrane, and the choriocapillaris, resulting in photoreceptor damage and death (86).

The pathogenesis of AMD is multifactorial: lipofuscin accumulation in the lysosomes of the RPE; extracellular drusen deposits between the RPE and the internal collagen layer of Bruch's membrane; oxidative damage; and chronic inflammation. Owing to their antioxidant and anti-inflammatory properties, estrogens might play a protective role in AMD (38). Beside these pathogenic factors there are genetic and environmental risk factors: age is perhaps the most important, in addition to smoking, obesity, atherosclerosis, hypertensions, hypercholesterolemia, unhealthy diet, and history of cataract surgery (81). Female sex is a weak risk factor (32, 87, 88) though exudative AMD is more common among women (34). These risk factors have been investigated in various studies. A case-control study (33) involved the participants in the Age-Related Eye Disease Study (AREDS) and used as controls subjects with fewer than 15 small drusen. Preliminary analysis showed that age was the main risk factor; subsequent analyses were accordingly adjusted for age to minimize its confounding with other factors. Smoking and hypertension both resulted as risk factors. Other correlated characteristics were Caucasian race, body-mass index, low educational level, hypermetropia, lens opacities, and female sex. A population-based study (89) identified alcohol abuse as another risk factor. Exposure to exogenous estrogens was a weakly protective factor against drusenoid deposit in AMD.

Spurred by the prospects of a protective action by estrogens against the development of AMD, researchers investigated the effect of HRT in postmenopausal women. Haan et al. (90) sought to determine whether HRT had a beneficial effect and whether different HRTs achieved different effects. They compared the efficacy of therapy based on conjugated equine estrogens (CEE) with CEE therapy combined with a progestinic. No association was found between the use of either therapy and the early development of AMD, suggesting that the early stages of AMD are not influenced by HRT. In contrast, conjugate therapy was more effective than CEE therapy alone in reducing the risk of developing both the drusenoid and neovascular forms of AMD.

In addition to investigating the protective effect of HRT on the development of certain types of AMD, Feskanich et al. (91) examined the potential role of estrogens as oral contraceptives during reproductive age. They observed a lower risk for the development of neovascular AMD in women receiving HRT. The risk was further reduced in those who, in addition to HRT, had also taken oral contraceptives. An unexpected result was the correlation between the risk of early AMD and HRT. The risk of early AMD was higher in the women who had received HRT; this contrasted with other studies that reported no correlation between the two factors. When the gynecological characteristics (age at menarche and menopause, number of pregnancies) were analyzed, none of these reproductive factors significantly modified the risk of developing AMD, except for a slight reduction associated with multiple pregnancies.

Velez Edwards et al. (92) investigated whether genetic factors could interact with HRT in modulating the risk of AMD and found that postmenopausal HRT and use of estrogen oral contraceptives during reproductive age had a protective effect against AMD. When, however, the study population was stratified by AMD severity, i.e., distinguishing between early AMD characterized by geographic atrophy and neovascular AMD, the lower risk remained only for neovascular AMD. During the second part of the study, genetic analyses were carried out on peripheral blood samples to determine whether single nucleotide polymorphisms (SNPs) in genes thought to increase the risk of AMD could modulate the risk of AMD in association with HRT or previous exposure to oral contraceptives. The study findings showed that two SNPs of the *ARMS2* gene (AMD 2) located on chromosome 10 enhanced the positive effect of HRT in preventing AMD.

The hypothesis for a link between HRT and lower AMD incidence was investigated by other studies which showed that estrogen exerted a protective effect only against certain types of AMD, like drusenoid AMD, demonstrating that this type of AMD is more prevalent among women with multiple pregnancies, whereas the correlation was not statistically significant when comparing early AMD and late AMD (93).

Other studies focusing attention on the role reproductive factors can have in the incidence of maculopathies. Blasiak et al. (37) reported a statistically significant reduction in the incidence of advanced AMD in women who had received HRT and a significantly higher risk of developing advanced AMD in women who began menarche late. These findings demonstrated that estrogen exposure, including exogenous estrogens, plays a beneficial role in reducing the risk of advanced AMD. The hypothesis that early

TABLE 1 | Role of sex hormones in ocular diseases.

++	+	+/–	/	–
Protective effect	**Modest correlation**	**Non-significant correlation**	**Non-associated factor**	**Inversely correlated factor**

Disease	E	P	T	Studies
AMD	+/–	/	/	Menopausal and reproductive factors and risk of age-related macular degeneration. Feskanich et al.
				The effect of the hormone therapy on the risk for age-related maculopathy in postmenopausal women. Abramov et al.
				Reproductive exposures, incident age-related cataracts, and age-related maculopathy in women: the Beaver Dam Eye Study. Klein et al.
				Female reproductive factors and eye disease in a rural south Indian population: the Aravind comprehensive eye survey. Nirmalan et al.
	/			Clinical risk factors for age-related macular degeneration: a systematic review and meta-analysis. Chakravarthy et al.
				Age-related macular degeneration guidelines for management. The Royal College of Ophthalmologists.
				Sex steroid and AMD in older French women: the POLA study. Defay et al.
AMD (drusenoid or neovascular)	++			Hormone therapy and age-related macular degeneration. The women's health initiative sight exam study. Haan et al.
				Inverse association of female hormone replacement therapy (HRT) with AMD and interaction with ARMS2 polymorphisms. Velez et al.
				HRT, reproductive factors, and age-related macular degeneration: the Salisbury Eye Evaluation Project. Freeman et al.
				Association between reproductive and hormonal factors and age-related maculopathy in postmenopausal women. Snow et al.
	+			Clinical risk factors for age-related macular degeneration: a systematic review and meta-analysis. Chakravarthy et al.
				Risk factors for age-related macular degeneration. Evans
				Five-year incidence of age-related maculopathy lesions: the Blue Mountains Eye Study. Mitchell et al.
				Risk factors associated with age-related macular degeneration: a case-control study in the age-related eye disease study (AREDS): AREDS report number 3. Group, AREDS research
				Smoking, alcohol intake, estrogen use, and AMD in Latinos: the Los Angeles Latino Eye Study. Fraser-Bell et al.
CSCR	/	/	–	The potential role of testosterone in central serous chorioretinopathy. Grieshaber et al.
				Central serous chorioretinitis associated with testosterone therapy. Ahad et al.
				Central serous chorioretinopathy in patients receiving exogenous testosterone therapy. Nudleman et al.
				Finasteride for chronic central serous chorioretinopathy. Foroogian et al.
	/	/	/	Serum cortisol and testosterone levels in chronic central serous chorioretinopathy. Tufan et al.
				Serous central chorioretinopathy and endogenous hypercortisolemia. Kapetanios et al.
MACULAR HOLE	++	/	/	Clinical features of idiopathic macular cysts and holes. McDonnell et al.
				Macular holes. James and Feman
				Estrogen antagonist and development of macular hole. Chung et al.
				Estrogen and macular holes: a postal questionnaire. Gray et al.
				Systemic risk factors for idiopathic macular holes: a case-control study. Evans et al.
	–	/	/	Vitreous estrogen levels in patients with an idiopathic macular hole. Inokuchi et al.
Retinitis Pigmentosa	/	++	/	Enhancing survival of photoreceptor cells *in vivo* using the sintetic progestin norgestrel. Doonan et al.
				Norgestrel may be a potential therapy for retinal degenerations. Doonan and Cotter
				Neuroprotective actions of progesterone in an *in vivo* model of retinitis pigmentosa. Sanchez-Vallejo et al.
Diabetic Retinopathy	/	/	+/–	The role of sex hormones in diabetic retinopathy. Grisby et al.
				Dehydroepiandrosterone protects bovine retinal capillary pericytes against glucose toxicity. Briganrdello et al.
	++ *If early stage* – *If late stage*		/	Gender and estrogen supplementation increases severity of experimental choroidal neovascularization. Espinosa-Heidmann et al.
				Effects of tamoxifen versus raloxifene on retinal capillary endothelial cell proliferation. Grigsby et al.
	/	/	/	Exogenous estrogen exposures and changes in diabetic retinopathy: the Wisconsin Epidemiologic Study of Diabetic Retinopathy. Klein et al.

(*Continued*)

TABLE 1 | Continued

++	+	+/–	/	–
Protective effect	**Modest correlation**	**Non-significant correlation**	**Non-associated factor**	**Inversely correlated factor**
Disease	**E**	**P**	**T**	**Studies**
Glaucoma	++	/	/	Is estrogen a therapeutic target for glaucoma? Dewundara et al. The obligatory role of endothelial cells in the relaxation of arterial smooth muscle by acetylcholine. Furchgott et al. Estrogen deficiency accelerates aging of the optic nerve. Vajaranant and Pasquae Primary open-angle glaucoma. Weinreb and Khaw The effect of the menstrual cycle on optic nerve had analysis in healthy women. Akar et al. Estrogen pathway polymorphisms in relation to primary open angle glaucoma: an analysis accounting for gender from the United States. Pasquale et al.

For and against evidences for each disease, with type of correlation.
AMD, age-related macular degeneration; CSRC, central serous chorioretinopathy; E, estrogens; P, progesterone; T, testosterone.

menopause (before age 45 years), because it reduces the duration of exposure to estrogens, could constitute a risk for the development of macular degeneration was evaluated by Vigerling et al. (94) who compared different samples of women, including those that had experienced spontaneous early menopause and others who had experienced iatrogenic early menopause following ovariectomy. The results showed no increased risk for AMD among the women who experienced spontaneous early menopause, whereas the risk of developing macular degeneration was significantly increased in those who had undergone ovariectomy before age 45 years.

Studies Showing No Protective Effect of Estrogens

While some studies have found a neuroprotective effect of estrogens, others have not, leaving the question of their potential neuroprotective effect open. The guidelines for the management of AMD issued by the Royal College of Ophthalmologists (95) state that, on the basis of a meta-analysis (32), female sex is not a factor associated with higher risk of AMD. The guidelines go on to state that the higher prevalence of AMD among women is largely due to their longer life expectancy (87).

Numerous studies cited by the guidelines report that reproductive characteristics, e.g., age at menarche and menopause, and exposure to HRT are inconsistently associated with AMD (50, 96–98). The POLA study, for example, found that advanced AMD and drusenoid AMD or AMD with pigment abnormalities were not associated with oophorectomy or hysterectomy or HRT exposure. The POLA study examined serum levels of diverse hormones and correlated molecules (estradiol, testosterone, DHEAS, sex hormone-binding globulin) and found a correlation, albeit weak, only for high DHEAS levels that appeared to be associated with an increased prevalence of drusenoid AMD. Other studies and a review corroborate the hypothesis for the lack of a correlation between estrogens and macular degeneration. A systematic review (32) of 18 population-based studies and 6 case-control studies on the strength of the relationship among factors, increasing the risk for AMD reported that the risk factors most strongly correlated with degenerative maculopathy were age, smoking (33, 99, 100), history of cataract surgery (101–103), and family history of AMD (104, 105). Moderately correlated factors were body-mass index (99), history of cardiovascular disease (99, 106), hypertension (99, 106, 107), and elevated plasma fibrinogen (108). Factors weakly or inconsistently correlated with AMD were sex (107, 109, 110), ethnic group (107, 111), color of iris (104), history of cardiovascular disease (99, 106) and serum levels of cholesterol (99, 106), and triglycerides (106). Female sex was not considered a risk factor, precluding the role of sex hormones in higher risk for the disease.

Central Serous Chorioretinopathy (CSCR)

Evidence of the Association between CSCR and Sex Hormones: Testosterone and Increased Risk of CSCR

Central serous chorioretinopathy is an acquired eye disease characterized by exudative detachment of the retinal and/or the

RPE. Its pathogenesis is not yet fully understood; however, it is thought that alterations in choroid circulation and RPE function may be implicated in the development of the disease. This notion is corroborated by findings from fluorangiography and OCT that document augmented capillary permeability and pressure of the choroid vessels (107, 108). Risk factors vary widely from psychosocial stress to type A personality, Cushing's syndrome, infections, smoking, alcohol, to pregnancy, and steroid therapy (109–111), all of which are characterized by elevated serum levels of glucocorticoids (112–114).

Given its higher prevalence among men, androgens have been directly implicated in the pathogenesis of CSCR (111, 115). In their study, Nudleman et al. (116) examined patients receiving exogenous testosterone therapy and who had no known risk factors for CSCR. The results showed that testosterone therapy is a probable independent risk factor for CSCR; moreover, disease symptoms and subretinal fluid accumulation resolved after discontinuation of testosterone therapy. Further evidence for the role of testosterone came from a case report of a woman who was not pregnant while receiving testosterone therapy (111), and another case report of a male population receiving testosterone therapy for hypogonadotropic hypogonadism (115), the latter of which demonstrated a temporal correlation between administration of therapy and the development of CSCR, indicating both testosterone and estrogen as the cause. Given the link between testosterone and CSCR, finasteride, an inhibitor of DHT synthesis, was considered as an alternative in the treatment of CSCR. Forooghian et al. (117) investigated the effect of finasteride administered for 6 months and monitored changes in visual acuity, macular thickness, subretinal fluid accumulation, OCT, serum DHT and testosterone, and cortisol levels in urine. Though no changes in visual acuity occurred, macular thickness and subretinal fluid level were lowest at 3 months in therapy before increasing slightly though remaining below basal reference limits. Furthermore, macular thickness and subretinal fluid both increased after therapy was discontinued in four patients and normalized in the patients who continued with therapy. These findings suggest a possible role for finasteride in the treatment of chronic CSCR.

Studies Showing an Absence of Association between CSCR and Testosterone

The study of Kapetanios et al. (114) reported a statistically significant association between elevated cortisol levels and the development of ICSCR, whereas no significant differences in testosterone levels were noted and levels remained within the normal range in both groups. A case-control study (118) of chronic ICSCR reported that cortisol and testosterone levels were similar in both groups. Though there appears to be a correlation between hormones and ICSCR, conflicting evidence leaves many questions about the etiopathogenesis and treatment of CSCR open.

Macular Hole

Evidence of Estrogen Protection in the Macular Hole

Macular hole is a major cause of diminished vision, especially in advanced age. Although in some cases the cause can be identified, e.g., contusive trauma (119), cystoid macular edema (120), or diabetes (121), it is idiopathic in the majority and thought to be due to circumferential vitreoretinal contraction (122). Macular hole affects women far more often than men (123). As in other eye diseases, it is thought that estrogens have a beneficial effect on macular health and protect against the development of macular hole. For example, estrogens stimulate the synthesis of collagen and hyaluronic acid in the skin, suggesting that a similar process might also occur in the eye. With the sudden drop in estrogen production after menopause, this protection is lost, posing the retina to a higher risk than that for men, in whom estrogen levels are generally low throughout life and do not change abruptly. In addition to menopause, early hysterectomy or HRT may influence estrogen activity in relation to the development of macular holes (124, 125). Current evidence indicates strong correlations between macular hole and female sex and postmenopausal age (126), as demonstrated by various studies. A population-based study showed a female-to-male ratio of 3.3:1 for full-thickness macular hole (127). In their case-control study, Evans et al. (128) found that 67% of persons with macular hole were women and that 74% of the women were aged 65 years or older. The study analyzed various risk factors, including ethnic origin, systemic comorbidities, current use and history of medications, alcohol intake, smoking, body weight and height, menstrual and obstetric history, age at menopause and severity of associated symptoms, and exposure to HRT. The study findings indicated few systemic factors associated with idiopathic full-thickness macular hole (IFTMH), and though sex-correlated, no association was found between the principal indicators of exposure to estrogens and the incidence of macular hole. Nonetheless, a role for estrogens was suggested by the fact that women with macular hole generally experienced a more difficult menopause and more bothersome climacteric symptoms such as hot flashes than healthy women. The results also suggested that the development of IFTMH may be more due to the sudden change in hormone levels that chronic exposure, as demonstrated by the higher risk is associated with menopause, hysterectomy, and oophorectomy.

Correlations have been found between tamoxifen and macular hole and its precursor lesions (129). Tamoxifen is an anti-estrogenic nonsteroid drug used in adjuvant therapy for breast cancer (130). In this case report, all three women were receiving tamoxifen therapy and presented with cystic changes of the foveal region and defects of the external retina suggestive of initial macular hole.

A Study Shows That Estrogen Could Have a Negative Effect on Macular Hole

Another study investigated whether there were differences between the estrogen levels in the vitreous of subjects with macular hole and in those with other retinal disorders, who served as controls (131). The estrogen concentration was significantly higher in those with macular hole ($p < 0.05$), implicating it in the pathogenesis of the disorder. Since estrogens activate collagenase, this could be correlated with the development of vitreous collagen disorders; however, owing to the small study sample (10 cases and 9 controls), no definitive conclusions could be drawn.

Retinitis Pigmentosa

Evidence of the Benefical Effect of Progestinic Therapy in Retinitis Pigmentosa

Retinitis pigmentosa refers to a group of inherited retinal degenerative disorders in which genetic mutations lead to the death of retinal photoreceptors (132). Although the mutations in several genes implicated in the development of the diseases are known, the mechanism by which they cause cell death is not fully understood and no effective treatment is currently available (133). Recent studies using mouse models have suggested Norgestrel, a synthetic analog of progesterone, as a potential agent (134). Norgestrel's protective action has been demonstrated on retinal explants *in vitro* and in two different *in vivo* models of retinal degeneration: the one involving mice exposed to photostress-induced damage and the other involving mice with genetic mutations characteristic of retinitis pigmentosa. Both models showed a reduction in cell loss, with improvement in cell survival of about 70% (calculated on the basis of photoreceptor number, structural integrity, and function), indicating that apoptosis was interrupted or slowed. Although the mechanism of action is not yet fully understood, it is thought that norgestrel activates a survival pathway probably based on the increased expression of fibroblast growth factor 2 (FGF-2), a powerful neurotrophic factor whose production is increased by retinal stress. Its action promotes cell survival and inhibits apoptosis by activating the intracellular cascades involving mitogen-activated protein kinase, PI3K, and protein kinase C (PKC). The involvement of FGF-2 was demonstrated by measuring its changes in the control subjects who were administered only the vehicle and in the subjects receiving norgestrel therapy: the finding of higher FDG-2 values after norgestrel administration confirmed the hypothesis. These findings were strengthened by the same research group in a subsequent study (135) in which they investigated the potential of norgestrel as therapy for retinal degeneration.

Other studies investigated the relationship between progesterone and progestrinics and retinitis pigmentosa (136) building on previous studies on progesterone in experimental models of acute brain damage in which the drug had shown a neuroprotective effect (137). The action of progesterone was analyzed to determine the number of surviving cells, as measured by electroretinography, and the potential protective effect of the drug owing to its ability to limit damage by free radicals or to increase antioxidant defenses. The results showed a reduction in cell death and gliosis, with a statistically significant reduction in glutamate and a significant increase in reduced glutathione and oxidized glutathione. The study underlined the beneficial action of progesterone which exerts *via* multiple modes of action in protecting the retina during retinitis pigmentosa, suggesting its use or that of its analogs in the treatment of the disease.

Diabetic Retinopathy

The Uncertain Role of Sex Hormones in Diabetic Retinopathy

Poor glycemic control ultimately results in macrovascular and microvascular complications, affecting the kidney and the eye in persons with diabetes. Diabetic retinopathy is most common complication (138) and is present in 34.6% of diabetics (139). Two forms are distinguished: nonproliferative or early stage diabetic retinopathy, and proliferative or late stage retinopathy in which retinal neovascularization is evident, leading to increased risk of loss of vision due to retinal detachment, neovascular glaucoma, and vitreous hemorrhaging. Another common cause of loss of vision is macular edema, which may arise in any stage of retinopathy (140). Studies investigating the possible links between sex hormones and diabetic retinopathy have analyzed the incidence of the condition by sex and produced conflicting results (49). One possible explanation for the discrepancies is the likely presence of confounding factors. Grisby et al. (141) compared the direct action of sex hormones on retinal cells and their action on vasculature, and found that various hormones are involved in the development and progression of retinopathy in diabetic patients. Androgens and androgen inhibitors appear to play both a causal and a protective role, since they increase blood pressure and the levels of adhesion molecules (ICAM and VCAM-1), with worsening of lipid levels. A low level is associated with the metabolic syndrome and may alter lipid, glycemic, and blood pressure values. Dehydroepiandrosterone has a proven protective effect against the damage of elevated glucose levels in pericytes (142). It is believed that the damage due to elevated glucose levels occurs mainly through oxidative mechanisms. The toxicity of glucose and subsequent vascular damage manifest in four ways: activation of the PKC cascade; activation of aldoso-reductase; protein glycosylation; and activation of the hexosamine pathway. According to the so-called unifying therapy, the formation of free oxygen radicals underlies the mechanisms leading to glucose damage (143, 144).

As oxidative stress is implicated in the development and progression of diabetic retinopathy, studies have investigated the role of estrogens, which possess antioxidant properties. Estrogens stimulate the ERβ receptor and protect retinal cells against oxidative stress through their ability to modulate the transcription of antioxidant genes and protect the mitochondria (145). Estrogens can exert a differential action depending on the stage of retinopathy: during the initial stages, the proliferation of endothelial cells induced by estradiol has a beneficial effect and protects the retina by inducing repair processes, whereas during the proliferative stage, this same effect exacerbates the disease (146, 147). Selective estrogen receptor modulators (SERMs), including tamoxifen and raloxifen, act as antagonists or agonists of estrogen depending on the type of receptor to which they bind. In the retina, both drugs strongly antagonize estrogen-induced angiogenesis (147). From the multitude of data collected so far it is clear that the use of sex hormones or their antagonists in the treatment of retinopathy must be personalized based on sex, age, and stage of disease. Stimulation or hormonal modulation may provide a novel therapeutic option.

Other studies have investigated differences in electroretinographic patterns in relation to neuroretinal function in men and women with type 2 diabetes, but not retinopathy to evaluate risk for neurodegenerative disease (148). The analysis showed that neuroretinal dysfunction leading to diabetic retinopathy was far more common among men than women, suggesting a sex-related protective mechanism. This finding was corroborated in a minireview issued by the Berkeley School of Optometry (49) that noted a more frequent incidence of abnormal neuroretinal function in men with type 2 diabetes. It was also observed that advanced proliferative retinopathy in type 1 diabetes more often affects men, that retinopathy is more likely present at diagnosis of diabetes in men, and that it is often more severe than in women.

HRT Does Not Influence Diabetic Retinopathy

A possible benefit of HRT for retinopathy in postmenopausal women has been studied (149); however, no connection between changes in retinopathy and the incidence of macular edema and exposure to exogenous estrogen could be established, indicating that, unlike its effects observed in other eye disorders, HRT has no effect on diabetic retinopathy.

Glaucoma

Benefical Effects of Estrogens in Glaucoma

Glaucoma, the second leading cause of blindness in the world (43), is a slow, progressive neurodegenerative disease characterized by gradual loss of RGC (150) and loss of vision (151). A recent review (152) examining possible correlations between glaucoma and estrogens reported that factors influencing the duration of estrogen exposure (e.g., age at menarche, use of oral contraceptives, bilateral ovariectomy, age at menopause) can raise the risk of POAG. A higher risk for POAG was associated with age at menarche over 13 years, as compared to age less than 12 years (153), and a 25% higher risk was noted in women who took oral contraceptives for more than 5 years (154). Bilateral ovariectomy before age 43 increased the risk of developing glaucoma (155), as did spontaneous menopause before age 45 years (156), whereas the risk was significantly lower in women over age 65 who entered menopause after age 54 years (154). Prolonged estrogen exposure reduced the risk of glaucoma or glaucoma-related conditions, as demonstrated by evidence that IOP is lower during pregnancy when estrogen levels are elevated, particularly during the third trimester (157, 158). Evidence for a protective effect of HRT against glaucoma is uneven (79, 159, 160).

Genetic factors may also play a role in increasing the risk for developing glaucoma. SNPs implicated in the estrogen metabolic pathway associated with women, but not men (161), and polymorphisms of the endothelial nitric oxide synthase gene encoding the enzyme regulated by estrogens are correlated with the development of open-angle glaucoma (162). Estrogen exposure may alter the pathogenesis of glaucoma and exert a neuroprotective action. A future area of focus is the use of estrogens in glaucoma treatment or prevention. Numerous studies have reported an association between estrogens and glaucoma; for example, estrogen deficiency was associated with the acceleration of aging of the optic nerve (163). Estrogens have also been implicated in aqueous humor production and drainage via receptors on the ciliary epithelium (10, 159). Changes in estrogen levels appear to influence IOP, which is responsible for optic nerve trophism (164). Epidemiology, clinical, and experimental evidence supports the hypothesis that early reduction of estrogen levels leads to premature aging of the optic nerve and increased susceptibility to glaucoma.

In their study on the role of estrogens in modulating the topography of the optic nerve head, Akar et al. (165) reported that, as observed in diabetic women, hormonal fluctuations during the menstrual cycle affect the central area and the margin of the optic nerve head. Genetic analysis to determine whether there exist associations between certain SNPs of genes involved in estrogen metabolism and the development of POAG (161) showed that SNPs were correlated with global POAG and POAG with elevated, but not with low IOP and no correlation of any type was noted for the men. Among the women, however, the gene that encodes the catechol-O-methyltransferase enzyme was found to be associated with open-angle glaucoma. Summarizing, links between SNPs of the estrogen pathways and the development of glaucoma were noted for certain types of glaucoma and only in women.

FUTURE PROSPECTS AND OPPORTUNITIES

A Place for HRT?

In light of the amount of research conducted so far on sex hormones and neuroretinal diseases, the question arises whether and how it can be applied to the identification and development of new drugs or to expanding indications for drugs already on the market. An emblematic case is that of HRT for the treatment of climacteric symptoms.

Despite the wealth of data, the question remains open. A study evaluated the efficacy of HRT with phytoestrogens on eye function, as measured with short-wavelength automated perimetry in postmenopausal women (166). Phytoestrogens are nonsteroids of plant origin with estrogen-like action in modulating vision sensitivity. Consistent with the theory of timing, which states that the benefits of HRT diminish the later the therapy is initiated, a loss of efficacy was noted in relation to the time between initiation of phytoestrogen therapy and onset of menopausal symptoms, with no benefit gained if the therapy was started in women over 60 years of age. No conclusions could be drawn from this study and no recommendations for the use of HRT for eye diseases could be made.

Implications for Future Study Design

The present review of the literature found evidence for a sex-related difference in the prevalence of certain eye diseases. A plausible explanation for the difference is the differential effect of sex hormones on the development and course of disease, which may be as meaningful as it is complex, though the underlying mechanisms are not yet fully understood.

The link between sex hormones and retinopathies opens new therapeutic horizons. To obtain a better understanding of the interactions between sex hormones and eye diseases, studies should be designed to determine the presence of an association between sex, hormones, and disease, and if such an association exists, the potential therapeutic correlates. To reach these objectives, key areas of focus are: epidemiological studies on the distribution of eye disease in a population, while taking sex and hormonal status into account; experimental studies on the changes in the incidence and/or course of disease in relation to hormone administration or deprivation; and preclinical animal studies comparing differences between the sexes.

AUTHOR CONTRIBUTIONS

All the authors have equally contributed to the search of the literature and cooperated to write the article.

REFERENCES

1. Rosner W, Hankinson SE, Sluss PM, Vesper HW, Wierman ME. Challenges to the measurement of estradiol: an endrocrine society position statement. *J Clin Endocrinol Metab* (2013) 98(4):1376–87. doi:10.1210/jc.2012-3780
2. Clarke BL, Khosla S. Female reproductive system and bone. *Arch Biochem Biophys* (2010) 503(1):118–28. doi:10.1016/j.abb.2010.07.006
3. Gillies GE, McArthur S. Estrogen actions in the brain and the basis for differential action in men and women: a case for a sex-specific medicines. *Pharmacol Rev* (2010) 62(2):155–98. doi:10.1124/pr.109.002071
4. Simpson ER. Sources of estrogen and their importance. *J Steroid Biochem Mol Biol* (2003) 86(3–5):225–30. doi:10.1016/S0960-0760(03)00360-1
5. Azcoitia I, Arevalo MA, De Nicola AF, Garcia-Segura LM. Neuroprotective actions of estradiol revisited. *Trends Endocrinol Metab* (2011) 22:467–73. doi:10.1016/j.tem.2011.08.002
6. Melcangi RC, Panzica G, Garcia-Segura LM. Neuroactive steroids: focus on human brain. *Neuroscience* (2011) 191:1–5. doi:10.1016/j.neuroscience.2011.06.024
7. Hutchinson CV, Walker JA, Davidson C. Oestrogen, ocular function and low-level vision. *J Endocrinol* (2014) 223(2):R9–18. doi:10.1530/JOE-14-0349
8. Wickham LA, Gao J, Toda I, Rocha EM, Ono M, Sullivan DA. Identification of androgen, estrogen and progesterone receptor mRNAs in the eye. *Acta Ophthalmol Scand* (2000) 78(2):146–53. doi:10.1034/j.1600-0420.2000.078002146.x
9. Gupta PD, Johar K, Nagpal K, Vasavada AR. Sex hormone receptors in the human eye. *Surv Ophthalmol* (2005) 50(3):274–84. doi:10.1016/j.survophthal.2005.02.005
10. Ogueta SB, Schwartz SD, Yamashita CK, Farber DB. Estrogen receptor in the human eye: influence of gender and age on gene expression. *Invest Ophthalmol Vis Sci* (1999) 40(9):1906–11.
11. Guarnieri P, Guarnieri R, Cascio C, Pavasant P, Piccoli F, Papadopoulos V. Neurosteoidogenesis in rat retina. *J Neurochem* (1994) 63(1):86–96. doi:10.1046/j.1471-4159.1994.63010086.x
12. Cascio C, Russo D, Drago G, Galizzi G, Passantino R, Guarnieri R, et al. 17b-estradiol synthesis in the adult male rat in retina. *Exp Eye Res* (2007) 85(1):166–72. doi:10.1016/j.exer.2007.02.008
13. Ishikawa M, Yoshitomi T, Zorumski CF, Izumi Y. Neurosteroids are endogenous neuroprotectants in an ex vivo glaucoma model. *Invest Ophthalmol Vis Sci* (2014) 55(12):8531–41. doi:10.1167/iovs.14-15624
14. Cascio C, Deidda I, Russo D, Guarnieri P. The estrogenic retina: the potential contribution to healthy aging and age-related neurodegenerative diseases of the retina. *Steroids* (2015) 103:31–41. doi:10.1016/j.steroids.2015.08.002
15. Fliesler SJ, Bretillon L. The ins and outs of cholesterol in the vertebrate retina. *J Lipid Res* (2010) 51(12):3399–413. doi:10.1194/jlr.R010538
16. Mellon SH, Griffin LD, Compagnone NA. Biosynthesis and action of neurosteroids. *Brain Res Brain Res Rev* (2001) 37(1–3):3–12. doi:10.1016/S0165-0173(01)00109-6
17. Chaychi S, Polosa A, Lachapelle P. Difference in retinal structure and function between aging male and female Sprague-Dawley rats are strongly influenced by the estrus cycle. *PLoS One* (2015) 10(8):e0136056. doi:10.1371/journal.pone.0136056
18. Ozawa GY, Bearse MA, Harrison WW, Bronson-Castain K, Schneck ME, Barez S, et al. Differences in neuroretinal function between adult males and females. *Optom Vis Sci* (2014) 91(6):602–7. doi:10.1097/OPX.0000000000000255
19. Zetterberg M. Age-related eye disease and gender. *Maturitas* (2016) 83:19–26. doi:10.1016/j.maturitas.2015.10.005
20. Kahn HA, Leibowitz HM, Ganley JP, Kini MM, Colton T, Nickerson RS, et al. The Framingham eye study. I. Outline and major prevalence findings. *Am J Epidemiol* (1977) 106(1):17–32. doi:10.1093/oxfordjournals.aje.a112428
21. Klein BE, Klein R, Linton KL. Prevalence of age-related lens opacities in a population. The Beaver Dam Eye study. *Ophthalmology* (1992) 99(4):546–52. doi:10.1016/S0161-6420(92)31934-7
22. Lundstrom M, Stenevi U, Thorburn W. Gender and cataract surgery in Sweden 1992–1997. A retrospective observational study based on the Swedish National Cataract Register. *Acta Ophthalmol Scand* (1999) 77(2):204–8. doi:10.1034/j.1600-0420.1999.770218.x
23. Lundstorm M, Stenevi U, Thorburn W. The Swedish National Cataract Register: a nine-year review. *Acta Ophthalmol Scand* (2002) 80(3):248–57. doi:10.1034/j.1600-0420.2002.800304.x
24. Freeman EE, Munoz B, Schein OD, West SK. Hormone replacement. *Arch Ophthalmol* (2001) 119(11):1687–92. doi:10.1001/archopht.119.11.1687
25. Klein BE. Lens opacities in women in Beaver Dam, Wisconsin: is there evidence of an effect of sex hormones. *Trans Am Ophthalmol Soc* (1993) 91:517–44.
26. Klein BE, Klein R, Ritter LL. Is there evidence of an estrogen effect on age-related lens opacities? The Beaver Dam Eye study. *Arch Ophthalmol* (1994) 112(1):85–91. doi:10.1001/archopht.1994.01090130095025
27. Younan C, Mitchell P, Cummin RG, Panchapakesan J, Rochtchina E, Hales AM. Hormone replacement therapy, reproductive factors, and the incidence of cataract and cataract surgery: the Blue Mountains Eye Study. *Am J Epidemiol* (2002) 155(11):997–1006. doi:10.1093/aje/155.11.997
28. Beebe DC, Holekamp NM, Shui YB. Oxidative damage and the prevention of age-related cataracts. *Ophthalmic Res* (2010) 44(3):155–65. doi:10.1159/000316481
29. Zettemberg M, Celojevic D. Gender and cataract – the role of estrogen. *Curr Eye Res* (2015) 40(2):176–90. doi:10.3109/02713683.2014.898774
30. Buch H, Nielsen NV, Vinding T, Jensen GB, Prause JU, la Cour M. 14-years incidence, progression and visual morbidity of age-related maculopathy: the Copenhagen City Eye study. *Ophthalmology* (2005) 112(5):787–98. doi:10.1016/j.ophtha.2004.11.040
31. Laitinen A, Laatikainen L, Harkanen T, Koskinen S, Reunanen A, Aromaa A. Prevalence of major eye diseases and causes of visual impairment in the adult Finnish population: a nationwide population-based survey. *Acta Ophthalmol* (2010) 88(4):463–71. doi:10.1111/j.1755-3768.2009.01566.x
32. Chakravarthy U, Wong TY, Fletcher A, Piault E, Evans C, Zlateva G, et al. Clinical risk factors for age-related macular degeneration: a systematic review and meta-analysis. *BMC Ophthalmol* (2010) 10:31. doi:10.1186/1471-2415-10-31
33. Age-Related Eye Disease Study Research Group. Risk factors associated with age-related macular degeneration. A case control study in the age-related eye disease study: age-related eye disease study report number 3. *Ophthalmology* (2000) 107(12):2224–32. doi:10.1016/S0161-6420(00)00409-7
34. Rudnicka AR, Jarrar Z, Wormald R, Cook DG, Fletcher A, Owen CG. Age and gender variations in age-related macular degeneration prevalence in populations of European ancestry: a meta-analysis. *Ophthalmology* (2012) 119(3):571–80. doi:10.1016/j.ophtha.2011.09.027
35. Smith W, Mitchell P, Wang JJ. Gender, oestrogen, hormone replacement and age-related macular degeneration: results from the Blue Mountains Eye study. *Aust N Z J Ophthalmol* (1997) 25(Suppl 1):S13–5. doi:10.1111/j.1442-9071.1997.tb01745.x
36. Snow KK, Cote J, Yang W, Davis NJ, Seddon JM. Association between reproductive and hormonal factors and age-related maculopathy in post-menopausal women. *Am J Ophthalmol* (2002) 134(6):842–8. doi:10.1016/S0002-9394(02)01755-5
37. Blasiak J, Petrovski G, Vereb Z, Facsko A, Kaarniranta K. Oxidative stress, hypoxia and autophagy in the neovascular process of age macular degeneration. *Biomed Res Int* (2014) 2014:768026. doi:10.1155/2014/768026
38. Kaarniranta K, Machalinska A, Vereb Z, Salminen A, Petrovski G, Kauppinen A. Estrogen signalling in the pathogenesis of age-related macular degeneration. *Curr Eye Res* (2015) 40(2):226–33. doi:10.3109/02713683.2014.925933
39. Quigley HA, Broman AT. The number of people with glaucoma worldwide in 2010 and 2020. *Br J Ophthalmol* (2006) 90(3):262–7. doi:10.1136/bjo.2005.081224
40. Rudnicka AR, Mt-Isa S, Owen CG, Cook DG, Ashby D. Variation in primary open-angle glaucoma prevalence by age, gender and race: a Bayesian meta-analysis. *Invest Ophthalmol Vis Sci* (2006) 47(10):4254–61. doi:10.1167/iovs.06-0299
41. Erie JC, Hodge DO, Gray DT. The incidence of primary angle-closure glaucoma in Olmsted County, Minnesota. *Arch Ophthalmol* (1997) 115(2):177–81. doi:10.1001/archopht.1997.01100150179005
42. Ng WS, Ang GS, Azuara-Blanco A. Primary angle closure glaucoma: a descriptive study in Scottish Caucasian. *Clin Exp Ophthalmol* (2008) 36(9):847–51. doi:10.1111/j.1442-9071.2008.01904.x
43. Tham YC, Li X, Wong TY, Quigley HA, Aung T, Cheng CY. Global prevalence of glaucoma and projections of glaucoma burden through 2040: a systematic review and meta-analysis. *Ophthalmology* (2014) 121(11):2081–90. doi:10.1016/j.ophtha.2014.05.013
44. Wandell PE, Carlsson AC. Time trends and gender differences in incidence and prevalence of type 1 diabetes in Sweden. *Curr Diabetes Rev* (2013) 9(4):342–9. doi:10.2174/15733998113099990064

45. Chaturvedi N, Sjoelie AK, Porta M, Aldington SJ, Fuller JH, Songini M, et al. Markers of insulin resistance are strong risk factors for retinopathy incidence in type 1 diabetes. *Diabetes Care* (2001) 24(2):284–9. doi:10.2337/diacare.24.2.284
46. Klein R, Knudtson MD, Lee KE, Gangnon R, Klein BE. The Wisconsin epidemiologic study of diabetic retinopathy XXIII: the twenty-five-years incidence of macular edema in persons with type 1 diabetes. *Ophthalmology* (2009) 116(3):497–503. doi:10.1016/j.ophtha.2008.10.016
47. Kostev K, Rathmann W. Diabetic retinopathy at diagnosis of type 2 diabetes in the UK: a database analysis. *Diabetologia* (2013) 56(1):109–11. doi:10.1007/s00125-012-2742-7
48. Looker HC, Nyangoma SO, Cromie D, Olson JA, Leese GP, Black J, et al. Diabetic retinopathy at diagnosis of type 2 diabetes in Scotland. *Diabetologia* (2012) 55(9):2335–42. doi:10.1007/s00125-012-2596-z
49. Ozawa GY, Bearse MA Jr, Adams AJ. Male-female differences in diabetic retinopathy? *Curr Eye Res* (2015) 40(2):234–46. doi:10.3109/02713683.2014.958500
50. Nirmalan PK, Katz J, Robin AL, Ramakrishnan R, Krishnadas R, Thulasiraj RD, et al. Female reproductive factors and eye disease in a rural south Indian population: the Aravind comprehensive eye survey. *Invest Ophthalmol Vis Sci* (2004) 45(12):4273–6. doi:10.1167/iovs.04-0285
51. Nixon E, Simpkins JW. Neuroprotective effects of nonfeminizing estrogen in retinal photoreceptor neurons. *Invest Ophthalmol Vis Sci* (2012) 53(8):4739–47. doi:10.1167/iovs.12-9517
52. Murphy TH, Miyamoto M, Sastre A, Schnaar RL, Coyle JT. Glutamate toxicity in a neuronal cell line involves inhibition of cystine transport leading to oxidative stress. *Neuron* (1989) 2(6):1547–58. doi:10.1016/0896-6273(89)90043-3
53. Bailey TA, Kanuga N, Romero IA, Greenwood J, Luthert PJ, Cheetham ME. Oxidative stress affects the junctional integrity of retinal pigment epithelial cells. *Invest Ophthalmol Vis Sci* (2004) 45(2):675–84. doi:10.1167/iovs.03-0351
54. Usui S, Oveson BC, Lee SY, Jo YJ, Yoshida T, Miki A, et al. NADPH oxidase plays a central role in cone cell death in retinitis pigmentosa. *J Neurochem* (2009) 110(3):1028–37. doi:10.1111/j.1471-4159.2009.06195.x
55. Mo MS, Li HB, Wang BY, Wang SL, Zhu ZL, Yu XR. PI3K/Akt and NF-kB activation following intravitreal administration of 17b-estradiol: neuroprotection of the rat retina from light-induced apoptosis. *Neuroscience* (2013) 228:1–12. doi:10.1016/j.neuroscience.2012.10.002
56. Kaja S, Yang SH, Wei J, Fujitani K, Liu R, Brun-Zinkernagel A, et al. Estrogen protects the inner retina from apoptosis and ischemia-induced loss of Vesl-1L/Homer 1c immunoreactive synaptic connections. *Invest Ophthalmol Vis Sci* (2003) 44(7):3155–62. doi:10.1167/iovs.02-1204
57. Moosmann B, Behl C. The antioxidant neuroprotective effects of estrogen and phenolic compounds are independent from their estrogenic proprieties. *Proc Natl Acad Sci U S A* (1999) 96(16):8867–72. doi:10.1073/pnas.96.16.8867
58. Nakazawa T, Takakashia H, Shimurac M. Estrogen has a neuroprotective effect on axotomized RGCs through ERK signal transduction pathway. *Brain Res* (2006) 1093(1):141–9. doi:10.1016/j.brainres.2006.03.084
59. Lai P, Li T, Yang J, Xie C, Zhu X, Xie H, et al. Upregulation of stromal cell-derived factor1 (SDF-1) expression in microvasculature endothelial cells in retina ischemia-reperfusion injury. *Graefes Arch Clin Exp Ophthalmol* (2008) 246(12):1707–13. doi:10.1371/journal.pone.0114564
60. Wang Y, Li X, Wang J, Shi H, Bi W, Hou W, et al. 17b-estradiol mediates upregulation of stromal cell-derived factor-1 in the retina through activation of estrogen receptor in an ischemia-reperfusion injury model. *Graefes Arch Clin Exp Ophthalmol* (2015) 253(1):17–23. doi:10.1007/s00417-014-2657-8
61. Kaldi I, Berta A. Progesterone administration fails to protect albino make rats against photostress-induced retinal degeneration. *Eur J Ophthalmol* (2004) 14(4):306–14. doi:10.1177/112067210401400405
62. Na KS, Jee DH, Han K, Park YG, Kim MS, Kim EC. The ocular benefits of estrogen replacement therapy: a population-based study in postmenopausal Korean women. *PLoS One* (2014) 9(9):e106473. doi:10.1371/journal.pone.0106473
63. Schmidl D, Schmetterer L, Garhofer G, Popa-Cherecheanu A. Gender differences in ocular blood flow. *Curr Eye Res* (2015) 40(2):201–12. doi:10.3109/02713683.2014.906625
64. Burgansky-Eliash Z, Barash H, Nelson D, Grinvald A, Sorkin A, Loewenstein A, et al. Retinal blood flow velocity in patient with age-related macular degeneration. *Curr Eye Res* (2014) 39(3):304–11. doi:10.3109/02713683.2013.840384
65. Grunwald JE, Metelitsina TI, Dupont JC, Ying GS, Maguire MG. Reduced foveolar choroidal blood flow in eyes with increasing AMD severity. *Invest Ophthalmol Vis Sci* (2005) 46(3):1033–8. doi:10.1167/iovs.04-1050
66. Friedman E, Krupsky S, Lane AM, Oak SS, Friedman ES, Egan K, et al. Ocular blood flow velocity in age-related macular degeneration. *Ophthalmology* (1995) 102(4):640–6. doi:10.1016/S0161-6420(95)30974-8
67. Fuchsjager-Mayrl G, Wally B, Georgopoulos M, Rainer G, Kircher K, Buehl W, et al. Ocular blood flow and systemic blood pressure in patients with primary open-angle glaucoma and ocular hypertension. *Invest Ophthalmol Vis Sci* (2004) 45(3):834–9. doi:10.1167/iovs.03-0461
68. Meng N, Zhang P, Huang H, Ma J, Zhang Y, Li H, et al. Color Doppler imaging analysis of retrobulbar blood flow velocities in primary open-angle glaucomatous eyes: a meta-analysis. *PLoS One* (2013) 8(5):e62723. doi:10.1371/journal.pone.0062723
69. Pemp B, Polska E, Garhofer G, Baverle-Eder M, Kautzky-Willer A, Schmetterer L. Retinal blood flow in type 1 diabetic patients with no or mild diabetic retinopathy during euglycemic clamp. *Diabetes Care* (2010) 33(9):2038–42. doi:10.2337/dc10-0502
70. Patel V, Rassam S, Newsom R, Wiek J, Kohner E. Retinal blood flow in diabetic retinopathy. *BMJ* (1992) 305(6855):678–83. doi:10.1136/bmj.305.6855.678
71. Gracner T. Ocular blood flow velocity determined by color Doppler imaging in diabetic retinopathy. *Ophthalmologica* (2004) 218(4):237–42. doi:10.1159/000078613
72. Toker E, Yenice O, Akpinar I, Aribal E, Kazokoglu H. The influence of sex hormones on ocular blood flow in women. *Acta Ophthalmol Scand* (2003) 81(6):617–24. doi:10.1111/j.1395-3907.2003.00160.x
73. Faria AF, de Souza MA, Geber S. Vascular resistance of central retinal artery is reduced in postmenopausal women after use of estrogen. *Menopause* (2011) 18(8):869–72. doi:10.1097/gme.0b013e31820cc60c
74. Dechenes MC, Descovic D, Moreau M, Granger L, Kuchel GA, Mikkola TS, et al. Postmenopausal hormone therapy increases retinal blood flow and protects the retinal nerve fiber layer. *Invest Ophthalmol Vis Sci* (2010) 51(5):2587–600. doi:10.1167/iovs.09-3710
75. Souza AM, Souza BM, Geber S. Progesterone increases resistance of ophthalmic and central retinal arteries in climacteric women. *Climacteric* (2013) 16(2):284–7. doi:10.3109/13697137.2012.720620
76. Viana LC, Faria M, Petternsen H, Sampaio M, Geber S. Menstrual phase-related differences in the pulsatility index on the central retinal artery suggest an oestrogen vasodilatation effect that antagonizes with progesterone. *Arch Gynecol Obstet* (2011) 283(3):569–73. doi:10.1007/s00404-010-1403-7
77. Harris-Yitzhak M, Harris A, Ben-Refael Z, Zarfati D, Garzozi HJ, Martin BJ. Estrogen-replacement therapy: effects on retrobulbar hemodynamics. *Am J Ophthalmol* (2000) 129(5):623–8. doi:10.1016/S0002-9394(99)00468-7
78. Jones TH. Testosterone deficiency: a risk factor for cardiovascular disease? *Trends Endocrinol Metab* (2010) 21(8):496–503. doi:10.1016/j.tem.2010.03.002
79. Toker E, Yenice O, Temel A. Influence of serum levels of sex hormones on intraocular pressure in menopausal women. *J Glaucoma* (2003) 12(5):436–40. doi:10.1097/00061198-200310000-00007
80. Malan NT, Smith W, von Kanel R, Hamer M, Schutte AE, Malan L. Low serum testosterone and increased diastolic ocular perfusion pressure: a risk for retinal microvasculature. *Vasa* (2015) 44(6):435–43. doi:10.1024/0301-1526/a000466
81. Kaarniranta K, Sinha D, Blasiak J, Kauppinen A, Vereb Z, Salminen A, et al. Autophagy and heterophagy dysregulation leads to retinal pigment epithelium dysfunction and development of age-related macular degeneration. *Autophagy* (2013) 9(7):973–84. doi:10.4161/auto.24546
82. Eisner A, Stoumbos VD, Klein ML, Fleming SA. Relations between fundus appearance and function. Eyes whose fellow eye has exudative age-related macular degeneration. *Invest Ophthalmol Vis Sci* (1991) 32(1):8–20.
83. Eisner A, Klein ML, Zilis JD, Watkins MD. Visual function and the subsequence development of exudative age-related macular degeneration. *Invest Ophthalmol Vis Sci* (1992) 33(11):3091–102.
84. Owsley C, McGwin G Jr, Jackson GR, Kallies K, Clark M. Cone- and rod-mediated dark adaptation impairment in age-related maculopathy. *Ophthalmology* (2007) 114(9):1728–35. doi:10.1016/j.ophtha.2006.12.023
85. Dimitrov PN, Robman LD, Varsamidis M, Aung KZ, Makeyeva G, Busija L, et al. Relationship between clinical macular changes and retinal function in age-related macular degeneration. *Invest Ophthalmol Vis Sci* (2012) 53(9):5213–20. doi:10.1167/iovs.11-8958

86. Bhutto I, Lutty G. Understanding age-related macular degeneration (AMD): relationships between the photoreceptor/ retinal pigment epithelium/Bruch's membrane/choriocapillaris complex. *Mol Aspects Med* (2012) 33(4):295–317. doi:10.1016/j.mam.2012.04.005
87. Evans JR. Risk factors for age-related macular degeneration. *Prog Retin Eye Res* (2001) 20(2):227–53. doi:10.1016/S1350-9462(00)00023-9
88. Mitchell P, Wang JJ, Foran S, Smith W. Five-year incidence of age-related maculopathy lesions: the Blue Mountains Eye study. *Ophthalmology* (2002) 109(6):1092–7. doi:10.1016/S0161-6420(02)01055-2
89. Fraser-Bell S, Wu J, Klein R, Azen SP, Varma R. Smoking, alcohol intake, estrogen use, and age-related macular degeneration in Latinos: the Los Angeles Latino Eye study. *Am J Ophthalmol* (2006) 141(1):79–87. doi:10.1016/j.ajo.2005.08.024
90. Haan MN, Klein R, Klein BE, Deng Y, Blythe LK, Seddon JM, et al. Hormone therapy and age-related macular degeneration – the women's health initiative sight exam study. *Arch Ophthalmol* (2006) 124(7):988–92. doi:10.1001/archopht.124.7.988
91. Feskanich D, Cho E, Schaumberg DA, Colditz GA, Hankinson SE. Menopausal and reproductive factors and risk of age-related macular degeneration. *Arch Ophthalmol* (2008) 126(4):519–24. doi:10.1001/archopht.126.4.519
92. Velez Edwards DE, Gallins P, Polk M, Ayala-Haedo G, Schwartz SG, Kovach JL, et al. Inverse association of female hormone replacement therapy with age-related macular degeneration and interaction with ARMS2 polymorphisms. *Invest Ophthalmol Vis Sci* (2010) 51(4):1873–9. doi:10.1167/iovs.09-4000
93. Freeman EE, Munoz B, Bressler SB, West SK. Hormone replacement therapy, reproductive factors and age-related macular degeneration: the Salisbury Eye Evaluation Project. *Ophthalmic Epidemiol* (2005) 12(1):37–45. doi:10.1080/09286580490907779
94. Virgerling JR, Dielemans I, Witteman JC, Hofman A, Grobbee DE, de Jong PT. Macular degeneration and early menopause: a case-control study. *BMJ* (1995) 310(6994):1570–1. doi:10.1136/bmj.310.6994.1570
95. The Royal College of Ophthalmologists. *Age-Related Macular Degeneration Guidelines for Management*. (2013).
96. Defay R, Pinchinat S, Lumbroso S, Sutan C, Delcourt C; Pola Study Group. Sex steroid and age-related macular degeneration in older French women: the POLA study. *Ann Epidemiol* (2004) 14(3):202–8. doi:10.1016/S1047-2797(03)00130-3
97. Abramov Y, Borik S, Yahalom C, Fatum M, Avgil G, Brzezinski A, et al. The effect of the hormone therapy on the risk for age-related maculopathy in postmenopausal women. *Menopause* (2004) 11(1):62–8. doi:10.1097/01.GME.0000074701.19603.11
98. Klein BE, Klein R, Lee KE. Reproductive exposures, incident age-related cataracts, and age-related maculopathy in women: the Beaver Dam Eye study. *Am J Ophthalmol* (2000) 130(3):322–6. doi:10.1016/S0002-9394(00)00474-8
99. Tomany SC, Wang JJ, Van Leeuwen R, Klein R, Mitchell P, Virgerling JR, et al. Risk factors for incident age-related macular degeneration: pooled findings from 3 continents. *Ophthalmology* (2004) 111(7):1280–7. doi:10.1016/j.ophtha.2003.11.010
100. Chakravarthy U, Augood C, Bentham GC, De Jong PT, Rahu M, Seland J, et al. Cigarette smoking and age-related macular degeneration in the EUREYE study. *Ophthalmology* (2007) 114(6):1157–63. doi:10.1016/j.ophtha.2006.09.022
101. Wang JJ, Klein R, Smith W, Klein BE, Tomany S, Mitchell P. Cataract surgery and the 5-years incidence of late-stage age-related maculopathy: pooled findings from the Beaver Dam and Blue Mountains eye studies. *Ophthalmology* (2003) 110(10):1960–7. doi:10.1016/S0161-6420(03)00816-9
102. Cugati S, Mitchell P, Rochtchina E, Tan AG, Smith W, Wang JJ. Cataract surgery and the 10-years incidence of age-related maculopathy: the Blue Mountains Eye study. *Ophthalmology* (2006) 113(11):2020–5. doi:10.1016/j.ophtha.2006.05.047
103. Klein R, Klein BE, Wong TY, Tomany SC, Cruickshanks KJ. The association of cataract and cataract surgery with the long-term incidence of age-related maculopathy: the Beaver Dam Eye study. *Arch Ophthalmol* (2002) 120(11):1551–8. doi:10.1001/archopht.120.11.1551
104. Hyman LG, Lilienfeld AM, Ferris FL III, Fine SL. Senile macular degeneration: a case-control study. *Am J Epidemiol* (1983) 118(2):213–27. doi:10.1093/oxfordjournals.aje.a113629
105. Klaver CC, Wolfs RC, Assink JJ, van Dujin CM, Hofman A, De Jong PT. Genetic risk of age-related maculopathy. Population-based familial aggregation study. *Arch Ophthalmol* (1998) 116(12):1646–51. doi:10.1001/archopht.116.12.1646
106. Tan JS, Mitchell P, Smith W, Wang JJ. Cardiovascular risk factors and the long-term incidence of the age-related macular degeneration: the Blue Mountains Eye study. *Ophthalmology* (2007) 114(6):1143–50. doi:10.1016/j.ophtha.2006.09.033
107. Iida T, Kishi S, Hagimura N, Shimizu K. Persistent and bilateral choroidal vascular abnormalities in central serous chorioretinopathy. *Retina* (1999) 19(6):508–12. doi:10.1097/00006982-199919060-00005
108. Prunte C, Flammer J. Choroidal capillary and venous congestion in central serous chorioretinopathy. *Am J Ophthalmol* (1996) 121(1):26–34. doi:10.1016/S0002-9394(14)70531-8
109. Liew G, Quin G, Gillies M, Fraser-Bell S. Central serous chorioretinopathy: a review of epidemiology and pathophysiology. *Clin Exp Ophthalmol* (2013) 41(2):201–14. doi:10.1111/j.1442-9071.2012.02848.x
110. Ross A, Ross AH, Mohamed Q. Review and update of central serous chorioretinopathy. *Curr Opin Ophthalmol* (2011) 22(3):166–73. doi:10.1097/ICU.0b013e3283459826
111. Grieshaber MC, Staub JJ, Flammer J. The potential role of testosterone in central serous chorioretinopathy. *Br J Ophthalmol* (2007) 91(1):118–9. doi:10.1136/bjo.2006.098277
112. Haimovici R, Rumelt S, Melby J. Endocrine abnormalities in patients with central serous chorioretinopathy. *Ophthalmology* (2003) 110(4):698–703. doi:10.1016/S0161-6420(02)01975-9
113. Zakir SM, Shukla M, Simi ZUR, Ahmad J, Sajid M. Serum cortisol and testosterone levels in idiopathic central serous chorioretinopathy. *Indian J Ophthalmol* (2009) 57(6):419–22. doi:10.4103/0301-4738.57143
114. Kapetanios AD, Donati G, Bouzas E, Mastorakos G, Pournaras CJ. Serous central chorioretinopathy and endogenous hypercortisolemia. *Klin Monbl Augenheilkd* (1998) 212(5):343–4. doi:10.1055/s-2008-1034901
115. Ahad AM, Chua CN, Evans NM. Central serous chorioretinis associated with testosterone therapy. *Eye (Lond)* (2006) 20(4):503–5. doi:10.1038/sj.eye.6701905
116. Nudleman E, Witmer MT, Kiss S, Wlliams GA, Wolfe JD. Central serous chorioretinopathy in patients receiving exogenous testosterone therapy. *Retina* (2014) 34(10):2128–32. doi:10.1097/IAE.0000000000000198
117. Forooghian F, Meleth AD, Cukras C, Chew EY, Wong WT, Meyerle CB. Finasteride for chronic central serous chorioretinopathy. *Retina* (2011) 31(4):766–71. doi:10.1097/IAE.0b013e3181f04a35
118. Tufan HA, Gencer B, Comez AT. Serum cortisol and testosterone levels in chronic central serous chorioretinopathy. *Graefes Arch Clin Exp Ophthalmol* (2013) 251(3):677–80. doi:10.1007/s00417-012-2075-8
119. La Cour M, Friis J. Macular holes: classification, epidemiology, natural history and treatment. *Acta Ophthalmol Scand* (2002) 80(6):579–87. doi:10.1034/j.1600-0420.2002.800605.x
120. Frangieh GT, Green WR, Engel HM. A histopathologic study of macular cyst and holes. *Retina* (1981) 1(4):311–36. doi:10.1097/00006982-198101040-00008
121. Morgan CM, Scha UH. Idiopathic macular holes. *Am J Ophthalmol* (1985) 99(4):437–44. doi:10.1016/0002-9394(85)90011-X
122. Gass JD. Idiopathic senile macular holes: its early stages and pathogenesis. *Arch Ophthalmol* (1988) 106(5):629–39. doi:10.1001/archopht.1988.01060130683026
123. Wylegała E, Woyna-Orlewicz A, Piłat J, Teper S, Ludyga A. Traction maculopathies – pathogenesis and diagnostics. *Klin Oczna* (2006) 108(10–12): 457–63.
124. McDonnell PJ, Fine SL, Hillis AI. Clinical features of idiopathic macular cysts and holes. *Am J Ophthalmol* (1982) 93(6):777–86. doi:10.1016/0002-9394(82)90474-3
125. James M, Feman SS. Macular holes. *Albrecht Von Graefes Arch Klin Exp Ophthalmol* (1980) 215(1):59–63. doi:10.1007/BF00413397
126. Gray RH, Gregor ZJ, Marsh M. Oestrogen and macular holes: a postal questionnaire. *Eye (Lond)* (1994) 8(3):368–9. doi:10.1038/eye.1994.83
127. McCannel CA, Ensminger JL, Diehl NN, Hodge DN. Population based incidence of macular holes. *Ophthalmology* (2009) 116(7):1366–9. doi:10.1016/j.ophtha.2009.01.052
128. Evans JR, Schwartz SD, McHugh JDA, Thamby-Rajah Y, Hodgson SA, Wormald RPL, et al. Systemic risk factors for idiopathic macular holes: a case-control study. *Eye (Lond)* (1998) 12(2):256–9. doi:10.1038/eye.1998.60
129. Chung SE, Kim SW, Chung HW, Kang SW. Estrogen antagonist and development of macular hole. *Korean J Ophthalmol* (2010) 24(5):306–9. doi:10.3341/kjo.2010.24.5.306

130. Bourla DH, Sarraf D, Schwartz SD. Peripheral retinopathy and maculopathy in high-dose tamoxifen therapy. *Am J Ophthalmol* (2007) 144(1):126–8. doi:10.1016/j.ajo.2007.03.023
131. Inokuchi N, Ikeda T, Nakamura K, Morishita S, Fukumoto M, Kida T, et al. Vitreous estrogen levels in patients with an idiopathic macular hole. *Clin Ophthalmol* (2015) 9:549–52. doi:10.2147/OPTH.S80754
132. Usui S, Komeima K, Lee SY, Jo YJ, Ueno S, Rogers BS, et al. Increased expression of catalase and superoxide dismutase 2 reduce con cell death in retinitis pigmentosa. *Mol Ther* (2009) 17(5):778–86. doi:10.1038/mt.2009.47
133. Kennan A, Aherne A, Humpries P. Light in retinitis pigmentosa. *Trends Genet* (2005) 21(2):103–10. doi:10.1016/j.tig.2004.12.001
134. Doonan F, O'Driscoll C, Kenna P, Cotter TG. Enhancing survival of photoreceptor cells in vivo using the synthetic progestin norgestrel. *J Neurochem* (2011) 118(5):915–27. doi:10.1111/j.1471-4159.2011.07354.x
135. Doonan F, Cotter TG. Norgestrel may be a potential therapy for retinal degenerations. *Expert Opin Investig Drugs* (2012) 21(5):579–81. doi:10.1517/13543784.2012.667400
136. Sanchez-Vallejo V, Benlloch-Navarro S, Lopez-Pedrajas R, Romero FJ, Miranda M. Neuroprotective actions of progesterone in an in vivo model of retinitis pigmentosa. *Pharmacol Res* (2015) 99:276–88. doi:10.1016/j.phrs.2015.06.019
137. Singh M, Su C. Progesterone and neuroprotection. *Horm Behav* (2013) 63(2):284–90. doi:10.1016/j.yhbeh.2012.06.003
138. Sivaprasad S, Gupta B, Crosby-Nwaobi R, Evans J. Prevalence of diabetic retinopathy in various ethnic groups: a worldwide perspective. *Surv Ophthalmol* (2012) 57(4):347–70. doi:10.1016/j.survophthal.2012.01.004
139. Yau JW, Rogers SL, Kawasaki R, Lamoureux EL, Kowalski JW, Bek T, et al. Global prevalence and major risk factors of diabetic retinopathy. *Diabetes Care* (2012) 35(3):556–64. doi:10.2337/dc11-1909
140. Romero P, Baget M, Mendez I, Fernandez J, Slavat M, Martinez I. Diabetic macular edema and its relationship to renal microangiopathy: a sample of type 1 diabetes mellitus patients in a 15-year follow up study. *J Diabetes Complications* (2007) 21(3):172–80. doi:10.1016/j.jdiacomp.2006.07.008
141. Grisby JG, Allen DM, Culbert RB, Escobedo G, Parvathaneni K, Betts BS, et al. The role of sex hormones in diabetic retinopathy. *Diabetic Retinopathy* (2012) 17:331–56. doi:10.5772/30643
142. Briganrdello E, Beltramo E, Molinatti PA, Aragno M, Gatto V, Tamagno E, et al. Dehydroepiandrosterone protects bovine retinal capillary pericytes against glucose toxicity. *J Endocrinol* (1998) 158(1):21–6. doi:10.1677/joe.0.1580021
143. Cunha-Vaz J. Diabetic retinopathy. Human and experimental studies. *Trans Ophthalmol Soc U K* (1972) 92:111–24.
144. Brownlee M. Biochemistry and molecular cell biology of diabetic complications. *Nature* (2001) 414(6865):813–20. doi:10.1038/414813a
145. Giddabasappa A, Bauler M, Yepuru M, Chaum E, Dalton JT, Eswaraka J. 17-β estradiol protects ARPE-19 cells from oxidative stress through estrogen receptor-β. *Invest Ophthalmol Vis Sci* (2010) 51(10):5278–87. doi:10.1167/iovs.10-5316
146. Espinosa-Heidmann DG, Marin-Castano ME, Pereira-Simon S, Hernandez EP, Elliot S, Cousins SW. Gender and estrogen supplementation increases severity of experimental choroidal neovascularization. *Exp Eye Res* (2005) 80(3):413–23. doi:10.1016/j.exer.2004.10.008
147. Grigsby JG, Parvathaneni K, Almaza MA, Botello AM, Mondragon AA, Allen DM, et al. Effects of tamoxifen versus raloxifene on retinal capillary endothelial cell proliferation. *J Ocul Pharmacol Ther* (2011) 27(3):225–33. doi:10.1089/jop.2010.0171
148. Ozawa GY, Bearse MA, Bronson-Castain KW, Harrison WW, Schneck ME, Barez S, et al. Neurodegenerative difference in the retinas of male and female patients with type 2 diabetes. *Invest Ophthalmol Vis Sci* (2012) 53(6):3040–6. doi:10.1167/iovs.11-8226
149. Klein BEK, Klein R, Moss SE. Exogenous estrogen exposures and changes in diabetic retinopathy: the Wisconsin epidemiologic study of diabetic retinopathy. *Diabetes Care* (1999) 22(12):1984–7. doi:10.2337/diacare.22.12.1984
150. Schmidt KG, Bergert H, Funk RH. Neurodegenerative disease of the retina and potential for protection and recovery. *Curr Neuropharmacol* (2008) 6(2):164–78. doi:10.2174/157015908784533851
151. Yucel YH, Zhang Q, Weinreb RN, Kaufman PL, Gupta N. Effects of retinal ganglion cell loss on magno-, parvo-, koniocellular pathways in the lateral geniculate nucleus and visual cortex in glaucoma. *Prog Retin Eye Res* (2003) 22(4):465–81. doi:10.1016/S1350-9462(03)00026-0
152. Dewundara SS, Wiggs JL, Sullivan DA, Pasquale LR. Is estrogen a therapeutic target for glaucoma? *Semin Ophthalmol* (2016) 31(1–2):140–6. doi:10.3109/08820538.2015.1114845
153. Lee AJ, Mitchell P, Rochtchina E, Healey PR; Blue Mountains Eye Study. Female reproductive factors and open angle glaucoma: the Blue Mountains Eye study. *Br J Ophthalmol* (2003) 87(11):1324–8. doi:10.1136/bjo.87.11.1324
154. Pasquale LR, Kang JH. Female reproductive factors and primary open-angle glaucoma in Nurses' Health study. *Eye (Lond)* (2011) 25(5):633–41. doi:10.1038/eye.2011.34
155. Vajaranant S, Grossardt BR, Maki PM, Pasquale LR, Sit AJ, Shuster LT, et al. Risk of glaucoma after early bilateral oophorectomy. *Menopause* (2014) 21(4):391–8. doi:10.1097/GME.0b013e31829fd081
156. Hulsman CA, Westendorp IC, Ramrattan RS, Wolfs RC, Witteman JC, Vingerling JR, et al. Is open-angle glaucoma associated with early menopause? The Rotterdam study. *Am J Epidemiol* (2001) 154(2):138–44. doi:10.1093/aje/154.2.138
157. Qureshi IA, Xi XR, Wu XD. Intraocular pressure trends in pregnancy and in the third trimester hypertensive patients. *Acta Obstet Gynecol Scand* (1996) 75(9):816–9. doi:10.3109/00016349609054709
158. Qureshi IA. Intraocular pressure: association with menstrual cycle, pregnancy and menopause in apparently healthy women. *Chin J Physiol* (1995) 38(4):229–34.
159. Altinta SO, Caglar Y, Yuksel N, Demirci A, Karabas L. The effects of menopause and hormone replacement therapy on quality and quantity of tear, intraocular pressure and blood flow. *Ophthalmologica* (2004) 218(2):120–9. doi:10.1159/000076148
160. Sator MO, Joura EA, Frigo P, Kurz C, Metka M, Hommer A, et al. Hormone replacement therapy and intraocular pressure. *Maturitas* (1997) 28(1):55–8. doi:10.1016/S0378-5122(97)00060-1
161. Pasquale LR, Loomis SJ, Weiner RN, Kang JH, Yaspan BL, Bailey JC, et al. Estrogen pathway polymorphisms in relation to primary open angle glaucoma: an analysis accounting for gender from the United States. *Mol Vis* (2013) 19:1471–81.
162. Furchgott RF, Zawaszki JV. The obligatory role of endothelial cells in the relaxation of arterial smooth muscle by acetylcholine. *Nature* (1980) 288(5789):373–6. doi:10.1038/288373a0
163. Vajaranant TS, Pasquae LR. Estrogen deficiency accelerates aging of the optic nerve. *Menopause* (2012) 19(8):942–7. doi:10.1097/gme.0b013e3182443137
164. Weinreb RN, Khaw PT. Primary open-angle glaucoma. *Lancet* (2004) 363(9422):1711–20. doi:10.1016/S0140-6736(04)16257-0
165. Akar ME, Taskin O, Yucel I, Akar Y. The effect of the menstrual cycle on optic nerve had analysis in healthy women. *Acta Ophthalmol Scand* (2004) 82(6):741–5. doi:10.1111/j.1600-0420.2004.00351.x
166. Eisner A, Demirel S. Variability in short-wavelength automated perimetry among peri- or postmenopausal women: a dependence on phyto-oestrogen consumption? *Acta Ophthalmol* (2011) 89(3):e217–24. doi:10.1111/j.1755-3768.2009.01799.x

6

Sex Differences in Medium Spiny Neuron Excitability and Glutamatergic Synaptic Input: Heterogeneity Across Striatal Regions and Evidence for Estradiol-Dependent Sexual Differentiation

*Jinyan Cao[1,2], Jaime A. Willett[1,2,3], David M. Dorris[1] and John Meitzen[1,2,4,5]**

[1] Department of Biological Sciences, North Carolina State University, Raleigh, NC, United States, [2] W.M. Keck Center for Behavioral Biology, North Carolina State University, Raleigh, NC, United States, [3] Graduate Program in Physiology, North Carolina State University, Raleigh, NC, United States, [4] Center for Human Health and the Environment, North Carolina State University, Raleigh, NC, United States, [5] Comparative Medicine Institute, North Carolina State University, Raleigh, NC, United States

***Correspondence:**
John Meitzen
jemeitze@ncsu.edu

Steroid sex hormones and biological sex influence how the brain regulates motivated behavior, reward, and sensorimotor function in both normal and pathological contexts. Investigations into the underlying neural mechanisms have targeted the striatal brain regions, including the caudate–putamen, nucleus accumbens core (AcbC), and shell. These brain regions are of particular interest to neuroendocrinologists given that they express membrane-associated but not nuclear estrogen receptors, and also the well-established role of the sex steroid hormone 17β-estradiol (estradiol) in modulating striatal dopamine systems. Indeed, output neurons of the striatum, the medium spiny neurons (MSNs), exhibit estradiol sensitivity and sex differences in electrophysiological properties. Here, we review sex differences in rat MSN glutamatergic synaptic input and intrinsic excitability across striatal regions, including evidence for estradiol-mediated sexual differentiation in the nucleus AcbC. In prepubertal animals, female MSNs in the caudate–putamen exhibit a greater intrinsic excitability relative to male MSNs, but no sex differences are detected in excitatory synaptic input. Alternatively, female MSNs in the nucleus AcbC exhibit increased excitatory synaptic input relative to male MSNs, but no sex differences in intrinsic excitability were detected. Increased excitatory synaptic input onto female MSNs in the nucleus AcbC is abolished after masculinizing estradiol or testosterone exposure during the neonatal critical period. No sex differences are detected in MSNs in prepubertal nucleus accumbens shell. Thus, despite possessing the same neuron type, striatal regions exhibit heterogeneity in sex differences in MSN electrophysiological properties, which likely contribute to the sex differences observed in striatal function.

Keywords: sex, estradiol, hormones, striatum, medium spiny neuron, nucleus accumbens, caudate–putamen, electrophysiology

INTRODUCTION

Steroid sex hormones and biological sex are important factors influencing neuron function (1–4). Historically, research into the roles of biological sex and hormones targeted brain regions directly involved in sex-specific reproduction-related behaviors in adult animals (5, 6). These regions display large sex differences in volume, neuron cellular anatomy, and/or electrophysiological properties. Examples of these regions include the spinal nucleus of the bulbocavernosus (7), the sexually dimorphic nucleus of the preoptic area (8), and the song control nuclei in sexually dimorphic songbirds (9). Years of work have built upon these early studies to make significant advances. Notable among these is the discovery that biological sex and steroid sex hormones can modulate brain regions not directly involved with sex-specific reproductive behaviors. Although the extent of the influence on biological sex in the nervous system remains vastly underexplored, especially since few studies documented experimental animal sex (10–12), contemporary research has detected sex differences in neural substrates across the brain (13–18). The newly appreciated role of sex in modulating neural substrate also includes the striatal brain regions, comprising the caudate–putamen (also called dorsal striatum), the nucleus accumbens core (AcbC) and the nucleus accumbens shell (AcbS).

Biological sex, exogenous 17β-estradiol (estradiol), and endogenously circulating hormones *via* the estrous or menstrual cycle can modulate striatal-mediated cognitive, locomotor, and sensorimotor behaviors, including those related to motivation and reward (19–30). Many striatal pathologies are sensitive to estradiol and/or show sex differences in incidence and/or phenotype. These include depression, Parkinson's disease, drug addiction, schizophrenia, tardive dyskinesia, Huntington's disease, ADHD, and Tourette's syndrome, among others (31–41). The majority of published research in this field probes the link between sex and estradiol-induced influences on striatal-mediated normal and pathological behaviors (20, 42–46), especially regarding critical neurotransmitter/modulator systems such as dopamine and acetylcholine (43, 47–64). This research has established that sex and estradiol can influence striatal function *via* action on neurotransmitter and modulator systems, especially since the striatal regions show no robust sex differences in regional volume, neuron density, or soma size (65, 66). One area that has historically received less attention is how sex and estradiol modulate the electrophysiological properties of striatal neurons, including both the output neuron of the striatum, the medium spiny neuron (MSN) (67), and striatal interneurons (68). The term MSN is synonymous with striatal projection neuron. This is unfortunate, given that to change striatal circuit output and ultimately function, estradiol and sex must in some respect influence the electrophysiology of the MSN. This mini-review will focus upon the current state of knowledge regarding sex differences in rat MSN electrophysiological properties across striatal regions, with a focus on glutamatergic inputs and intrinsic excitability.

MSNs IN ADULT CAUDATE–PUTAMEN SHOW SEX-SPECIFIC AND ESTRADIOL-INDUCED DIFFERENCES IN EXCITABILITY *IN VIVO*

This research began in the 1980s, when Vincent and colleagues discovered that estradiol exposure increased *in vivo* spontaneous action potential generation and dopamine sensitivity in striatal neurons in ovariectomized adult female rat caudate–putamen (69). Tansey and colleagues then identified that the striatal neurons showing increased *in vivo* spontaneous action potential generation in response to high estradiol levels included nigrostriatal MSNs (other MSN subtypes and striatal interneurons were not examined). This increase in spontaneous action potential generation was induced either *via* exogenous estradiol exposure in ovariectomized animals or endogenously during specific phases of the estrous cycle (70). MSN spontaneous action potential firing rates were elevated in females compared with males only during the phases of the estrous cycle associated with the effects of increased estradiol and progesterone (proestrus and estrus). MSNs outside of the caudate–putamen were not examined in either study. The next breakthrough in targeting MSN electrophysiology came in the mid-1990s, when Mermelstein and colleagues established that estradiol rapidly decreases L-type calcium channel currents in both prepubertal and adult female rat caudate–putamen MSNs (71). In this case, estradiol acted within seconds in a steroid- and dose-dependent method on a membrane-associated estrogen receptor. The receptor was eventually identified as membrane-associated estrogen receptor β (72). Later research encompassing both the caudate–putamen and the nucleus accumbens established the presence of membrane-associated estrogen receptors α, β, and GPER-1 in MSNs, striatal interneurons, presynaptic terminals, and glia (72–78). The presence of aromatase, the enzyme that converts testosterone into estradiol, was also confirmed (79–82). There is little to no evidence of nuclear estrogen receptors in the striatal regions in adult rodents (83–85), although an exhaustive search across development, estrus cycle stages, and relevant species has not been performed.

These studies established several foundational themes for more recent research on the influences of estradiol and sex on MSN electrophysiology. First, estradiol can act *directly* on MSNs to modulate electrophysiological properties in addition to *indirectly* acting on MSNs by manipulating neuromodulatory influences such as those encompassed by the dopaminergic and cholinergic systems. Second, MSN sensitivity to estradiol can occur in a sex-specific fashion. Third, estradiol can manipulate MSN excitability, and in particular can increase MSN excitability in adult female animals. This sex-specific increase in MSN excitability could be potentially induced by multiple cellular mechanisms, broadly grouped into two types: mechanisms inducing alterations in synaptic input onto MSNs and mechanisms inducing alterations in the intrinsic electrophysiological properties of MSN. These mechanisms are not necessarily mutually exclusive and are not necessarily active in every striatal region. Recent research has uncovered that both mechanism types can influence MSN excitability, with heterogeneity across striatal regions (**Table 1**).

EXCITATORY SYNAPSE NUMBER IS INCREASED ONTO FEMALE COMPARED WITH MALE AcbC MSNs, AND THESE SYNAPSES ARE MODULATED BY ESTRADIOL IN ADULTHOOD

Regarding the AcbC, in the early part of this decade, Woolley and colleagues formulated the hypothesis that excitatory synapses onto MSNs in this region are increased in females compared with males (86). Anatomical studies employing electron microscopy, immunocytochemistry, and other techniques established that increased excitatory synapses are present on MSNs in the AcbC of adult rat females in proestrus compared with gonad-intact males (86–88). Alterations in excitatory synapse activity instruct AcbC function in many contexts (89–93), including the responsiveness to drugs of abuse (94). Even minor sex differences in these excitatory synaptic inputs are potentially influential on AcbC function.

One neuroanatomical correlate of increased excitatory synapse number onto female compared with male rat AcbC MSNs was concomitant increased dendritic spine density (87, 88). This sex difference in dendritic spine density was also identified in adult human AcbC, with increased dendritic spine density on female compared with male MSNs (95). In other brain regions, dendritic spine density has long been documented to be sensitive to estradiol exposure, either *via* endogenous exposure *via* the estrous or menstrual cycles, or exogenous (96–98). Regarding the AcbC, Staffend et al. elucidated that a 2-day exposure to exogenous estradiol altered dendritic spine density on MSNs in gonadectomized female hamsters (99). This exogenous estradiol-induced change in spine density is also detected in gonadectomized rat females and is dependent upon estradiol activating mGluR5 and endocannabinoid signaling *via* CB1 receptors (100, 101). This estrogen receptor/mGluR5 signaling pathway in the AcbC is speculated to induce an increased drive for sex (23), although this has not been tested in the context of the estrous cycle. Regarding neurological disorders, this pathway is implicated as one mechanism underlying estradiol-induced potentiation of cocaine-induced locomotor sensitization and cocaine self-administration (102, 103). This estradiol-induced change in dendritic spine density seems specific to the AcbC, at least in the absence of other interacting variables. No estradiol-induced changes in dendritic spine density were measured in the caudate–putamen, and only one of three experiments showed an estradiol-induced change in spine density in the AcbS (99, 101). There is select evidence that postsynaptic excitatory synapse markers are also increased in female AcbS (86), but this is not a robust finding (88, 104). There is evidence that sex differences in excitatory synapse in the AcbS are induced by the effects of stress and potentially other environmental factors (105). In AcbS MSNs, a stress paradigm induced sex-specific alterations in presynaptic but not postsynaptic excitatory synapse markers (106). Investigating the interactions between sex, hormones, and environmental inputs such as stress or environmental chemical exposure is an essential future line of research. Regarding male MSNs, another possibility is that testosterone regulates excitatory synaptic input onto nucleus accumbens neurons, as suggested by experiments analyzing dendritic spine density in response to week-long exogenous testosterone exposure in gonad-intact male rats (107), and the role of androgens in reward-related behaviors (108).

INCREASED EXCITATORY SYNAPSE ACTIVITY IN FEMALE AcbC MSNs IS PRESENT BEFORE PUBERTY AND IS BLOCKED BY NEONATAL EXPOSURE TO ESTRADIOL

This body of data indicates that excitatory synapse number is increased onto adult female compared with male MSNs in the AcbC. Whether these differences in excitatory synapse number are functional has been assessed by analyzing miniature excitatory postsynaptic current (mEPSC) properties (**Table 1**). Wissman and colleagues discovered increased mEPSC frequency in adult gonad-intact female compare to male rat AcbC MSN, with estrous cycle not formally assessed (88). No differences were detected in mEPSC amplitude, decay, or in paired pulse properties, consistent with a model of increased excitatory synapse number in female compared with male AcbC, although sex differences in synaptic release probability

TABLE 1 | Development of sex differences in MSN electrophysiological properties varies by striatal region.

Electrophysiological property	Developmental stage	Caudate–putamen	Nucleus Accumbens Core	Nucleus Accumbens Shell
Intrinsic neuronal excitability	Prepubertal	Female > male	Female = male	Female = male
	Adult	?[a]	?	?
Excitatory synaptic Input	Prepubertal	Female = male	Female > male	Female = male
	Adult	?[a]	Female > male[b]	Female = male?[b,c]

[a]*Adult caudate–putamen medium spiny neurons (MSNs) show increased excitability in vivo in females compared with males, but the mechanisms underlying this phenomenon remains unknown and are not included in this table.*

[b]*Animals were gonad intact, but female estrous cycle stage has not been comprehensively examined.*

[c]*Most but not all accumbens shell (AcbS) literature shows no evidence of sex differences or estrogen sensitivity in excitatory synaptic input in adult animals unexposed to adverse environmental stimuli.*

?—Data not available or complex.

Color signifies the presence of a sex difference.

remain possible. This increase in excitatory synaptic input could potentially be generated either in puberty or during the early natal sensitive period, and then modulated in adult females by the estrous cycle. Cao and coauthors addressed this question in three respects (109). First, increased mEPSC frequency onto female compared with male MSN in the rat AcbC was present prepuberty, determining that sex differences in excitatory synapse are generated before puberty and adulthood. Second, MSNs from females exposed to masculinizing levels of estradiol or testosterone during the neonatal sensitive period to organizational hormone action lacked increased mEPSC frequency compared with control females or males. This finding shows that neonatal masculinization/defeminization *via* estrogen exposure is sufficient to permanently downregulate excitatory synaptic input onto MSNs, an endocrine process which would normally occur only in male animals. This suggests an overall model that sex differences in AcbC excitatory synapse number are organized by steroid sex hormone action during early development, with estrogen exposure in males permanently decreasing AcbC synapse number and possibly adult estrogen sensitivity. Finally, Cao and colleagues found no evidence that MSN intrinsic membrane or action potential properties differed by sex, including those mediating intrinsic excitability. These findings tentatively focus the working model explaining sex differences in AcbC function toward the neuroanatomical inputs onto MSNs, most prominently glutamatergic synapse, but also dopamine inputs. Intriguing possibilities include interactions between sex, estradiol, glutamate, and dopamine. Consistent with this speculation, female compared with male AcbC MSNs demonstrate an increased proportion of large-head dendritic spines adjacent to dopaminergic terminals (87). Estradiol may also differentially modulate dopamine signaling across striatal regions, as anatomical studies revealed membrane-associated estrogen receptor α and GPER-1 expression in dopaminergic terminals in the nucleus accumbens, but not the caudate–putamen (73, 74). Dysregulation of sex differences in glutamatergic and dopaminergic signaling may potentially induce sex differences in the phenotype and incidence of AcbC-related disorders.

The anatomical source of increased excitatory input into the AcbC is unknown. One possibility of many is that the AcbC receives a sex-specific excitatory input distinct from other striatal regions. Consistent with this possibility, the AcbC receives a different set of glutamatergic inputs than other striatal regions (110, 111). These differential inputs are consistent with the AcbC mediating separate aspects of behavior than other striatal regions, including locomotor behaviors (112, 113), but also maternal, social, reward, learning, sensorimotor, and sex-related behaviors (112–121). Relatively new transgenic techniques could potentially be applied to address gaps in anatomical knowledge (122). However, inbred laboratory mice may not be effective tools to address the role of sex in modulating AcbC properties, as domestication induced female mice to lose sex- and AcbC-relevant behaviors compared with non-domesticated mice (123). In addition, many drug-abuse and other reward-mediated behaviors regulated by the nucleus accumbens are difficult or impossible to observe in mice (124). Regarding other avenues of investigation, it is unknown whether excitatory synaptic input, intrinsic excitability, and other components such as estrogen receptor α and β gene expression are modulated across estrous cycle stage. This should be a future avenue of research given the differences in striatal-mediated behaviors across the estrous and menstrual cycles. Another unknown is how GABA receptor activation and sex interact in MSNs. This question is interesting given that in select cases GABA receptor activation can facilitate MSN action potential generation (125), and that estradiol exposure can decrease extracellular GABA concentration in adult female rat caudate–putamen (126).

NO EVIDENCE FOR SEX DIFFERENCES IN EXCITATORY SYNAPTIC INPUT ONTO MSNs IN THE PREPUBERTAL AcbS AND CAUDATE–PUTAMEN

Prepubertal sex differences in excitatory synaptic input seem specific to the AcbC. MSNs in prepubertal male and female AcbS and caudate–putamen show no evidence of sex differences in mEPSC frequency, amplitude or decay (104, 127). Although there is no evidence of sex differences in excitatory synaptic properties so far, it is always a possibility that sex or estradiol modulates unexamined aspects of glutamatergic or other neurotransmission, including but not limited to NMDA/AMPA ratios/function, synaptic plasticity, and/or silent synapse formation. At this point it is unknown whether MSNs in adult AcbS or caudate–putamen exhibit sex differences in excitatory synaptic input, although one study used anterograde but not retrograde tracing methods to provide evidence of increased projections from the orbital frontal cortex to the caudate–putamen in adult gonad-intact female compared with male rats (128). Regarding synaptic plasticity, a recent study established that pharmacological inhibition of aromatase blocked the induction of long-term potentiation of glutamatergic excitatory inputs onto MSNs in adult gonad-intact male rat caudate–putamen neurons (81). This study did not include females, but increased estradiol concentrations in adult female caudate–putamen compared with estradiol concentrations in circulating plasma levels (129), along with the presence of aromatase in caudate–putamen and nucleus accumbens (79–82) hint that aromatase may be locally active across the striatum in both sexes.

MSNs SHOW INCREASED INTRINSIC EXCITABILITY IN FEMALE COMPARED WITH MALE PREPUBERTAL CAUDATE–PUTAMEN BUT NOT THE AcbC OR AcbS

Up to this point, this review has focused on sex differences in excitatory synaptic input. Alternatively, sex differences could occur in the intrinsic electrophysiological properties of MSNs, including alterations in action potential properties, the frequency of evoked action potentials to injected current properties, and passive (membrane) properties. Intrinsic electrophysiological properties regulate action potential generation in response to synaptic input (130), making these values integral in producing the functional output of MSNs. For example, augmented MSN intrinsic excitability would increase the number of action potentials that an MSN generates in response to a unit current. Alterations in MSN intrinsic excitability have been implicated in a number of striatal functions and disorders, including the responsivity to abused drugs, homeostatic plasticity, and striatal neuron subtypes (94, 131–136).

Female MSNs in prepubertal caudate–putamen show increased intrinsic excitability compared with male MSNs (127), unlike MSNs in the AcbC and AcbS (104, 109). This excitability is manifested in several respects. Female MSNs on average produce more action potentials than male MSNs for similar moderate amounts of injected positive current. This difference in action potential to current ratio is generated by an increased initial action potential firing rate in female compared with male MSNs, along with a decreased action potential after hyperpolarization peak and a mildly hyperpolarized action potential threshold. No sex differences were detected in passive membrane properties such as input resistance or in mEPSC properties. This lack of difference in mEPSC properties is essential for interpreting sex differences in MSN intrinsic excitability, as intrinsic excitability can be altered either independently or in concert with other attributes such as changes in excitatory synaptic input (94, 137–140). These findings support a model where increased excitability in prepubertal caudate–putamen MSNs is driven by internal changes to MSN electrical properties, rather than changes in excitatory synaptic input. Elucidating the ionic and receptor basis underlying this increased intrinsic excitation in female MSNs will be critical future experiments, along with assessments of adult MSNs, possible regional differences between dorsolateral and dorsomedial caudate–putamen, and the rostral–caudal axis. Changes in intrinsic excitability may be responsible for the increased excitability of female compared with male MSNs *in vivo* recorded in adult caudate–putamen (50, 69, 70). However, it is possible that intrinsic excitability and/or excitatory synaptic input in the caudate–putamen may be reorganized during puberty, such as glutamatergic synaptic input in the medial amygdala (141, 142), or striatal dopamine receptors (31, 143, 144). Either or both of these properties may be modulated by estrous cycle stage (145, 146), as suggested by *in vivo* recordings of caudate–putamen MSNs (69, 70). Overall, data from caudate–putamen MSNs support the theme of increased excitability in female compared with male MSNs, but indicate that the mechanism underlying these differences varies by striatal region.

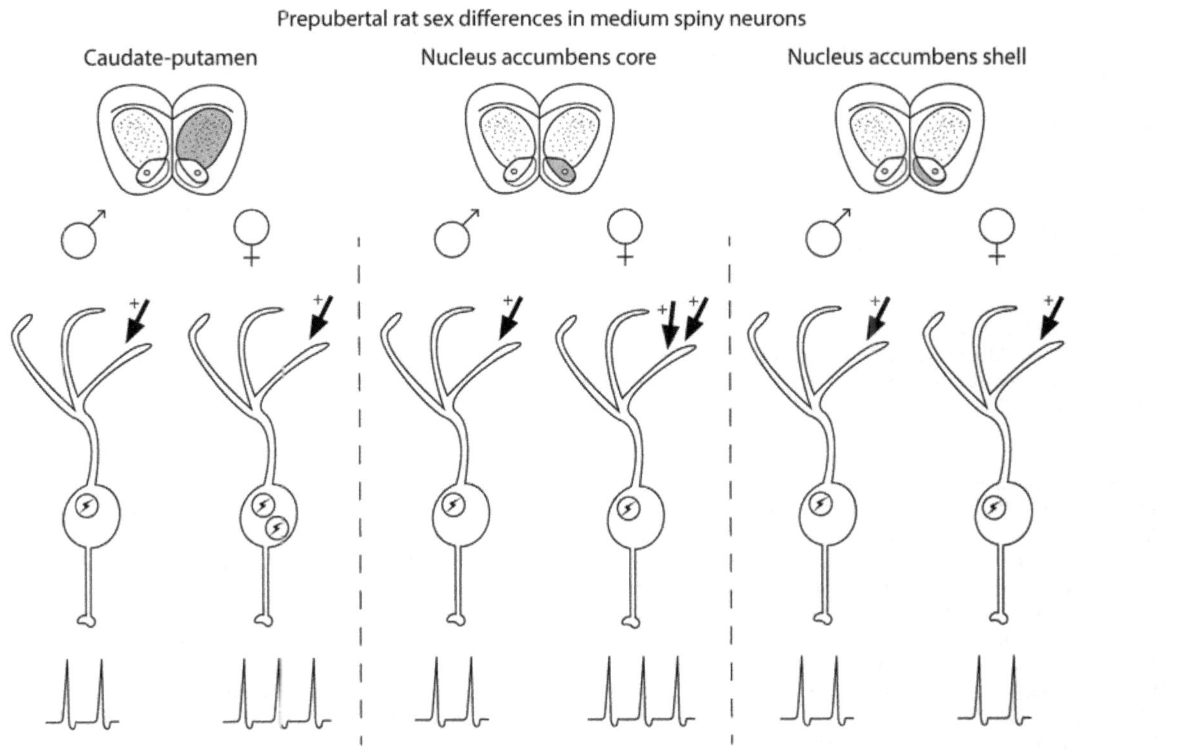

FIGURE 1 | Schematic of sex differences in medium spiny neurons (MSNs) in prepubertal rat caudate–putamen, nucleus accumbens core (AcbC), and nucleus accumbens shell (AcbS). In general, MSNs recorded from prepubertal female rats exhibit increased excitation compared with male MSNs in the caudate–putamen and nucleus AcbC. However, the exact nature of the increased excitability in female MSNs differs by striatal region, encompassing changes in either intrinsic excitability (indicated in the schematic with an encircled lightning bolt) or excitatory synaptic input (indicated with arrows with plus signs). Differences in intrinsic excitability and excitatory synaptic input are indicated with more or less lightning bolts and arrows, respectively. Caudate–putamen MSNs show increased intrinsic excitability in prepubertal females compared with males. Nucleus AcbC MSNs receive augmented excitatory synaptic input in prepubertal females compared with males. Nucleus AcbS MSNs exhibit little evidence for sex differences in either intrinsic excitability or excitatory synaptic input in prepubertal animals.

CONCLUSION

Medium spiny neuron electrophysiological properties are sensitive to sex and steroid sex hormone action in a striatal region-specific manner (**Figure 1**). In prepubertal caudate–putamen, MSNs show on average increased intrinsic excitation in females compared with males. In adult caudate–putamen, MSNs likewise show increased excitability in females compared with males, but the mechanism underlying this difference remains unknown. In both prepubertal and adult AcbC, MSNs receive augmented excitatory synaptic input in females compared with males, and early-life exposure to estradiol is instrumental in the sexual differentiation of this property. In the AcbS, there is little evidence for sex differences in intrinsic excitability or excitatory synaptic input in prepubertal animals unexposed to adverse environmental stimuli. These data argue for heterogeneity across striatal regions in the sensitivity to MSNs to sex and steroid sex hormones and the relative amount and nature of masculinization and feminization in MSN electrophysiological properties differs by striatal region. These findings highlight the importance of differentiating between striatal regions, developmental stage, sex, and estrous cycle. These data extend earlier mosaic models of brain sexuality, in that not only individual brain regions but also individual neuron types, in this instance MSNs, show differential degrees of masculinization, feminization, and homogeny (147, 148). These sex differences and similarities in MSN electrophysiological properties, along with developmental, individual, subtype, and the other documented variables in MSN properties, induce a dizzying variety *within the same neuron type* both between and within males and females.

AUTHOR CONTRIBUTIONS

JM wrote the manuscript; DD prepared the figure; and JC, JW, DD, and JM edited and approved the manuscript and figure.

FUNDING

We acknowledge NIH MH109471 to JM and P30ES025128 (Center for Human Health and the Environment).

REFERENCES

1. Cahill L. Fundamental sex difference in human brain architecture. *Proc Natl Acad Sci U S A* (2014) 111(2):577–8. doi:10.1073/pnas.1320954111
2. de Vries GJ, Forger NG. Sex differences in the brain: a whole body perspective. *Biol Sex Differ* (2015) 6:15. doi:10.1186/s13293-015-0032-z
3. McEwen BS, Milner TA. Understanding the broad influence of sex hormones and sex differences in the brain. *J Neurosci Res* (2017) 95(1–2):24–39. doi:10.1002/jnr.23809
4. McCarthy MM, Woolley CS, Arnold AP. Incorporating sex as a biological variable in neuroscience: what do we gain? *Nat Rev Neurosci* (2017) 18(12):707–8. doi:10.1038/nrn.2017.137
5. Breedlove SM, Hampson E. Sexual differentiation of the brain and behavior. In: Becker JB, Breedlove SM, Crews D, McCarthy MM, editors. *Behavioral Endocrinology*. London: MIT Press (2002). p. 75–114.
6. De Vries GJ. Minireview: sex differences in adult and developing brains: compensation, compensation, compensation. *Endocrinology* (2004) 145(3): 1063–8. doi:10.1210/en.2003-1504
7. Breedlove SM, Arnold AP. Sexually dimorphic motor nucleus in the rat lumbar spinal cord: response to adult hormone manipulation, absence in androgen-insensitive rats. *Brain Res* (1981) 225(2):297–307. doi:10.1016/0006-8993(81)90837-4
8. Gorski RA, Gordon JH, Shryne JE, Southam AM. Evidence for a morphological sex difference within the medial preoptic area of the rat brain. *Brain Res* (1978) 148(2):333–46. doi:10.1016/0006-8993(78)90723-0
9. Nottebohm F, Arnold AP. Sexual dimorphism in vocal control areas of the songbird brain. *Science* (1976) 194(4261):211–3. doi:10.1126/science.959852
10. Beery AK, Zucker I. Sex bias in neuroscience and biomedical research. *Neurosci Biobehav Rev* (2011) 35(3):565–72. doi:10.1016/j.neubiorev.2010.07.002
11. Will TR, Proano SB, Thomas AM, Kunz LM, Thompson KC, Ginnari LA, et al. Problems and progress regarding sex bias and omission in neuroscience research. *eNeuro* (2017) 4(6):ENEURO.0278-17.2017. doi:10.1523/ENEURO.0278-17.2017
12. Shansky RM, Woolley CS. Considering sex as a biological variable will be valuable for neuroscience research. *J Neurosci* (2016) 36(47):11817–22. doi:10.1523/JNEUROSCI.1390-16.2016
13. Oberlander JG, Woolley CS. 17beta-estradiol acutely potentiates glutamatergic synaptic transmission in the hippocampus through distinct mechanisms in males and females. *J Neurosci* (2016) 36(9):2677–90. doi:10.1523/JNEUROSCI.4437-15.2016
14. Blume SR, Freedberg M, Vantrease JE, Chan R, Padival M, Record MJ, et al. Sex- and estrus-dependent differences in rat basolateral amygdala. *J Neurosci* (2017) 37(44):10567–86. doi:10.1523/JNEUROSCI.0758-17.2017
15. Salvatore M, Wiersielis K, Luz S, Waxler D, Bhatnagar S, Bangasser DA. Sex differences in circuits activated by corticotropin releasing factor in rats. *Horm Behav* (2018) 97:145–53.
16. Farrell MR, Holland FH, Shansky RM, Brenhouse HC. Sex-specific effects of early life stress on social interaction and prefrontal cortex dendritic morphology in young rats. *Behav Brain Res* (2016) 310:119–25. doi:10.1016/j.bbr.2016.05.009
17. Laman-Maharg A, Trainor BC. Stress, sex, and motivated behaviors. *J Neurosci Res* (2017) 95(1–2):83–92. doi:10.1002/jnr.23815
18. Terasaki LS, Gomez J, Schwarz JM. An examination of sex differences in the effects of early-life opiate and alcohol exposure. *Philos Trans R Soc Lond B Biol Sci* (2016) 371(1688):20150123. doi:10.1098/rstb.2015.0123
19. Beatty WW. Gonadal hormones and sex differences in nonreproductive behaviors in rodents: organizational and activational influences. *Horm Behav* (1979) 12(2):112–63. doi:10.1016/0018-506X(79)90017-5
20. Becker JB. Hormonal influences on sensorimotor function. In: Becker JB, Breedlove SM, Crews D, McCarthy MM, editors. *Behavioral Endocrinology*. Cambridge: MIT Press (2002). p. 497–525.
21. Carroll ME, Anker JJ. Sex differences and ovarian hormones in animal models of drug dependence. *Horm Behav* (2010) 58(1):44–56. doi:10.1016/j.yhbeh.2009.10.001
22. Yoest KE, Cummings JA, Becker JB. Estradiol, dopamine and motivation. *Cent Nerv Syst Agents Med Chem* (2014) 14(2):83–9. doi:10.2174/18715249 14666141226103135
23. Tonn Eisinger KR, Larson EB, Boulware MI, Thomas MJ, Mermelstein PG. Membrane estrogen receptor signaling impacts the reward circuitry of the female brain to influence motivated behaviors. *Steroids* (2018) 133:53–9.
24. Becker JB, Snyder PJ, Miller MM, Westgate SA, Jenuwine MJ. The influence of estrous cycle and intrastriatal estradiol on sensorimotor performance in the female rat. *Pharmacol Biochem Behav* (1987) 27(1):53–9. doi:10.1016/0091-3057(87)90476-X
25. Smith SS. Female sex steroid hormones: from receptors to networks to performance – actions on the sensorimotor system. *Prog Neurobiol* (1994) 44(1):55–86. doi:10.1016/0301-0082(94)90057-4
26. Hampson E, Kimura D. Reciprocal effects of hormonal fluctuations on human motor and perceptual-spatial skills. *Behav Neurosci* (1988) 102(3):456–9. doi:10.1037/0735-7044.102.3.456
27. Hampson E. Estrogen-related variations in human spatial and articulatory-motor skills. *Psychoneuroendocrinology* (1990) 15(2):97–111. doi:10.1016/0306-4530(90)90018-5
28. Simic N, Tokic A, Pericic M. Performance of fine motor and spatial tasks during the menstrual cycle. *Arh Hig Rada Toksikol* (2010) 61(4):407–14. doi:10.2478/10004-1254-61-2010-2055

29. Jennings PJ, Janowsky JS, Orwoll E. Estrogen and sequential movement. *Behav Neurosci* (1998) 112(1):154–9. doi:10.1037/0735-7044.112.1.154
30. Zoghi M, Vaseghi B, Bastani A, Jaberzadeh S, Galea MP. The effects of sex hormonal fluctuations during menstrual cycle on cortical excitability and manual dexterity (a Pilot Study). *PLoS One* (2015) 10(8):e0136081. doi:10.1371/journal.pone.0136081
31. Andersen SL, Teicher MH. Sex differences in dopamine receptors and their relevance to ADHD. *Neurosci Biobehav Rev* (2000) 24(1):137–41. doi:10.1016/S0149-7634(99)00044-5
32. Bosse R, DiPaolo T. The modulation of brain dopamine and GABAA receptors by estradiol: a clue for CNS changes occurring at menopause. *Cell Mol Neurobiol* (1996) 16(2):199–212. doi:10.1007/BF02088176
33. Dluzen DE, McDermott JL. Gender differences in neurotoxicity of the nigrostriatal dopaminergic system: implications for Parkinson's disease. *J Gend Specif Med* (2000) 3(6):36–42.
34. Elbaz A, Bower JH, Maraganore DM, McDonnell SK, Peterson BJ, Ahlskog JE, et al. Risk tables for parkinsonism and Parkinson's disease. *J Clin Epidemiol* (2002) 55(1):25–31. doi:10.1016/S0895-4356(01)00425-5
35. Lynch WJ, Roth ME, Carroll ME. Biological basis of sex differences in drug abuse: preclinical and clinical studies. *Psychopharmacology* (2002) 164(2):121–37. doi:10.1007/s00213-002-1183-2
36. Pauls DL, Cohen DJ, Heimbuch R, Detlor J, Kidd KK. Familial pattern and transmission of Gilles de la Tourette syndrome and multiple tics. *Arch Gen Psychiatry* (1981) 38(10):1091–3. doi:10.1001/archpsyc.1981.01780350025002
37. Bode FJ, Stephan M, Suhling H, Pabst R, Straub RH, Raber KA, et al. Sex differences in a transgenic rat model of Huntington's disease: decreased 17beta-estradiol levels correlate with reduced numbers of DARPP32+ neurons in males. *Hum Mol Genet* (2008) 17(17):2595–609. doi:10.1093/hmg/ddn159
38. Roos RA, Vegter-van der Vlis M, Hermans J, Elshove HM, Moll AC, van de Kamp JJ, et al. Age at onset in Huntington's disease: effect of line of inheritance and patient's sex. *J Med Genet* (1991) 28(8):515–9. doi:10.1136/jmg.28.8.515
39. Becker JB, McClellan ML, Reed BG. Sex differences, gender and addiction. *J Neurosci Res* (2017) 95(1–2):136–47. doi:10.1002/jnr.23963
40. Quinn NP, Marsden CD. Menstrual-related fluctuations in Parkinson's disease. *Mov Disord* (1986) 1(1):85–7. doi:10.1002/mds.870010112
41. Castrioto A, Hulliger S, Poon YY, Lang AE, Moro E. A survey on the impact of the menstrual cycle on movement disorders severity. *Can J Neurol Sci* (2010) 37(4):478–81. doi:10.1017/S0317167100010490
42. Bobzean SA, DeNobrega AK, Perrotti LI. Sex differences in the neurobiology of drug addiction. *Exp Neurol* (2014) 259:64–74. doi:10.1016/j.expneurol.2014.01.022
43. Davis DM, Jacobson TK, Aliakbari S, Mizumori SJ. Differential effects of estrogen on hippocampal- and striatal-dependent learning. *Neurobiol Learn Mem* (2005) 84(2):132–7. doi:10.1016/j.nlm.2005.06.004
44. Fattore L, Melis M, Fadda P, Fratta W. Sex differences in addictive disorders. *Front Neuroendocrinol* (2014) 35:272–84. doi:10.1016/j.yfrne.2014.04.003
45. Pavon JM, Whitson HE, Okun MS. Parkinson's disease in women: a call for improved clinical studies and for comparative effectiveness research. *Maturitas* (2010) 65(4):352–8. doi:10.1016/j.maturitas.2010.01.001
46. Zurkovsky L, Brown SL, Boyd SE, Fell JA, Korol DL. Estrogen modulates learning in female rats by acting directly at distinct memory systems. *Neuroscience* (2007) 144(1):26–37. doi:10.1016/j.neuroscience.2006.09.002
47. Gordon JH, Borison RL, Diamond BI. Modulation of dopamine receptor sensitivity by estrogen. *Biol Psychiatry* (1980) 15(3):389–96.
48. Hruska RE, Silbergeld EK. Increased dopamine receptor sensitivity after estrogen treatment using the rat rotation model. *Science* (1980) 208(4451):1466–8. doi:10.1126/science.7189902
49. Becker JB, Ramirez VD. Sex differences in the amphetamine stimulated release of catecholamines from rat striatal tissue in vitro. *Brain Res* (1981) 204(2):361–72. doi:10.1016/0006-8993(81)90595-3
50. Demotes-Mainard J, Arnauld E, Vincent JD. Estrogens modulate the responsiveness of in vivo recorded striatal neurons to lontophoretic application of dopamine in rats: role of D and D2 receptor activation. *J Neuroendocrinol* (1990) 2(6):825–32. doi:10.1111/j.1365-2826.1990.tb00647.x
51. Gordon JH, Perry KO. Pre- and postsynaptic neurochemical alterations following estrogen-induced striatal dopamine hypo- and hypersensitivity. *Brain Res Bull* (1983) 10(4):425–8. doi:10.1016/0361-9230(83)90137-5
52. Clopton J, Gordon JH. In vivo effects of estrogen and 2-hydroxyestradiol on D-2 dopamine receptor agonist affinity states in rat striatum. *J Neural Transm* (1986) 66(1):13–20. doi:10.1007/BF01262954
53. Levesque D, Gagnon S, Di Paolo T. Striatal D1 dopamine receptor density fluctuates during the rat estrous cycle. *Neurosci Lett* (1989) 98(3):345–50. doi:10.1016/0304-3940(89)90426-6
54. Levesque D, Di Paolo T. Rapid conversion of high into low striatal D2-dopamine receptor agonist binding states after an acute physiological dose of 17 beta-estradiol. *Neurosci Lett* (1988) 88(1):113–8. doi:10.1016/0304-3940(88)90324-2
55. Tonnaer JA, Leinders T, van Delft AM. Ovariectomy and subchronic estradiol-17 beta administration decrease dopamine D1 and D2 receptors in rat striatum. *Psychoneuroendocrinology* (1989) 14(6):469–76. doi:10.1016/0306-4530(89)90046-2
56. Bazzett TJ, Becker JB. Sex differences in the rapid and acute effects of estrogen on striatal D2 dopamine receptor binding. *Brain Res* (1994) 637(1–2):163–72. doi:10.1016/0006-8993(94)91229-7
57. Becker JB. Direct effect of 17 beta-estradiol on striatum: sex differences in dopamine release. *Synapse* (1990) 5(2):157–64. doi:10.1002/syn.890050211
58. Walker QD, Rooney MB, Wightman RM, Kuhn CM. Dopamine release and uptake are greater in female than male rat striatum as measured by fast cyclic voltammetry. *Neuroscience* (2000) 95(4):1061–70. doi:10.1016/S0306-4522(99)00500-X
59. Calipari ES, Juarez B, Morel C, Walker DM, Cahill ME, Ribeiro E, et al. Dopaminergic dynamics underlying sex-specific cocaine reward. *Nat Commun* (2017) 8:13877. doi:10.1038/ncomms13877
60. Becker JB. Sex differences in addiction. *Dialogues Clin Neurosci* (2016) 18(4):395–402.
61. Euvrard C, Labrie F, Boissier JR. Effect of estrogen on changes in the activity of striatal cholinergic neurons induced by DA drugs. *Brain Res* (1979) 169(1):215–20. doi:10.1016/0006-8993(79)90392-5
62. Becker JB, Perry AN, Westenbroek C. Sex differences in the neural mechanisms mediating addiction: a new synthesis and hypothesis. *Biol Sex Differ* (2013) 3(1):14. doi:10.1186/2042-6410-3-14
63. Di Paolo T. Modulation of brain dopamine transmission by sex steroids. *Rev Neurosci* (1994) 5(1):27–41. doi:10.1515/REVNEURO.1994.5.1.27
64. Walker QD, Ray R, Kuhn CM. Sex differences in neurochemical effects of dopaminergic drugs in rat striatum. *Neuropsychopharmacology* (2006) 31(6):1193–202. doi:10.1038/sj.npp.1300915
65. Wong JE, Cao J, Dorris DM, Meitzen J. Genetic sex and the volumes of the caudate-putamen, nucleus accumbens core and shell: original data and a review. *Brain Struct Funct* (2016) 221(8):4257–67. doi:10.1007/s00429-015-1158-9
66. Meitzen J, Pflepsen KR, Stern CM, Meisel RL, Mermelstein PG. Measurements of neuron soma size and density in rat dorsal striatum, nucleus accumbens core and nucleus accumbens shell: differences between striatal region and brain hemisphere, but not sex. *Neurosci Lett* (2011) 487(2):177–81. doi:10.1016/j.neulet.2010.10.017
67. Mai JK, Paxinos G. *The Human Nervous System*. 3rd ed. London: Academic Press (2012).
68. Rapanelli M, Frick LR, Xu M, Groman SM, Jindachomthong K, Tamamaki N, et al. Targeted interneuron depletion in the dorsal striatum produces autism-like behavioral abnormalities in male but not female mice. *Biol Psychiatry* (2017) 82(3):194–203. doi:10.1016/j.biopsych.2017.01.020
69. Arnauld E, Dufy B, Pestre M, Vincent JD. Effects of estrogens on the responses of caudate neurons to microiontophoretically applied dopamine. *Neurosci Lett* (1981) 21(3):325–31. doi:10.1016/0304-3940(81)90225-1
70. Tansey EM, Arbuthnott GW, Fink G, Whale D. Oestradiol-17 beta increases the firing rate of antidromically identified neurones of the rat neostriatum. *Neuroendocrinology* (1983) 37(2):106–10. doi:10.1159/000123527
71. Mermelstein PG, Becker JB, Surmeier DJ. Estradiol reduces calcium currents in rat neostriatal neurons via a membrane receptor. *J Neurosci* (1996) 16(2):595–604. doi:10.1523/JNEUROSCI.16-02-00595.1996
72. Grove-Strawser D, Boulware MI, Mermelstein PG. Membrane estrogen receptors activate the metabotropic glutamate receptors mGluR5 and mGluR3 to bidirectionally regulate CREB phosphorylation in female rat striatal neurons. *Neuroscience* (2010) 170:1045–55. doi:10.1016/j.neuroscience.2010.08.012

73. Almey A, Filardo EJ, Milner TA, Brake WG. Estrogen receptors are found in glia and at extranuclear neuronal sites in the dorsal striatum of female rats: evidence for cholinergic but not dopaminergic colocalization. *Endocrinology* (2012) 153(11):5373–83. doi:10.1210/en.2012-1458
74. Almey A, Milner TA, Brake WG. Estrogen receptors in the central nervous system and their implication for dopamine-dependent cognition in females. *Horm Behav* (2015) 74:125–38. doi:10.1016/j.yhbeh.2015.06.010
75. Almey A, Milner TA, Brake WG. Estrogen receptor alpha and G-protein coupled estrogen receptor 1 are localised to GABAergic neurons in the dorsal striatum. *Neurosci Lett* (2016) 622:118–23. doi:10.1016/j.neulet.2016.04.023
76. Bourque M, Morissette M, Di Paolo T. Raloxifene activates G protein-coupled estrogen receptor 1/Akt signaling to protect dopamine neurons in 1-methyl-4-phenyl-1,2,3,6-tetrahydropyridine mice. *Neurobiol Aging* (2014) 35(10):2347–56. doi:10.1016/j.neurobiolaging.2014.03.017
77. Schultz KN, von Esenwein SA, Hu M, Bennett AL, Kennedy RT, Musatov S, et al. Viral vector-mediated overexpression of estrogen receptor-alpha in striatum enhances the estradiol-induced motor activity in female rats and estradiol-modulated GABA release. *J Neurosci* (2009) 29(6):1897–903. doi:10.1523/JNEUROSCI.4647-08.2009
78. Kuppers E, Beyer C. Expression of estrogen receptor-alpha and beta mRNA in the developing and adult mouse striatum. *Neurosci Lett* (1999) 276(2):95–8. doi:10.1016/S0304-3940(99)00815-0
79. Foidart A, Harada N, Balthazart J. Aromatase-immunoreactive cells are present in mouse brain areas that are known to express high levels of aromatase activity. *Cell Tissue Res* (1995) 280(3):561–74. doi:10.1007/BF00318360
80. Stanic D, Dubois S, Chua HK, Tonge B, Rinehart N, Horne MK, et al. Characterization of aromatase expression in the adult male and female mouse brain. I. Coexistence with oestrogen receptors alpha and beta, and androgen receptors. *PLoS One* (2014) 9(3):e90451. doi:10.1371/journal.pone.0090451
81. Tozzi A, de Iure A, Tantucci M, Durante V, Quiroga-Varela A, Giampa C, et al. Endogenous 17beta-estradiol is required for activity-dependent long-term potentiation in the striatum: interaction with the dopaminergic system. *Front Cell Neurosci* (2015) 9:192. doi:10.3389/fncel.2015.00192
82. Kuppers E, Beyer C. Expression of aromatase in the embryonic and postnatal mouse striatum. *Brain Res Mol Brain Res* (1998) 63(1):184–8. doi:10.1016/S0169-328X(98)00279-4
83. Warembourg M, Jolivet A, Milgrom E. Immunohistochemical evidence of the presence of estrogen and progesterone receptors in the same neurons of the guinea pig hypothalamus and preoptic area. *Brain Res* (1989) 480(1–2):1–15. doi:10.1016/0006-8993(89)91561-8
84. Lauber AH, Romano GJ, Pfaff DW. Gene expression for estrogen and progesterone receptor mRNAs in rat brain and possible relations to sexually dimorphic functions. *J Steroid Biochem Mol Biol* (1991) 40(1–3):53–62. doi:10.1016/0960-0760(91)90167-4
85. Milner TA, Thompson LI, Wang G, Kievits JA, Martin E, Zhou P, et al. Distribution of estrogen receptor beta containing cells in the brains of bacterial artificial chromosome transgenic mice. *Brain Res* (2010) 1351:74–96. doi:10.1016/j.brainres.2010.06.038
86. Forlano PM, Woolley CS. Quantitative analysis of pre- and postsynaptic sex differences in the nucleus accumbens. *J Comp Neurol* (2010) 518(8):1330–48. doi:10.1002/cne.22279
87. Wissman AM, May RM, Woolley CS. Ultrastructural analysis of sex differences in nucleus accumbens synaptic connectivity. *Brain Struct Funct* (2012) 217(2):181–90. doi:10.1007/s00429-011-0353-6
88. Wissman AM, McCollum AF, Huang GZ, Nikrodhanond AA, Woolley CS. Sex differences and effects of cocaine on excitatory synapses in the nucleus accumbens. *Neuropharmacology* (2011) 61:217–27. doi:10.1016/j.neuropharm.2011.04.002
89. Huang YH, Schluter OM, Dong Y. Silent synapses speak up: updates of the neural rejuvenation hypothesis of drug addiction. *Neuroscientist* (2015) 21(5):451–9. doi:10.1177/1073858415579405
90. Grueter BA, Rothwell PE, Malenka RC. Integrating synaptic plasticity and striatal circuit function in addiction. *Curr Opin Neurobiol* (2012) 22(3):545–51. doi:10.1016/j.conb.2011.09.009
91. Robinson TE, Kolb B. Structural plasticity associated with exposure to drugs of abuse. *Neuropharmacology* (2004) 47:33–46. doi:10.1016/j.neuropharm.2004.06.025
92. Roitman MF, Na E, Anderson G, Jones TA, Bernstein IL. Induction of a salt appetite alters dendritic morphology in nucleus accumbens and sensitizes rats to amphetamine. *J Neurosci* (2002) 22(11):RC225.
93. Meisel RL, Mullins AJ. Sexual experience in female rodents: cellular mechanisms and functional consequences. *Brain Res* (2006) 1126(1):56–65. doi:10.1016/j.brainres.2006.08.050
94. Wolf ME. The Bermuda Triangle of cocaine-induced neuroadaptations. *Trends Neurosci* (2010) 33(9):391–8. doi:10.1016/j.tins.2010.06.003
95. Sazdanovic M, Slobodanka M, Zivanovic-Macuzic I, Jeremic D, Tanaskovic I, Milosavljevic Z, et al. Sexual dimorphism of medium-sized neurons with spines in human nucleus accumbens. *Arch Biol Sci Belgrade* (2013) 65(3):1149–55. doi:10.2298/ABS1303149S
96. Meisel RL, Luttrell VR. Estradiol increases the dendritic length of ventromedial hypothalamic neurons in female Syrian hamsters. *Brain Res Bull* (1990) 25(1):165–8. doi:10.1016/0361-9230(90)90269-6
97. Gould E, Woolley CS, Frankfurt M, McEwen BS. Gonadal steroids regulate dendritic spine density in hippocampal pyramidal cells in adulthood. *J Neurosci* (1990) 10(4):1286–91. doi:10.1523/JNEUROSCI.10-04-01286.1990
98. Woolley CS, McEwen BS. Estradiol mediates fluctuation in hippocampal synapse density during the estrous cycle in the adult rat. *J Neurosci* (1992) 12(7):2549–54. doi:10.1523/JNEUROSCI.12-07-02549.1992
99. Staffend NA, Loftus CM, Meisel RL. Estradiol reduces dendritic spine density in the ventral striatum of female Syrian hamsters. *Brain Struct Funct* (2011) 215(3–4):187–94. doi:10.1007/s00429-010-0284-7
100. Peterson BM, Martinez LA, Meisel RL, Mermelstein PG. Estradiol impacts the endocannabinoid system in female rats to influence behavioral and structural responses to cocaine. *Neuropharmacology* (2016) 110:118–24. doi:10.1016/j.neuropharm.2016.06.002
101. Peterson BM, Mermelstein PG, Meisel RL. Estradiol mediates dendritic spine plasticity in the nucleus accumbens core through activation of mGluR5. *Brain Struct Funct* (2015) 220:2415–22. doi:10.1007/s00429-014-0794-9
102. Martinez LA, Gross KS, Himmler BT, Emmitt NL, Peterson BM, Zlebnik NE, et al. Estradiol facilitation of cocaine self-administration in female rats requires activation of mGluR5. *eNeuro* (2016) 3(5):ENEURO.0140-16.2016. doi:10.1523/ENEURO.0140-16.2016
103. Martinez LA, Peterson BM, Meisel RL, Mermelstein PG. Estradiol facilitation of cocaine-induced locomotor sensitization in female rats requires activation of mGluR5. *Behav Brain Res* (2014) 271:39–42. doi:10.1016/j.bbr.2014.05.052
104. Willett JA, Will TR, Hauser CA, Dorris DM, Cao J, Meitzen J. No evidence for sex differences in the electrophysiological properties and excitatory synaptic input onto nucleus accumbens shell medium spiny neurons. *eNeuro* (2016) 3(1):ENEURO.0147-15.2016. doi:10.1523/ENEURO.0147-15.2016
105. Hodes GE, Pfau ML, Purushothaman I, Ahn HF, Golden SA, Christoffel DJ, et al. Sex differences in nucleus accumbens transcriptome profiles associated with susceptibility versus resilience to subchronic variable stress. *J Neurosci* (2015) 35(50):16362–76. doi:10.1523/JNEUROSCI.1392-15.2015
106. Brancato A, Bregman D, Ahn HF, Pfau ML, Menard C, Cannizzaro C, et al. Sub-chronic variable stress induces sex-specific effects on glutamatergic synapses in the nucleus accumbens. *Neuroscience* (2017) 350(14 May):180–9. doi:10.1016/j.neuroscience.2017.03.014
107. Wallin-Miller K, Li G, Kelishani D, Wood RI. Anabolic-androgenic steroids decrease dendritic spine density in the nucleus accumbens of male rats. *Neuroscience* (2016) 330:72–8. doi:10.1016/j.neuroscience.2016.05.045
108. Frye CA, Rhodes ME, Rosellini R, Svare B. The nucleus accumbens as a site of action for rewarding properties of testosterone and its 5alpha-reduced metabolites. *Pharmacol Biochem Behav* (2002) 74(1):119–27. doi:10.1016/S0091-3057(02)00968-1
109. Cao J, Dorris DM, Meitzen J. Neonatal masculinization blocks increased excitatory synaptic input in female rat nucleus accumbens core. *Endocrinology* (2016) 157(8):3181–96. doi:10.1210/en.2016-1160
110. Groenewegen HJ, Wright CI, Beijer AV, Voorn P. Convergence and segregation of ventral striatal inputs and outputs. *Ann N Y Acad Sci* (1999) 877:49–63. doi:10.1111/j.1749-6632.1999.tb09260.x
111. Britt JP, Benaliouad F, McDevitt RA, Stuber GD, Wise RA, Bonci A. Synaptic and behavioral profile of multiple glutamatergic inputs to the nucleus accumbens. *Neuron* (2012) 76(4):790–803. doi:10.1016/j.neuron.2012.09.040
112. Ito R, Robbins TW, Everitt BJ. Differential control over cocaine-seeking behavior by nucleus accumbens core and shell. *Nat Neurosci* (2004) 7(4):389–97. doi:10.1038/nn1217

113. Pulvirenti L, Berrier R, Kreifeldt M, Koob GF. Modulation of locomotor activity by NMDA receptors in the nucleus accumbens core and shell regions of the rat. *Brain Res* (1994) 664(1–2):231–6. doi:10.1016/0006-8993(94)91977-1
114. Bradley KC, Boulware MB, Jiang H, Doerge RW, Meisel RL, Mermelstein PG. Changes in gene expression within the nucleus accumbens and striatum following sexual experience. *Genes Brain Behav* (2005) 4(1):31–44. doi:10.1111/j.1601-183X.2004.00093.x
115. Henschen CW, Palmiter RD, Darvas M. Restoration of dopamine signaling to the dorsal striatum is sufficient for aspects of active maternal behavior in female mice. *Endocrinology* (2013) 154(11):4316–27. doi:10.1210/en.2013-1257
116. Pena CJ, Neugut YD, Calarco CA, Champagne FA. Effects of maternal care on the development of midbrain dopamine pathways and reward-directed behavior in female offspring. *Eur J Neurosci* (2014) 39(6):946–56. doi:10.1111/ejn.12479
117. O'Connell LA, Hofmann HA. The vertebrate mesolimbic reward system and social behavior network: a comparative synthesis. *J Comp Neurol* (2011) 519(18):3599–639. doi:10.1002/cne.22735
118. West AE, Carelli RM. Nucleus accumbens core and shell differentially encode reward-associated cues after reinforcer devaluation. *J Neurosci* (2016) 36(4):1128–39. doi:10.1523/JNEUROSCI.2976-15.2016
119. Corbit LH, Balleine BW. The general and outcome-specific forms of Pavlovian-instrumental transfer are differentially mediated by the nucleus accumbens core and shell. *J Neurosci* (2011) 31(33):11786–94. doi:10.1523/JNEUROSCI.2711-11.2011
120. Corbit LH, Muir JL, Balleine BW. The role of the nucleus accumbens in instrumental conditioning: evidence of a functional dissociation between accumbens core and shell. *J Neurosci* (2001) 21(9):3251–60.
121. Willett JA, Johnson AG, Vogel AR, Patisaul HB, McGraw LA, Meitzen J. Nucleus accumbens core medium spiny neuron electrophysiological properties and partner preference behavior in the adult male prairie vole, *Microtus ochrogaster*. *J Neurophysiol* (2018). doi:10.1152/jn.00737.2017
122. Lerner TN, Ye L, Deisseroth K. Communication in neural circuits: tools, opportunities, and challenges. *Cell* (2016) 164(6):1136–50. doi:10.1016/j.cell.2016.02.027
123. Chalfin L, Dayan M, Levy DR, Austad SN, Miller RA, Iraqi FA, et al. Mapping ecologically relevant social behaviours by gene knockout in wild mice. *Nat Commun* (2014) 5:4569. doi:10.1038/ncomms5569
124. Parker CC, Chen H, Flagel SB, Geurts AM, Richards JB, Robinson TE, et al. Rats are the smart choice: rationale for a renewed focus on rats in behavioral genetics. *Neuropharmacology* (2014) 76(Pt B):250–8. doi:10.1016/j.neuropharm.2013.05.047
125. Bracci E, Panzeri S. Excitatory GABAergic effects in striatal projection neurons. *J Neurophysiol* (2006) 95(2):1285–90. doi:10.1152/jn.00598.2005
126. Hu M, Watson CJ, Kennedy RT, Becker JB. Estradiol attenuates the K+-induced increase in extracellular GABA in rat striatum. *Synapse* (2006) 59(2):122–4. doi:10.1002/syn.20221
127. Dorris DM, Cao J, Willett JA, Hauser CA, Meitzen J. Intrinsic excitability varies by sex in pre-pubertal striatal medium spiny neurons. *J Neurophysiol* (2015) 113(3):720–9. doi:10.1152/jn.00687.2014
128. Bayless DW, Daniel JM. Sex differences in myelin-associated protein levels within and density of projections between the orbital frontal cortex and dorsal striatum of adult rats: implications for inhibitory control. *Neuroscience* (2015) 300:286–96. doi:10.1016/j.neuroscience.2015.05.029
129. Morissette M, Garcia-Segura LM, Belanger A, Di Paolo T. Changes of rat striatal neuronal membrane morphology and steroid content during the estrous cycle. *Neuroscience* (1992) 49(4):893–902. doi:10.1016/0306-4522(92)90365-9
130. Hille B. *Ion Channels of Excitable Membranes*. Sunderland, MA: Sinauer Associates (2001).
131. Ishikawa M, Mu P, Moyer JT, Wolf JA, Quock RM, Davies NM, et al. Homeostatic synapse-driven membrane plasticity in nucleus accumbens neurons. *J Neurosci* (2009) 29(18):5820–31. doi:10.1523/JNEUROSCI.5703-08.2009
132. Kourrich S, Thomas MJ. Similar neurons, opposite adaptations: psychostimulant experience differentially alters firing properties in accumbens core versus shell. *J Neurosci* (2009) 29(39):12275–83. doi:10.1523/JNEUROSCI.3028-09.2009
133. Mu P, Moyer JT, Ishikawa M, Zhang Y, Panksepp J, Sorg BA, et al. Exposure to cocaine dynamically regulates the intrinsic membrane excitability of nucleus accumbens neurons. *J Neurosci* (2010) 30(10):3689–99. doi:10.1523/JNEUROSCI.4063-09.2010
134. Zhang XF, Hu XT, White FJ. Whole-cell plasticity in cocaine withdrawal: reduced sodium currents in nucleus accumbens neurons. *J Neurosci* (1998) 18(1):488–98. doi:10.1523/JNEUROSCI.18-01-00488.1998
135. Gertler TS, Chan CS, Surmeier DJ. Dichotomous anatomical properties of adult striatal medium spiny neurons. *J Neurosci* (2008) 28(43):10814–24. doi:10.1523/JNEUROSCI.2660-08.2008
136. Planert H, Berger TK, Silberberg G. Membrane properties of striatal direct and indirect pathway neurons in mouse and rat slices and their modulation by dopamine. *PLoS One* (2013) 8(3):e57054. doi:10.1371/journal.pone.0057054
137. Otaka M, Ishikawa M, Lee BR, Liu L, Neumann PA, Cui R, et al. Exposure to cocaine regulates inhibitory synaptic transmission in the nucleus accumbens. *J Neurosci* (2013) 33(16):6753–8. doi:10.1523/JNEUROSCI.4577-12.2013
138. Schulz DJ. Plasticity and stability in neuronal output via changes in intrinsic excitability: it's what's inside that counts. *J Exp Biol* (2006) 209(Pt 24):4821–7. doi:10.1242/jeb.02567
139. Suska A, Lee BR, Huang YH, Dong Y, Schluter OM. Selective presynaptic enhancement of the prefrontal cortex to nucleus accumbens pathway by cocaine. *Proc Natl Acad Sci U S A* (2013) 110(2):713–8. doi:10.1073/pnas.1206287110
140. Zakon HH. The effects of steroid hormones on electrical activity of excitable cells. *Trends Neurosci* (1998) 21(5):202–7. doi:10.1016/S0166-2236(97)01209-5
141. Cooke BM. Synaptic reorganisation of the medial amygdala during puberty. *J Neuroendocrinol* (2011) 23(1):65–73. doi:10.1111/j.1365-2826.2010.02075.x
142. Cooke BM, Woolley CS. Effects of prepubertal gonadectomy on a male-typical behavior and excitatory synaptic transmission in the amygdala. *Dev Neurobiol* (2009) 69(2–3):141–52. doi:10.1002/dneu.20688
143. Andersen SL, Rutstein M, Benzo JM, Hostetter JC, Teicher MH. Sex differences in dopamine receptor overproduction and elimination. *Neuroreport* (1997) 8(6):1495–8. doi:10.1097/00001756-199704140-00034
144. Andersen SL, Thompson AP, Krenzel E, Teicher MH. Pubertal changes in gonadal hormones do not underlie adolescent dopamine receptor overproduction. *Psychoneuroendocrinology* (2002) 27(6):683–91. doi:10.1016/S0306-4530(01)00069-5
145. Woolley CS. Acute effects of estrogen on neuronal physiology. *Annu Rev Pharmacol Toxicol* (2007) 47:657–80. doi:10.1146/annurev.pharmtox.47.120505.105219
146. Wu WW, Adelman JP, Maylie J. Ovarian hormone deficiency reduces intrinsic excitability and abolishes acute estrogen sensitivity in hippocampal CA1 pyramidal neurons. *J Neurosci* (2011) 31(7):2638–48. doi:10.1523/JNEUROSCI.6081-10.2011
147. Joel D, McCarthy MM. Incorporating sex as a biological variable in neuropsychiatric research: where are we now and where should we be? *Neuropsychopharmacology* (2017) 42(2):379–85. doi:10.1038/npp.2016.79
148. Cahill L. Why sex matters for neuroscience. *Nat Rev Neurosci* (2006) 7(6):477–84. doi:10.1038/nrn1909

7

Secretoneurin A Directly Regulates the Proteome of Goldfish Radial Glial Cells *In Vitro*

Dillon F. Da Fonte[1], Chris J. Martyniuk[2], Lei Xing[1†] and Vance L. Trudeau[1*]

[1] Department of Biology, University of Ottawa, Ottawa, ON, Canada, [2] Department of Physiological Sciences, College of Veterinary Medicine, UF Genetics Institute, University of Florida, Gainesville, FL, United States

***Correspondence:**
Vance L. Trudeau
trudeauv@uottawa.ca

Radial glial cells (RGCs) are the main macroglia in the teleost brain and have established roles in neurogenesis and neurosteroidogenesis. They are the only brain cell type expressing aromatase B (*cyp19a1b*), the enzyme that synthesizes estrogens from androgen precursors. There are few studies on the regulation of RGC functions, but our previous investigations demonstrated that dopamine stimulates *cyp19a1b* expression in goldfish RGCs, while secretoneurin A (SNa) inhibits the expression of this enzyme. Here, we determine the range of proteins and cellular processes responsive to SNa treatments in these steroidogenic cells. The focus here is on SNa, because this peptide is derived from selective processing of secretogranin II in magnocellular cells embedded within the RGC-rich preoptic nucleus. Primary cultures of RGCs were treated (24 h) with 10, 100, or 1,000 nM SNa. By using isobaric tagging for relative and absolute quantitation and a Hybrid Quadrupole Obritrap Mass Spectrometry system, a total of 1,363 unique proteins were identified in RGCs, and 609 proteins were significantly regulated by SNa at one or more concentrations. Proteins that showed differential expression with all three concentrations of SNa included H1 histone, glutamyl-prolyl-tRNA synthetase, Rho GDP dissociation inhibitor γ, vimentin A2, and small nuclear ribonucleoprotein-associated protein. At 10, 100, and 1,000 nM SNa, there were 5, 195, and 489 proteins that were downregulated, respectively, whereas the number of upregulated proteins were 72, 44, and 51, respectively. Subnetwork enrichment analysis of differentially regulated proteins revealed that processes such as actin organization, cytoskeleton organization and biogenesis, apoptosis, mRNA processing, RNA splicing, translation, cell growth, and proliferation are regulated by SNa based on the proteomic response. Moreover, we observed that, at the low concentration of SNa, there was an increase in the abundance of proteins involved in cell growth, proliferation, and migration, whereas higher concentration of SNa appeared to downregulate proteins involved in these processes, indicating a dose-dependent proteome response. At the highest concentration of SNa, proteins linked to the etiology of diseases of the central nervous system (brain injuries, Alzheimer disease, Parkinson's disease, cerebral infraction, brain ischemia) were also differentially regulated. These data implicate SNa in the control of cell proliferation and neurogenesis.

Keywords: secretogranin II, secretoneurin, radial glial cells, aromatase, neurogenesis

INTRODUCTION

Radial glial cells (RGCs) are a macroglial subtype present during central nervous system (CNS) development of all vertebrates and are characterized by their bipolar morphology (1) and stem-like progenitor properties (2). The cell bodies of radial glia line the brain ventricles and have an elongated radial fiber terminating on the walls of blood vessels or at the pial surface with end feet (3). Due to this unique morphology, their radial processes are used as scaffolds for the migration of newborn neurons (4, 5). As stem-like cells, RGCs are capable of undergoing neurogenesis and/or gliogenesis to produce neurons or other glial cells (6). RGC populations are transient in mammals as they differentiate into astrocytes at the end of cortical development. In contrast, RGCs are abundant throughout the adult brain in teleost fish, supporting the ability for unsurpassed high levels of neurogenesis and regeneration (7, 8). In addition, teleost RGCs express various steroidogenic enzymes (9, 10) and are the exclusive cell type to express the estrogen-synthesizing enzyme, aromatase B (*cyp19a1b*) (11–13), and thus, they are neuroendocrine cells that produce neuroestrogens and other steroids in the CNS. Although RGCs in fish have established roles in neurogenesis and neurosteroidogenesis, little is known about other functions of these cells and the factors that regulate them. As RGCs are the main macroglia in fish CNS (14), they share close interactions with different neurons and can express neurotransmitters, neuropeptides, and hormone receptors (15). Therefore, these cells may be under functional control through neuronal–glial interactions.

We previously reported on the close neuroanatomical relationship between the soma of secretoneurin A (SNa)-immunoreactive magnocellular preoptic neurons and RGCs along the third ventricle in goldfish (16). The neuropeptide SN is generated from endoproteolytic processing of its precursor protein secretogranin II (SgII) and has well-established functions in endocrine, nervous, and immune systems (17, 18). Currently, there are two known SgII paralogs, SgIIa and SgIIb, that likely arose from the genome duplication events in teleost fish, and these paralogs produce SNa and SNb peptides, respectively (19). Both *in vivo* and *in vitro*, SNa reduces *cyp19a1b* mRNA levels in goldfish RGCs, implicating SNa in the control of neuroestrogen production (16). Furthermore, data from transcriptome sequencing of cultured goldfish RGCs revealed that gene networks related to immune responses and CNS physiology were responsive to 1,000 nM SNa (15). Altogether, these anatomical and transcriptomic data propose that SNa is a regulator of RGC functions. The objectives of this study were to (1) characterize the RGC proteome, (2) determine the differentially regulated proteins over a range of SNa concentrations, and (3) identify protein networks responsive to SNa regulation.

MATERIALS AND METHODS

Experimental Animals

All procedures were approved by the University of Ottawa Protocol Review Committee and followed standard Canadian Council on Animal Care guidelines on the use of animals in research. Common adult female goldfish (*Carassius auratus*) were purchased from a commercial supplier (Mt. Parnell Fisheries Inc., Mercersburg, PA, USA) and allowed to acclimate for at least 3 weeks prior to experimentation. Goldfish were maintained at 18°C under a stimulated natural photoperiod and fed standard flaked goldfish food. Sexually mature female goldfish (18–35 g) were anesthetized using 3-aminobenzoic acid ethyl ester (MS222) for all handling and dissection procedures.

Cell Culture and Exposure

The direct effects of SNa on RGCs were tested using a previously established and validated cell culture method (20). In short, the hypothalamus and telencephalon were dissected from female goldfish and rinsed twice with Hanks Balanced Salt Solution (HBSS; 400 mg KCl, 600 mg KH_2PO_4, 350 mg $NaHCO_3$, 8 g NaCl, 48 mg Na_2HPO_4, and 1 g D-Glucose in 1 L ddH_2O) with Antibiotic-Antimycotic solution (Gibco) and minced into small explants. RGCs were dissociated with trypsin (0.25%; Gibco) and cultured in Leibovitz's L-15 medium (Gibco) with 15% fetal bovine serum (Gibco) and Antibiotic-Antimycotic solution. Cell culture medium was changed 4–7 days after isolation and then once a week thereafter. RGCs were subcultured by trypsinization (0.125%) for three passages and then used for experimentation. Goldfish SNa was synthesized as reported previously (21). Stock solutions of synthetic goldfish SNa peptide were made in water and stored at −20°C until use. Aliquots were thawed on ice then diluted to desired concentrations in serum-free media. Cells were exposed for 24 h to one of the three concentrations of goldfish SNa or the water control.

Protein Extraction, Isobaric Tagging for Relative and Absolute Quantitation (iTRAQ), and LC-MS/MS

Proteins were extracted as previously described (22) prior to labeling and dissolved in denaturant buffer [0.1% SDS (w/v)] and dissolution buffer (0.5 M triethylammonium bicarbonate, pH 8.5) in the iTRAQ Reagents 8-plex kit (AB Sciex Inc., Foster City, CA, USA). For each sample, 100 μg of protein were reduced, alkylated, trypsin-digested, and labeled according to the manufacturer's instructions (AB Sciex Inc.). Two 8-plex iTRAQ labeling reactions were conducted, each with two biological replicates. Peptides from the control group were labeled with either iTRAQ tags 113 or 114. The three treatments were labeled as follows: 10 nM SNa (115, 116), 100 nM SNa (117, 118), and 1,000 nM SNa (119, 121). This labeling scheme was repeated in a second experiment, so the data are derived from a sample size of $n = 4$ biological replicates per group.

Labeled peptides were combined for each iTRAQ experiment, desalted with C18-solid phase extraction, and dissolved in strong cation exchange solvent A [25% (v/v) acetonitrile, 10 mM ammonium formate, and 0.1% (v/v) formic acid, pH 2.8]. The peptides were fractionated using an Agilent HPLC 1260 with a polysulfoethyl A column (2.1 mm × 100 mm, 5 μm, 300 Å; PolyLC, Columbia, MD, USA). Peptides were eluted with a linear gradient of 0–20% solvent B [2 5% (v/v) acetonitrile and 500 mM ammonium formate, pH 6.8] over 50 min., followed by ramping up to 100% solvent B in 5 min. The absorbance at 280 nm was monitored, and a total of 14 fractions were collected. The fractions were lyophilized and resuspended in LC solvent A [0.1% formic acid in 97% water (v/v), 3% acetonitrile (v/v)]. A hybrid quadrupole Orbitrap (Q Exactive) MS system (Thermo Fisher Scientific) was used with high-energy collision dissociation in each MS and MS/MS cycle. The MS system was interfaced with an automated Easy-nLC 1000 system (Thermo Fisher Scientific). Each sample fraction was loaded onto an Acclaim Pepmap 100 pre-column (20 mm × 75 μm; 3 μm-C18) and separated using a PepMap RSLC analytical column (250 mm × 75 μm; 2 μm-C18) at a flow rate at 350 nL/min during a linear gradient from solvent A [0.1% formic acid (v/v)] to 25% solvent B [0.1% formic acid (v/v) and 99.9% acetonitrile (v/v)] for 80 min and to 100% solvent B for an additional 15 min.

The raw MS/MS data files were processed by a thorough database searching approach considering biological modification and amino acid substitution against the National Center for Biotechnology Information Cyprinidae database (downloaded on March 23, 2016) using the ProteinPilot v4.5 with the Fraglet and Taglet searches under ParagonTM algorithm (23). The following parameters were considered for all the searching: fixed modification of methylmethane thiosulfonate-labeled cysteine, fixed iTRAQ modification of amine groups in the *N*-terminus, lysine, and variable iTRAQ modifications of tyrosine. The MS/MS spectra that (1) were unique to a specific protein and (2) showed a sum of the signal-to-noise ratios for all the peak pairs greater than 9 were used for quantification. A protein was quantified if it was represented with at least three unique spectra in at least two of the biological replicates, along with a Fisher's combined probability of <0.05 and a fold change of <0.5 or >1.5.

Gene Ontology (GO) and Pathway Analysis

Gene ontology terms were assigned using protein annotation through evolutionary relationships to classify all proteins identified in RGC cultures (24). GO categories for biological processes, molecular functions, cellular components, protein classes, and pathways were used to identify the distribution of proteins within each GO category. Pathway Studio 9.0 (Elsevier) and ResNet 10.0 were used to build a protein interaction network for SNa effects in RGCs. Official gene symbols were manually retrieved using Gene Cards (http://www.genecards.org) to map proteins into Pathway Studio. The number of proteins that successfully mapped to Pathway Studios using Name + Alias was as follows: 10 nM SNa = 99, 100 nM SNa = 231, and 1,000 nM SNa = 499. Interaction networks were based on expression, binding, and regulatory interactions in the database and were constructed using direct connections with one neighbor. Subnetwork enrichment analysis (SNEA) for cell processes was performed in Pathway Studio to determine if differentially expressed proteins were related to specific biological functions. *P* value for gene seeds was set at < 0.05 and the criterion of >5 members per cell process or group was required for inclusion as a significantly regulated gene network.

RESULTS

Identification and GO Classification of RGC Proteins

A complete list of proteins (n = 1,363) that were identified in this study is provided in Table S1 in Supplementary Material. The annotated proteins were assigned GO terms and classified in three main GO categories: biological function, molecular function, and cellular component (**Figure 1**). A variety of biological functions were identified with 1,546 unique biological processes classified into 12 functional groups. The most represented biological functions included the categories of cellular process (438 proteins), metabolic process (414), and cellular component organization or biogenesis (199). Other important biological function allocations included the categories of developmental process (86 proteins), response to stimulus (65), immune system process (30), and biological adhesion (11). A broad array of 893 molecular functions was categorized into 9 functional groups. The molecular functions most represented in the RGC proteome were binding (334 proteins), catalytic (299), structural molecule (177), and transporter (38) activities. When organized by cellular component, RGC proteins were enriched in the categories of cell part (379 proteins), organelle (238), and macromolecular complex (165). Most proteins identified in RGCs were further classified into protein class, with nucleic acid binding (187 proteins), cytoskeletal proteins (147), and enzyme molecular (90) being the most represented classes detected in RGCs (**Figure 2**). Finally, a total of 535 proteins were represented by 102 pathways. The top 25 represented pathway ontologies are shown in **Table 1**. Proteins were most enriched in relation to Parkinson disease (31 proteins), integrin signaling pathway (28), ubiquitin proteasome pathway (26), cytoskeletal regulation by Rho GTPase (26), Huntington disease (25), and inflammation mediate by chemokine and cytokine signaling (24) (**Table 1**). Comparison of the assigned pathway ontologies identified by transcriptomics (15) and proteomics reveals high similarity. For example, of the top 25 pathways from transcriptomic and proteomic datasets, 18 (72%) were identical (**Table 1**). A full list of GO classifications can be found in Table S2 in Supplementary Material.

Quantitative Proteomic Responses in Radial Glia to SNa *In Vitro*

A total of 609 proteins differed in abundance following SNa treatment (**Figure 3**), and there were 17 unique expression patterns recognized within the data set (**Table 2**). At 10, 100, and 1,000 nM SNa, there were 5, 195, and 489 downregulated proteins, respectively, whereas the numbers of upregulated proteins were 72, 44, and 51, respectively. There were more downregulated proteins observed as the concentration of SNa increased in the cultures. The overlap of the differentially regulated proteins between concentrations is shown in **Figure 4**. A total of 10 common proteins were regulated in all three concentrations, and some examples include H1 histone, glutamyl-prolyl-tRNA synthetase, Rho GDP dissociation inhibitor γ, vimentin A2, and small nuclear ribonucleoprotein-associated protein. **Table 3** highlights the top

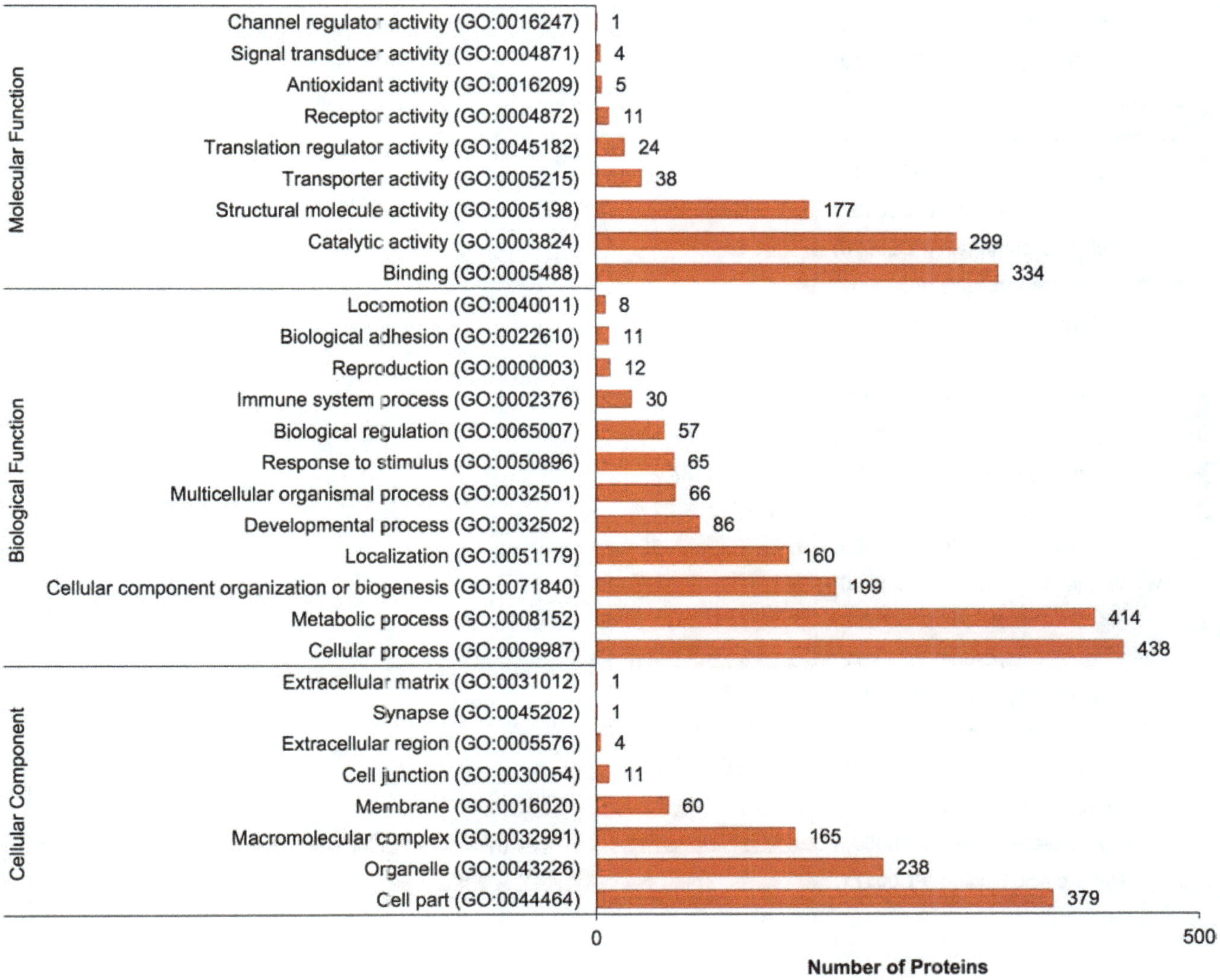

FIGURE 1 | Gene ontology classification of *Carassius auratus* radial glial cell (RGC) proteins into molecular function, biological function, and cellular component categories. The number of proteins ascribed to each classification, along with accession number, is provided.

20 proteins that were most regulated by each concentration of SNa based on the *P* value.

Identifying Cellular Processes Affected by SNa Using SNEA

The major objective of this study is to identify cellular processes that were responsive to SNa through the analysis of significantly regulated RGC proteins. Processes that were regulated by all concentrations of SNa included actin organization, cytoskeleton organization and biogenesis, apoptosis, mRNA processing, RNA splicing, translation, cell growth, and proliferation. At the low 10 nM SNa dose, proteins that were increased are related to processes such as blood vessel development, actin organization, cytoskeleton organization and biogenesis, cell proliferation, growth, and migration (**Figure 5**). The proteins affected by 100 nM SNa control similar processes such as cell proliferation and growth; however, proteins involved in these processes were downregulated compared to 10 nM SNa (**Figure 6.**). Similarly, 1,000 nM SNa treatment resulted in the downregulation of proteins related to cell processes that include actin organization, cytoskeleton organization and biogenesis, cell proliferation, growth, and migration. In addition, protein responses at 1,000 nM SNa suggested enrichment of processes related to neurite outgrowth and nerve fiber regeneration (**Figure 7A**) and tight and gap junction assembly (**Figure 7B**). Both 100 and 1,000 nM SNa caused changes in proteins involved in cell cycle, mitochondrial function (mitochondrial membrane permeability, depolarization, damage), and RNA processing (RNA metabolism, processing, splicing).

In addition, SNEA was used to determine if regulated proteins were known to be associated with human diseases. Major themes in disease networks that were associated with proteins altered by 1,000 nM SNa included diseases of the CNS (brain

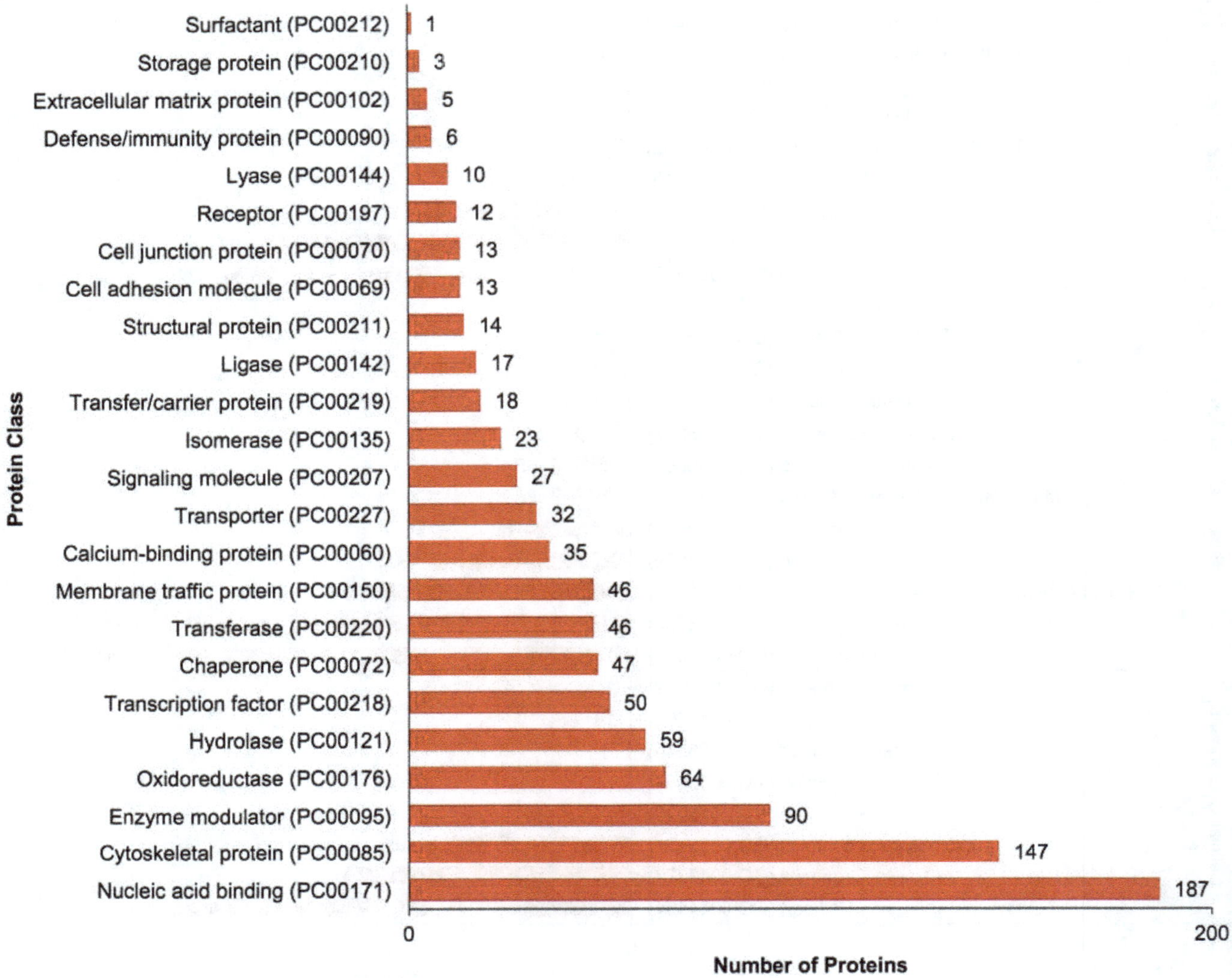

FIGURE 2 | Gene ontology classification of *Carassius auratus* radial glial cell (RGC) proteins by protein class. The number of proteins ascribed to each classification, along with accession number, is provided.

injuries, Alzheimer disease, Parkinson disease, cerebral infraction, brain ischemia), diseases of the cardiovascular system (heart failure, cardiomyopathies, heart injury, cardiac hypertrophy), and neoplasms (lung, ovarian, colorectal, pancreatic, prostatic, breast, endometrial). An example of a network associated with Alzheimer, Parkinson, and neurodegenerative diseases is shown in **Figure 8**. All the identified subnetworks are presented in Table S3 in Supplementary Material.

DISCUSSION

This study used quantitative proteomics to determine the response of RGCs to SNa in an *in vitro* cell culture system. This effort to characterize the goldfish RGC proteome identified 1,363 unique proteins and adds to those previously reported (25). A total of 609 proteins showed changes in relative abundance across three concentrations of SNa, with higher doses eliciting a greater suppressive response in protein abundance. In each concentration, SNa regulated proteins that have a role in cell processes including actin organization, cell growth, proliferation, and migration. Previous research on the effects of SN in the CNS focused on neurons (26), so our work on the effects of SNa on the RGC transcriptome (15) and proteome (current study) is the first to characterize the effects of SNa in any glial cell type.

Assigning pathway ontologies to the identified proteins revealed many relationships to the immune system, including chemokine and cytokine signaling, T cell activation, TGFβ signaling, toll receptor signaling pathway, B cell activation, and interleukin signaling pathway. While the role of RGCs *per se* in neuroinflammation is not well studied, both the transcriptomic and proteomic data support the hypothesis that RGCs contribute to immune-related functions in fish. In the mammalian CNS, this is more typically associated with astrocytes, which possess both pro- and anti-inflammatory functions, depending on the mode of injury (27). In fish brain, RGCs are the main macroglia due to the lack of typical stellate

TABLE 1 | Top 25 pathway ontologies associated with *Carassius auratus* RGC proteins based on number of protein identified in each pathway.

Pathway name	Pathway accession	# of proteins identified
Parkinson disease[a]	P00049	31
Integrin signaling pathway[a]	P00034	28
Ubiquitin proteasome pathway	P00060	26
Cytoskeletal regulation by Rho GTPase[a]	P00016	26
Huntington disease[a]	P00029	25
Inflammation mediated by chemokine and cytokine signaling pathway[a]	P00031	24
FGF signaling pathway[a]	P00021	15
EGF receptor signaling pathway[a]	P00018	15
CCKR signaling map[a]	P06959	14
Wnt signaling pathway[a]	P00057	14
Angiogenesis[a]	P00005	13
Gonadotropin-releasing hormone receptor pathway[a]	P06664	12
Cadherin signaling pathway[a]	P00012	12
Alzheimer disease-presenilin pathway[a]	P00004	10
T cell activation[a]	P00053	10
Nicotinic acetylcholine receptor signaling pathway	P00044	10
Ras pathway[a]	P04393	10
Glycolysis	P00024	10
Cell cycle	P00013	10
Apoptosis signaling pathway[a]	P00006	8
TGF-beta signaling pathway[a]	P00052	7
De novo purine biosynthesis	P02738	7
PDGF signaling pathway[a]	P00047	7
Dopamine receptor-mediated signaling pathway	P05912	7
Axon guidance mediated by Slit/Robo	P00008	6

[a]These pathways were also identified in the de novo transcriptome assembly data in Ref. (15).

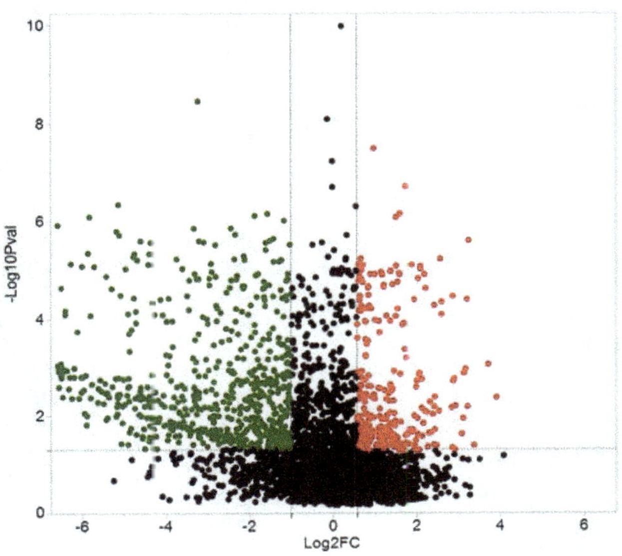

FIGURE 3 | Volcano plots for protein expression in *Carassius auratus* radial glial cells (RGCs) treated with three concentrations of secretoneurin A. Significantly regulated proteins were determined using a cut off of >1.5 or <0.5 and $P < 0.05$. Red and green dots represent proteins that are upregulated and downregulated, respectively.

TABLE 2 | Expression patterns of the differentially regulated proteins in *Carassius auratus* RGCs treated with various concentrations of SNa compared to control.

Expression pattern	10 nM	100 nM	1000 nM	Number of protein IDs
I	↑	↑	↑	5
II	↑	↑	–	9
III	↑	–	↑	3
IV	↑	–	–	31
V	↑	–	↓	20
VI	↑	↓	↓	4
VII	–	↑	↑	11
VIII	–	↑	–	18
IX	–	↑	↓	1
X	–	–	↑	25
XI	–	–	–	757
XII	–	–	↓	288
XIII	–	↓	↑	6
XIV	–	↓	–	7
XV	–	↓	↓	176
XVI	↓	–	–	3
XVII	↓	↓	↑	1
XVIII	↓	↓	–	1

RGC, radial glial cell.

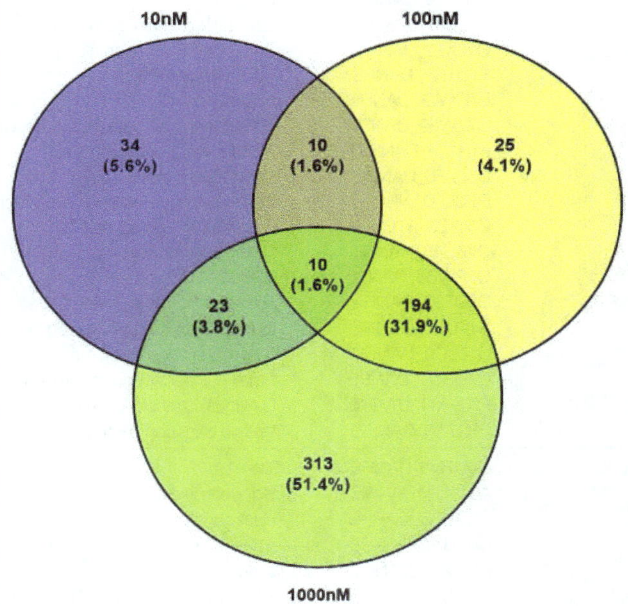

FIGURE 4 | Venn diagram showing the overlap of differentially expressed proteins following secretoneurin A (10–1,000 nM) treatment in *Carassius auratus* radial glial cells.

astrocytes, thus RGCs likely share some functions with mammalian astrocytes in brain homeostasis (14). In addition, many neurotransmitter (5-HT, DA, ACh, glutamate, GABA, histamine) and hormone (thyrotrophin-release hormone, oxytocin, corticotropin-releasing factor) receptor-mediated pathways were identified, providing further evidence that neuronal–glial interactions are important in the control of this cell type. Our proteomic data show the presence of several well-characterized RGC markers including brain lipid binding protein (BLBP),

TABLE 3 | Top 20 proteins identified by iTRAQ as different in abundance among groups in *Carassius auratus* RGCs treated with one of three concentrations of SNa.

Concentration (nM)	Accession	Protein	% coverage protein ID	Fold change	*P* value
10	A7MCL7_DANRE	Cystatin 14a, tandem duplicate 2	47	3.34	2.02E−07
	Q6DN21_CARAU	Calmodulin long form	99.33	5.94	6.11E−06
	A0A0C5Q0E9_MEGAM	Fibroblast growth factor receptor 1b	11.62	1.54	7.76E−06
	E7F1X7_DANRE	Serine and arginine repetitive matrix 1	33.69	1.65	8.06E−06
	VIM2_CARAU	Vimentin A2	44.03	3.72	8.07E−06
	F1QNJ3_DANRE	Testin LIM domain protein	25.51	4.29	8.58E−06
	F1Q5X0_DANRE	Synaptosome associated protein 29 kDa	44.74	4.29	9.73E−06
	B0UXN7_DANRE	C-Abl oncogene 2, non-receptor tyrosine kinase	20.18	3.00	1.19E−05
	C0LYZ3_9TELE	High-mobility group box 1	55.44	2.02	1.23E−05
	A0A0R4IMX7_DANRE	SH3 and PX domains 2B	25.68	1.87	1.23E−05
	X1WGZ7_DANRE	Glutamyl-prolyl-tRNA synthetase	25.03	4.57	1.25E−05
	E7F354_DANRE	Tyrosine 3-monooxygenase/tryptophan 5-monooxygenase	57.89	3.03	1.25E−05
	Q802W6_DANRE	Arhgdia protein	39.41	2.70	2.01E−05
	Q6Y3R4_CARAU	H1 histone	34.03	4.66	2.43E−05
	B3DGP9_DANRE	Protein tyrosine kinase 2aa	11.29	1.58	3.44E−05
	Q6NYA1_DANRE	Heterogeneous nuclear ribonucleoprotein A/Bb	36.25	7.30	3.53E−05
	Q802Y1_DANRE	Serine/arginine-rich splicing factor 4	39.34	1.57	4.18E−05
	143BA_DANRE	Tyrosine 3-monooxygenase/tryptophan 5-monooxygenase activation protein beta	77.46	0.15	6.06E−05
	RBM8A_DANRE	RNA-binding protein 8A	22.99	1.90	6.22E−05
	F1QG80_DANRE	Ribosomal protein L22	34.75	1.60	7.03E−05
100	Q5U7N6_DANRE	Talin 1	18.95	0.45	9.82E−07
	Q4U0S2_DANRE	Myosin, heavy chain 11a, smooth muscle	24.77	0.49	3.08E−06
	E7FEK9_DANRE	Golgin A4	40.17	0.04	4.72E−06
	F1QIN6_DANRE	CAP-GLY domain containing linker protein 2	43.21	0.05	4.76E−06
	Q1LXT2_DANRE	Eukaryotic translation elongation factor 2a, tandem duplicate 1	26.11	1.60	5.96E−06
	F1QTN7_DANRE	Acidic leucine-rich nuclear phosphoprotein 32 family member A	27.38	0.13	7.51E−06
	E7EYW2_DANRE	Epsin 2	16.27	0.02	8.56E−06
	Q7ZW39_DANRE	Phosphoribosyl pyrophosphate synthetase 1A	22.33	0.08	9.34E−06
	F1R1J9_DANRE	AHNAK nucleoprotein	53.03	2.60	1.08E−05
	Q502F6_DANRE	Zgc:112271 protein	75.58	0.29	1.20E−05
	EIF3L_DANRE	Eukaryotic translation initiation factor 3 subunit L	22.57	0.28	1.30E−05
	C0LYZ3_9TELE	High-mobility group box 1	55.44	1.57	1.35E−05
	Q7ZU46_DANRE	Heat shock protein 4a	28.45	0.14	1.36E−05
	Q0PWB8_DANRE	PDZ and LIM domain 3b	32.7	0.11	1.51E−05
	Q9DF20_DANRE	Fragile X mental retardation 1	40.77	0.10	1.51E−05
	A4FUN5_DANRE	ISY1 splicing factor homolog	57.54	0.32	1.75E−05
	Q1LYC9_DANRE	Calpain, small subunit 1 a	47.69	0.35	2.04E−05
	Q6DRC1_DANRE	Small nuclear ribonucleoprotein F	48.84	0.17	2.90E−05
	F1QYM4_DANRE	Eukaryotic translation initiation factor 4 h	55.08	0.50	3.11E−05
	F1Q7S0_DANRE	Vesicle transport through interaction with t-SNAREs 1A	41.94	0.03	3.32E−05
1,000	Q5U7N6_DANRE	Talin 1	18.95	0.11	3.56E−09
	A0JMJ1_DANRE	Scinderin like a	33.06	0.03	4.60E−07
	Q0GC55_CARAU	Heat shock protein 47 kDa	24.81	0.34	7.06E−07
	Q6PBR5_DANRE	ATPase, H+ transporting, V1 subunit G isoform 1	80.51	3.05	7.17E−07
	F1RDG4_DANRE	si:dkey-222f2.1	55.02	0.28	7.79E−07
	Q7ZTZ6_DANRE	STIP1 homology and U-Box containing protein 1	34.51	0.02	8.19E−07
	F1R1J9_DANRE	AHNAK nucleoprotein	53.03	2.86	8.48E−07
	Q804W1_DANRE	Parvalbumin isoform 4b	45.87	0.01	1.22E−06
	F1QFN1_DANRE	ELKS/RAB6-interacting/CAST family member 1b	31.20	0.19	1.41E−06
	EIF3L_DANRE	Eukaryotic translation initiation factor 3 subunit L	22.57	0.10	1.42E−06
	Q7SXA1_DANRE	Ribosomal protein L26	55.17	0.03	1.63E−06
	E7F049_DANRE	Kinectin 1	26.47	0.20	1.90E−06
	Q7ZW39_DANRE	Phosphoribosyl pyrophosphate synthetase 1A	22.33	0.03	1.96E−06
	Q803A9_DANRE	DnaJ (Hsp40) homolog, subfamily B, member 11	11.94	0.38	2.32E−06
	A0A0R4I9C6_DANRE	Ubiquitin-fold modifier 1	73.33	0.35	2.55E−06
	B8JJS6_DANRE	Programmed cell death protein 10-B	32.86	9.51	2.58E−06
	F1QTN7_DANRE	Acidic leucine-rich nuclear phosphoprotein 32 family member A	27.38	0.04	2.58E−06
	A4FUN5_DANRE	ISY1 splicing factor homolog	57.54	0.11	2.59E−06
	Q502F6_DANRE	zgc:112271	75.58	0.12	2.74E−06
	Q9W792_DANRE	T-complex polypeptide 1	26.98	0.05	2.78E−06

All fold changes are relative to control.

iTRAQ, isobaric tagging for relative and absolute quantitation; RGC, Radial glial cell; SNa, secretoneurin A.

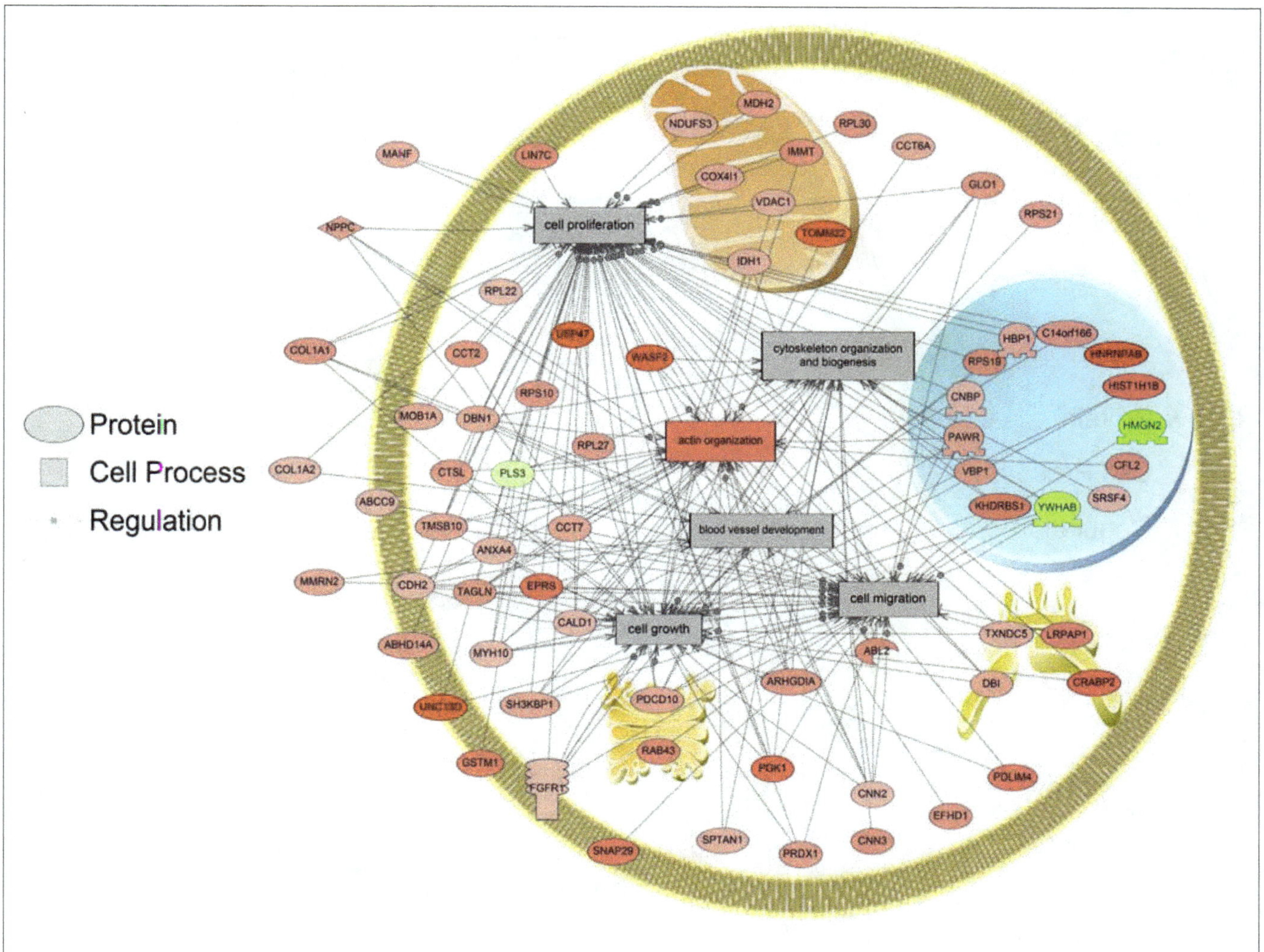

FIGURE 5 | Cellular processes of blood vessel development, actin organization, cytoskeleton organization and biogenesis, cell proliferation, growth, and migration were enriched in primary *Carassius auratus* radial glial cell culture after 10 nM secretoneurin A treatment ($P < 0.05$) based on the protein profiles. Red indicates that the protein is increased, and green indicates that the protein is decreased in abundance relative to the control group. All abbreviations are provided in Table S4 in Supplementary Material.

glial fibrillary acidic protein (GFAP), tight junction protein ZO-1, Sox2, and vimentin (28, 29), confirming that these cultured cells are indeed RGCs. Furthermore, analysis of the differentially regulated proteins shows that SNa can regulate these classical protein markers of RGCs. At each concentration, SNa increased the expression of the intermediate filament protein vimentin. While vimentin is implicated in several glial processes, it has also been shown to be involved in the initial stages of neurite outgrowth in rat hippocampal neurons *in vitro* (30). However, the 1,000 nM SNa treatment decreased BLBP and ZO-1. These proteins are lost when RGCs differentiate into neurons. Moreover, SNa decreases the expression of aromatase B (*cyp19a1b*) in RGCs *in vivo* and *in vitro* in a dose-dependent manner (16). Taken together, these data suggest that SNa downregulates some of the genes related to the progenitor-like characteristics of this cell type.

A low dose of 10 nM SNa upregulated proteins known to be involved in processes of blood vessel development, actin organization, cytoskeleton organization and biogenesis, cell growth, migration, and proliferation. It has been previously established that SN can induce mouse angiogenesis and vasculogenesis (31, 32), which supports our data that 10 nM SNa increases the expression of proteins associated with blood vessel development. Mouse RGCs have been shown to regulate angiogenesis in the brain through their interactions with blood vessels (33). Since SNa can regulate proteins involved in blood vessel formation, this may control the function of RGCs to regulate angiogenesis. As a chemoattractant, SN has the ability to stimulate the migration of various cell types. SN can stimulate the migration of human monocytes both *in vivo* and *in vitro* at nanomolar concentrations (34). Similarly, SN induces eosinophil (35), dendritic cell (36), and fibroblast (37) chemotaxis. These studies indicate that the chemotactic activity of SN is dose dependent with maximal affects between 0.1 and 100 nM, and higher doses elicit an inhibitory affect. Interestingly, here, we report that proteins involved in cell migration are decreased by a high concentration of 1,000 nM

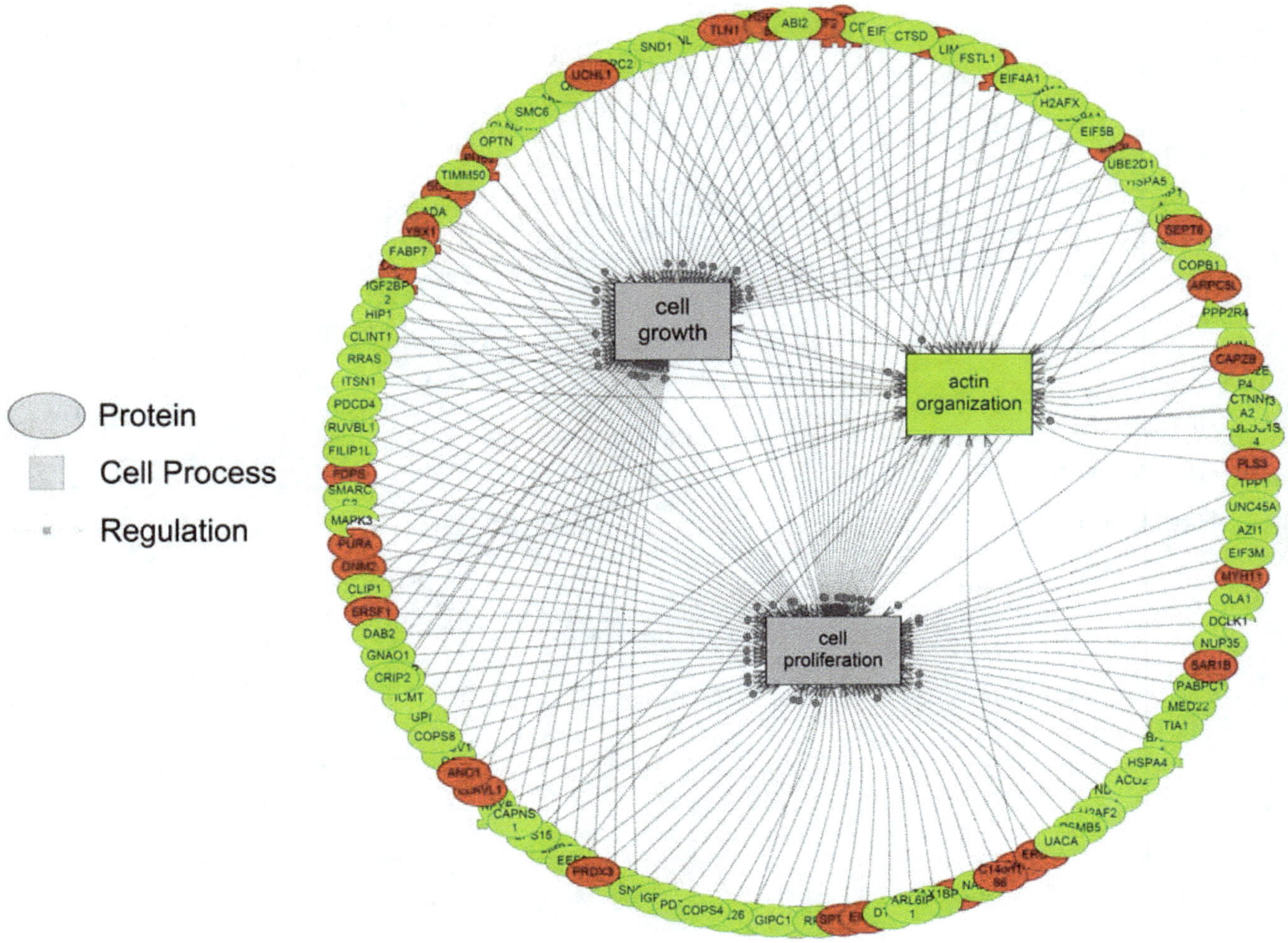

FIGURE 6 | Cellular processes of actin organization, cell proliferation, and growth were significantly enriched in primary *Carassius auratus* radial glial cell culture after 100 nM secretoneurin A treatment ($P < 0.05$) based on the protein profiles. Red indicates that the protein is increased, and green indicates that the protein is decreased in abundance relative to the control group. All abbreviations are provided in Table S4 in Supplementary Material.

SNa, indicating that SNa may regulate proteins involved in cell migration in a dose-dependent manner. In addition, both 100 and 1,000 nM concentrations regulated actin organization, cell growth, and cell proliferation protein networks; however, these higher concentrations decreased expression of proteins involved in these cell processes.

Following treatment with 1,000 nM SNa, subnetworks related to tight junction and gap junction assembly were enriched based on the proteins regulated. These cell processes were also identified by gene set enrichment analysis of transcriptomic data and were increased by SNa at the gene network level (15). Unlike the transcriptomic response, proteins involved in tight junction and gap junction assembly were downregulated, indicating that there is a complex regulation of the transcriptome and proteome that control these processes. Among the adherens junctions that were regulated by SNa, *N*-cadherin (cadherin 2) is a calcium-dependent adhesion molecule (38), and it is expressed to uphold RGC apical–basal polarity while anchoring adjacent RGCs to each other to create stem cell niches (39–42). *N*-cadherin controls mouse RGC function in neuronal migration and directing axon formation (42, 43). Furthermore, *N*-cadherin through its interactions with its effector β-catenin regulates RGC proliferation and differentiation (44–46). Reduction in mouse *N*-cadherin causes RGCs to migrate from the stem cell niche and stimulate neuronal differentiation (46). In our study, *N*-cadherin levels were increased at 10 nM and decreased at 1,000 nM SNa. Therefore, our data on *N*-cadherin expression indicate a role for SNa in the regulation of RGC-mediated neuronal migration, as well as RGC proliferation and differentiation.

Proteins involved in cellular processes such as neurite outgrowth and nerve fiber regeneration were also altered in abundance in RGCs following treatment with 1,000 nM SNa. The high dose of SNa significantly decreased the abundance of proteins known to be involved in neurite outgrowth. Although this cellular process was not enriched at lower doses, these data indicate that SNa has inhibitory effects on proteins that regulate neurite outgrowth. In contrast, SN stimulates neurite outgrowth in mouse cerebellar granule cells with a maximal concentration

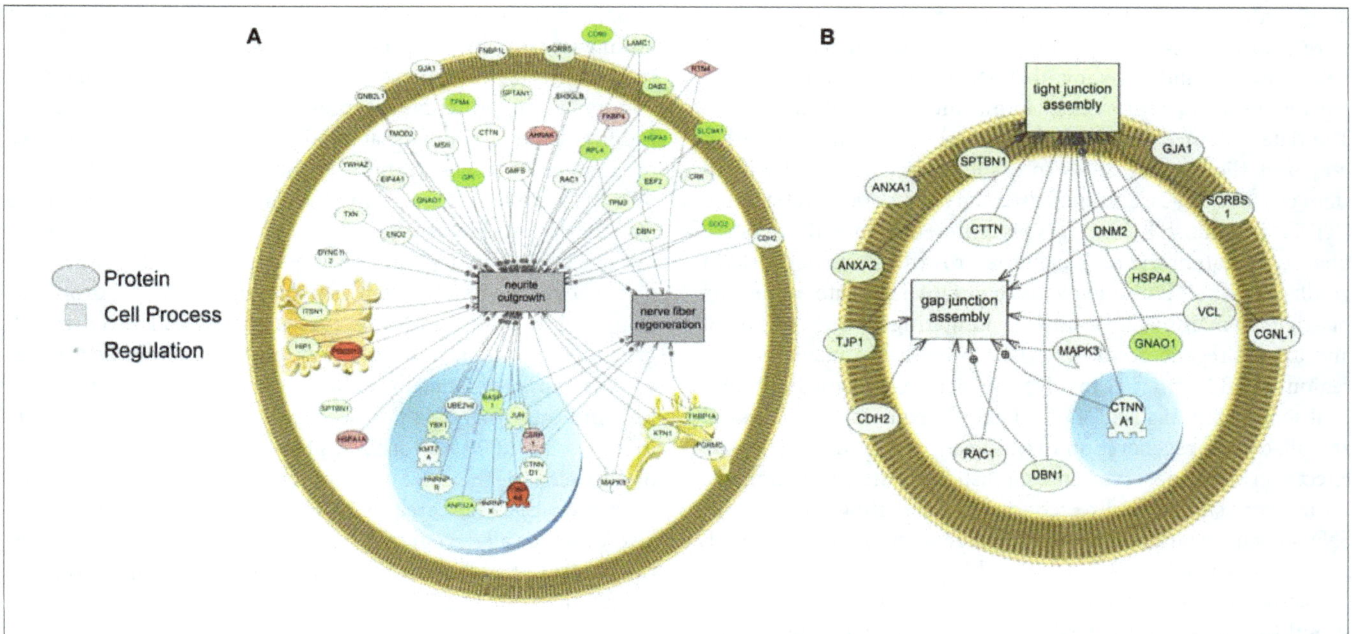

FIGURE 7 | Cellular processes of **(A)** neurite outgrowth and nerve fiber regeneration and **(B)** tight and gap junction assembly were enriched in primary *Carassius auratus* radial glial cell culture after 1,000 nM secretoneurin A treatment ($P < 0.05$) based on the protein profiles. Red indicates that the protein is increased, and green indicates that the protein is decreased in abundance relative to the control group. All abbreviations are provided in Table S4 in Supplementary Material.

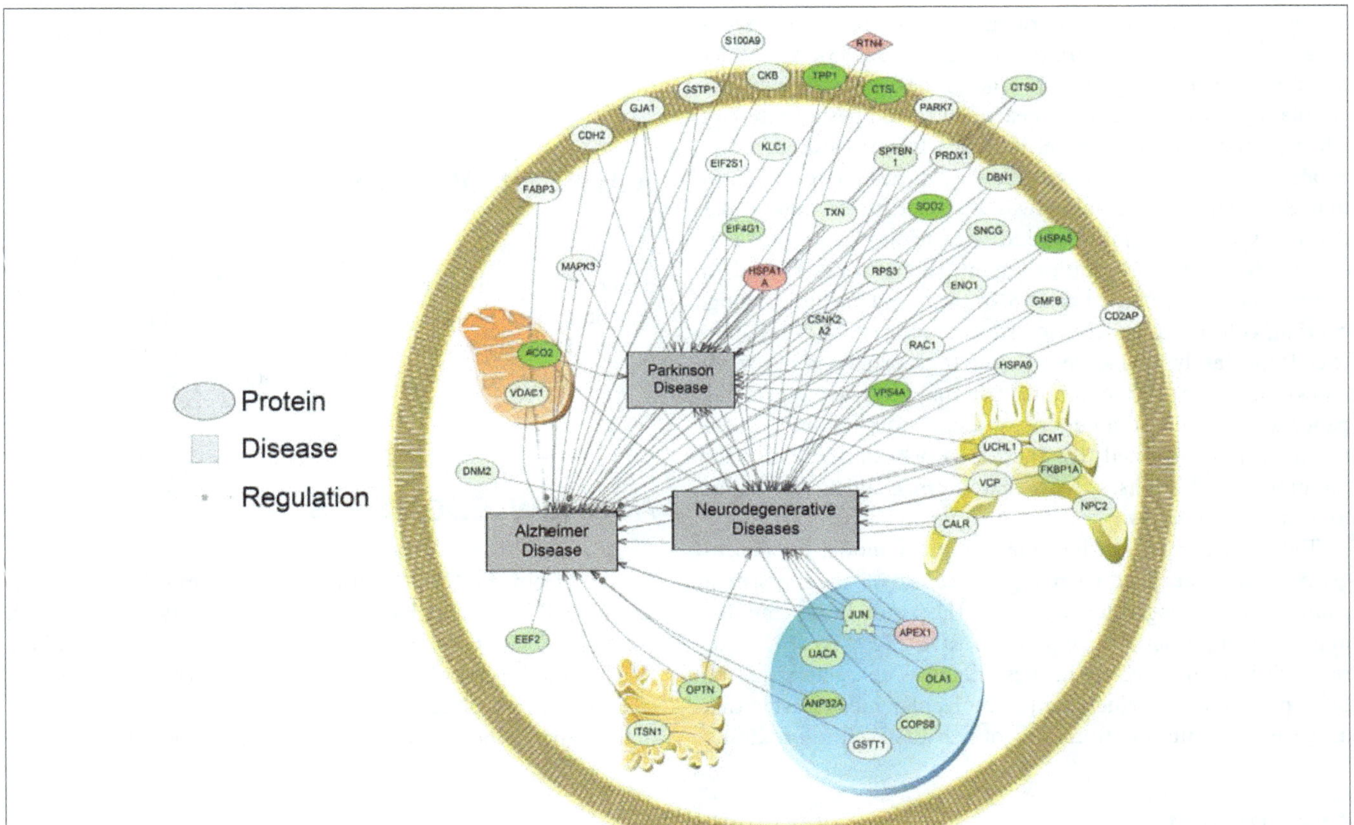

FIGURE 8 | Alzheimer, Parkinson, and neurodegenerative disease pathways were enriched in primary *Carassius auratus* radial glial cell culture after 1,000 nM secretoneurin A treatment ($P < 0.05$) based on the protein profiles. Red indicates that the protein is increased, and green indicates that the protein is decreased in abundance relative to the control group. All abbreviations are provided in Table S4 in Supplementary Material.

of 100 nM (47). Proteins related to nerve fiber regeneration were also decreased in goldfish RGCs exposed to 1,000 nM SNa. Previous findings show that SN treatment induces neural regeneration and neurogenesis in murine models of stroke (48). The data obtained from goldfish reveal protein networks that may underlie the role of SN in tissue repair and specifically in stem cell-like RGCs. SNa increased the expression of reticulon 4 (RTN4) in goldfish RGCs. RTN4 is represented in both the nerve fiber regeneration and the neurite outgrowth protein networks in goldfish RGCs. It is also known as a negative regulator of neurite plasticity in mammalian models by inhibiting neurite outgrowth and axonal regeneration (49–51). However, the major protein region of RTN4 that is involved in neurite growth inhibition is absent in zebrafish RTN4 (52) and is required for successful zebrafish axon regeneration (53). Therefore, given the opposite effects of RTN4 observed in zebrafish compared to mammals, future work should be directed toward elucidating the effects of SNa on neurite outgrowth and axon regeneration in fish through mechanisms involving RTN4.

Many proteome subnetworks were identified that correspond to diseases of the CNS and cardiovascular system along with several neoplasms. Protein networks in RGCs related to Alzheimer disease, Parkinson disease, brain ischemia, and brain injury were all regulated by 1,000 nM SNa. Changes in these networks are consistent with previous studies that have associated SN with these neuropathological conditions. SN is differentially regulated in brain ischemia (48, 54, 55), Alzheimer disease (56–58), and epilepsy (59, 60). It has been reported that circulating SN increases after heart failure and has a protective effect by reducing myocardial ischemia injury, cardiomyocyte apoptosis, and inducing angiogenesis (61, 62). Here, we show that SNa can regulate subnetworks related to cardiovascular diseases such as cardiomyopathies, heart injury, cardiomegaly, and heart failure. In addition, many subnetworks related to neoplasms were enriched after SNa treatment including lung, ovarian, colorectal, pancreatic, prostatic, breast, and endometrial. Importantly, SN has been shown to be expressed in several types of neuroendocrine tumors including prostate, lung, rectal, pancreatic, thyroid, duodenum, and appendix (63–65). Taken together, it is suggested that these networks underlie, in part, the molecular responses to SN that are mechanistically linked to these disease states.

The teleost brain has become a popular model for neurogenesis and neuroendocrinology because of the persistent abundance of progenitor RGCs in the adult brain and the high aromatase activity present in RGCs (29, 66, 67). Our research has implications in these fields as characterizing the RGC proteome can elucidate the molecular mechanisms that underlie these unique functions of fish RGCs. The proximity of SNa-immunoreactive magnocellular preoptic neurons with aromatase B/GFAP expressing RGCs prompted our efforts to characterize the effects of SNa on the transcriptome (15) and now the proteome of these multifunctional cells. For the first time, we show that the RGC proteome is responsive to nanomolar concentrations of SNa. Proteins regulated by SNa are implicated in many cell processes including those associated with blood vessel development, actin organization, cytoskeleton organization and biogenesis, neurite outgrowth, nerve fiber regeneration, cell growth, migration, and proliferation. At lower doses, SNa increased proteins involved in cell growth, migration, and proliferation, whereas higher doses of SNa downregulated proteins involved in these processes. This indicates that SNa has dose-dependent regulatory effects in RGCs. At 1,000 nM of SNa, proteins linked to the etiology of diseases of the CNS (brain injuries, Alzheimer disease, Parkinson disease, cerebral infraction, brain ischemia) were also differentially regulated. These data implicate that SNa in the control of pathways is important in cell proliferation and neurogenesis through direct actions on RGCs.

ETHICS STATEMENT

The study was carried out in accordance with the Canadian Council on Animal Care and approved by the University of Ottawa animal care and veterinary services.

AUTHOR CONTRIBUTIONS

DD performed experiments, analyzed the data, and wrote the paper. CM performed experiments, analyzed the data, and contributed to writing the paper. LX performed experiments, analyzed the data, and contributed to writing the paper. VT helped design experiments and co-wrote the paper.

ACKNOWLEDGMENTS

Funding from the NSERC Discovery program (VLT), NSERC-CGSM (DDF), and Michael Smith Foreign Study Award (DDF), University of Ottawa Research Chair in Neuroendocrinology (VLT), and the Ontario Trillium Scholarship (LX) are acknowledged with appreciation. Some of the results presented are part of the research thesis of DDF at the University of Ottawa (68).

REFERENCES

1. Schmechel DE, Rakic P. A Golgi study of radial glial cells in developing monkey telencephalon: morphogenesis and transformation into astrocytes. *Anat Embryol (Berl)* (1979) 156:115–52. doi:10.1007/BF00300010
2. Florio M, Huttner WB. Neural progenitors, neurogenesis and the evolution of the neocortex. *Development* (2014) 141:2182–94. doi:10.1242/dev.090571
3. Barry DS, Pakan JMP, McDermott KW. Radial glial cells: key organisers in CNS development. *Int J Biochem Cell Biol* (2014) 46:76–9. doi:10.1016/j.biocel.2013.11.013
4. Rakic P. Guidance of neurons migrating to the fetal monkey neocortex. *Brain Res* (1971) 33:471–6. doi:10.1016/0006-8993(71)90119-3
5. Silver J, Lorenz SE, Wahlsten D, Coughlin J. Axonal guidance during development of the great cerebral commissures: descriptive and experimental

studies, in vivo, on the role of preformed glial pathways. *J Comp Neurol* (1982) 210:10–29. doi:10.1002/cne.902100103

6. Radakovits R, Barros CS, Belvindrah R, Patton B, Müller U. Regulation of radial glial survival by signals from the meninges. *J Neurosci* (2009) 29:7694–705. doi:10.1523/JNEUROSCI.5537-08.2009
7. Almarestani L, Waters SM, Krause JE, Bennett GJ, Ribeiro-da-Silva A. Morphological characterization of spinal cord dorsal horn lamina I neurons projecting to the parabrachial nucleus in the rat. *J Comp Neurol* (2007) 504:287–97. doi:10.1002/cne.21410
8. Strobl-Mazzulla PH, Nuñez A, Pellegrini E, Gueguen M-M, Kah O, Somoza GM. Progenitor radial cells and neurogenesis in pejerrey fish forebrain. *Brain Behav Evol* (2010) 76:20–31. doi:10.1159/000316022
9. Diotel N, Do Rego J-L, Anglade I, Vaillant C, Pellegrini E, Gueguen M-M, et al. Activity and expression of steroidogenic enzymes in the brain of adult zebrafish. *Eur J Neurosci* (2011) 34:45–56. doi:10.1111/j.1460-9568.2011.07731.x
10. Xing L, Goswami M, Trudeau VL. Radial glial cell: critical functions and new perspective as a steroid synthetic cell. *Gen Comp Endocrinol* (2014) 203:181–5. doi:10.1016/j.ygcen.2014.03.010
11. Forlano PM, Deitcher DL, Myers DA, Bass AH. Anatomical distribution and cellular basis for high levels of aromatase activity in the brain of teleost fish: aromatase enzyme and mRNA expression identify glia as source. *J Neurosci* (2001) 21:8943–55.
12. Pellegrini E, Menuet A, Lethimonier C, Adrio F, Gueguen M-M, Tascon C, et al. Relationships between aromatase and estrogen receptors in the brain of teleost fish. *Gen Comp Endocrinol* (2005) 142:60–6. doi:10.1016/j.ygcen.2004.12.003
13. Tong S-K, Mouriec K, Kuo M-W, Pellegrini E, Gueguen M-M, Brion F, et al. A cyp19a1b-gfp (aromatase B) transgenic zebrafish line that expresses GFP in radial glial cells. *Genesis* (2009) 47:67–73. doi:10.1002/dvg.20459
14. Grupp L, Wolburg H, Mack AF. Astroglial structures in the zebrafish brain. *J Comp Neurol* (2010) 518:4277–87. doi:10.1002/cne.22481
15. Da Fonte DF, Martyniuk CJ, Xing L, Pelin A, Corradi N, Hu W, et al. Secretoneurin A regulates neurogenic and inflammatory transcriptional networks in goldfish (*Carassius auratus*) radial glia. *Sci Rep* (2017) 7:14930. doi:10.1038/s41598-017-14930-8
16. Da Fonte DF, Xing L, Mikwar M, Trudeau VL. Secretoneurin-A inhibits aromatase B (cyp19a1b) expression in female goldfish (*Carassius auratus*) radial glial cells. *Gen Comp Endocrinol* (2017) 257:106–12. doi:10.1016/j.ygcen.2017.04.014
17. Fischer-Colbrie R, Laslop A, Kirchmair R. Secretogranin II: molecular properties, regulation of biosynthesis and processing to the neuropeptide secretoneurin. *Prog Neurobiol* (1995) 46:49–70.
18. Zhao E, Zhang D, Basak A, Trudeau VL. New insights into granin-derived peptides: evolution and endocrine roles. *Gen Comp Endocrinol* (2009) 164:161–74. doi:10.1016/j.ygcen.2009.01.011
19. Zhao E, Hu H, Trudeau VL. Secretoneurin as a hormone regulator in the pituitary. *Regul Pept* (2010) 165:117–22. doi:10.1016/j.regpep.2009.11.019
20. Xing L, McDonald H, Da Fonte DF, Gutierrez-Villagomez JM, Trudeau VL. Dopamine D1 receptor activation regulates the expression of the estrogen synthesis gene aromatase B in radial glial cells. *Front Neurosci* (2015) 9:1–12. doi:10.3389/fnins.2015.00310
21. Zhao E, Basak A, Trudeau VL. Secretoneurin stimulates goldfish pituitary luteinizing hormone production. *Neuropeptides* (2006) 40:275–82. doi:10.1016/j.npep.2006.05.002
22. Koh J, Chen S, Zhu N, Yu F, Soltis PS, Soltis DE. Comparative proteomics of the recently and recurrently formed natural allopolyploid *Tragopogon mirus* (Asteraceae) and its parents. *New Phytol* (2012) 196:292–305. doi:10.1111/j.1469-8137.2012.04251.x
23. Shilov IV, Seymour SL, Patel AA, Loboda A, Tang WH, Keating SP, et al. The Paragon algorithm, a next generation search engine that uses sequence temperature values and feature probabilities to identify peptides from tandem mass spectra. *Mol Cell Proteomics* (2007) 6:1638–55. doi:10.1074/mcp.T600050-MCP200
24. Mi H, Poudel S, Muruganujan A, Casagrande JT, Thomas PD. PANTHER version 10: expanded protein families and functions, and analysis tools. *Nucleic Acids Res* (2016) 44:D336–42. doi:10.1093/nar/gkv1194
25. Xing L, Martyniuk CJ, Esau C, Da Fonte DF, Trudeau VL. Proteomic profiling reveals dopaminergic regulation of progenitor cell functions of goldfish radial glial cells in vitro. *J Proteomics* (2016) 144:123–32. doi:10.1016/j.jprot.2016.05.003
26. Troger J, Theurl M, Kirchmair R, Pasqua T, Tota B, Angelone T, et al. Granin-derived peptides. *Prog Neurobiol* (2017) 154:37–61. doi:10.1016/j.pneurobio.2017.04.003
27. Liddelow SA, Barres BA. Reactive astrocytes: production, function, and therapeutic potential. *Immunity* (2017) 46:957–67. doi:10.1016/j.immuni.2017.06.006
28. Mack AF, Tiedemann K. Cultures of astroglial cells derived from brain of adult cichlid fish. *J Neurosci Methods* (2013) 212:269–75. doi:10.1016/j.jneumeth.2012.11.003
29. Than-Trong E, Bally-Cuif L. Radial glia and neural progenitors in the adult zebrafish central nervous system. *Glia* (2015) 63:1406–28. doi:10.1002/glia.22856
30. Boyne LJ, Fischer I, Shea TB. Role of vimentin in early stages of neuritogenesis in cultured hippocampal neurons. *Int J Dev Neurosci* (1996) 14:739–48. doi:10.1016/S0736-5748(96)00053-6
31. Kirchmair R, Egger M, Walter DH, Eisterer W, Niederwanger A, Woell E, et al. Secretoneurin, an angiogenic neuropeptide, induces postnatal vasculogenesis. *Circulation* (2004) 110:1121–7. doi:10.1161/01.CIR.0000139884.81390.56
32. Kirchmair R, Gander R, Egger M, Hanley A, Silver M, Ritsch A, et al. The neuropeptide secretoneurin acts as a direct angiogenic cytokine in vitro and in vivo. *Circulation* (2004) 109:777–83. doi:10.1161/01.CIR.0000112574.07422.C1
33. Ma S, Kwon HJ, Johng H, Zang K, Huang Z. Radial glial neural progenitors regulate nascent brain vascular network stabilization via inhibition of Wnt signaling. *PLoS Biol* (2013) 11(1):e1001469. doi:10.1371/journal.pbio.1001469
34. Reinisch N, Kirchmair R, Kähler CM, Hogue-Angeletti R, Fischer-Colbrie R, Winkler H, et al. Attraction of human monocytes by the neuropeptide secretoneurin. *FEBS Lett* (1993) 334:41–4. doi:10.1016/0014-5793(93)81676-Q
35. Dunzendorfer S, Meierhofer C, Wiedermann CJ. Signaling in neuropeptide-induced migration of human eosinophils. *J Leukoc Biol* (1998) 64:828–34. doi:10.1002/jlb.64.6.828
36. Dunzendorfer S, Kaser A, Meierhofer C, Tilg H, Wiedermann CJ. Cutting edge: peripheral neuropeptides attract immature and arrest mature blood-derived dendritic cells. *J Immunol* (2001) 166:2167–72. doi:10.4049/jimmunol.166.4.2167
37. Kahler C, Bellmann R, Reinisch N, Schratzberger P, Gruber B, Wiedermann CJ. Stimulation of human skin fibroblast migration by the neuropeptide secretoneurin. *Eur J Pharmacol* (1996) 304(1–3):135–9.
38. Takeichi M. Morphogenetic roles of classic cadherins. *Curr Opin Cell Biol* (1995) 7:619–27. doi:10.1016/0955-0674(95)80102-2
39. Hatta K, Takagi S, Fujisawa H, Takeichi M. Spatial and temporal expression pattern of N-cadherin cell adhesion molecules correlated with morphogenetic processes of chicken embryos. *Dev Biol* (1987) 120:215–27. doi:10.1016/0012-1606(87)90119-9
40. Kadowaki M, Nakamura S, Machon O, Krauss S, Radice GL, Takeichi M. N-cadherin mediates cortical organization in the mouse brain. *Dev Biol* (2007) 304:22–33. doi:10.1016/j.ydbio.2006.12.014
41. Rago L, Beattie R, Taylor V, Winter J. MiR379-410 cluster miRNAs regulate neurogenesis and neuronal migration by fine-tuning N-cadherin. *EMBO J* (2014) 33:906–20. doi:10.1002/embj.201386591
42. Shikanai M, Nakajima K, Kawauchi T. N-cadherin regulates radial glial fiber-dependent migration of cortical locomoting neurons. *Commun Integr Biol* (2011) 4:326–30. doi:10.4161/cib.4.3.14886
43. Xu C, Funahashi Y, Watanabe T, Takano T, Nakamuta S, Namba T, et al. Radial glial cell-neuron interaction directs axon formation at the opposite side of the neuron from the contact site. *J Neurosci* (2015) 35:14517–32. doi:10.1523/JNEUROSCI.1266-15.2015
44. Machon O, Van Den Bout CJ, Backman M, Kemler R, Krauss S. Role of beta-catenin in the developing cortical and hippocampal neuroepithelium. *Neuroscience* (2003) 122:129–43. doi:10.1016/S0306-4522(03)00519-0
45. Woodhead GJ, Mutch CA, Olson EC, Chenn A. Cell-autonomous beta-catenin signaling regulates cortical precursor proliferation. *J Neurosci* (2006) 26:12620–30. doi:10.1523/JNEUROSCI.3180-06.2006
46. Zhang J, Woodhead GJ, Swaminathan SK, Noles SR, McQuinn ER, Pisarek AJ, et al. Cortical neural precursors inhibit their own differentiation via N-cadherin maintenance of beta-catenin signaling. *Dev Cell* (2010) 18:472–9. doi:10.1016/j.devcel.2009.12.025
47. Gasser MC, Berti I, Hauser KF, Fischer-Colbrie R, Saria A. Secretoneurin promotes pertussis toxin-sensitive neurite outgrowth in cerebellar granule cells. *J Neurochem* (2003) 85:662–9. doi:10.1046/j.1471-4159.2003.01677.x

48. Shyu W-C, Lin S-Z, Chiang M-F, Chen D-C, Su C-Y, Wang H-J, et al. Secretoneurin promotes neuroprotection and neuronal plasticity via the Jak2/Stat3 pathway in murine models of stroke. *J Clin Invest* (2008) 118:133–48. doi:10.1172/JCI32723
49. Chen MS, Huber AB, van der Haar ME, Frank M, Schnell L, Spillmann AA, et al. Nogo-A is a myelin-associated neurite outgrowth inhibitor and an antigen for monoclonal antibody IN-1. *Nature* (2000) 403:434–9. doi:10.1038/35000219
50. GrandPré T, Nakamura F, Vartanian T, Strittmatter SM. Identification of the Nogo inhibitor of axon regeneration as a reticulon protein. *Nature* (2000) 403:439–44. doi:10.1038/35000226
51. Oertle T, van der Haar ME, Bandtlow CE, Robeva A, Burfeind P, Buss A, et al. Nogo-A inhibits neurite outgrowth and cell spreading with three discrete regions. *J Neurosci* (2003) 23:5393–406.
52. Diekmann H, Klinger M, Oertle T, Heinz D, Pogoda HM, Schwab ME, et al. Analysis of the reticulon gene family demonstrates the absence of the neurite growth inhibitor Nogo-A in fish. *Mol Biol Evol* (2005) 22:1635–48. doi:10.1093/molbev/msi158
53. Welte C, Engel S, Stuermer CAO. Upregulation of the zebrafish Nogo-A homologue, Rtn4b, in retinal ganglion cells is functionally involved in axon regeneration. *Neural Dev* (2015) 10:6. doi:10.1186/s13064-015-0034-x
54. Hasslacher J, Lehner GF, Harler U, Beer R, Ulmer H, Kirchmair R, et al. Secretoneurin as a marker for hypoxic brain injury after cardiopulmonary resuscitation. *Intensive Care Med* (2014) 40:1518–27. doi:10.1007/s00134-014-3423-4
55. Martí E, Ferrer I, Blasi J. Differential regulation of chromogranin A, chromogranin B and secretoneurin protein expression after transient forebrain ischemia in the gerbil. *Acta Neuropathol* (2001) 101:159–66. doi:10.1007/s004010000280
56. Kaufmann WA, Barnas U, Humpel C, Nowakowski K, DeCol C, Gurka P, et al. Synaptic loss reflected by secretoneurin-like immunoreactivity in the human hippocampus in Alzheimer's disease. *Eur J Neurosci* (1998) 10:1084–94. doi:10.1046/j.1460-9568.1998.00121.x
57. Lechner T, Adlassnig C, Humpel C, Kaufmann WA, Maier H, Reinstadler-Kramer K, et al. Chromogranin peptides in Alzheimer's disease. *Exp Gerontol* (2004) 39:101–13. doi:10.1016/j.exger.2003.09.018
58. Marksteiner J, Kaufman WA, Gurka P, Humpel C. Synaptic proteins in Alzheimer's disease. *J Mol Neurosci* (2002) 18(1–2):53. doi:10.1385/JMN:18:1-2:53
59. Marti E, Blasi J, Ferrer I. Early induction of secretoneurin expression following kainic acid administration at convulsant doses in the rat and gerbil hippocampus. *Hippocampus* (2002) 12:174–85. doi:10.1002/hipo.1103
60. Pirker S, Czech T, Baumgartner C, Novak HM, Fürtinger S, Fischer-Colbrie R, et al. Chromogranins as markers of altered hippocampal circuitry in temporal lobe epilepsy. *Ann Neurol* (2001) 50:216–26. doi:10.1002/ana.1079
61. Albrecht-Schgoer K, Schgoer W, Holfeld J, Theurl M, Wiedemann D, Steger C, et al. The angiogenic factor secretoneurin induces coronary angiogenesis in a model of myocardial infarction by stimulation of vascular endothelial growth factor signaling in endothelial cells. *Circulation* (2012) 126:2491–501. doi:10.1161/CIRCULATIONAHA.111.076950
62. Røsjø H, Stridsberg M, Florholmen G, Stensløkken KO, Ottesen AH, Sjaastad I, et al. Secretogranin II; a protein increased in the myocardium and circulation in heart failure with cardioprotective properties. *PLoS One* (2012) 7(5):e37401. doi:10.1371/journal.pone.0037401
63. Ischia R, Culig Z, Eder U, Bartsch G, Winkler H, Fischer-Colbrie R, et al. Presence of chromogranins and regulation of their synthesis and processing in a neuroendocrine prostate tumor cell line. *Prostate Suppl* (1998) 8:80–7. doi:10.1002/(SICI)1097-0045(1998)8+<80::AID-PROS12>3.0.CO;2-N
64. Portela-Gomes GM, Grimelius L, Stridsberg M. Secretogranin III in human neuroendocrine tumours. A comparative immunohistochemical study with chromogranins A and B and secretogranin II. *Regul Pept* (2010) 165:30–5. doi:10.1016/j.regpep.2010.06.002
65. Weiler R, Fisher-Colbrie R, Schmid KW, Feichtinger H, Bussolati G, Grimelius L, et al. Immunological studies on the occurrence and properties of chromogranin A and B and secretogranin II in endocrine tumors. *Am J Surg Pathol* (1988) 12:877–84. doi:10.1097/00000478-198811000-00008
66. Diotel N, Le Page Y, Mouriec K, Tong S-K, Pellegrini E, Vaillant C, et al. Aromatase in the brain of teleost fish: expression, regulation and putative functions. *Front Neuroendocrinol* (2010) 31:172–92. doi:10.1016/j.yfrne.2010.01.003
67. Zupanc GKH. Neurogenesis and neuronal regeneration in the adult fish brain. *J Comp Physiol A Neuroethol Sens Neural Behav Physiol* (2006) 192:649–70. doi:10.1007/s00359-006-0104-y
68. Da Fonte, D.F. *Transcriptomic and Proteomic Characterizations of Goldfish (Carassius auratus) Radial Glia Reveal Complex Regulation by the Neuropeptide Secretoneurin. [Dissertation/Master's Thesis]*. Ottawa (ON): University of Ottawa (2016).

8

Steroids and Brain, a Rising Bio-Medical Domain

*Etienne-Emile Baulieu**

INSERM UMR 1195, Université Paris-Saclay, Hôpital Le Kremlin Bicêtre, Val de Marne, France

***Correspondence:**
Etienne-Emile Baulieu
etienne.baulieu@inserm.fr

Some newly described steroid-related compounds, also found in the rest of the body, are formed and active in the central nervous system, particularly in the brain. Some are of pharmacological and physiopathological interest. We specifically report on two compounds, "MAP4343," a new neurosteroid very efficient antidepressant, and "FKBP52," a protein component of hetero-oligomeric steroid receptors that we found involved in cerebral function, including in Alzheimer's disease.

Keywords: brain steroids, neurosteroids, Alzheimer's disease, tauopathies, pregnenolone, MAP4343, FKBP52, RU486

INTRODUCTION

Some cholesterol found in brain and spinal cord is biologically largely independent of that found in the rest of the body (**Figure 1**). It gives rise to "neurosteroids" (1) and we mention in this short "Perspective" some of their pharmacological and pathophysiological properties. In particular, we report the therapeutic antidepressant activity of a new neurosteroid drug "MAP4343," derivative of pregnenolone (PREG) (2). Very differently, we mention the cloning (3) and the function of a protein, "FKBP52," which is a component of hetero-oligomeric steroid receptors and that, with Chambraud et al. (4), we found involved in the function of the cerebral Tau protein, including in Alzheimer's disease. Thus, we take care of two novel and distinct active steroid-related compounds of medical interest.

First, among "neurosteroids" (1), PREG (6) is rather important quantitatively, and MAP4343, its synthetic derivative 3β-methoxy-Δ5-pregnene-20 one [**Figure 2**; (7)], is remarkably active to treat depressive states and addiction to ethanol (in preparation with G. Koob and O. George); it is currently studied in human beings.

Second, "FKBP52" is a protein complexed with hetero-oligomeric steroid receptors that we found to have an unforeseen interaction (4) with the Tau protein centrally involved in Alzheimer's disease and other dementias. The profound decrease of FKBP52 in several tauopathies (9) suggests its possible therapeutic importance.

NEUROSTEROIDS: MAP4343, A THERAPEUTICALLY ACTIVE DERIVATIVE OF PREG

The synthesis of cholesterol in the nervous system has been described by Bloch (10). Its metabolic steroids synthetized in the central and the peripheral nervous systems (11, 12) are called neurosteroids (1, 13); their syntheses in vertebrate brains (14) occurs in neurons and glial cells, sometimes from some imported steroidal precursors. Neurosteroids include several 3β-hydroxy-Δ5 compounds, such as PREG (6, 15) and dehydroepiandrosterone (DHEA) (16–19), and their sulfate esters (20, 21). Moreover, there are Δ4-3oxo steroid hormones (progesterone is quite abundant) (22), and some of their reduced metabolites, such as one of the tetrahydroderivatives

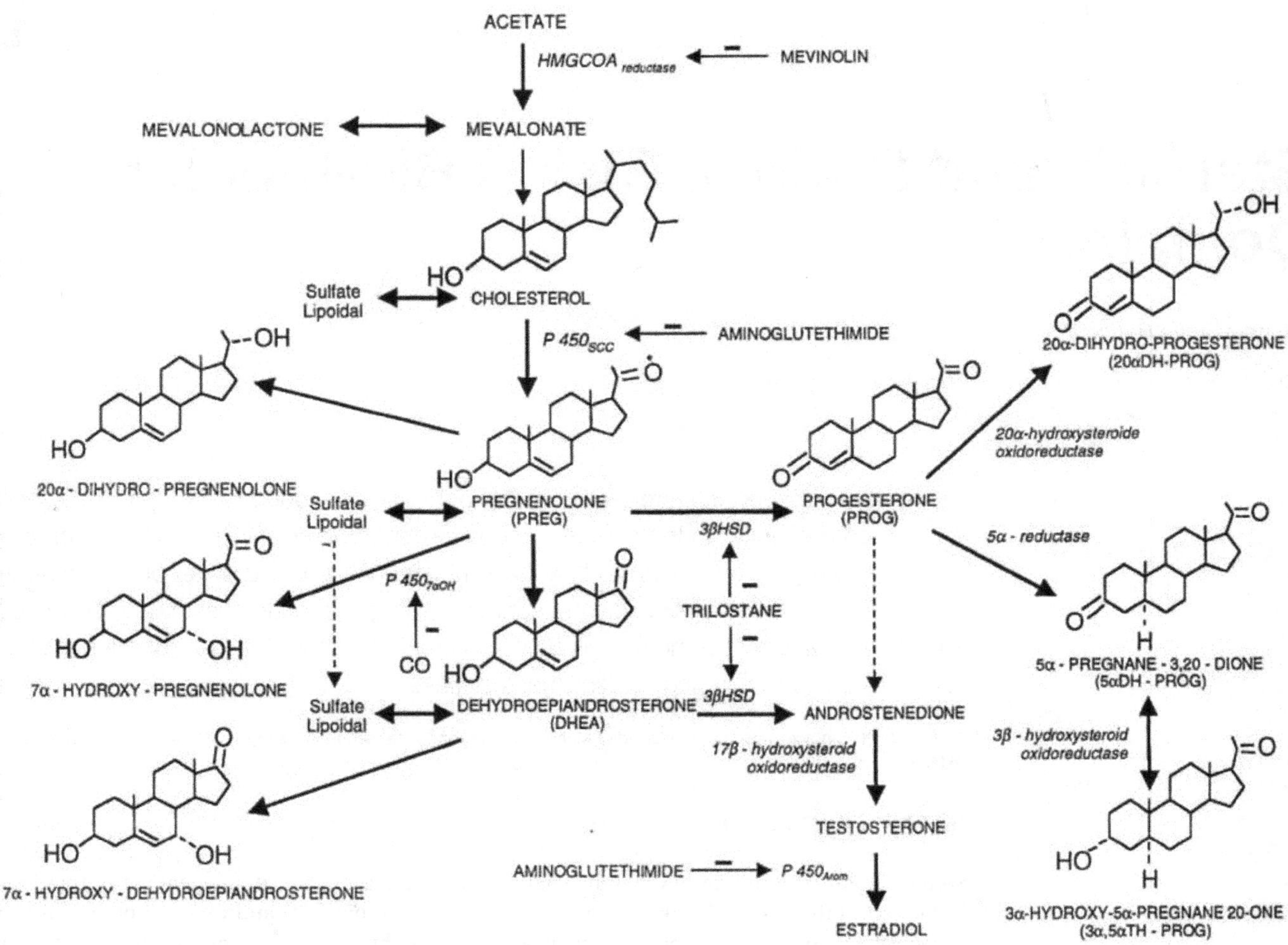

FIGURE 1 | Some metabolic pathways of physiological steroids. All steroids are cholesterol derivatives. The P450scc cytochrome (scc for side chain cleavage) cut the 6 carbon chain of cholesterol, and pregnenolone thus synthetized is precursor of all steroid hormones (3β-HSD, 3β-hydroxysteroid dehydrogenase; 3α-HSOR, 3α-hydroxysteroid oxidoreductase; 17β-HSOR, 17β-hydroxysteroid oxidoreductase). Negative signs (–) indicate the lack of the enzymatic function corresponding to the indicated product. Figure from Baulieu (5).

of progesterone (3αhydroxy-5αpregnan-20one, also called allopregnanolone) (23, 24). Several neurosteroids can act as modulators of neurotransmitter receptors, in particular those of $GABA_A$ (25), NMDA, and sigma-1. Frequently, 3β-hydroxy-Δ5 steroids are metabolized to Δ4-3oxo steroids in brain by 3βHSD (3β-hydroxysteroid dehydrogenase). Δ4-3oxo neurosteroids act *via* classical nuclear steroid receptors (26). Recent studies with progesterone indicate the possibility of distinct hormonal derivatives (27). 3β-hydroxy-Δ5 compounds themselves can also bind to the microtubule-associated protein MAP2 (28). With different locations through the brain, neurosteroids may have several concentrations and/or display diverse activities with various roles on environment and behavior (5).

The oxidative transformation of PREG to progesterone and the metabolism of progesterone to other active neurosteroids (including androgens and corticosteroids) have led us to avoid the metabolism in the brain of 3β-hydroxy-Δ5 neurosteroids to oxydated 3oxo compounds; for this reason, we synthetized and used 3β-methoxy-Δ5 steroids which are not metabolizable to Δ4-3oxo steroids of unnecessary or even pathogenically activity: for instance, an appropriate synthetic derivative of PREG is the methoxylated compound MAP4343 [**Figure 2**; (7)]. Interestingly, both PREG and its 3β-methoxy derivative can bind to protein MAP2 and they display the same activity on the microtubular system through their association to this protein (29). The interaction of MAP2 with PREG (natural neurosteroid) or MAP4343 (synthetic derivative) modifies the function of microtubules in target cells, stimulates their assembly, and is then responsible of positive improvement of behavior: not metabolizable to Δ4-3oxo steroids contrarily to PREG (which therefore cannot be safely administered as such). MAP4343 is very active and therefore medically convenient. Experimentally, MAP4343 increases anxiolytic and anti-depressive activities (30) in rats submitted to a specific psychosocial condition (31), in stressed tree shrews (32), and in Kyoto rats resistant to currently available antidepressants (to be submitted by Villey et al. in 2018). MAP4343 is therapeutically rapid and remarkably safe.

There are other results making 3βhydroxy-Δ5 steroids interesting to study. Their deficit in hippocampus of aged rodents may be responsible for some cognitive alteration (33); however, a similar effect has not yet been demonstrated in human beings. It is also worthwhile to analyze the possible effect of cerebral DHEA and its sulfate (34), unevenly distributed in the human brain.

Progesterone is a steroid difficult to study in the central nervous system (CNS) both qualitatively and metabolically. Progesterone is particularly involved in protection/repair after traumatisms of the CNS (35–37) and it plays a fundamental role in (re)myelination (**Figures 3** and **4**). After cryolesion of peripheral nerves, we have analyzed the function of progesterone synthetized by Schwann cells (38, 39).

A particular transcription factor "Krox-20," expressed in Schwann cells and stimulated by progesterone, plays an important role in myelination of regenerating sciatic nerve and sensory neurons (40, 41). The blockade of progesterone stimulation by RU486 suggests a function as for a classical progesterone receptor. There is also another membrane-associated progesterone-binding protein initially called 25Dx and currently known as PGRMC [progesterone receptor membrane compound; (42)].

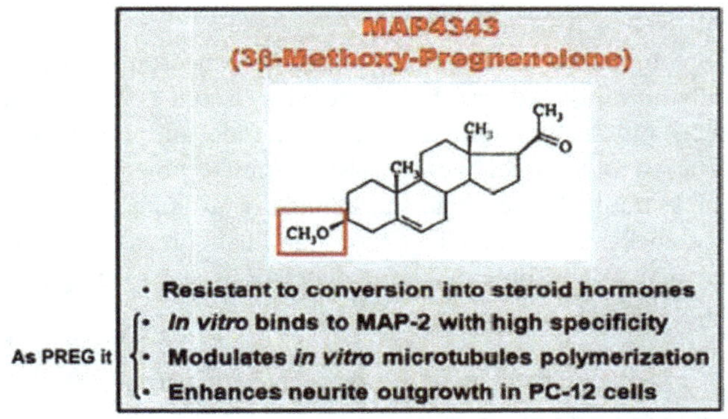

FIGURE 2 | MAP4343, a pregnenolone derivative. Data from Baulieu (8).

Moreover, besides genomic mechanism, membrane actions of progesterone in the CNS have been described (27). Several membrane progesterone receptor(s) have been discovered (27, 43–47). It is also interesting to note that the reduced tetrahydro-metabolite of progesterone (allopregnanolone), at nanomolar concentration, can modify GABA evoked current (45). Several other neurosteroids modify functionally the activity of neuromediator receptors.

It is clear that the pharmacological function of some neurosteroids such as progesterone is diversified and this may be the reason for which it is not easy to rationalize the medical usage of post-menopausal hormone replacement (48). In addition, there are a number of synthetic progesterone analogs, multiplying the variety of compounds displaying some selective function(s) of progestins (49).

There are also a number of different neuroestrogens which, as estradiol (50), include a phenolic nucleus equivalent to the Δ4-3oxo structure of other steroid hormones and have distinct metabolic properties (51).

Δ4-3oxo neuroandrogens, the best known and active being testosterone, are partly derived from neurosteroidal 3β-hydroxy-Δ5 compounds such as DHEA, but androgenic neurosteroids synthetized in the brain have not yet been properly quantified. The androgen receptor is decisive in the spontaneous regeneration of myelin (52).

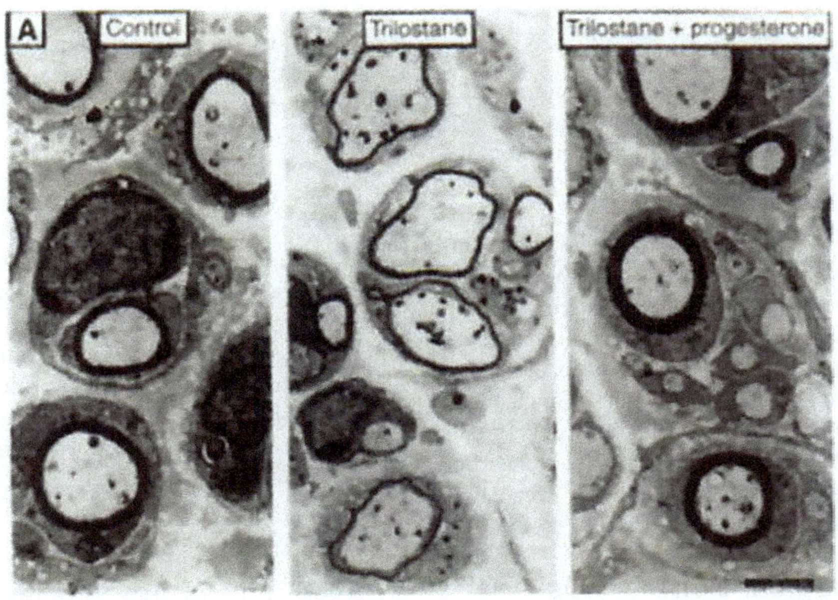

FIGURE 3 | Role of neurosteroids in the formation of myelin sheaths. The thickness of myelin sheaths (number of lamellae) was quantified by electron microscopy of cross section of sciatic nerves from male mice 15 days after cryolesion. Effect of trilostane in the absence (center panel) or presence (right panel) of progesterone on the thickness of myelin sheaths, relative to that in control nerves (left panel). Scale bar, 2 μm. Data from Koenig et al. (38).

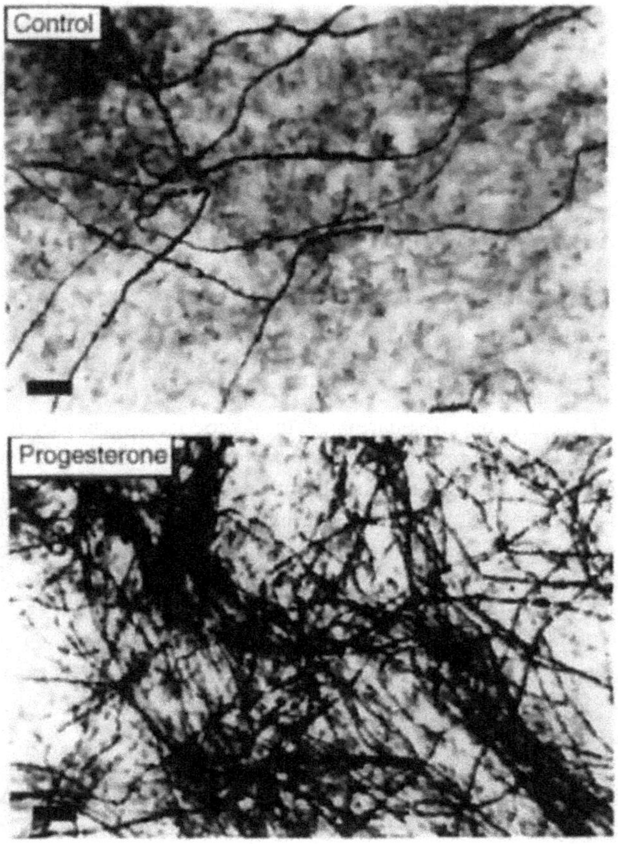

FIGURE 4 | Effect of progesterone on myelin formation in DRG cultures. Cells were cultured for 2 weeks in myelination-promoting medium in the absence (top) or presence (bottom) of 20 nM progesterone. Myelinated fibers were stained with Sudan black and the number of myelin segments was determined. Only myelinated fibers are visible on these photographs. Scale bars, 40 μm. Data from Koenig et al. (38).

It is not yet known if, in the brain, there are neurosteroids with glucocorticosteroid properties active by themselves, or if there are, in the brain, only corticosteroids transferred from the body and participating to the quantitative regulation of their own production.

In summary, not only PREG, DHEA, as well as their sulfates, may by themselves be active in the brain, they also are potential precursors in the CNS of Δ4-3oxo steroids which are biologically active *via* binding to nuclear receptors. There are also, making it even more varied, well-known hormonal steroids certainly imported at least in part into the brain from glands of the body which have a function of physiologically quantitative importance on the development and the activities of neurons and myelination. They are not really "neurosteroids," even if they are intimately linked to the function of the CNS.

Other Pharmacological Compounds With Activities Related to Neurosteroids

An Enantiomeric Form of PREG Sulfate (53–55)

This synthetic compound (56) is curiously much promnesic than PREG sulfate itself, and this effect opens a new field of research to compare activity between natural and enantiomeric structures of hormonal steroids [parenthetically, the natural PREG and PREG sulfate both are themselves active on memory; (21)].

Lithium

It has neuroprotective activity, particularly for remyelination of peripheral nerves (57). The results open perspectives in treatments by an inhibitor of glycogen synthase kinase 3β such as lithium.

Etifoxine (58, 59)

This neurostimulant of estrogens and progestins is active on experimental autoimmune encephalomyelitis, a model of multiple sclerosis (60, 61). However, attempts to decrease post-partum relapses in sick women (62) have not shown a significant success.

RU486 (Mifepristone, an Efficient Anti-Progesterone) (63)

The compound, which is also antiglucocorticosteroid, can be orally administered and has demonstrated anti-neurosteroidal effects on inappropriate neuroprogesterone and neuroglucocorticosteroid pathologies. It also permits protective effects against traumatic neuronal alterations [for example, protection of cerebellar Purkinje cells (64, 65)] and has shown therapeutically activity on some psychotic depressions and meningiomas (unpublished).

ALZHEIMER'S DISEASE: FKBP52, A CONSTITUENT OF HETERO-OLIGOMERIC STEROID HORMONE RECEPTORS, INTERACTS WITH TAU STRUCTURE AND FUNCTION

In human beings, the most frequent and severe human senile dementia, the Alzheimer's disease, currently is not biochemically explained nor treated in order to recover. However, there are several recent progresses for the diagnostic, biomarkers and imagery of the sick brain (66). Since the publication of Alois Alzheimer in 1907, two proteins remain of greatest interest (67). Up to now, the most studied has been "amyloid-β" (Aβ), essentially observed between neurons but its study has still not been successful in any therapeutic approach. The other protein, the structure and the cloning of which have been only precisely analyzed since the 1980 period, is "Tau" (68–70). Besides association to microtubules, the Tau protein is involved in several other cellular functions, including gene regulation (71). In human patients, Tau is present within neuronal cells, and the six isoforms, hyperphosphorylated (72) according to a well-defined pattern (73), are also partly truncated by caspase activity (74). Isomerization and oligomerization of Tau due to FKBP52 are independent processes (75). These modifications are largely responsible for fibrillation and aggregation, and they contribute to establish intracellular neurodegeneration in transgenic animals. It is accepted that modified Tau can be responsible for altered function of nerves, even if details of the mechanism of pathological function of abnormal Tau are not well explained.

Distinct from Alzheimer's disease, there are dementias which are exclusively tauopathy (69), supporting the belief that Tau abnormalities are directly responsible of dementia activity of the brain in Alzheimer's disease (72); the tauopathic diseases without Aβ abnormality could be called "pure tauopathies": some are FTDP17: frontotemporal dementias and parkinsonism linked to chromosome 17; progressive supra-nuclear palsy; Pick diseases, etc.

Consequently, Tau, mostly in aggregated forms, is clearly involved principally in terms of neurodegeneration, and pathological Tau may be most appropriate as potential target for treating Alzheimer (76). The pure tauopathies, human and experimental in animals, are very severe diseases and matters of a large number of studies: in particular, the diseases due to P301L mutation of Tau have been very much studied as convenient models. In genetically P301L mutated zebrafishes, the Tau is much oligomerized and abnormally phosphorylated (77).

In studying steroid receptors in human beings, we had analyzed some of their hetero-oligomeric variants (78, 79). They differ according to diseases, but often include the protein FKBP52. In Alzheimer's disease, this protein colocalizes with the autophagic-endolysosomal system (**Figure 5**). The FKBP structure includes an N-terminal domain (FK1) which harbors a sequence with enzymatic PPIase activity (peptidyl-*cis*/*trans*-prolyl-isomerase), thus classifying FKBP52 among the immunophilins which may bind many small molecular ligands (80, 81). The second domain of FKBP52, FK2, is architecturally similar to the FK1 but does not have a PPIase activity. The rest of the

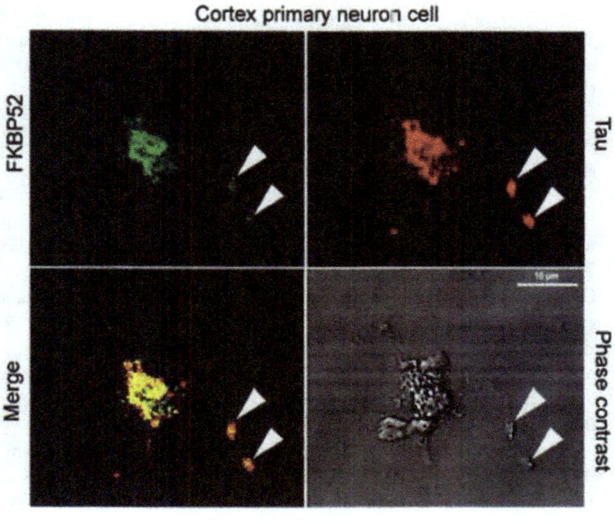

FIGURE 5 | Colocalization of FKBP52 and Tau in primary cortical neurons and PC12 cells. Immunofluorescence staining of primary cortical neurons and PC12 cells treated with 50 nM NGF for 5 days. Double staining for Tau and FKBP52 was performed after cytosol extraction to reveal cytoskeletal association. Arrows indicate preferential colocalization of both proteins in the distal part of the nerve cell axon and at the extremity of PC12 cell neurites. Confocal images of primary cortical neurons. Analysis of 0.5-μm slices confirms the preferential colocalization in the distal part of the axon (arrowheads). Data from Chambraud et al. (4).

FKBP52 protein includes three TetratricoPeptid Repeats' (TPR) sequences and binds to hsp90, which itself interacts with an hormonal steroid molecule, completing the hetero-oligomeric composition of steroid receptors. After TPR, there is a C terminal sector-binding calmodulin. It is therefore *via* FKBP52 that the hetero-oligomeric steroid hormones could interact functionally with a neuro-protein such as Tau.

Indeed, we had, additionally and very importantly, discovered an interaction of FKBP52 with Tau [(4); **Figures 5** and **6**], completing the description of steroid–FKBP52–Tau sequence(s) never described till now, and that have not been studied in functional terms.

Experiments with zebrafishes under the direction of Dr. Marcel Tawk (77) utilizing transgenic animals expressing the human Tau P301L, severely suffering of abnormal escape behavior and with some change of Tau phosphorylation, indicated, *in vivo* and *in vitro* studies, the functional abnormalities due to the pathogenic mutation of Tau.

This is the basis of a strategy leading to look for a treatment of tauopathies, including Alzheimer's disease and other dementias. FKBP52 may serve for inducing qualitatively and anti-pathological Tau activity and/or directly decreases Tau: considering that Tau is centrally involved in the pathophysiology of Alzheimer, we look for modifying the function of FKBP52 to obtain an actively anti-pathological Tau effect. There is a very profound decrease and/or a reduced function of FKBP52 that we have described in pathological circumstances: in Alzheimer's disease, FTDP17 (9), and other tauopathies. Our hypothesis is based on the concept that the function of Tau is decisively pathological in dementias, and we hypothesize a FKBP 52 induced change quantitatively and/or qualitatively, which could be profitable to the patients (**Figure 7**) treated as early as possible after the beginning of the disease. In summary, appropriate modification of FKBP52 induced by some ligand(s) may help to normalize Tau activity and consequently be able to improve the cerebral function.

It is not excluded that several brain steroids may modify the function of parameters implied in this novel approach for treating

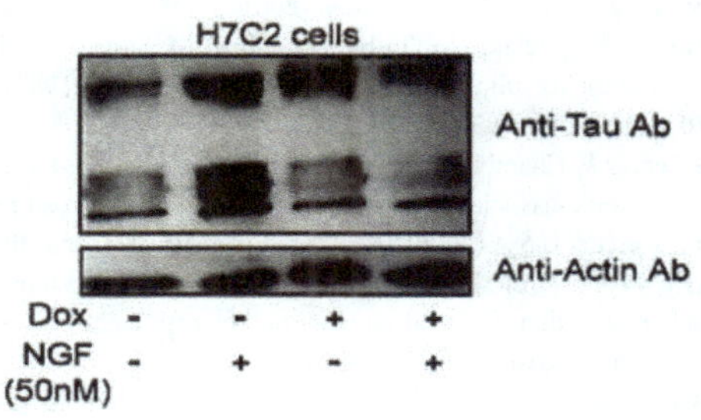

FIGURE 6 | Effect of FKBP52 overexpression on Tau protein accumulation. H7C2 cells: stably transformed PC12 cells by an FKBP52-inducible expression system based on a tetracycline responsive element (82). NGF: 5 days—Dox: 7 days. H7C2 and PC12 cells were treated or not with NGF for 5 days in the presence or absence of DOX for 1 week; 50 μg of extracts was subjected to SDS-PAGE and immunoblotted with anti-Tau (antibody clone DC25). Actin was used as the loading control. Data from Chambraud et al. (4).

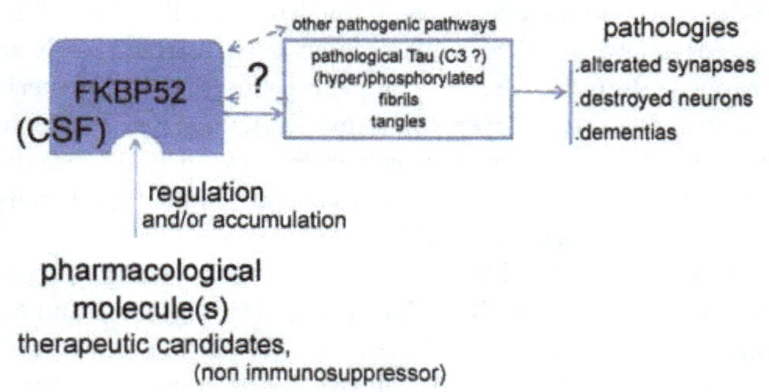

FIGURE 7 | Schema of the working hypothesis and strategy for prevention/treatment of dementias *via* the novel target FKBP52. FKBP52 is measurable in CSF. Data from Baulieu (8).

cerebral abnormality. Other approaches may help to understand alterations of the Tau protein: for instance, studies of synaptic structure (83, 84) and activity (in preparation), and experiments of deep cerebral stimulation can be involved in methods including autophagic-lysosomal protection (85).

Our therapeutic approach centered on effect of FKBP52 on Tau (dys)function may be still far to be operationally favorable to treat dementias (**Figure 7**). Working on Tau with new modified/liganded FKBP52 function and steroid activities, we will obtain novel results. Will they be valuable?

SUMMARY

In this "Perspective," we have treated two distinct examples concerning steroid associated molecules involved in activities of the CNS. They exemplify typical compounds of (1) neurosteroid derivatives and (2) components of hetero-oligomeric steroid receptors. We are happy that, in a number of other laboratories, many publications (not reported in this "Perspective"), have followed our two original studies. This paper is not a review, but we hope to draw attention to the versatile involvement of the steroidal structure and thus in important physiopathological derivatives.

AUTHOR CONTRIBUTIONS

The author confirms being the sole contributor of this work and approved it for publication.

ACKNOWLEDGMENTS

I thank Christine Broussot-Charbonnier for her remarkable administrative assistance.

FUNDING

No funding for this "Perspective." Support for the work in each cited paper to which I collaborated is detailed in the corresponding reference.

REFERENCES

1. Baulieu EE. Neurosteroids: a new function in the brain. *Biol Cell* (1991) 71:3–10. doi:10.1016/0248-4900(91)90045-O
2. Bianchi M, Baulieu EE. 3β-Methoxy-pregnenolone (MAP4343) as an innovative therapeutic approach for depressive disorders. *Proc Natl Acad Sci U S A* (2012) 109:1713–8. doi:10.1073/pnas.1121485109
3. Lebeau MC, Massol N, Herrick J, Faber LE, Renoir JM, Radanyi C, et al. P59, an hsp 90-binding protein. Cloning and sequencing of its cDNA and preparation of a peptide-directed polyclonal antibody. *J Biol Chem* (1992) 267:4281–4.
4. Chambraud B, Sardin E, Giustiniani J, Dounane O, Schumacher M, Goedert M, et al. A role for FKBP52 in Tau protein function. *Proc Natl Acad Sci U S A* (2010) 107:2658–63. doi:10.1073/pnas.0914957107
5. Baulieu EE. [Neurosteroids, their role in brain physiology: neurotrophicity, memory, aging…]. *Bull Acad Natl Med* (2001) 185:349–69; discussion 370–2.
6. Corpéchot C, Synguelakis M, Talha S, Axelson M, Sjövall J, Vihko R, et al. Pregnenolone and its sulfate ester in the rat brain. *Brain Res* (1983) 270:119–25. doi:10.1016/0006-8993(83)90797-7
7. Fontaine-Lenoir V, Chambraud B, Fellous A, David S, Duchossoy Y, Baulieu EE, et al. Microtubule-associated protein 2 (MAP2) is a neurosteroid receptor. *Proc Natl Acad Sci U S A* (2006) 103:4711–6. doi:10.1073/pnas.0600113103
8. Baulieu EE. From steroid hormones to depressive states and senile dementias: new mechanistic, therapeutical and predictive approaches. *C R Biol* (2015) 338:613–6. doi:10.1016/j.crvi.2015.06.003
9. Giustiniani J, Sineus M, Sardin E, Dounane O, Panchal M, Sazdovitch V, et al. Decrease of the immunophilin FKBP52 accumulation in human brains of Alzheimer's disease and FTDP-17. *J Alzheimers Dis* (2012) 29:471–83. doi:10.3233/JAD-2011-111895
10. Bloch K. The biological synthesis of cholesterol. *Science* (1965) 150:19–28. doi:10.1126/science.150.3692.19
11. Le Goascogne C, Robel P, Gouézou M, Sananès N, Baulieu EE, Waterman M. Neurosteroids: cytochrome P-450scc in rat brain. *Science* (1987) 237:1212–5. doi:10.1126/science.3306919
12. Ibanez C, Guennoun R, Liere P, Eychenne B, Pianos A, El-Etr M, et al. Developmental expression of genes involved in neurosteroidogenesis: 3β-hydroxysteroid dehydrogenase/Δ5-Δ4 isomerase in the rat brain. *Endocrinology* (2003) 144:2902–11. doi:10.1210/en.2002-0073
13. Baulieu EE, Robel P, Schumacher M. Neurosteroids: beginning of the story. *Int Rev Neurobiol* (2001) 46:1–32. doi:10.1016/S0074-7742(01)46057-0
14. Tsutsui K, Ukena K, Takase M, Kohchi C, Lea RW. Neurosteroid biosynthesis in vertebrate brains. *Comp Biochem Physiol C Pharmacol Toxicol Endocrinol* (1999) 124:121–9. doi:10.1016/S0742-8413(99)00065-1
15. Hu ZY, Bourreau E, Jung-Testas I, Robel P, Baulieu EE. Neurosteroids: oligodendrocyte mitochondria convert cholesterol to pregnenolone. *Proc Natl Acad Sci U S A* (1987) 84:8215–9. doi:10.1073/pnas.84.23.8215
16. Corpéchot C, Robel P, Lachapelle F, Baumann N, Axelson M, Sjövall J, et al. Free and sulfo-conjugated dehydroepiandrosterone in the brain of mice with myelin biosynthesis disorders. *C R Seances Acad Sci III* (1981) 292: 231–4.
17. Corpéchot C, Robel P, Axelson M, Sjövall J, Baulieu EE. Characterization and measurement of dehydroepiandrosterone sulfate in rat brain. *Proc Natl Acad Sci U S A* (1981) 78:4704–7. doi:10.1073/pnas.78.8.4704
18. Majewska MD, Demirgören S, Spivak CE, London ED. The neurosteroid dehydroepiandrosterone sulfate is an allosteric antagonist of the GABAA receptor. *Brain Res* (1990) 526:143–6. doi:10.1016/0006-8993(90)90261-9
19. Zwain IH, Yen SS. Dehydroepiandrosterone: biosynthesis and metabolism in the brain. *Endocrinology* (1999) 140:880–7. doi:10.1210/endo.140.2.6528
20. Schumacher M, Liere P, Akwa Y, Rajkowski K, Griffiths W, Bodin K, et al. Pregnenolone sulfate in the brain: a controversial neurosteroid. *Neurochem Int* (2008) 52:522–40. doi:10.1016/j.neuint.2007.08.022
21. Ladurelle N, Eychenne B, Denton D, Blair-West J, Schumacher M, Robel P, et al. Prolonged intracerebroventricular infusion of neurosteroids affects cognitive performances in the mouse. *Brain Res* (2000) 858:371–9. doi:10.1016/S0006-8993(00)01953-3
22. Guennoun R, Fiddes RJ, Gouézou M, Lombès M, Baulieu EE. A key enzyme in the biosynthesis of neurosteroids, 3 beta-hydroxysteroid dehydrogenase/delta 5-delta 4-isomerase (3 beta-HSD), is expressed in rat brain. *Brain Res Mol Brain Res* (1995) 30:287–300. doi:10.1016/0169-328X(95)00016-L
23. El-Etr M, Akwa Y, Fiddes RJ, Robel P, Baulieu EE. A progesterone metabolite stimulates the release of gonadotropin-releasing hormone from GT1-1

hypothalamic neurons via the gamma-aminobutyric acid type A receptor. *Proc Natl Acad Sci U S A* (1995) 92:3769–73. doi:10.1073/pnas.92.9.3769
24. Guennoun R, Labombarda F, Gonzalez-Deniselle MC, Liere P, De Nicola AF, Schumacher M. Progesterone and allopregnanolone in the central nervous system: response to injury and implication for neuroprotection. *J Steroid Biochem Mol Biol* (2015) 146:48–61. doi:10.1016/j.jsbmb.2014.09.001
25. Paul SM, Purdy RH. Neuroactive steroids. *FASEB J* (1992) 6:2311–22. doi:10.1096/fasebj.6.6.1347506
26. Evans RM. The steroid and thyroid hormone receptor superfamily. *Science* (1988) 240:889–95. doi:10.1126/science.3283939
27. Schumacher M, Coirini H, Robert F, Guennoun R, El-Etr M. Genomic and membrane actions of progesterone: implications for reproductive physiology and behavior. *Behav Brain Res* (1999) 105:37–52. doi:10.1016/S0166-4328(99)00081-9
28. Murakami K, Fellous A, Baulieu EE, Robel P. Pregnenolone binds to microtubule-associated protein 2 and stimulates microtubule assembly. *Proc Natl Acad Sci U S A* (2000) 97:3579–84. doi:10.1073/pnas.97.7.3579
29. Baulieu EE, Robel P, Fellous A, Duchossoy Y, Fontaine-Lenoir V, David S. Mapreg: toward a novel approach of neuroprotection and treatment of Alzheimer's disease. *J Mol Neurosci* (2004) 24:63–5. doi:10.1385/JMN:24:1:063
30. Akwa Y, Ladurelle N, Teixeira-Silva N, Sananès N, Weill-Engerer S, Baulieu EE. Neurostéroïdes: rôle dans l'anxiété et la mémoire. In: Ferreri M, editor. *Anxiété, anxiolytiques et troubles cognitifs*. Paris: Elsevier Masson (2004). p. 59–70.
31. Bianchi M, Fone KF, Azmi N, Heidbreder CA, Hagan JJ, Marsden CA. Isolation rearing induces recognition memory deficits accompanied by cytoskeletal alterations in rat hippocampus. *Eur J Neurosci* (2006) 24:2894–902. doi:10.1111/j.1460-9568.2006.05170.x
32. Parésys L, Hoffmann K, Froger N, Bianchi M, Villey I, Baulieu EE, et al. Effects of the synthetic neurosteroid: 3β-methoxypregnenolone (MAP4343) on behavioral and physiological alterations provoked by chronic psychosocial stress in tree shrews. *Int J Neuropsychopharmacol* (2016) 19:1–12. doi:10.1093/ijnp/pyv119
33. Vallée M, Mayo W, Darnaudéry M, Corpéchot C, Young J, Koehl M, et al. Neurosteroids: deficient cognitive performance in aged rats depends on low pregnenolone sulfate levels in the hippocampus. *Proc Natl Acad Sci U S A* (1997) 94:14865–70. doi:10.1073/pnas.94.26.14865
34. Weill-Engerer S, David JP, Sazdovitch V, Liere P, Schumacher M, Delacourte A, et al. In vitro metabolism of dehydroepiandrosterone (DHEA) to 7α-hydroxy-DHEA and Δ5-androstene-3β, 17β-diol in specific regions of the aging brain from Alzheimer's and non-demented patients. *Brain Res* (2003) 969:117–25. doi:10.1016/S0006-8993(03)02288-1
35. Gonzalez-Deniselle MC, Lopez Costa JJ, Gonzalez SL, Labombarda F, Garay L, Guennoun R, et al. Basis of progesterone protection in spinal cord neurodegeneration. *J Steroid Biochem Mol Biol* (2002) 83:199–209. doi:10.1016/S0960-0760(02)00262-5
36. Labombarda F, Gonzalez SL, Lima A, Roig P, Guennoun R, Schumacher M, et al. Effects of progesterone on oligodendrocyte progenitors, oligodendrocyte transcription factors, and myelin proteins following spinal cord injury. *Glia* (2009) 57:884–97. doi:10.1002/glia.20814
37. De Nicola AF, Labombarda F, Gonzalez-Deniselle MC, Gonzalez SL, Garay L, Meyer M, et al. Progesterone neuroprotection in traumatic CNS injury and motoneuron degeneration. *Front Neuroendocrinol* (2009) 30:173–87. doi:10.1016/j.yfrne.2009.03.001
38. Koenig HL, Schumacher M, Ferzaz B, Do Thi AN, Ressouches A, Guennoun R, et al. Progesterone synthesis and myelin formation by Schwann cells. *Science* (1995) 268:1500–3. doi:10.1126/science.7770777
39. Robert F, Guennoun R, Désarnaud F, Do-Thi A, Benmessahel Y, Baulieu EE, et al. Synthesis of progesterone in Schwann cells: regulation by sensory neurons. *Eur J Neurosci* (2001) 13:916–24. doi:10.1046/j.0953-816x.2001.01463.x
40. Jung-Testas I, Schumacher M, Robel P, Baulieu EE. Demonstration of progesterone receptors in rat Schwann cells. *J Steroid Biochem Mol Biol* (1996) 58:77–82. doi:10.1016/0960-0760(96)00009-X
41. Guennoun R, Benmessahel Y, Delespierre B, Gouézou M, Rajkowski KM, Baulieu EE, et al. Progesterone stimulates Krox-20 gene expression in Schwann cells. *Brain Res Mol Brain Res* (2001) 90:75–82. doi:10.1016/S0169-328X(01)00094-8
42. Guennoun R, Meffre D, Labombarda F, Gonzalez SL, Gonzalez-Deniselle MC, Stein DG, et al. The membrane-associated progesterone-binding protein 25-Dx: expression, cellular localization and up-regulation after brain and spinal cord injuries. *Brain Res Rev* (2008) 57:493–505. doi:10.1016/j.brainresrev.2007.05.009
43. Zhu Y, Bond J, Thomas P. Identification, classification, and partial characterization of genes in humans and other vertebrates homologous to a fish membrane progestin receptor. *Proc Natl Acad Sci U S A* (2003) 100:2237–42. doi:10.1073/pnas.0436133100
44. Thomas P. Characteristics of membrane progestin receptor alpha (mPRalpha) and progesterone membrane receptor component 1 (PGMRC1) and their roles in mediating rapid progestin actions. *Front Neuroendocrinol* (2008) 29:292–312. doi:10.1016/j.yfrne.2008.01.001
45. Schumacher M, Mattern C, Ghoumari A, Oudinet JP, Liere P, Labombarda F, et al. Revisiting the roles of progesterone and allopregnanolone in the nervous system: resurgence of the progesterone receptors. *Prog Neurobiol* (2014) 113:6–39. doi:10.1016/j.pneurobio.2013.09.004
46. Schumacher M, Guennoun R, Mercier G, Désarnaud F, Lacor P, Bénavides J, et al. Progesterone synthesis and myelin formation in peripheral nerves. *Brain Res Brain Res Rev* (2001) 37:343–59. doi:10.1016/S0165-0173(01)00139-4
47. Schumacher M, Ghoumari A, Guennoun R, Labombarda F, Gonzalez SL, Gonzalez-Deniselle MC, et al. Progestins and antiprogestins: mechanisms of action, neuroprotection and myelination. In: Kordon C, Gaillard RC, editors. *Hormones and the Brain*. Berlin, Heidelberg: Springer-Verlag (2005). p. 111–54.
48. Schumacher M, Guennoun R, Ghoumari A, Massaad C, Robert F, El-Etr M, et al. Novel perspectives for progesterone in hormone replacement therapy, with special reference to the nervous system. *Endocr Rev* (2007) 28:387–439. doi:10.1210/er.2006-0050
49. Schumacher M, Akwa Y, Guennoun R, Robert F, Labombarda F, Desarnaud F, et al. Steroid synthesis and metabolism in the nervous system: trophic and protective effects. *J Neurocytol* (2000) 29:307–26. doi:10.1023/A:1007152904926
50. Naftolin F, Ryan KJ, Davies IJ, Reddy VV, Flores F, Petro Z, et al. The formation of estrogens by central neuroendocrine tissues. *Recent Prog Horm Res* (1975) 31:295–319.
51. Toran-Allerand CD. Minireview: a plethora of estrogen receptors in the brain: where will it end? *Endocrinology* (2004) 145:1069–74. doi:10.1210/en.2003-1462
52. Bielecki B, Mattern C, Ghoumari AM, Javaid S, Smietanka K, Ghanem CA, et al. Unexpected central role of the androgen receptor in the spontaneous regeneration of myelin. *Proc Natl Acad Sci U S A* (2016) 113:14829–34. doi:10.1073/pnas.1614826113
53. Akwa Y, Ladurelle N, Covey DF, Baulieu EE. The synthetic enantiomer of pregnenolone sulfate is very active on memory in rats and mice, even more so than its physiological neurosteroid counterpart: distinct mechanisms? *Proc Natl Acad Sci U S A* (2001) 98:14033–7. doi:10.1073/pnas.241503698
54. Petit GH, Tobin C, Krishnan K, Moricard Y, Covey DF, Rondi-Reig L, et al. Pregnenolone sulfate and its enantiomer: differential modulation of memory in a spatial discrimination task using forebrain NMDA receptor deficient mice. *Eur Neuropsychopharmacol* (2011) 21:211–5. doi:10.1016/j.euroneuro.2010.09.010
55. El Bitar F, Meunier J, Villard V, Alméras M, Krishnan K, Covey DF, et al. Neuroprotection by the synthetic neurosteroid enantiomers *ent*-PREGS and *ent*-DHEAS against $A\beta_{25-35}$ peptide-induced toxicity in vitro and in vivo in mice. *Psychopharmacology* (2014) 231:3293–312. doi:10.1007/s00213-014-3435-3
56. Covey DF. ent-Steroids: novel tools for studies of signaling pathways. *Steroids* (2009) 74:577–85. doi:10.1016/j.steroids.2008.11.019
57. Makoukji J, Belle M, Meffre D, Stassart R, Grenier J, Shackleford GG, et al. Lithium enhances remyelination of peripheral nerves. *Proc Natl Acad Sci U S A* (2012) 109:3973–8. doi:10.1073/pnas.1121367109
58. Verleye M, Akwa Y, Liere P, Ladurelle N, Pianos A, Eychenne B, et al. The anxiolytic etifoxine activates the peripheral benzodiazepine receptor and increases the neurosteroid levels in rat brain. *Pharmacol Biochem Behav* (2005) 82:712–20. doi:10.1016/j.pbb.2005.11.013
59. Girard C, Liu S, Cadepond F, Adams D, Lacroix C, Verleye M, et al. Etifoxine improves peripheral nerve regeneration and functional recovery. *Proc Natl Acad Sci U S A* (2008) 105:20505–10. doi:10.1073/pnas.0811201106
60. El-Etr M, Vukusic S, Gignoux L, Durand-Dubief F, Achiti I, Baulieu EE, et al. Steroid hormones in multiple sclerosis. *J Neurol Sci* (2005) 233:49–54. doi:10.1016/j.jns.2005.03.004
61. El-Etr M, Ghoumari A, Sitruk-Ware R, Schumacher M. Hormonal influences in multiple sclerosis: new therapeutic benefits for steroids. *Maturitas* (2011) 68:47–51. doi:10.1016/j.maturitas.2010.09.014

62. Vukusic S, El-Etr M, Cornu C, Cucherat M, Gignoux L, Durand-Dubieg F, et al. POPART'MUS: un essai de phase III de prévention des poussées du post-partum dans la sclérose en plaques par les hormones sexuelles. *Rev Neurol* (2005) 161(1):1S38. doi:10.1016/S0035-3787(05)85017-9
63. Herrmann W, Wyss R, Riondel A, Philibert D, Teutsch G, Sakiz E, et al. The effects of an antiprogesterone steroid in women: interruption of the menstrual cycle and of early pregnancy. *C R Seances Acad Sci III* (1982) 294:933–8.
64. De Nicola AF, Gonzalez SL, Labombarda F, Gonzalez-Deniselle MC, Garay L, Guennoun R, et al. Progesterone treatment of spinal cord injury: effects on receptors, neurotrophins, and myelination. *J Mol Neurosci* (2006) 28:3–15. doi:10.1385/JMN:28:1:3
65. Rakotomamonjy J, Levenes C, Baulieu EE, Schumacher M, Ghoumari AM. Novel protective effect of mifepristone on detrimental $GABA_A$ receptor activity to immature Purkinje neurons. *FASEB J* (2011) 25:3999–4010. doi:10.1096/fj.11-183384
66. Hane FT, Robinson M, Lee BY, Bai O, Leonenko Z, Albert MS. Recent progress in Alzheimer's disease research, part 3: diagnosis and treatment. *J Alzheimers Dis* (2017) 57:645–65. doi:10.3233/JAD-160882
67. Ittner LM, Götz J. Amyloid-β and tau – a toxic pas de deux in Alzheimer's disease. *Nat Rev Neurosci* (2011) 12:65–72. doi:10.1038/nrn2967
68. Goedert M, Wischik CM, Crowther RA, Walker JE, Klug A. Cloning and sequencing of the cDNA encoding a core protein of the paired helical filament of Alzheimer disease: identification as the microtubule-associated protein tau. *Proc Natl Acad Sci U S A* (1988) 85:4051–5. doi:10.1073/pnas.85.11.4051
69. Goedert M, Spillantini MG, Jakes R, Rutherford D, Crowther RA. Multiple isoforms of human microtubule-associated protein Tau: sequences and localization in neurofibrillary tangles of Alzheimer's disease. *Neuron* (1989) 3:519–26. doi:10.1016/0896-6273(89)90210-9
70. Spillantini MG, Goedert M. Tau pathology and neurodegeneration. *Lancet Neurol* (2013) 12:609–22. doi:10.1016/S1474-4422(13)70090-5
71. Lebouvier T, Pasquier F, Buée L. Update on tauopathies. *Curr Opin Neurol* (2017) 30:589–98. doi:10.1097/WCO.0000000000000502
72. Buée L, Bussière T, Buée-Scherrer V, Delacourte A, Hof PR. Tau protein isoforms, phosphorylation and role in neurodegenerative disorders. *Brain Res Brain Res Rev* (2000) 33:95–130. doi:10.1016/S0165-0173(00)00019-9
73. Despres C, Byrne C, Qi H, Cantrelle FX, Huvent I, Chambraud B, et al. Identification of the Tau phosphorylation pattern that drives its aggregation. *Proc Natl Acad Sci U S A* (2017) 114:9080–5. doi:10.1073/pnas.1708448114
74. Rissman RA, Poon WW, Blurton-Jones M, Oddo S, Torp R, Vitek MP, et al. Caspase-cleavage of Tau is an early event in Alzheimer disease tangle pathology. *J Clin Invest* (2004) 114:121–30. doi:10.1172/JCI200420640
75. Kamah A, Cantrelle FX, Huvent I, Giustiniani J, Guillemeau K, Byrne C, et al. Isomerization and oligomerization of truncated and mutated Tau forms by FKBP52 are independent processes. *J Mol Biol* (2016) 428:1080–90. doi:10.1016/j.jmb.2016.02.015
76. Li C, Götz J. Tau-based therapies in neurodegeneration: opportunities and challenges. *Nat Rev Drug Discov* (2017) 16:863–83. doi:10.1038/nrd.2017.155
77. Giustiniani J, Chambraud B, Sardin E, Dounane O, Guillemeau K, Nakatani H, et al. Immunophilin FKBP52 induces Tau-P301L filamentous assembly in vitro and modulates its activity in a model of tauopathy. *Proc Natl Acad Sci U S A* (2014) 111:4584–9. doi:10.1073/pnas.1402645111
78. Baulieu EE, Binart N, Cadepond F, Catelli MG, Chambraud B, Garnier J, et al. Do receptor-associated nuclear proteins explain earliest steps of steroid hormone function? In: Carlstedt-Duke J, Eriksson H, Gustafsson JA, editors. *The Steroid/Thyroid Hormone Receptor Family and Gene Regulation. Proceedings of the 2nd International CBT Symposium; 1988 Nov 4-5*. Stockholm, Sweden (1989). p. 301–18.
79. Schiene-Fischer C, Yu C. Receptor accessory folding helper enzymes: the functional role of peptidyl prolyl cis/trans isomerases. *FEBS Lett* (2001) 495:1–6. doi:10.1016/S0014-5793(01)02326-2
80. Steiner JP, Hamilton GS, Ross DT, Valentine HL, Guo H, Connolly MA, et al. Neurotrophic immunophilin ligands stimulate structural and functional recovery in neurodegenerative animal models. *Proc Natl Acad Sci U S A* (1997) 94:2019–24. doi:10.1073/pnas.94.5.2019
81. Blackburn EA, Walkinshaw MD. Targeting FKBP isoforms with small-molecule ligands. *Curr Opin Pharmacol* (2011) 11:365–71. doi:10.1016/j.coph.2011.04.007
82. Gossen M, Bujard H. Tight control of gene expression in mammalian cells by tetracycline-responsive promoters. *Proc Natl Acad Sci U S A* (1992) 89:5547–51. doi:10.1073/pnas.89.12.5547
83. Doudna JA, Charpentier E. Genome editing. The new frontier of genome engineering with CRISPR-Cas9. *Science* (2014) 346:1258096. doi:10.1126/science.1258096
84. Incontro S, Asensio CS, Edwards RH, Nicoll RA. Efficient, complete deletion of synaptic proteins using CRISPR. *Neuron* (2014) 83:1051–7. doi:10.1016/j.neuron.2014.07.043
85. Akwa Y, Gondard E, Mann A, Capetillo-Zarate E, Alberdi E, Matute C, et al. Synaptic activity protects against AD and FTD-like pathology via autophagic-lysosomal degradation. *Mol Psychiatry* (2017) 1–11. doi:10.1038/mp.2017.142

9

Hashimoto's Encephalopathy and Seizure Disorders

Jie Li [1,2*] *and Fengzhen Li* [1]

[1] *Department of Neurology, The First Affiliated Hospital of Xinxiang Medical University, Weihui, China,*

[2] *Xinxiang Medical University, Xinxiang, China*

***Correspondence:**
Jie Li
l.j.lijie@163.com

Hashimoto's encephalopathy (HE) is a rare, clinically heterogeneous condition associated with positive thyroid autoantibodies. It is increasingly recognized as an important and treatable cause of autoimmune encephalopathy. Thyroid-associated antibodies such as thyroperoxidase (TPO) antibody, thyroglobulin (TG) antibody, and thyrotropin receptor (TR) antibody were found in HE patients with seizure disorders. Although antithyroid antibodies are required for the diagnosis of HE, their role in the pathogenesis of HE remains uncertain. Instead of playing a key role in the pathophysiology processes of HE, it is suggested that thyroid-associated antibodies are hallmarks of HE. Seizure disorders were found in approximately two-thirds of HE patients, and common anticonvulsant therapy alone is usually ineffective. Some patients did not respond to any antiepileptic drugs. The use of immunotherapy can effectively control seizure disorders. Electroencephalography and imaging findings are not specific to HE patients and can also be seen in other causes of encephalopathies. However, the prognosis in the majority of patients with HE was usually good if it is diagnosed and treated correctly.

Keywords: Hashimoto's encephalopathy, seizure, immunotherapy, autoimmune encephalopathy, diagnosis

INTRODUCTION

Hashimoto's encephalopathy (HE) is a rare clinical condition first described by Lord Brain (1). The prevalence of HE in the adult population is estimated to be 2.1/100,000 subjects in a study examining patients with unexplained encephalopathy with detectable antithyroid antibodies (2). It has become increasingly recognized in the last few years as an important and treatable cause of autoimmune encephalopathy.

The incidence of HE is higher in female (about 70–88% of female patients). The average age of onset is about 40 years old (3). Clinically, there may be various manifestations such as seizure disorders, rapidly progressive cognitive impairment, and stroke-like attack. The course of the disease may be recurrence–remission or gradual progression. Characteristically, these patients usually have high titers of thyroperoxidase antibody (TPOAb) and respond well to corticosteroid therapy. Because of these features, an acronym, steroid-responsive encephalopathy associated with autoimmune thyroiditis (SREAT), was used in some research articles (4, 5). It was also called NAIM (non-vasculitic autoimmune inflammatory meningoencephalitis) because of the absence of cerebral vasculitis seen on brain biopsies in affected individuals (6). In fact, HE lacks a clear definition, and the symptoms often overlap with other neuronal antibody-associated autoimmune encephalopathies (7).

HE can be regarded as a possible immune encephalopathy due to its possible immune-mediated mechanism. The diagnosis criteria for HE remain a diagnosis of exclusion because its antibodies are not specific to HE patients. Thyroid antibodies and α-enolase antibodies (anti-NAE) have been detected in healthy people and patients with other autoimmune diseases. Although hundreds of HE patients have been reported in the literature, the specific mechanism of HE is not fully understood.

It is suggested that HE is better termed autoimmune encephalopathy associated with thyroid antibodies because antithyroid antibodies are essential laboratory features of the diagnosis of HE (8). Seizure disorders were seen in about 60–70% patients, and many of them showed as the first manifestation of the disease. HE was often misdiagnosed with other diseases by the neurologist and pediatrician, especially doctors not majored in epilepsy. Awareness of HE has increased in the last few years, but it is still rather uncommon. HE is easy to be misdiagnosed because of the low incidence and the atypical symptoms. However, if it is diagnosed and treated correctly, the prognosis of the disease is good. Therefore, it is important to recognize the characteristics of HE. In this article, we review the characteristics of seizure disorders and the diagnostics of HE.

CLINICAL PRESENTATION OF SEIZURE DISORDERS IN HE

HE is a rare, clinically heterogeneous condition with increased antithyroid autoantibodies (9). One report divided HE into two classes: vasculitic type and indolent progressive type; the former manifested with repetitive stroke-like events, such as transient hemiparesis, aphasia, and ataxia with no or only slightly cognitive impairment. The latter shows an insidious onset of altered consciousness, seizure attacks, hallucinations, or psychotic disorders. Seizures, tremors, myoclonus, and stupor can occur in both types (10). Unusual presentations of HE like headache and peripheral neuropathy were also reported in some cases (7, 11).

Seizures are common in patients with HE. Approximately two-thirds of patients of HE experience seizure disorders. Seizure presentations include progressive focal or generalized onset seizures and new-onset status epilepticus (SE) (12–14). SE includes epilepsia partialis continua (EPC), and non-convulsive SE (NCSE) has been reported in 12% of HE patients (9, 14, 15). The most common seizure pattern was focal onset seizures with secondary generalization (4, 16). Seizure disorders are more common in children (present with seizures about 80%) than in adults and change in level of consciousness (17, 18). The type of epileptic manifestation may be generalized or focal, convulsive as well as myoclonic. EPC, a form of SE characterized by recurrent seizures that can last for hours, days, or even longer can also be found in HE individuals (19). Varassi et al. (20) describe a man with recurrent episodes of unilateral left-sided auditory hallucinations. The patient did not respond to antiepileptic drugs, such as diazepam, levetiracetam, lacosamide, and phenytoin. The patient later developed a refractory NCSE presenting with a stuporous state. Visual hallucinations were also reported before the onset of seizures in HE patients (21). Presentation of faciobrachial dystonic seizures was reported in a 58-year-old patient diagnosed with HE. Screening of autoimmune antibodies especially voltage-gated potassium channels (VGKCs)/leucine-rich glioma inactivated 1 (LGI1) antibodies were negative. Instead, the finding of high titer of serum antithyroid and the dramatic response to steroid therapy led to the diagnosis of HE (9).

POSSIBLE MECHANISMS OF SEIZURE DISORDERS IN HASHIMOTO'S ENCEPHALOPATHY

The mechanisms of seizure disorders in HE are still not fully understood. Possible mechanisms including autoimmune mechanisms may play a variety of roles in the pathophysiology of epilepsy because HE belongs to a spectrum of autoimmune encephalitis (22). Thyroid-associated antibodies such as TPOAb, thyroglobulin antibody (TgAb), thyrotropin [thyroid-stimulating hormone (TSH)] receptor antibody (TRAb or TSHRAb), and α-enolase antibody targets for cortical neurons and endothelial cells were found in HE patients with epilepsy. Although antithyroid antibodies are important when HE is diagnosed, the role in the underlying pathogenesis mechanism remains unclear, and no direct correlation between serum antibody titers and clinical state of disease severity is found. The pathogenic roles of antibodies in HE have been questioned. Rather than playing a direct role in the pathophysiology of HE, it is suggested that thyroid-associated anti-TPO is a hallmark of HE (23). Yuceyar et al. reported a case with a family history, and they hypothesized that a genetic factor may participate in the pathogenesis of HE (24). Besides, other research suggested that toxic effects of TSH, brain hypoperfusion, and edema-induced cerebral dysfunction due to autoimmune-mediated vasculitis may also play a role in the mechanisms of seizure disorders (8, 25).

EVALUATION OF SEIZURE DISORDERS IN PATIENTS WITH SUSPECTED HE

For patients with suspected HE, diagnostic testing of blood and cerebrospinal fluid (CSF), electroencephalography, and neuroimaging such as brain computed tomography (CT) scan and magnetic resonance imaging (MRI) are important in differential diagnosis from other causes of neurologic disease, such as inflammation diseases, electrolyte and metabolic disturbances, multiple sclerosis, toxins, and tumors.

LABORATORY

Thyroid hormone dysfunction ranging from hypothyroid to thyrotoxic was found in HE. Most cases occur under euthyroid and hypothyroid metabolic conditions. TPOAb in serum is one of the most frequent signs of HE, ranging from several times to several 100 times higher than normal controls. Serum TgAb also increased (71%) in some patients; however, high-titer thyroid antibodies are not HE specific. They present in about 13% of healthy subjects and even higher (27%) in white women older than 60 years. Thyroid antibodies were also found increased in patients with other autoimmune encephalitis. Some scholars found NAE autoantibodies in the serum of patients with HE and considered that it may be a specific serological biomarker for the diagnosis of HE (25).

CSF examination may be needed in order to exclude other infectious or autoimmune encephalitis. Ilias et al. found that about 75% of individuals with HE presented with CSF antibodies, which are absent in the healthy individuals (26). The main changes of cerebrospinal fluid in patients were mild to moderate increase in protein and normal or elevated cerebrospinal fluid pressure. The increased rates in two studies were 78 and 66%, respectively (27). Lymphocytes can be slightly higher, sometimes with oligoclonal bands. Some patients might have other antibodies in addition to anti-TPC. Thus, it is necessary to detect all autoimmune antibody such as gamma-aminobutyric acid A receptor (GABAAR), N-methyl-D-aspartate receptor (NMDAR), LGi1, and antinuclear antibodies (ANA) (28).

NEUROIMAGING

MRI findings of HE varied from normal to diversified appearance, including ischemic lesions, white matter demyelination, and focal vasogenic edema (29). Many studies showed that the CT/MRI imaging of HE may sometimes simulate an ischemic stroke, multiple tumors, granulomas, or even a degenerative disease (30–32). The diverse neuroimaging features of HE may be due to different or diverse pathological process stages of HE when performing CT/MRI scan. Various and mostly unspecific abnormalities were found by MR and/or CT in about 50%. Single photon emission computed tomography (SPECT) examinations showed attenuated cerebral perfusion in cortical areas or basal ganglia (33).

ELECTROENCEPHALOGRAPHY

The etiology of epileptic seizures includes structural metabolism, immunity, inflation, trauma, and endocrine and degeneration causes, among others. To clarify the causes of seizure disorders in patients with suspected HE, electroencephalography (EEG), laboratory examination of serum and CSF, MRI, SPECT, and neuropsychological examinations need to be used.

EEG is a useful tool in the evaluation of patients suspected of HE. Abnormal EEG results were recorded in 98% of patients with HE (27). Repeated EEG or long-term video EEG increased the positive rate of examination. EEG findings usually show moderate to severe abnormalities, which are often in parallel with clinical improvement after appropriate treatment (34). The EEG abnormalities seen in HE include non-specific diffuse slowing of the background activity (delta or theta frequency wave), interictal epileptiform discharges, repetitive focal spikes or sharps, photomyogenic response, photoparoxysmal response, and generalized biphasic or triphasic waves (35). Diffuse slowing of the background activity is the most common abnormality in HE individuals. The location of epileptic activity is not always consistent with the site of lesions shown on neuroimaging or physical examination (33, 36). Myoclonus seizures were found in about half of the patients with steroid-responsive encephalopathy associated with autoimmune thyroiditis in one study (36). None of these EEG findings were specific for the diagnosis of HE and can be seen in encephalopathy due to other causes. Because of the non-specificity of the EEG examination, it seems to be a limited tool in differential diagnosis of seizure disorders and/or encephalopathy with other possible causes of encephalopathy (37). However, EEG is helpful in reflecting changes in brain functions during hospitalization and follow-up.

DIAGNOSIS

Generally, the diagnostic criteria of HE are based on the clinical features with elevated antithyroid antibodies and good response to steroids (9).

When there are unexplained episodes of focal or generalized seizures, refractory to common antiepileptic drugs, with cognitive impairment and/or neuropsychiatric symptoms, Hashimoto encephalopathy may be considered. Before the diagnosis of HE is suspected on a patient with seizure disorders, detection of neural autoantibodies, lumbar puncture for CSF examination, and brain MRI/CT are needed to exclude other etiologies such as metabolic, infectious, vascular, and other inflammatory etiologies.

We should know that positive thyroid peroxidase antibodies and good response to steroid therapy are not sufficient criteria to establish the diagnosis of HE. Diagnostic criteria of HE have been proposed by Graus et al. (38) (**Table 1**) and Castillo et al. (4). These two criteria suggested that the diagnosis of HE remains a diagnosis of exclusion.

DIFFERENTIAL DIAGNOSIS

Seizures are an extremely common symptom in HE and deserve consideration in the differential diagnosis of patients with newly onset epileptic seizures.

As all the diagnostic criteria have suggested, if the patients were diagnosed with HE, all the specific clinical syndromes of autoimmune encephalitis (with and without positive autoantibodies) and those accompanied by well-defined autoantibodies should be excluded. Due to the diversity of clinical manifestations of HE, some patients are prone to be misdiagnosed as having viral encephalitis because of their prominent psychiatric symptoms. Prominent symptoms of cognitive dysfunction, tremor, and seizure are easily misdiagnosed as Creutzfeldt-Jakob disease (CJD). If HE is characterized by a stroke-like episode, it needs to be differentiated from central nervous system vasculitis. Therefore, when clinically highly suspected to be CJD, the possibility of HE should be considered. In the literature, 53% of patients initially diagnosed with CJD were eventually diagnosed with HE (8); at the same time, HE should be distinguished from primary mental disease, metabolism, poisoning, and paraneoplastic encephalopathy. If the patients combined with peripheral nerve

TABLE 1 | Diagnostic criteria for Hashimoto's encephalopathy, from Graus et al. (38).

Diagnosis can be made when all six of the following criteria have been met:
1. Encephalopathy with seizures, myoclonus, hallucinations, or stroke-like episodes
2. Subclinical or mild overt thyroid disease (usually hypothyroidism)
3. Brain MRI normal or with non-specific abnormalities
4. Presence of serum thyroid (thyroid peroxidase, thyroglobulin) antibodies
5. Absence of well-characterized neuronal antibodies in serum and CSF
6. Reasonable exclusion of alternative causes

damage, Guillain–Barre syndrome should be excluded. Patients with HE may also have a positive ANA, thus often causing confusion with neuropsychiatric involvement in systemic lupus erythematosus. We should pay attention to the fact that psychiatric symptoms can also occur in patients diagnosed with hypothyroidism.

TREATMENT

Once the diagnosis of HE is made, immunotherapy usually brings a dramatic recovery. Seizure disorders accompanied with HE are usually refractory to antiepileptic drugs unless immunotherapy was used. Common anticonvulsant therapy alone is usually ineffective; some patients did not respond to any antiepileptic drugs, including valproic acid, phenytoin, levetiracetam, lacosamide, topiramate, midazolam, and even propofol (20). The use of immunotherapy in the acute stage of HE not only can effectively control seizure disorders but also can assist in the diagnosis of immune epilepsy.

High-dose glucocorticoids and intravenous immunoglobulin are the first-line treatment of HE. First-line treatment also includes plasma exchange. When the first-line treatment regimen is ineffective or has a poor response, second-line treatment (including rituximab and cyclophosphamide) can be used. Patients who received early immunotherapy usually had a better prognosis. Study showed that patients receiving second-line treatment also had a better prognosis than those who did not receive second-line treatment when the first-line treatment was ineffective (7). When the disease is in a stable state, the immunosuppressive agent will be kept in the lowest effective dose for a while and then tapered slowly (39). Steroid treatment leads to complete neurological recovery in most patients, but patients will not always be responsive to corticosteroids. For these patients, other alternative forms of immunity therapy should be tried.

Seizures and other neurological features can also improve dramatically after intravenous immunoglobulin and plasmapheresis, alone or in combination (9, 33). Cyclophosphamide or rituximab can be used as a second-line medication when it is encountered in patients with refractory epilepsy. In recent years, it has been found that T cell inhibitors (cyclosporine A, tacrolimus, and sirolimus) successfully applied to control seizures. Others such as methotrexate, azathioprine, and hydroxychloroquine also showed effectiveness in reported cases (40).

Often, antiepileptic drug therapies that control seizures do not need to be used in the long term in patients with HE. It should be mentioned that seizure disorders can recur especially when steroids were tapered; hence, in some patients, maintenance immunotherapy is necessary (21). For patients with recurrent symptoms, reuse of glucocorticoids, plasma exchange, or immunoglobulin therapy is still effective (33). In order to prevent recurrence, it is recommended that glucocorticoid therapy should be done in sufficient maintenance doses and tapered slowly. Second-line immunosuppressant drugs mentioned above can be used if necessary. It is inappropriate to use serum TPOAb as a marker to determine when steroid therapy should be stopped because the effect of corticosteroids on TPOAb serum levels remains controversial (2, 41). For those patients with severe sequelae, including cognitive impairment and refractory seizures, immunotherapy, and antiepileptic drugs should be used longer (42, 43). Use of immunotherapy requires a close follow-up and regular measures for prevention of side effects.

CONCLUSION

Seizure disorders are common manifestations of HE. The diagnosis of HE still mainly depends on clinical presentation and supplementary examinations (including EEG, CT and/or MRI, and neuroelectrophysiology). The exact molecular mechanism that leads to seizures is still not clear. This type of immune-related seizures is not sensitive to conventional antiepileptic drugs, but has obvious effects on immunomodulatory therapy. Immunosuppressive therapy should be used in addition to antiepileptic drugs to control seizure disorders when HE is diagnosed. However, a better prognosis can be achieved when diagnosed early and treated with immunotherapy. We suggest that the diagnosis of HE should be considered in patients with unexplained encephalopathy presenting with uncontrolled seizures because steroid therapy is highly efficacious in these patients and is reversible.

The clinical spectrum of autoimmune epilepsy syndromes is expanding. HE is a rare, progressive, and relapsing multiform disease. Numerous challenges remain with the diagnosis and exploring the mechanisms of HE. A better understanding of the specific mechanisms underlying autoimmune epilepsy in HE is needed in the future.

AUTHOR CONTRIBUTIONS

All authors listed have made a substantial, direct and intellectual contribution to the work, and approved it for publication.

FUNDING

This work was supported by National Natural Science Foundation of China (No. 81671289).

REFERENCES

1. Brain L, Jellinek EH, Ball K. Hashimoto's disease and encephalopathy. *Lancet.* (1966) 2:512–4.
2. Ferracci F, Moretto G, Candeago RM, Cimini N, Conte F, Gentile M, et al. Antithyroid antibodies in the CSF: their role in the pathogenesis of Hashimoto's encephalopathy. *Neurology.* (2003) 60:712–4.
3. Ferracci F, Carnevale A. The neurological disorder associated with thyroid autoimmunity. *J Neurol.* (2006) 253:975–84. doi: 10.1007/s00415-006-0170-7
4. Castillo P, Woodruff B, Caselli R, Vernino S, Lucchinetti C, Swanson J, et al. Steroid-responsive encephalopathy associated with autoimmune thyroiditis. *Arch Neurol.* (2006) 63:197–202. doi: 10.1001/archneur.63.2.197
5. Mahad DJ, Staugaitis S, Ruggieri P, Parisi J, Kleinschmidt-Demasters BK, Lassmann H, et al. Steroid-responsive encephalopathy associated with

autoimmune thyroiditis and primary CNS demyelination. *J Neurol Sci.* (2005) 228:3–5. doi: 10.1016/j.jns.2004.08.015

6. Caselli RJ, Boeve BF, Scheithauer BW, O'Duffy JD, Hunder GG. Non-vasculitic autoimmune inflammatory meningoencephalitis (NAIM): a reversible form of encephalopathy. *Neurology.* (1999) 53:1579–81.
7. Montagna G, Imperiali M, Agazzi P, D'Aurizio F, Tozzoli R, Feldt-Rasmussen U, et al. Hashimoto's encephalopathy: a rare proteiform disorder. *Autoimmun Rev.* (2016) 15:466–76. doi: 10.1016/j.autrev.2016.01.014
8. Chaudhuri A, Behan PO. The clinical spectrum, diagnosis, pathogenesis and treatment of Hashimoto's encephalopathy (recurrent acute disseminated encephalomyelitis). *Curr Med Chem.* (2003) 10(19):1945–53. doi: 10.2174/0929867033456873
9. Gul Mert G, Horoz OO, Herguner MO, Incecik F, Yildizdas RD, Onenli Mungan N, et al. Hashimoto's encephalopathy: four cases and review of literature. *Int J Neurosci.* (2014) 124:302–6. doi: 10.3109/00207454.2013.836706
10. Kothbauer-Margreiter I, Sturzenegger M, Komor J, Baumgartner R, Hess CW. Encephalopathy associated with Hashimoto thyroiditis: diagnosis and treatment. *J Neurol.* (1996) 243:585–93.
11. Beckmann YY, Top D, Yigit T. Unusual presentations of Hashimoto's encephalopathy: trigeminal neuralgiaform headache, skew deviation, hypomania. *Endocrine.* (2011) 40:495–6. doi: 10.1007/s12020-011-9506-x
12. Aydin-Ozemir Z, Tuzun E, Baykan B, Akman-Demir G, Ozbey N, Gurses C, et al. Autoimmune thyroid encephalopathy presenting with epilepsia partialis continua. *Clin EEG Neurosci.* (2006) 37:204–9. doi: 10.1177/155005940603700308
13. Arya R, Anand V, Chansoria M. Hashimoto encephalopathy presenting as progressive myoclonus epilepsy syndrome. *Eur J Paediatr Neurol.* (2013) 17:102–4. doi: 10.1016/j.ejpn.2012.07.001
14. Chaigne B, Mercier E, Garot D, Legras A, Dequin PF, Perrotin D. Hashimoto's encephalopathy in the intensive care unit. *Neurocrit Care.* (2013) 18:386–90. doi: 10.1007/s12028-013-9834-1
15. Mocellin R, Walterfang M, Velakoulis D. Hashimoto's encephalopathy: epidemiology, pathogenesis and management. *CNS Drugs.* (2007) 21:799–811. doi: 10.2165/00023210-200721100-00002
16. Devinsky O, Schein A, Najjar S. Epilepsy associated with systemic autoimmune disorders. *Epilepsy Curr.* (2013) 13:62–8. doi: 10.5698/1535-7597-13.2.62
17. Alink J, de Vries TW. Unexplained seizures, confusion or hallucinations: think Hashimoto encephalopathy. *Acta Paediatr.* (2008) 97:451–3. doi: 10.1111/j.1651-2227.2008.00686.x
18. Vasconcellos E, Pina-Garza JE, Fakhoury T, Fenichel GM. Pediatric manifestations of Hashimoto's encephalopathy. *Pediatr Neurol.* (1999) 20:394–8.
19. Monti G, Pugnaghi M, Ariatti A, Mirandola L, Giovannini G, Scacchetti S, et al. Non-convulsive status epilepticus of frontal origin as the first manifestation of Hashimoto's encephalopathy. *Epileptic Disord.* (2011) 13:253–8. doi: 10.1684/epd.2011.0457
20. Varrasi C, Vecchio D, Magistrelli L, Strigaro G, Tassi L, Cantello R. Auditory seizures in autoimmune epilepsy: a case with anti-thyroid antibodies. *Epileptic Disord.* (2017) 19:99–103. doi: 10.1684/epd.2017.0904
21. Lee MJ, Lee HS, Hwang JS, Jung DE. A case of Hashimoto's encephalopathy presenting with seizures and psychosis. *Korean J Pediatr.* (2012) 55:111–3. doi: 10.3345/kjp.2012.55.3.111
22. Ong MS, Kohane IS, Cai T, Gorman MP, Mandl KD. Population-level evidence for an autoimmune etiology of epilepsy. *JAMA Neurol.* (2014) 71:569–74. doi: 10.1001/jamaneurol.2014.188
23. Mamoudjy N, Korff C, Maurey H, Blanchard G, Steshenko D, Loiseau-Corvez MN, et al. Hashimoto's encephalopathy: identification and long-term outcome in children. *Eur J Paediatr Neurol.* (2013) 17:280–7. doi: 10.1016/j.ejpn.2012.11.003
24. Yuceyar N, Karadeniz M, Erdogan M, Copur A, Akgun A, Kumral E, et al. Thyrotoxic autoimmune encephalopathy in a female patient: only partial response to typical immunosuppressant treatment and remission after thyroidectomy. *Clin Neurol Neurosurg.* (2007) 109:458–62. doi: 10.1016/j.clineuro.2007.02.006
25. Yoneda M, Fujii A, Ito A, Yokoyama H, Nakagawa H, Kuriyama M. High prevalence of serum autoantibodies against the amino terminal of alpha-enolase in Hashimoto's encephalopathy. *J Neuroimmunol.* (2007) 185:195–200. doi: 10.1016/j.jneuroim.2007.01.018
26. Ilias I, Karagiorga V, Paraskevas G, Bougea A, Bourbouli M, Pappa A, et al. Thyroid autoantibodies in the cerebrospinal fluid of subjects with and without thyroid disease: implications for Hashimoto's encephalopathy. *J Thyroid Res.* (2015) 2015:819072. doi: 10.1155/2015/819072
27. Chong JY, Rowland LP, Utiger RD. Hashimoto encephalopathy: syndrome or myth? *Arch Neurol.* (2003) 60:164–71. doi: 10.1001/archneur.60.2.164
28. Lancaster E, Martinez-Hernandez E, Dalmau J. Encephalitis and antibodies to synaptic and neuronal cell surface proteins. *Neurology.* (2011) 77:179–89. doi: 10.1212/WNL.0b013e318224afde
29. Kelley BP, Patel SC, Marin HL, Corrigan JJ, Mitsias PD, Griffith B. Autoimmune encephalitis: pathophysiology and imaging review of an overlooked diagnosis. *AJNR Am J Neuroradiol.* (2017) 38:1070–8. doi: 10.3174/ajnr.A5086
30. Chen N, Qin W, Wei C, Wang X, Li K. Time course of Hashimoto's encephalopathy revealed by MRI: report of two cases. *J Neurol Sci.* (2011) 300:169–72. doi: 10.1016/j.jns.2010.09.019
31. Su TH, Jin EH, He W. Hashimoto encephalopathy: a case report with proton MR spectroscopic findings. *Chin Med J.* (2011) 124:3420–2. doi: 10.3760/cma.j.issn.0366-6999.2011.20.039
32. Song YM, Seo DW, Chang GY. MR findings in Hashimoto encephalopathy. *AJNR Am J Neuroradiol.* (2004) 25:807–8.
33. Pari E, Rinaldi F, Premi E, Codella M, Rao R, Paghera B, et al. A follow-up (1)(8)F-FDG brain PET study in a case of Hashimoto's encephalopathy causing drug-resistant status epilepticus treated with plasmapheresis. *J Neurol.* (2014) 261:663–7. doi: 10.1007/s00415-013-7228-0
34. Marshall GA, Doyle JJ. Long-term treatment of Hashimoto's encephalopathy. *J Neuropsychiatry Clin Neurosci.* (2006) 18:14–20. doi: 10.1176/jnp.18.1.14
35. Ma RC, Leung H, Kwan P, So WY, Yap F, Chow CC. A 50-year-old woman with recurrent generalised seizures. *PLoS Med.* (2008) 5:e186. doi: 10.1371/journal.pmed.0050186
36. Schauble B, Castillo PR, Boeve BF, Westmoreland BF. EEG findings in steroid-responsive encephalopathy associated with autoimmune thyroiditis. *Clin Neurophysiol.* (2003) 114:32–7. doi: 10.1016/s1388-2457(02)00343-7
37. Baysal-Kirac L, Tuzun E, Altindag E, Ekizoglu E, Kinay D, Bilgic B, et al. Are there any specific EEG findings in autoimmune epilepsies? *Clin EEG Neurosci.* (2016) 47:224–34. doi: 10.1177/1550059415595907
38. Graus F, Titulaer MJ, Balu R, Benseler S, Bien CG, Cellucci T, et al. A clinical approach to diagnosis of autoimmune encephalitis. *Lancet Neurol.* (2016) 15:391–404. doi: 10.1016/S1474-4422(15)00401-9
39. Maroz N, Bernhardt N, Chow RD. Autoimmune encephalopathy associated with thyroid autoantibodies as the cause of reversible cognitive impairment. *J Community Hosp Intern Med Perspect.* (2012) 2. doi: 10.3402/jchimp.v2i1.11453
40. Fatourechi V. Hashimoto's encephalopathy: myth or reality? An endocrinologist's perspective. *Best Pract Res Clin Endocrinol Metab.* (2005) 19:53–66. doi: 10.1016/j.beem.2004.11.006
41. Fatemi S, Bedri J, Nicoloff JT. Encephalopathy associated with Hashimoto's thyroiditis: use of serum immunoglobulin G as a marker of disease activity. *Thyroid.* (2003) 13:227–8. doi: 10.1089/105072503321319576
42. Watemberg N, Greenstein D, Levine A. Encephalopathy associated with Hashimoto thyroiditis: pediatric perspective. *J Child Neurol.* (2006) 21:1–5. doi: 10.1177/08830738060210010201
43. Berger I, Castiel Y, Dor T. Paediatric Hashimoto encephalopathy, refractory epilepsy and immunoglobulin treatment—unusual case report and review of the literature. *Acta Paediatr.* (2010) 99:1903–5. doi: 10.1111/j.1651-2227.2010.01967.x

10

Pediatric Autoimmune Encephalitis: Case Series from Two Chinese Tertiary Pediatric Neurology Centers

Jianzhao Zhang[1†], Taoyun Ji[1†], Qian Chen[2], Yanan Jiang[1], Huan Cheng[1], Ping Zheng[2], Wenqiang Ma[1], Ting Lei[1], Yao Zhang[1], Yiwen Jin[1], Cuijie Wei[1], Ye Wu[1], Xingzhi Chang[1], Xinhua Bao[1], Yuehua Zhang[1], Hui Xiong[1], Xinna Ji[2], Shuo Feng[2], Haitao Ren[3], Jian Yang[2] and Yuwu Jiang[1]**

[1] Division of Pediatric Neurology, Pediatrics Department, Peking University First Hospital, Beijing, China, [2] Department of Pediatric Neurology, Children's Hospital Affiliated to the Capital Institute of Pediatrics, Beijing, China, [3] Department of Neurology, Peking Union Medical College Hospital, Chinese Academy of Medical Science, Beijing, China

***Correspondence:**
Jian Yang
yangjian1306@sina.com
Yuwu Jiang
jiangyuwu@bjmu.edu.cn

† These authors have contributed equally to this work

Background and purpose: We retrospectively analyzed the clinical characteristics of children with autoimmune encephalitis (AE) in two Chinese tertiary pediatric neurology centers. We also compared anti-NMDAR encephalitis with and without co-positive MOG antibody, as well as specific autoantibody-positive AE and autoantibody-negative but probable AE.

Methods: A retrospective study of children (0–18 years old) with AE in Peking University First Hospital and Children's Hospital Affiliated to Capital Institute of Pediatrics was carried out from May 2012 to January 2017. Demographics, clinical features, laboratory, and imaging findings, outcome, and co-positivity with MOG antibody were analyzed.

Results: A total of 103 children had AE, 89 (86.4%) had anti-NMDAR encephalitis, 2 (1.9%) had anti-LGI1 encephalitis, 1 (0.9%) had anti-CASPR2 encephalitis, and 11 (10.7%) were diagnosed as autoantibody-negative but probable AE. Among the 89 children with anti-NMDAR encephalitis, 35 were males and 54 were females. The follow-up time was 1–3 years. A total of 15 cases (15/89, 16.9%) with anti-NMDAR encephalitis had co-positive MOG antibody (serum or cerebrospinal fluid or both). These patients were more likely to experience relapse later in life ($P = 0.014$). We had two cases with anti-LGI1 encephalitis, that is, one with sleep disorder onset, and the other one with seizure onset, both of whom recovered after treatment. One case with anti-CASPR2 encephalitis was treated with an antiepileptic drug and fully recovered. There were 11 cases diagnosed as autoantibody-negative but probable AE who had relatively poorer outcome than those with autoantibody-positive AE (15.2%, 14/89). However, the difference was not significant ($P = 0.08$). Only one 12-year-old girl with NMDAR-antibody AE had ovarian teratoma.

Conclusion: Most subjects with AE in our Chinese cohort had anti-NMDAR AE, which had relatively good prognosis. Children with anti-LGI1 or anti-CASPR2 encephalitis were rare and showed good response on immunotherapy. Co-positive MOG antibody was relatively common in anti-NMDAR encephalitis, which was related to high relapse rate. In our study, the prognosis of autoantibody-negative but probable AE seemed worse than that of specific autoantibody-positive AE.

Keywords: NMDAR, autoimmune encephalitis, child, prognosis, MOG

INTRODUCTION

Autoimmune encephalitis (AE) is a brain disease caused by antibodies targeting neurons in the central nervous system to generate specific immune responses. Although immune encephalitis can occur at all ages, children's AE has unique characteristics. AE associated with cell surface antigens is more common in children, the most common of which is anti-NMDAR encephalitis, and other types of AE, such as LGI1 antibody-related AE, have also been reported (1–3). The common clinical manifestations of AE include abnormal mental behavior, seizure, abnormal memory and cognitive function, and motor and consciousness disorders. Cerebrospinal fluid and serum antibody detection is crucial to determine the specific type of AE. However, some patients were diagnosed with AE clinically but were autoantibody negative. In 2016, the new diagnostic criteria about autoantibody-negative but probable AE was established (4). The immunotherapy should be given as early as possible for AE. Although there is much in the literature about AE (5–7), regarding specifically for children's AE it is still limited. Therefore, we analyze the clinical characteristics, treatment, and prognosis of children with AE in two Chinese tertiary pediatric neurology centers herein.

SUBJECTS AND METHODS

Subjects

The study was approved by the Ethics Committee of the Peking University First Hospital.

The data of children with AE who were hospitalized from May 2012 to January 2017 in the of Peking University First Hospital and children's hospital affiliated to the Capital Institute of Pediatrics were collected.

Methods

The diagnostic criteria for autoantibody-negative but probable AE and definite antibody encephalitis was proposed by Graus et al. (4) in 2016. AE was diagnosed by pediatric neurologists in each hospital on the basis of clinical findings and the presence of specific antibodies in CSF. The flow diagram of this study is shown in **Figure 1**.

The serum and CSF samples of each patient were sent to Oumeng Biotechnology Corporation, Beijing, China, or Neurological Lab, Peking University First Hospital, China, for the antibodies against the NMDA receptor and other AE-related antibodies. All samples were analyzed by indirect immunofluorescence assay using the EU 90 cells transfected method (BIOCHIPs, Euroimmun AG, Lubek, Germany).

We summarized the symptoms, such as psychiatric symptoms, seizures, speech disturbance, sleep disturbance, dyskinesia, and movement disorders, consciousness disturbance, memory deficit, and autonomic instability. Clinical data including age, gender, symptoms, CSF analysis, brain magnetic resonance imaging (MRI), electroencephalography (EEG), treatment, and follow-up were reviewed. First-line immunotherapy included intravenous (IV) methylprednisolone or intravenous immunoglobulins (IVIG), or a combination of these. Rituximab or cyclophosphamide treatment was defined as second-line immunotherapy.

All patients were followed for at least 1 year (in the range of 1–5). Epilepsy was diagnosed when seizure lasted for more than 24 months after the encephalitis (post-encephalitis epilepsy). Good outcome was defined as no sequela, and poor outcome as having any sequela.

Statistical Analysis

Statistical analysis was conducted using SPSS 25.0. Data conformance to normal distribution is described by mean ± SE. Fisher's exact test was used to compare the categorical data. All predictors were tested in univariate models, the statistically significant indicators of the univariate analysis were added to the multivariate analysis, and the indicators considered probably to be clinically meaningful based on previous literature were also included in the multivariate analysis.

Associations were described as odds ratio used in developing the outcome in patients with each predictor relative to those without the predictor with 95% confidence interval and *P*-value. $P < 0.05$ was considered statistically significant.

RESULTS

Clinical Demographics

A total of 103 children with AE, including 89 with anti-NMDAR encephalitis, two with anti-LGI1 encephalitis, one with anti-CASPR2 encephalitis, and 11 with autoantibody-negative but probable AE, were followed up (**Figure 2**).

Characteristics of Children With Anti-NMDAR Encephalitis (Table 1)

The characteristics of anti-NMDAR encephalitis are as follows: 72 patients (80.9%) presented psychiatric symptoms, 65 (73.0%) experienced seizures, 65 (73.0%) had movement disorders, 60 (67.4%) had language disorders, 57 (64.0%) had memory disorders, and 43 (48.3%) had sleep disorders, followed by consciousness disturbance, paralysis, ataxia, sensory disturbance, and central hypoventilation. All patients underwent cranial MRI.

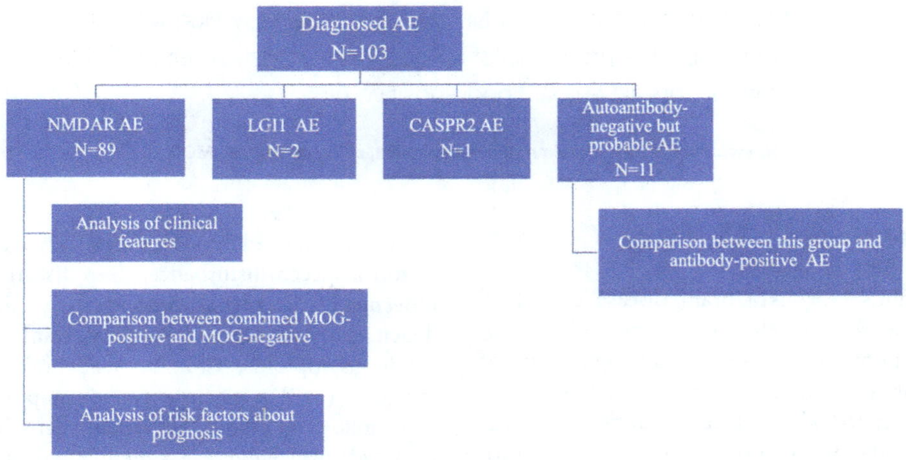

FIGURE 1 | Flow diagram of study.

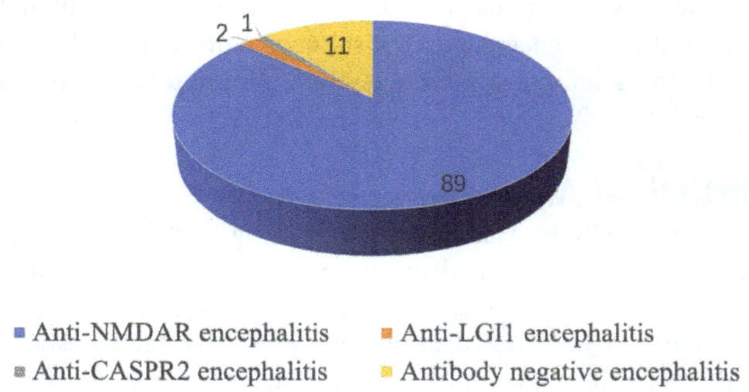

FIGURE 2 | Autoimmune encephalitis classification in children.

Radiologists reported that 29 patients (32.6%) were abnormal. The abnormal locations of cranial MRI in 21 (23.6%), 7 (7.9%), 7 (7.9%), and 5 patients (5.6%) were found in the temporal lobe, frontal lobe, parietal lobe, and basal ganglia, respectively. EEG was performed in all patients, and 79 patients (88.8%) obtained abnormal findings; 42 patients (47.2%) had generalized slow-wave, 33 (37.1%) had focal slow-wave, 55 (61.8%) had epileptic discharge, and 15 patients (16.8%) exhibited extreme delta brush. The CSF of all patients was positive for NMDAR-IgG, but 60 patients (67.4%) had positive NMDAR-IgG in serum. A total 41 patients (46.1%) had CSF leukocytosis ($>5/mm^3$). A total of 52 patients (58.4%) had oligoclonal band positive in CSF. MOG-positive serum or CSF was found in 15 patients (16.9%). For treatment, glucocorticoid therapy was performed in 87 patients (97.8%), intravenous immunoglobulin (IVIG) treatment was performed in 77 patients (86.5%), second-line drugs (rituximab and cyclophosphamide) were used in 32 patients (35.9%), and two children (2.2%) did not use immunotherapy because their parents refused to use it. Prognosis showed that 75 patients (84.3%) had complete recovery, six patients (6.7%) had epilepsy, six (6.7%) had cognitive dysfunction, one (1.1%) exhibited ataxia, and one (1.1%) died. A total of 12 patients (13.5%) experienced relapse.

Analysis of Factors Regarding Anti-NMDAR Encephalitis Outcome (Tables 2, 3)

The results of univariate analysis are shown in **Table 2**. On multivariate regression analysis, the factors associated with anti-NMDAR encephalitis outcome were admission to ICU (P = 0.016) and status epilepticus (P = 0.023, **Table 3**).

Comparison Between Combined MOG Antibody-Positive and -Negative Children With Anti-NMDAR Encephalitis (Table 4)

A higher proportion of precursor infection and relapse was found in MOG antibody-positive children than those in MOG antibody-negative ones, and the difference was statistically significant ($P < 0.05$).

Clinical Analysis of Children With Anti-LGI1 Encephalitis (Table 5)

Two patients had anti-LGI1 encephalitis, one of which was an 8-year-old boy with clinical manifestation mainly for insomnia. The cranial MRI of this patient showed left hippocampal lesions and showed positive CSF and serum LGI1 antibody. Without ICU admission, video EEG showed focal slow waves. The number of cerebrospinal fluid cells was normal. After 2 weeks of treatment with IVIG, the clinical manifestations and cranial MRI significantly improved. The second patient was a 15-year-old boy with seizure. Anti-LGI1-IgG antibody was positive (1:100) in the serum. No memory loss, cognitive impairment, mental disorder, sleep disorder, or movement disorders were reported. The prognosis was good by using IVIG (2 g/kg, for 5 days) and levetiracetam for 1 year.

TABLE 1 | Clinical characteristics of children with anti-NMDAR encephalitis.

Demographic and clinical characteristics	0–3 years old	3–6 years old	6–12 years old	12–18 years old	Total
Total	11	24	39	15	89
Seizures	8 (72.7%)	20(83.3%)	27 (69.2%)	10 (66.7%)	65(73.0%)
Seizures as initial symptom	6 (54.5%)	15(62.5%)	13 (33.3%)	7 (46.7%)	41(46.1%)
Psychiatric symptom	8 (72.7%)	21(87.5%)	31 (79.5%)	12 (80.0%)	72(80.9%)
Psychiatric as initial symptom	3 (27.3%)	8 (33.3%)	14 (35.9%)	6 (40.0%)	31(34.8%)
Movement disorders	7 (63.6%)	20(83.3%)	27 (69.2%)	11 (73.3%)	65(73.0%)
Movement disorder as initial symptom	1 (9.1%)	2 (8.3%)	4 (10.3%)	2 (13.3%)	9 (10.1%)
Speech dysfunction	3 (27.3%)	17(70.8)	30 (76.9%)	10 (66.7%)	60(67.4%)
Speech dysfunction as initial symptom	0	2 (8.3%)	5 (12.8%)	2 (13.3%)	9 (10.1%)
Sleep disorder	4 (36.4%)	14(58.3)	18 (46.2%)	7 (46.7%)	43(48.3%)
Memory disorder	5 (45.5%)	13(54.2%)	28 (71.8%)	11 (73.3%)	57(64.0%)
Consciousness disturbance	5 (45.5%)	7 (29.2%)	11 (28.2%)	6 (40.0%)	29(32.6%)
Ataxia	1 (9.1%)	4 (16.7%)	8 (20.5%)	2 (13.3%)	15(16.9%)
Sensory disorder	0	0	4 (10.3%)	0	4 (4.5%)
Paralysis	6 (54.5%)	5 (20.8%)	5 (12.8%)	1 (6.7%)	17(19.1%)
Hypoventilation	0	0	2 (5.1%)	0	2 (2.2%)
Cranial MRI with abnormal findings			29 (32.6%)		
Temporal lobe	1 (9.1%)	6 (25.0%)	12 (30.8%)	2 (13.3%)	21(23.6%)
Frontal lobe	1 (9.1%)	2 (8.3%)	4 (10.3%)	0	7 (7.9%)
Parietal lobe	0	2 (8.3%)	5 (12.8%)	0	7 (7.9%)
Basal ganglia	1 (9.1%)	2 (8.3%)	2 (5.1%)	0	5 (5.6%)
Brain stem	0	1 (4.2%)	2 (5.1%)	1 (6.7%)	4 (4.5%)
Cerebellum	0	1 (4.2%)	1 (2.6%)	1 (6.7%)	3 (3.4%)
Thalamus	0	0	1 (2.6%)	1 (6.7%)	2 (2.2%)
Occipital lobe	0	0	2 (5.1%)	0	2 (2.2%)
Deep white matter	2 (18.2%)	4 (16.7%)	1 (2.6%)	1 (6.7%)	8 (9.0%)
Subcortical white matter	1 (9.1%)	5 (20.8%)	3 (7.7%)	1 (6.7%)	10(11.2%)
EEG with abnormal findings			79 (88.8%)		
Focal slowing	2 (18.2%)	8 (33.3%)	16 (41.0%)	7 (46.7%)	33(37.1%)
Generalized slowing	6 (54.5%)	12(50.0%)	18 (46.2%)	6 (40.0%)	42(47.2%)
Epileptic form discharge	7 (63.6%)	16(66.7%)	24 (61.5%)	8 (53.3%)	55(61.8%)
Extreme delta brush	4 (36.4%)	3 (12.5%)	5 (12.8%)	3 (20.0%)	15(16.9%)
CSF pleocytosis (>5/mm^3)	2 (18.2%)	11(45.8%)	21 (53.8%)	7 (46.7%)	41(46.1%)
CSF Oligoclonal band	8 (72.7%)	13(54.2%)	24 (61.5%)	7 (46.7%)	52(58.4%)
MOG-positive (serum or CSF)	2 (18.2%)	5 (20.8%)	7 (17.9%)	1 (6.7%)	15(16.9%)
Immunotherapy					
Steroid only	10(90.9)	24(100%)	39 (100.0%)	14 (93.3%)	87(97.8%)
IVIG only	8 (72.7%)	20(83.3%)	35 (89.7%)	14 (93.3%)	77(86.5%)
Second-line drugs (rituximab or cyclophosphamide)	5 (45.5%)	11(45.8%)	14 (35.9%)	2 (13.3%)	32(35.9%)
No immunotherapy	1 (9.1%)	0	0	1 (6.7%)	2 (2.2%)
Relapse	1 (9.1%)	2 (8.3%)	7 (17.9%)	2 (13.3%)	12(13.5%)
Prognosis					
Complete recovery	10(90.9%)	17(70.8%)	35 (89.7%)	13 (86.7%)	75(84.3%)
Epilepsy	0	4 (16.7%)	0	2 (13.3%)	6 (6.7%)
Cognitive dysfunction	1 (9.1%)	2 (8.3%)	3 (7.7%)	0	6 (6.7%)
Ataxia	0	0	1 (2.6%)	0	1 (1.1%)
Death	0	1 (4.2%)	0	0	1 (1.1%)

Anti-CASPR 2 Encephalitis (Table 5)

One of the children was a 5-year-old boy who was admitted to the hospital for 1 day due to paroxysmal headache and vomiting for 2 months was diagnosed with anti-CASPR 2 encephalitis. During the course of the disease, convulsions lasted for 1 h and 30 min. Cranial MRI showed no abnormality, and EEG indicated slow waves in the occipital region. CSF test was normal, and serum anti-CASPR 2-IgG was positive. There was no ICU admission.

TABLE 2 | Factors associated with outcome of anti-NMDAR encephalitis: univariate analysis.

	Complete recovery	Incomplete recovery	OR (95% CI) or *t*-value	*P*-value
Potential predictors	75	14		
Age (mean ± SE, year)	7.92 ± 3.89	6.85 ± 4.96	−1.112	0.664
Female (%)	45 (60.0%)	9 (64.3%)	0.881 (0.269–2.891)	0.835
Status epilepticus	22 (29.3%)	9 (64.3%)	4.336 (1.305–14.411)	0.017
Consciousness disturbance	22 (29.3%)	7 (50.0%)	4.07 (1.228–13.489)	0.022
Movement disorder	52 (69.3%)	13 (92.9%)	5.396 (0.665–43.795)	0.115
CSF pleocytosis (≧5/mm^3)	34 (45.3%)	7 (50.0%)	1.072 (0.327–3.522)	0.908
Anti-NMDAR body titer ≧100	30 (40.0%)	10 (71.4%)	3.75 (1.076–13.065)	0.038
Abnormal cranial MRI	23 (30.7%)	6 (42.8%)	1.594 (0.497–5.106)	0.433
EEG with abnormal findings (slow wave or epileptic form discharge)	66 (88.0%)	13 (92.8%)	1.773 (0.207–15.217)	0.602
Extreme delta brush	12 (16.0%)	3 (21.4%)	1.97 (0.460–8.435)	0.361
ICU admission	3 (4.0%)	4 (28.6%)	9.6 (1.869)	0.007

TABLE 3 | Factors associated with anti-NMDAR encephalitis outcome: multivariate analysis.

	Odds ratio	95% CI	*P*-value
Status epilepticus	5.329	1.26–22.529	0.023
Consciousness disturbance	1.235	0.319–22.529	0.760
Movement disorder	2.944	0.302–28.696	0.353
Abnormal cranial MRI	1.455	0.331–6.388	0.619
Abnormal EEG	2.113	0.177–25.219	0.554
Anti-NMDAR antibody titer ≧ 100	1.821	0.447–7.415	0.403
ICU admission	11.494	1.569–84.2	0.016

No convulsions were observed for more than 2 years after the levetiracetam treatment, and the cognitive function of this patient was normal. Parents refused immunotherapy for this child.

Analysis of Autoantibody-Negative but Probable AE

A total of 11 patients were diagnosed with autoantibody-negative but probable AE. All patients were followed up for 1–2 years. Six patients were female, and their mean age was 6.18 ± 2.09 years old. Seizures were observed in all patients, mental symptoms were found in nine patients, and dyskinesia was presented in two patients. EEG showed generalized or focal slow-wave in all patients. Five patients exhibited epilepsy discharge, and all patients had cranial MRI abnormalities. Two patients did not receive immunotherapy. In terms of prognosis, two patients experienced epilepsy, one patient had dyskinesia, and one patient exhibited irritability. In this group, seven patients were cured, and four had sequelae.

Comparison Between Children With Autoantibody-Negative but Probable AE and With Antibody-Positive AE (Table 6)

In contrast to the antibody-positive encephalitis group, the proportions of movement disorders and CSF oligoclonal band were higher than those of the antibody-negative group ($P < 0.05$). The number of cluster seizures in the autoantibody-negative but probable AE group was higher than that in the antibody-positive encephalitis group ($P < 0.05$).

AE in Children With Tumor

All the children underwent chest- and abdomen-enhanced CT examination, and the boys underwent testicular ultrasound examination. Only one 12-year-old girl with anti-NMDAR encephalitis had ovarian teratoma (0.9%, 1/103). No tumors were found in children younger than 12 years old, and no patient with other AE had a tumor.

DISCUSSION

With the discovery of relevant antibodies, the etiology of some unknown causes of encephalitis has been clarified, and AE has become a topic receiving considerable interest in research. However, most of the published works on AE focus upon adult patients. Studies on children with AE are relatively few, or the analysis was not specific enough (5–8). Therefore, we analyze the cases of AE (including AE with known and unknown antibodies) in two Chinese tertiary pediatric neurology centers, of which both hospitals had patients from all over the country, thereby representing Chinese children with AE to some extent.

The most common clinical features of anti-NMDAR AE as the initial symptoms in our study were seizures, psychiatric symptoms, language disorders, movement disorders, and sleep disorders. Seizure is also the most common symptom in children, which is consistent with much literature (4, 5, 9–11). Children always manifested with neurological symptoms onset, adults with psychiatric symptoms (11). In the children's anti-NMDAR AE, the onset of epilepsy as the initial symptom reached 72%, and the form of epileptic attack was the most common (58%) and comprehensive attack (42%) (11). In adult patients, only 14% (12, 13) of patients are onset of seizures presented as the initial symptom. Other symptoms, such as psychiatric

TABLE 4 | Comparison between combined MOG antibody-positive and -negative children with anti-NMDAR encephalitis.

	MOG-positive	MOG-negative	X^2 or t-value	P-value
Total	15	74		
Age (mean ± SE, year)	6.31 ± 3.82	7.60 ± 3.92	−1.162	0.248
Preceding infection	8 (53.3%)	18 (24.3%)	5.075	0.024
Status epilepticus	5 (33.3%)	26 (35.1%)	1.103	0.218
Consciousness disturbance	6 (40.0%)	23 (31.1%)	0.452	0.502
CSF pleocytosis (≧5/mm^3)	7 (46.7%)	34 (43.2%)	0.002	0.964
Anti-NMDAR antibody titer ≧100	7 (46.7%)	33 (44.6%)	0.003	0.959
CSF Oligoclonal band	9 (60.0%)	43 (58.1%)	0.018	0.892
Cranial MRI with abnormal white matter	4 (26.7%)	14 (18.9%)	0.464	0.496
Extreme delta brush	1 (6.7%)	14 (18.9%)	1.336	0.248
ICU admission	1 (6.7%)	6 (8.1%)	0.036	0.850
Relapse	5 (33.3%)	7 (9.5%)	6.094	0.014
Second-line immunology	6 (40.0%)	26 (35.1%)	0.066	0.797
Sequela	2 (13.3%)	12 (16.2%)	0.078	0.780

TABLE 5 | Clinical characteristics of anti-LGI1 and anti-CASPR2 AE.

Patients	Anti-LGI1 patient 1	Anti-LGI1 patient 2	Anti-CASPR2
Age	8 years old	15 years old	5 years old
Gender	Male	Male	Male
Seizures	No	Yes	Yes
Status epilepticus	No	No	No
Psychiatric symptom	No	No	No
Movement disorders	No	No	No
Speech dysfunction	No	No	No
Sleep disorder	Yes	No	No
Memory disorder	No	No	No
Ataxia	No	No	No
Paralysis	No	No	No
Hypoventilation	No	No	No
Cranial MRI with abnormal findings	Yes	No	No
EEG with abnormal findings	Yes (focal slow waves)	Yes (focal slow waves and Epileptic form discharge)	Yes (focal slow waves)
CSF pleocytosis (>5/mm^3)	No	No	No
CSF Oligoclonal band	No	No	No
MOG-positive (serum or CSF)	No	No	No
Immunotherapy			
Steroid	No	No	No
IVIG	Yes	Yes	No
Second-line drugs (rituximab or cyclophosphamide)	No	No	No
Anti-epilepsy drugs	No	Yes	Yes
ICU admission	No	No	No
Complete recovery	Yes	Yes	Yes

symptoms, involuntary movements, language disorders, and sleep disturbances, are as common as reported in other literature.

The predictors of poor outcome were status epilepticus and ICU admission. In previous studies, the predictors of poor outcome included delayed treatment, young age, decreased consciousness, memory deficiency, high antibody titers, and ICU admission (11, 14, 15). ICU admission was a predictor of poor outcome, which was consistent with our study, whereas the status epilepticus as a predictor of poor outcome in our study is different from previous literature.

The concomitancy of anti-NMDAR antibody and MOG antibody has been reported recently (16, 17). In our cases, one patient was diagnosed with acute disseminated encephalomyelitis due to acute multiple demyelinating disease, and the test showed that the patient was NMDAR antibody-positive. Thus, we should pay attention in identifying demyelinating or acute demyelinating diseases combined with anti-NMDAR encephalitis. In the study of Titulaer et al. (18), the cohorts were divided into three groups. Group 1 included 12 patients whose anti-NMDAR encephalitis was preceded or followed by independent neuromyelitis or demyelinating syndromes (seven cases, all anti-MOG antibody-positive). Group 2 included 11 patients whose anti-NMDAR encephalitis occurred with MRI abnormality and symptoms compatible with demyelination (two MOG antibody-positive cases). Group 3 included 50 randomly selected patients with typical anti-NMDAR encephalitis (three MOG antibody-positive cases). In our cohort, MOG antibody-positive serum or CSF in 15 (16.9%) patients in anti-NMDAR encephalitis was higher than those in other reports. The reason may be that measuring positive for MOG-antibody is considerably high in children. The incidence of MOG-Ab often occurs in East Asia (19). Our patients also had increased risk of relapse later in life ($P = 0.014$) and a high proportion of preceding infection ($P = 0.024$). MOG is a specific glycoprotein in the white matter of the central nervous system. Anti-MOG antibodies can cause demyelinating lesions. In this study, 18 patients had MRI demyelinating lesions, of which 4 were positive for MOG antibodies, but 14 patients did not find any demyelinating related antibodies, including MOG and AQP4. In addition, there were 11 patients with positive MOG antibodies, but no demyelinating lesions were found on MRI. The mechanism by which MOG antibodies and NMDA antibodies are simultaneously positive is still unknown.

TABLE 6 | Comparison between children with autoantibody-negative but probable AE and antibody-positive AE.

	Negative	Positive	X^2 or *t*-value	*P*-value
Total	11	92		
Age (mean ± SE year)	6.20 ± 2.26	7.29 ± 2.87	0.017	0.334
Female (%)	6 (54.5%)	54 (58.7%)	0.227	0.634
Psychiatric symptom	8 (72.7%)	72 (78.3%)	0.109	0.742
Movement disorder	4 (36.3%)	65 (70.7%)	4.828	0.028
Cluster seizures	9 (81.8%)	42 (45.7%)	5.141	0.023
Status epilepticus	4 (36.4%)	31 (33.7%)	0.063	0.802
Consciousness disturbance	4 (36.4%)	29 (31.5%)	0.106	0.745
CSF pleocytosis (≧5/mm^3)	5 (45.5%)	41(44.6%)	0.003	0.955
CSF Oligoclonal band	2 (18.2%)	52 (56.5%)	5.791	0.016
ICU admission	1 (9.1%)	7 (7.6%)	0.03	0.862
Relapse	1 (9.1%)	12 (13.0%)	0.057	0.746
Second-line immunology	3 (27.3%)	32 (34.8%)	0.247	0.619
Sequelae	4 (36.4%)	14 (15.2%)	3.046	0.081

A previous study Dalmau et al. (9) reported that 55% of those with anti-NMDAR encephalitis had abnormal cranial MRI, and the lesions were located in the temporal lobe, hippocampus, corpus callosum, cerebellum/cerebellum cortex, basal ganglia, and brainstem. A multicenter study Schimmel et al. (1) of 540 patients with anti-NMDAR encephalitis showed that 33% of the patients had cranial MRI abnormalities, and 80% of the abnormal signals were found in the temporal and frontal lobes. A total of 29 cases (32.6%) of children with cranial MRI abnormalities located in the temporal, frontal, and parietal lobes were reported in our study. The high proportion of basal ganglia, the incidence of cranial MRI abnormalities, and lesions in the study of this area were consistent with the results in the literature, but the pathological feature and specificity of the lesion site are lacking. A total of 79 out of the 89 patients had abnormal EEGs (88.7%), which were mainly composed of diffused slow-wave, followed by focal slow-wave. However, the extreme delta brush was rare. This finding was also reported in some previous studies (6, 20).

Autoimmune encephalitis (AE) therapy mainly includes first-line and the second-line immunotherapy. A previous work Zekeridou et al. (12) and this study showed that glucocorticoid is still the most frequently used first-line drug. Second-line drugs are always used in children with severe illness or relapse, around 20–30% of total patients. Most of the children with anti-NMDAR encephalitis had relatively good prognosis. Seventy-five patients (84.3%) achieved good outcomes, while 15 patients had poor outcomes in our study. The ratio of good outcomes was lower than those in previous research because we considered cognitive impairment an indicator of poor outcome, which was less used in previous studies. Only one (1.1%) patient died in our study, which was similar to that in previous studies, that is, the death rate in young children is low (2.7%) (11). This finding may be associated with the low proportion of cancer and autonomic instability. Twelve patients (13.5%) relapsed and improved after second-line treatment, which was consistent with the results of a previous report (12%) (11). Relapse rate can also reach 20–24% (21, 22), but the patients in those studies were adults only or both adults and children.

Our study found two cases with anti-LGI1 encephalitis and one case with anti-CASPR2 encephalitis. For two cases with LGI1 encephalitis, their first symptom was only sleep disturbance or seizure, their cranial MRI had typical characteristics, and they both responded well to immunotherapy. Only one case with anti-CASPR2 encephalitis was found, which was mainly manifested as consciousness disturbance and seizure. The seizure was controlled after antiepileptic treatment.

Some patients can be diagnosed with AE in clinical manifestation without specific antibodies. According to the proposed diagnosis criteria (4) for autoantibody-negative but probable AE, we diagnosed 11 patients [10.7% (11/103)], which was higher than that reported previously (7%) (23). These patients were given immunotherapy and were observed for 1–2 years. The outcomes showed that two cases had epilepsy, one had dyskinesia, and one had a sharp temper. The comparison between antibody-positive and -negative encephalitis groups showed that the proportion of dyskinesia and CSF oligoclonal band was higher than those of the autoantibody-negative but probable AE group ($P < 0.05$). The cluster seizures in the autoantibody-negative but probable AE group were more frequent than in the antibody-positive encephalitis group ($P < 0.05$), which were not reported in the previous study. Compared with the other AE types in this study, the prognosis of patients with autoantibody-negative but probable AE was poor. Regarding the pathogenesis of antibody-negative encephalitis, some antibodies may have not yet been discovered. However, these patients may not be associated with autoantibody but related to abnormal cellular or innate immune process (24).

In all children with AE in our study, only one 12-year-old girl had ovarian teratoma in anti-NMDAR encephalitis, thereby suggesting that children were less likely to develop tumors than older people, which was consistent with the results of a previous report on a multicenter study (9) showing that the incidence of teratoma in patients with an age of >18 years old is 56%, thereby accounting for 31% of women with the age of <18 years old and 9% in women with the age of <14 years old. In our study, we only had one case of teratoma (1.1%). Thus, in the children with AE, the incidence of tumors is low, especially for young children. Therefore, according to the characteristics of childhood illness, infectious factors may be a major inducing factor in children.

In conclusion, AE in children has its own characteristics regardless of the first sign of the disease or the condition of tumor concomitant. The shortcoming of this study is that it is not a prospective study and does not use mRS to evaluate the function. Additional research, especially prospective studies to clarify the diagnosis and treatment of anti-NMDAR encephalitis in some subgroup of children, such as the treatment of anti-NMDAR encephalitis-related epileptic seizures, is still needed in the future.

ETHICS STATEMENT

Ethics approval for this study was obtained from the Ethics Committee of the Peking University First Hospital. The parents of the patients signed written informed consent and agreed with the participation of their children in this study and allowed the use of the relevant data and information for scientific research.

AUTHOR CONTRIBUTIONS

JZ and TJ contributed in preparing the draft manuscript of this article and prepared the text. PZ and XJ prepared the figure. YJia and JY were responsible for all supervision and are the guarantor of the article. HR was responsible for the detection of specimens. Other authors have been involved in the management of the children.

ACKNOWLEDGMENTS

We thank all the physicians, patients, and families who provided clinical information.

REFERENCES

1. Schimmel M, Frühwald MC, Bien CG. Limbic encephalitis with LGI1 antibodies in a 14-year-old boy. *Eur J Paediatr Neurol.* (2018) 22:190–3. doi: 10.1016/j.ejpn.2017.08.004
2. Steriade C, Mirsattari SM, Murray BJ, Wennberg R. Subclinical temporal EEG seizure pattern in LGI1-antibody-mediated encephalitis. *Epilepsia.* (2016) 57:e155–60. doi: 10.1111/epi.13436
3. Gadoth A, Pittock SJ, Dubey D, McKeon A, Britton JW, Schmeling JE, et al. Expanded phenotypes and outcomes among 256 LGI1/CASPR2-IgG-positive patients. *ANN Neurol.* (2017) 82:79–92. doi: 10.1002/ana.24979
4. Graus F, Titulaer MJ, Balu R, Benseler S, Bien CG, Cellucci T, et al. A clinical approach to diagnosis of autoimmune encephalitis. *Lancet Neurol.* (2016) 15:391–404. doi: 10.1016/S1474-4422(15)00401-9
5. Ho AC, Chan SH, Chan E, Wong SS, Fung ST, Cherk SW, et al. Anti-N-methyl-D-aspartate receptor encephalitis in children: incidence and experience in Hong Kong. *Brain Dev.* (2018) 40:473–9. doi: 10.1016/j.braindev.2018.02.005
6. Wang Y, Zhang W, Yin J, Lu Q, Yin F, He F, et al. Anti-N-methyl-D-aspartate receptor encephalitis in children of Central South China: clinical features, treatment, influencing factors, and outcomes. *J Neuroimmunol.* (2017) 312:59–65. doi: 10.1016/j.jneuroim.2017.09.005
7. de Bruijn MAAM, Aarsen FK, van Oosterhout MP, van der Knoop MM, Catsman-Berrevoets CE, Schreurs MWJ, et al. Long-term neuropsychological outcome following pediatric anti-NMDAR encephalitis. *Neurology.* (2018) 90:e1997–2005. doi: 10.1212/WNL.0000000000005605
8. Granata T, Matricardi S, Ragona F, Freri E, Zibordi F, Andreetta F., et al. Pediatric NMDAR encephalitis: a single center observation study with a closer look at movement disorders. *Eur J Paediatr Neurol.* (2018) 22:301–7. doi: 10.1016/j.ejpn.2018.01.012
9. Dalmau J, Lancaster E, Martinez-Hernandez E, Rosenfeld MR, Balice-Gordon R. Clinical experience and laboratory investigations in patients with anti-NMDAR encephalitis. *Lancet Neurol.* (2011) 10:63–74. doi: 10.1016/S1474-4422(10)70253-2
10. Favier M, Joubert B, Picard G, Rogemond V, Thomas L, Rheims S, et al. Initial clinical presentation of young children with N-methyl-D-aspartate receptor encephalitis. *Euro J Paediatr Neurol.* (2018) 22:404–11. doi: 10.1016/j.ejpn.2017.12.014
11. Titulaer MJ, McCracken L, Gabilondo I, Armangué T, Glaser C, Iizuka T, et al. Treatment and prognostic factors for long-term outcome in patients with anti-N-Methyl-D-Aspartate (NMDAR) receptor encephalitis: a cohort study. *Lancet Neurol.* (2013) 12:157–65. doi: 10.1016/S1474-4422(12)70310-1
12. Zekeridou A, Karantoni E, Viaccoz A, Ducray F, Gitiaux C, Villega F, et al. Treatment and outcome of children and adolescents with N-methyl-D-aspartate receptor encephalitis. *J Neurol.* (2015) 262:1859–66. doi: 10.1007/s00415-015-7781-9
13. Viaccoz A, Desestret V, Ducray F, Picard G, Cavillon G, Rogemond V., et al. Clinical specificities of adult male patients with NMDA receptor antibodies encephalitis. *Neurology.* (2014) 82:556–63. doi: 10.1212/WNL.0000000000000126
14. Lim JA, Lee ST, Jung KH, Kim S, Shin JW, Moon J., et al. Anti-N-methyl-D-aspartate receptor encephalitis in Korea: clinical features, treatment, and outcome. *J. Clin. Neurol.* (2014) 10:157–61. doi: 10.3988/jcn.2014.10.2.157
15. Gresa-Arribas N, Titulaer MJ, Torrents A, Aguilar E, McCracken L, Leypoldt F, et al. Antibody tiers at diagnosis and during follow-up of anti-NMDA receptor encephalitis: a retrospective study. *Lancet Neurol.* (2014) 13:167–77. doi: 10.1016/S1474-4422(13)70282-5
16. Zhou J, Tan W, Tan SE, Hu J, Chen Z, Wang K. An unusual case of anti-MOG CNS demyelination with concomitant mild anti-NMDAR encephalitis. *J Neuroimmunol.* (2018) 320:107–10. doi: 10.1016/j.jneuroim.2018.03.019
17. Zhou L, Zhang B, Li X, Li X, Huang Y, Wang M, et al. Cerebral cortical encephalitis followed by recurrent CNS demyelination in a patient with concomitant anti-MOG and anti-NMDAR receptor antibodies. *Mult Scler Relat Disord.* (2017) 18:90–2. doi: 10.1016/j.msard.2017.09.023
18. Titulaer MJ, Höftberger R, Iizuka T, Leypoldt F, McCracken L, Cellucci T., et al. Overlapping demyelinating syndromes and anti-N-methyl-D-aspartate receptor encephalitis. *Ann Neurol.* (2014) 75:411–28. doi: 10.1002/ana.24117
19. Asgari N, Owens T, Frøkiaer J, Stenager E, Lillevang ST, Kyvik KO. Neuromyelitis optica (NMO)-an autoimmune disease of the central nervous system (CNS). *Acta Neurol Scand.* (2011) 123:369–84. doi: 10.1111/j.1600-0404.2010.01416.x
20. da Silva-Júnior FP, Castro LH, Andrade JQ, Bastos CG, Moreira CH, Valério RM, et al. Serial and prolonged EEG monitoring in anti-N-methyl-D-aspartate receptor encephalitis. *Clin Neurophysiol.* (2014) 125:1541–4. doi: 10.1016/j.clinph.2014.01.001
21. Irani SR, Bera K, Waters P, Zuliani L, Maxwell S, Zandi MS., et al. N-methyl-D-aspartate antibody encephalitis: temporal progression of clinical and paraclinical observations in a predominantly non-paraneoplastic

disorder of both sexes. *Brain*. (2010) 133:1655–67. doi: 10.1093/brain/awq113

22. Gabilondo I, Saiz A, Galán L, González V, Jadraque R, Sabater L., et al. Analysis of relapses in anti-NMDAR encephalitis. *Neurology*. (2011) 77:996–9. doi: 10.1212/WNL.0b013e31822cfc6b
23. Graus F, Escudero D, Oleaga L, Bruna J, Villarejo-Galende A, Ballabriga J., et al. Syndrome and outcome of antibody-negative limbic encephalitis. *Eur J Neurol*. (2018) 25:1011–6. doi: 10.1111/ene.13661
24. Dale RC, Gorman MP, Lim M. Autoimmune encephalitis in children: clinical phenomenology, therapeutics, and emerging challenges. *Curr Opin Neurol*. (2017) 30:334–44. doi: 10.1097/WCO.0000000000000443

11

Androgen Regulation of the Mesocorticolimbic System and Executive Function

Daniel J. Tobiansky[1,2], Kathryn G. Wallin-Miller[3†], Stan B. Floresco[1,2], Ruth I. Wood[4] and Kiran K. Soma[1,2,5]*

[1] Department of Psychology, University of British Columbia, Vancouver, BC, Canada, [2] Djavad Mowafaghian Centre for Brain Health, University of British Columbia, Vancouver, BC, Canada, [3] Neuroscience Graduate Program, University of Southern California, Los Angeles, CA, United States, [4] Department of Integrative Anatomical Sciences, Keck School of Medicine of the University of Southern California, Los Angeles, CA, United States, [5] Department of Zoology, University of British Columbia, Vancouver, BC, Canada

***Correspondence:**
Daniel J. Tobiansky
djtobiansky@gmail.com

Multiple lines of evidence indicate that androgens, such as testosterone, modulate the mesocorticolimbic system and executive function. This review integrates neuroanatomical, molecular biological, neurochemical, and behavioral studies to highlight how endogenous and exogenous androgens alter behaviors, such as behavioral flexibility, decision making, and risk taking. First, we briefly review the neuroanatomy of the mesocorticolimbic system, which mediates executive function, with a focus on the ventral tegmental area (VTA), nucleus accumbens (NAc), medial prefrontal cortex (mPFC), and orbitofrontal cortex (OFC). Second, we present evidence that androgen receptors (AR) and other steroid receptors are expressed in the mesocorticolimbic system. Using sensitive immunohistochemistry and quantitative polymerase chain reaction (qPCR) techniques, ARs are detected in the VTA, NAc, mPFC, and OFC. Third, we describe recent evidence for local androgens ("neuroandrogens") in the mesocorticolimbic system. Steroidogenic enzymes are expressed in mesocorticolimbic regions. Furthermore, following long-term gonadectomy, testosterone is nondetectable in the blood but detectable in the mesocorticolimbic system, using liquid chromatography tandem mass spectrometry. However, the physiological relevance of neuroandrogens remains unknown. Fourth, we review how anabolic-androgenic steroids (AAS) influence the mesocorticolimbic system. Fifth, we describe how androgens modulate the neurochemistry and structure of the mesocorticolimbic system, particularly with regard to dopaminergic signaling. Finally, we discuss evidence that androgens influence executive functions, including the effects of androgen deprivation therapy and AAS. Taken together, the evidence indicates that androgens are critical modulators of executive function. Similar to dopamine signaling, there might be optimal levels of androgen signaling within the mesocorticolimbic system for executive functioning. Future studies should examine the regulation and functions of neurosteroids in the mesocorticolimbic system, as well as the potential deleterious and enduring effects of AAS use.

Keywords: 3β-hydroxysteroid dehydrogenase, aromatase, cognition, Cyp17a1, estradiol, neurosteroid, dehydroepiandrosterone, LC–MS/MS

INTRODUCTION

Berthold first reported the masculinizing effects of a bloodborne "substance" produced by the testes in male chicks (1). This substance is now known to belong to a class of steroids called androgens, which are synthesized by the male gonads and released into the circulatory system to regulate development, physiology, and behavior. Endogenous androgens are 19-carbon (C_{19}) steroids and include testosterone (T) and its metabolite 5α-dihydrotestosterone (DHT), which have the most pronounced androgenic effects. Other C_{19} steroids include T precursors such as dehydroepiandrosterone (DHEA) and androstenedione (**Figure 1**). Androgen synthesis from cholesterol occurs in the Leydig cells of the testes, stromal, and thecal cells of the ovaries, and the zona reticularis of the adrenal cortices in some mammalian species (2, 3).

Numerous studies examining the effects of gonadectomy (GDX), androgen receptor (AR) antagonists, androgen synthesis inhibitors, androgen replacement, and administration of supraphysiological amounts of androgens [i.e., anabolic-androgenic steroids (AAS)] demonstrate that androgens are critical for reproductive behavior [reviewed in Ref. (7)] and aggressive behavior [reviewed in Ref. (8, 9)]. However, recent research has revealed that more complex behaviors and cognitive processes, such as executive function, are also regulated by androgens. We will review research that examines the role of androgens in regulating the neural circuitry that mediates executive function and behaviors associated with executive function.

In the first section "The mesocorticolimbic system and executive function," we give a brief overview of the mesocorticolimbic system and its involvement in various executive functions. In the second section, we describe evidence for the presence of sex steroid receptors in the mesocorticolimbic system. In the third section, we summarize recent work that provides strong evidence for local synthesis of androgens and estrogens within the mesocorticolimbic system. In the fourth section, we discuss how AAS modulate the mesocorticolimbic system. In the fifth section, we explore how androgens alter neurochemical signaling and cytoarchitecture in nodes of the mesocorticolimbic system. Finally, in the last section, we review preclinical and clinical studies demonstrating that GDX, AAS, and perhaps local production of androgens influence executive functions such as behavioral flexibility and inhibitory control. Like many other neuromodulator systems, androgen signaling levels are likely maintained at particular levels within different brain regions to achieve optimal executive function.

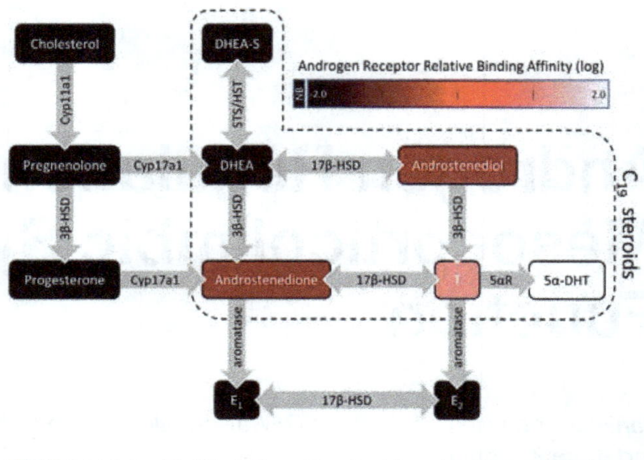

FIGURE 1 | A simplified illustration of the steroidogenic pathway with a focus on C_{19} steroids. For C_{19} steroids, fill color represents the relative binding affinity to the androgen receptor (4–6). Steroidogenic enzymes are represented by the gray arrows. Abbreviations: 3β-HSD, 3β-hydroxysteroid dehydrogenase/isomerase; 5αR, 5α-reductase; 5α-DHT, 5α-dihydrotestosterone; 17β-HSD, 17β-hydroxysteroid dehydrogenase; DHEA, dehydroepiandrosterone; DHEA-S, dehydroepiandrosterone sulfate; E_1, estrone; E_2, 17β-estradiol; HST, hydroxysteroid sulfotransferase; STS, steroid sulfatase; NB, no binding.

THE MESOCORTICOLIMBIC SYSTEM AND EXECUTIVE FUNCTION

Executive functions are a collection of cognitive operations that interact to facilitate selection and implementation of behaviors to attain chosen goals. More basic operations include selective attention, inhibitory control, and working memory (i.e., temporary maintenance and manipulation of information). These operations work in concert with those processed by other mnemonic, affective, and motivational systems to regulate more complex processes such as cognitive flexibility and cost/benefit decision making. It is well established from lesion and functional imaging studies in humans and non-human animals that various aspects of executive functioning are critically dependent on different regions of the prefrontal cortex (PFC) and its interactions with striatal regions, including the nucleus accumbens (NAc; **Figure 2**).

The PFC and the NAc receive dopamine (DA) input from the ventral tegmental area (VTA) in the midbrain, and DA transmission within these regions plays a key role in facilitating both basic and more complex functions mediated by these circuits. Thus, the seminal findings of Brozoski et al. (10) revealed that DA depletion in the frontal lobes of monkeys markedly impairs

---

Abbreviations: 17β-HSD, 17β-hydroxysteroid dehydrogenase; 3β-HSD, 3β-hydroxysteroid dehydrogenase/isomerase; 5αR, 5α-reductase; AAS, anabolic androgenic steroids; ACC, anterior cingulate cortex; ADT, androgen deprivation therapy; AR, androgen receptor; CPP, conditioned place preference; D_1R, dopamine receptor D_1; D_2R, dopamine receptor D_2; DA, dopamine; DAT, dopamine transporter; DHEA, dehydroepiandrosterone; DHEA-S, dehydroepiandrosterone sulfate; DHT, 5α-dihydrotestosterone; E_2, 17β-estradiol; ER, estrogen receptor; ERα, estrogen receptor α; ERβ, estrogen receptor β; GABA, γ-aminobutyric acid; $GABA_AR$, Type A γ-aminobutyric acid receptor; GDX, gonadectomy; GPER1, G protein–coupled estrogen receptor 1; GPRC6A, G protein–coupled receptor family C group 6 member A; HST, hydroxysteroid sulfotransferase 2A1; i.c.v., intracerebroventricular; i.v., intravenous; IGT, Iowa Gambling Task; ir, immunoreactivity; mAR, membrane-associated androgen receptor; mER, membrane-associated estrogen receptor; mPFC, medial prefrontal cortex; mPFC-PL, prelimbic medial prefrontal cortex; NAc, nucleus accumbens; NAcC, nucleus accumbens core; NAcS, nucleus accumbens shell; NMDA-R, *N*-methyl-D-aspartate receptor; OFC, orbitofrontal cortex; PCR, polymerase chain reaction; PFC, prefrontal cortex; POA/HYP, preoptic area/hypothalamus; PPI, prepulse inhibition; qPCR, quantitative polymerase chain reaction; StAR, steroidogenic acute regulatory protein; T, testosterone; TH, tyrosine hydroxylase; TSA, tyramide signal amplification; VTA, ventral tegmental area; ZIP9, Zrt- and Irt-like protein 9.

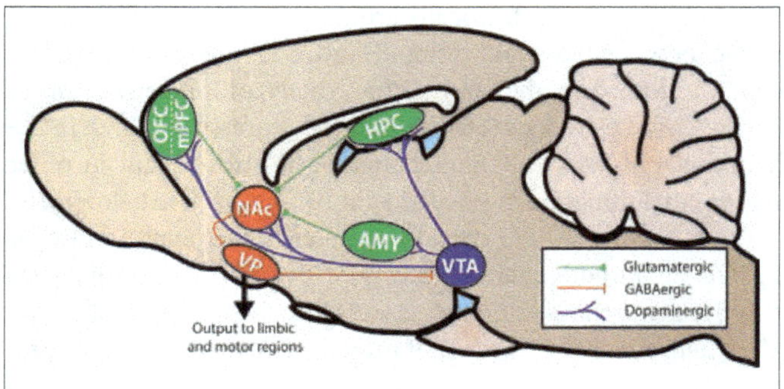

FIGURE 2 | A simplified diagram of the mesocorticolimbic system and associated structures in the rodent brain (sagittal view). Abbreviations: AMY, amygdala; HPC, hippocampus; NAc, nucleus accumbens; mPFC, medial prefrontal cortex; OFC, orbitofrontal cortex; VP, ventral pallidum; VTA, ventral tegmental area.

working memory, and subsequent psychopharmacological studies revealed that these functions are dependent primarily on PFC D_1 receptor (D_1R) activity [reviewed in Ref. (11)]. Different forms of cognitive flexibility are also dependent on DA activity within the frontal lobes and/or striatal regions. For example, shifts between strategies, rules, or attentional sets are dependent on DA transmission in both the medial prefrontal cortex (mPFC) and NAc. D_2 receptors (D_2R) in the PFC facilitate suppression of old strategies, whereas D_1R in the PFC and NAc facilitate establishment and maintenance of new strategies (11–14). In comparison, reversal learning is a simpler form of cognitive flexibility, entailing a shift between stimulus-reinforcement associations (i.e., use the same basic strategy, but approach a different stimulus). The orbitofrontal cortex (OFC) plays a key role in mediating reversal learning in both primates and rats (15, 16). Reversal learning is generally unimpaired by global depletion of PFC DA (17), and DA input to dorsal striatal regions appears more crucial to this form of flexibility (18, 19).

Dopamine transmission in prefrontal–striatal circuitry also mediates evaluative functions entailing a choice between a smaller, readily available reward vs. a larger/more palatable reward associated with some form of cost, which can diminish the subjective value of objectively larger or more-preferred rewards. These forms of decision making are exquisitely sensitive to manipulation of DA transmission, in that systemic treatment with DA antagonists reduces preference for larger rewards associated with a greater effort cost or uncertainty (20–22). However, the mechanisms through which DA regulates choice behavior can vary across different nodes of the mesocorticolimbic circuit. For example, blockade of D_1R, but not D_2R, in the NAc reduces risky choice (23), whereas blockade of either receptor in the NAc diminishes preference for more preferred rewards associated with a greater effort cost (24). Likewise, blockade of D_1R, but not D_2R, in different subregions of the mPFC shifts preference away from more costly rewards (25, 26) and also makes animals more risk-averse (27). Yet, blockade of PFC D_2R impairs modifications of decision biases in response to changes in risk/reward contingencies (27, 28). Collectively, these studies indicate that DA transmission within different nodes of the mesocorticolimbic system helps to refine different types of decision making by promoting choice toward larger, yet more costly, rewards, and modifying decision biases when cost/benefit contingencies change. The critical involvement of DA in various executive functions suggests that other signals that can influence DA signaling, such as sex steroids, may also influence these functions.

THE MESOCORTICOLIMBIC SYSTEM CONTAINS SEX-STEROID RECEPTORS

Multiple lines of evidence indicate that receptors for sex steroids are present in the VTA, NAc, mPFC, and OFC. Here, we focus on the classical AR, the estrogen receptors (ER)α and ERβ, and more recently discovered membrane-associated androgen receptors (mAR) and ER (mER). We briefly discuss androgen metabolites that can act *via* allosteric binding sites on neurotransmitter receptors.

Androgens can act on target cells by binding to intracellular AR. Of the endogenous androgens, T and DHT have the highest binding affinities for AR, while DHEA, androstenedione, and androstenediol have weak binding affinities for AR [(4–6); **Figure 1**]. AAS have a wide range of binding affinities for AR, and users select different AAS according to the balance of desired anabolic (myotrophic) actions and unwanted side-effects (e.g., gynecomastia).

Androgens are lipophilic and non-polar, and thus they can pass through the blood–brain barrier and then the plasma membrane of cells to bind with AR in the cytosol. This ligand–receptor complex then dimerizes, is phosphorylated, and translocates to the cell nucleus, where the DNA-binding domain binds to a specific sequence of DNA called the hormone response element and acts as a transcription factor (29). Such genomic effects are responsible for many of the peripheral effects of androgens, such as enhancing muscle growth (30). ARs are also found in multiple brain regions. Generally, ARs are found in the highest concentrations in hypothalamic and limbic regions that regulate homeostatic functions, reproductive behaviors, and aggressive behaviors (31). For example, male mice with reduced AR in the nervous system show decreases in mating and aggression (32).

One way in which androgens might influence executive function is through direct actions on the mesocorticolimbic system. ARs are expressed in regions of the mesocorticolimbic system, albeit at lower levels than in the hypothalamus. In particular, the VTA, NAc, and mPFC express low to moderate levels of AR in male and female rodents (33–37), non-human primates (38, 39), and humans (40). Using microdissected tissue from mesocorticolimbic nodes, we recently demonstrated AR mRNA in the VTA, NAc, and mPFC using sensitive and specific probe-based quantitative polymerase chain reaction (qPCR) assays (36). The presence of AR protein immunoreactivity (AR-ir) in these regions has also been reported; however, the number of AR per cell is low, which results in immunohistochemical staining that is faint, challenging to quantify, and easy to overlook (41). One reason is that, in extrahypothalamic regions, androgen receptor immunoreactivity (AR-ir) is often located in neuronal processes and not concentrated in neuronal nuclei. Nonetheless, there are many processes and nuclei that express AR in the cerebral cortex, which has been verified by immunoelectron microscopy (35, 41). By adding a Tyramide Signal Amplification (TSA) step in the immunohistochemistry protocol, we recently showed that AR-ir cells are present in the VTA, NAc, mPFC, and OFC [(33); **Figures 3** and **4**]. Double-label immunofluorescence coupled with confocal microscopy demonstrates that AR-ir cells in the PFC are neurons (**Figure 3**). In the VTA, AR-ir cells express tyrosine hydroxylase (TH), a marker of DA-synthetic neurons (42). Furthermore, perikarya in the VTA that project to the NAc and mPFC express AR (43). Of the VTA neurons that project to the prelimbic mPFC (mPFC-PL), the proportion of DAergic (TH-positive) efferents containing AR is higher in male rats than female rats (~30 vs <5%), but the proportion of TH-negative efferents containing AR is similar between males and females (44). Thus, androgens can influence the male mPFC *via* actions on these DAergic projection neurons (42). Taken together, these data suggest that AR are well positioned to modulate executive function.

In addition, T can be locally aromatized to E_2 and bind to ER in the mesocorticolimbic system (**Figure 1**). Many brain regions contain aromatase, the enzyme that catalyzes the conversion of androgens to estrogens (36). Aromatase expression is high in the hypothalamus (46, 47), and aromatase is also present in other regions including the mesocorticolimbic system (see below). The VTA, NAc, and mPFC contain some cells that express ERα or ERβ in female and male rats (48, 49). However, the VTA neurons that project to the NAc do not express ERβ. Instead, in both sexes, VTA neurons that express ERβ project principally to the ventral caudate putamen and amygdala (43). VTA neurons that project to mPFC-PL (TH-positive and TH-negative) lack ERα and less than 10% contain ERβ (44). In general, in female and male rodents, the NAc also has little intracellular ERα and ERβ (49–51).

In addition, androgens can modulate the mesocorticolimbic system through other mechanisms. First, hypothalamic nuclei that have high concentrations of AR, ERα, and ERβ directly innervate

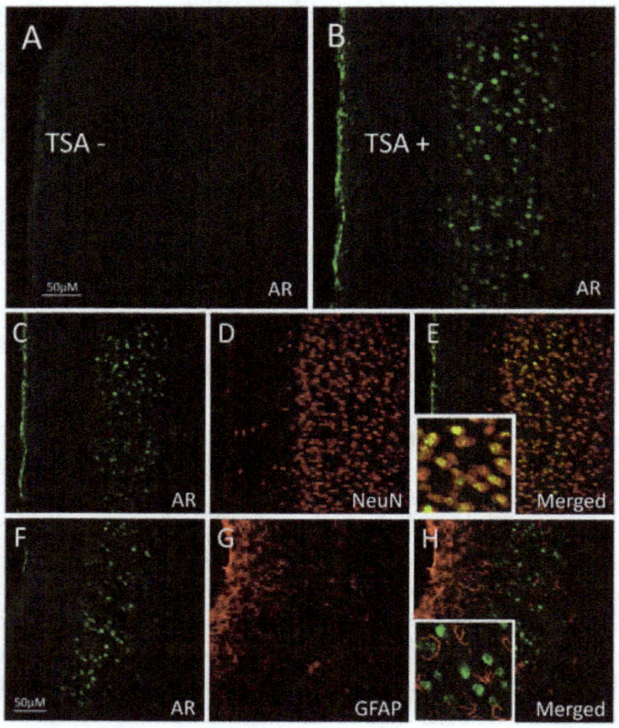

FIGURE 3 | Androgen receptor (AR), neuronal nuclei (NeuN, neuronal marker), and glial fibrillary acidic protein (GFAP; glial marker) immunoreactivity (ir) in the medial prefrontal cortex (mPFC) of adult male rats. **(A,B)** Pseudocolored confocal photomicrographs of androgen receptor immunoreactivity (AR-ir) in coronal hemisections of the mPFC **(A)** without tyramide signal amplification (TSA−) and **(B)** with tyramide signal amplification (TSA+). TSA-enhanced detection of AR in the mPFC of male rats. **(C–E)** Confocal photomicrographs of mPFC with **(C)** AR-ir cells (green), **(D)** NeuN-ir cells (red), and **(E)** AR-ir and NeuN-ir cells merged. Cells that co-express AR-ir and NeuN-ir appear orange–yellow, suggesting that AR is primarily expressed in neurons. **(F–H)** Confocal photomicrographs of **(F)** AR-ir cells (green), **(G)** GFAP-ir cells (red), and **(H)** AR-ir and GFAP-ir cells merged. AR-ir is not co-expressed with GFAP. Adapted from Ref. (33); Reprinted by permission of SAGE Publications.

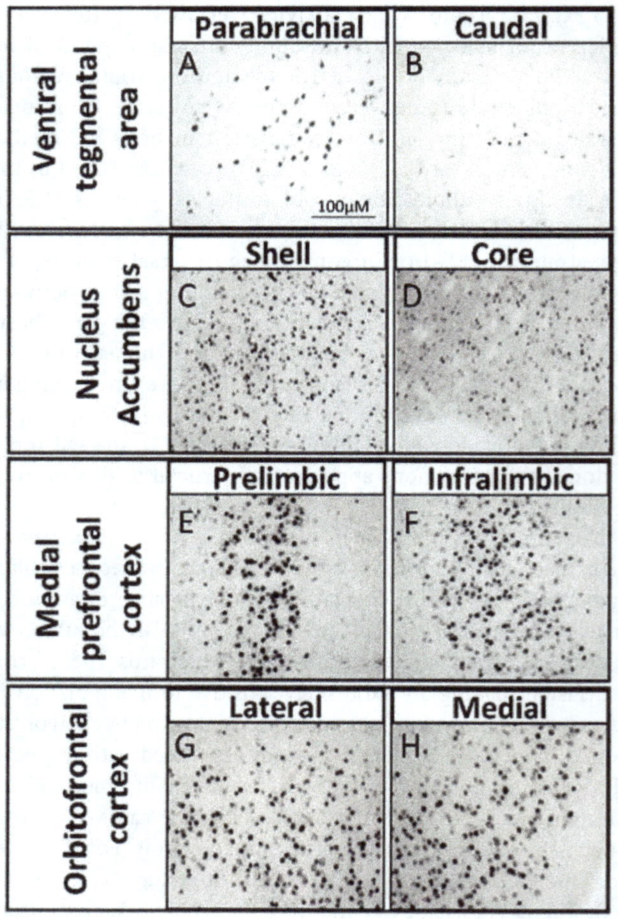

FIGURE 4 | Brightfield photomicrographs depicting androgen receptor immunoreactivity (AR-ir) with tyramide signal amplification in nodes of the mesocorticolimbic system of adult male rats. AR-ir in the **(A)** parabrachial pigmented nucleus of the ventral tegmental area (VTA), **(B)** caudal VTA, **(C)** shell of the nucleus accumbens (NAc), **(D)** core of the NAc, **(E)** prelimbic subregion of the medial prefrontal cortex (mPFC), **(F)** infralimbic subregion of the mPFC, **(G)** lateral subregion of the orbitofrontal cortex (OFC), and **(H)** medial subregion of the OFC. Adapted from Ref. (45).

mesocorticolimbic nodes and influence DA release. For example, the medial preoptic area is rich in AR and ERs and projects to the VTA and modulates DAergic neurons (52–54). Second, mAR and mER might mediate the rapid, nongenomic effects of androgens in the mesocorticolimbic circuit. Two possible candidates for mAR are ZIP9 and GPRC6A (55–57). However, no studies have examined ZIP9 or GPRC6A in mesocorticolimbic nodes, and whole-brain analyses have not reported either transcript in the VTA, NAc, or mPFC in mice (58, 59) or humans (40). In addition, AR variants have been found in neuronal lipid rafts (60). Alternatively, the G protein–coupled estrogen receptor 1 (GPER1; formerly known as GPR30) is present in the VTA, NAc, and, to a lesser extent, the PFC in rats and humans (61–63). Thus, systemic and locally synthesized estrogens could act on the mesocorticolimbic system *via* GPER1. Third, some C_{19} steroids can rapidly (milliseconds to seconds) modulate neuronal excitability *via* allosteric binding sites on neurotransmitter receptors, voltage-gated channels, and neurotrophin receptors [reviewed in Ref. (64)]. For example, the γ-aminobutyric acid (GABA)-gated chloride channel $GABA_A$ receptor ($GABA_AR$) and the glutamate-gated sodium/calcium channel *N*-methyl-D-aspartate receptor are sensitive to allosteric regulation by DHEA, DHEA-S, and 3α-androstanediol (65, 66).

THE MESOCORTICOLIMBIC SYSTEM LOCALLY SYNTHESIZES ANDROGENS

Our understanding of the role of androgens in the brain changed dramatically with the first suggestion of steroid synthesis in the rodent brain. Baulieu, Robel, and colleagues (67, 68) originally suggested that levels of DHEA and pregnenolone and their sulfoconjugates were higher in grossly dissected regions of the male rat brain (i.e., divided into the "anterior" and "posterior" brain) than in the serum. Moreover, GDX and adrenalectomy did not eliminate these steroids in the brain. Later, Liere and colleagues described how these findings were actually artifacts resulting from sample preparation, including oxidation of cholesterol in brain tissue (69). Recent studies, however, have shown that androgens are present at higher levels in several brain regions than in the blood in male rats [e.g., (36)], are directly synthesized in the brain in female and male rats [e.g., (70, 71)], or metabolized in the brain [e.g., (72)]. Local production of neurosteroids serves to influence gene expression or neuron excitability in an intracrine, paracrine, autocrine, or synaptocrine manner under normal physiological conditions (73) or as a compensatory mechanism when circulating steroid levels are low (74).

The steroidogenic capacity of the brain is further corroborated by studies demonstrating that steroidogenic enzymes are present in the brain. In many of the initial studies, the lower sensitivity of Northern blots, *in situ* hybridization, immunohistochemistry, and even PCR was insufficient to detect some steroidogenic enzymes in the brain. For example, Goascogne and colleagues (75) attempted to detect Cyp17a1 (**Figure 1**), which catalyzes conversion of progestins into androgens, in the rodent brain *via* immunostaining, but it was not until 1995 that several groups detected *Cyp17a1* transcripts and protein in the brain (76–78), and even then only at very low levels or only in embryonic brains. Several labs did find other steroidogenic enzymes in the brain, including Cyp11a1 (76, 79) and aromatase (78). Guennoun and colleagues (80) detected mRNA and protein of 3β-hydroxysteroid dehydrogenase/isomerase (3β-HSD) in the hippocampus (HPC), hypothalamus, cerebellum, and cerebral cortex. Current techniques, particularly PCR, can detect all the enzymes necessary for androgen synthesis and metabolism in multiple regions in the male and female rat brain (81–84) and human brain (85, 86).

Little is known about the androgenic capacity of the mesocorticolimbic system, and even less about the physiological relevance of these locally produced steroids. Most studies have measured steroidogenic enzymes in gross neuroanatomical regions (e.g., cerebral cortex, HPC), without specific attention to mesocorticolimbic regions [e.g., (81, 87, 88)]. Specifically, Cyp11a1, Cyp17a1, and aromatase have been reported in the frontal cortex and midbrain or tegmentum of birds (89, 90), rodents (79), and humans [reviewed in Ref. (85)]. However, these reports have low spatial resolution, so steroidogenic enzyme levels specifically in the mPFC or VTA are unclear. Raab and colleagues (91) detected aromatase mRNA in the VTA of male and female rats, but only during early development. More recently, one study showed a behavioral effect of Cyp11a1 overexpression in the VTA, but not in the NAc (92). These results suggest that, if present in the VTA, Cyp11a1 affects reward-seeking behavior, but they did not demonstrate the importance of endogenous Cyp11a1 in the VTA. In the NAc, 3α-HSD and 5α-reductase type I, both involved in synthesizing DHT, are present in GABAergic medium spiny neurons of male mice (93). The steroidogenic acute regulatory protein (StAR), which is essential for *de novo* steroid synthesis, is also present in the NAc of mice (84).

We have recently shown expression of *Cyp17a1*, *Cyp19a1* (aromatase), and *Hsd3b1* (3β-HSD type I) mRNA in microdissected mesocorticolimbic nodes in the adult male rat using exon-spanning, probe-based qPCR assays that are specific and sensitive [(36); **Figure 5**]. The VTA, NAc, and mPFC contained low levels of *Cyp17a1* mRNA, compared to the preoptic area/hypothalamus (POA/HYP). In the VTA, GDX decreased *Cyp17a1* mRNA at the 2 weeks time point. Compared to the VTA, the NAc and the mPFC contained much higher levels of aromatase mRNA. While GDX decreased aromatase mRNA in the POA/HYP, GDX had no effect on aromatase in VTA, NAc, or mPFC. 3β-HSD type I was expressed in trace amounts in the VTA, but was nondetectable in the NAc and mPFC. This is further evidence that the mesocorticolimbic system can synthesize androgens *de novo* from cholesterol or from circulating steroids (DHEA, progesterone).

Using the contralateral side of the brain of the same subjects described above, we also examined steroid concentrations in mesocorticolimbic nodes *via* specific and ultra-sensitive liquid chromatography tandem mass spectrometry. Several results suggested local T synthesis. First, in sham-operated animals, T levels were 2–4× higher in the VTA, NAc and mPFC than in the blood (**Figure 5B**). Second, in all GDX subjects, T was nondetectable in the blood at 2 and 6 wks postoperatively (**Figure 6**). In the VTA, NAc and mPFC, T levels were lowered by GDX but nonetheless still detectable in ~50% of GDX subjects at 2 and 6 wks postoperatively (**Figures 6A–D**). Third, in subjects with detectable T, VTA T levels were similar in sham-operated and GDX subjects. Fourth, in GDX subjects, local T levels in the VTA might be driven by 3β-HSD type I, as *Hsd3b1* mRNA was positively correlated with T levels ($r = 0.316$). We did not detect other significant correlations between local T concentrations and steroidogenic enzymes in GDX animals, but we did not examine all androgenic enzymes (e.g., 17β-HSD, 3β-HSD type 2). Overall, these data suggest that androgen synthesis occurs in mesocorticolimbic nodes and partially compensates for the loss of circulating T in GDX animals. Moreover, the fact that T remains at physiologically relevant levels long after GDX suggests that it exerts a significant physiological effect. Future studies should examine how other androgenic enzyme isoforms may contribute to regulation of local androgen synthesis, as well as the physiological relevance of neurally produced androgens.

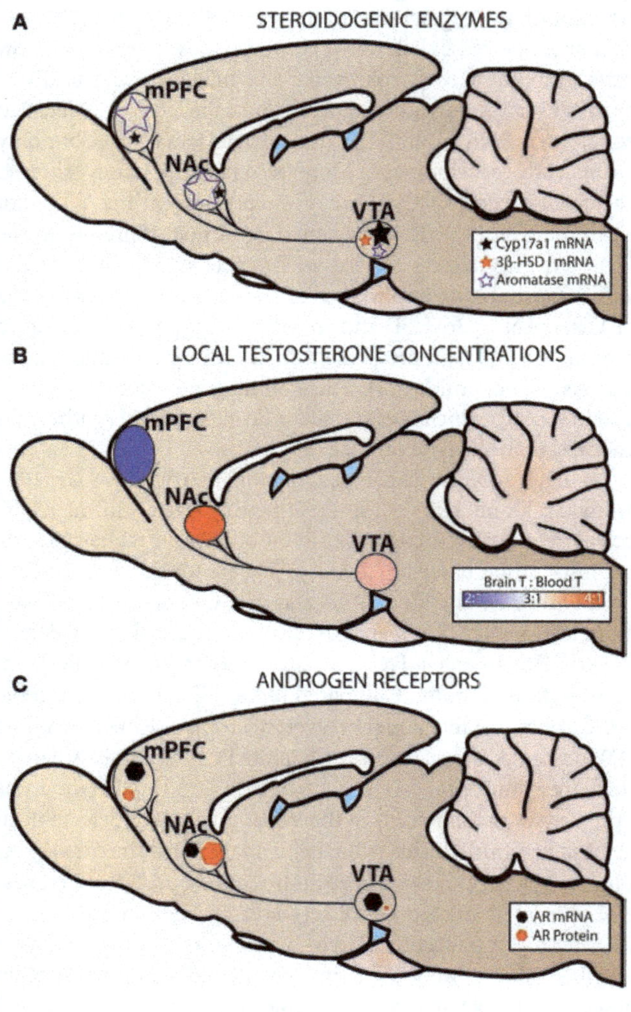

FIGURE 5 | Steroidogenic enzymes, local testosterone concentrations, and androgen receptors (AR) in the mesocorticolimbic system of adult male rats. **(A)** Levels of steroidogenic enzyme mRNA are based on probe-based quantitative polymerase chain reaction (qPCR) assays (36). **(B)** Local testosterone (T) concentrations are based on Brain T: Blood T ratios in intact adult male rats [fed *ad libitum* or calorie restricted (36)]. **(C)** Levels of AR mRNA are based on probe-based qPCR assays (36), and levels of AR protein are based on immunohistochemistry (33). Levels of AR mRNA and AR protein are not shown relative to one another.

The presence of steroidogenic enzyme mRNA or protein does not necessarily indicate steroidogenic enzyme activity. Few studies have demonstrated steroidogenic enzyme activity in brain cells *in vitro* or *in vivo*. In male rats, T in the cerebral cortex and tegmentum (including the VTA) is metabolized

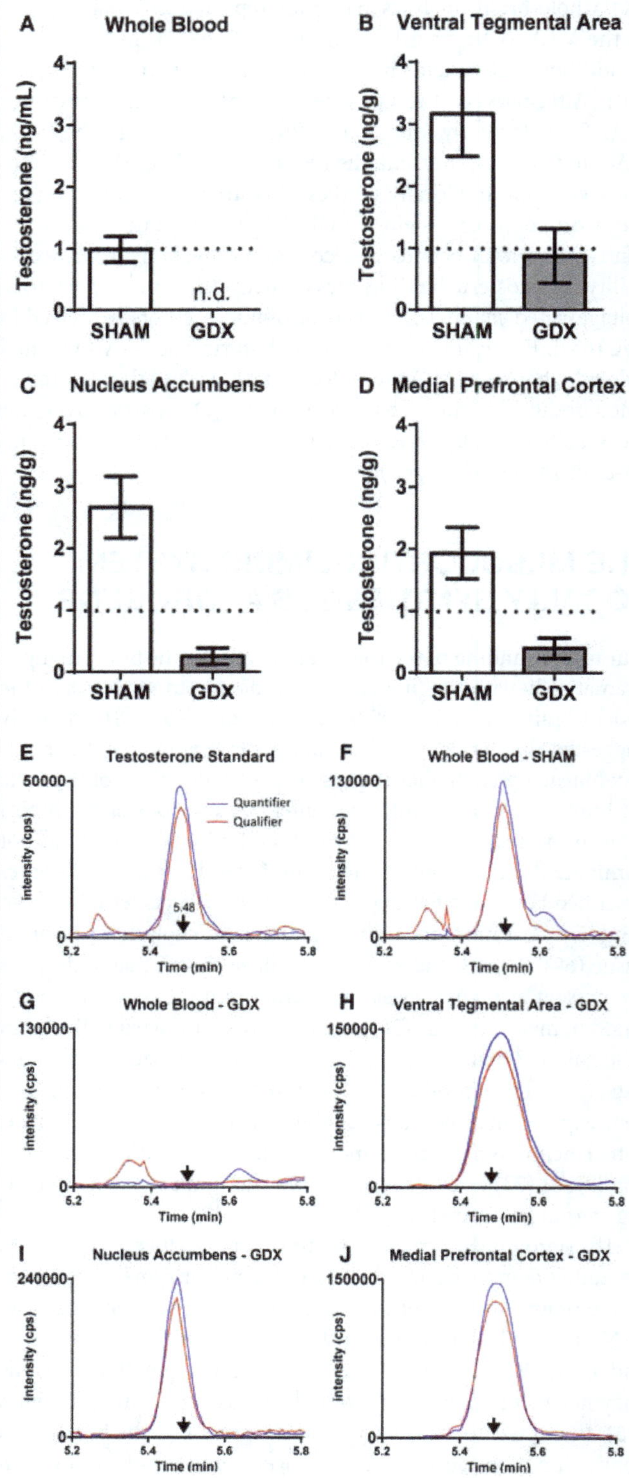

FIGURE 6 | Continued

FIGURE 6 | Testosterone is present in microdissected nodes of the mesocorticolimbic system of adult male rats at 6 weeks after GDX using LC–MS/MS. **(A–D)** Testosterone concentrations at 6 weeks after either SHAM surgery (n = 18–20) or GDX (n = 18–20) in the **(A)** whole blood, **(B)** ventral tegmental area (VTA), **(C)** nucleus accumbens (NAc), and **(D)** medial prefrontal cortex (mPFC). Values presented as mean ± SEM. **(E–J)** Representative chromatograms of testosterone quantifier ion (blue) and qualifier ion (red) for **(E)** testosterone standard (2 pg), **(F)** whole blood in a SHAM subject, **(G)** whole blood in a GDX subject, **(H)** VTA in a GDX subject, **(I)** NAc in a GDX subject, and **(J)** mPFC in a GDX subject. Arrows denote the retention time for testosterone. Note the differences in the intensity (counts per second, cps) on the y-axes. In **(G–J)**, samples are from different subjects, as not all GDX subjects had detectable testosterone in all brain regions. Adapted from Ref. (36). Abbreviations: GDX, gonadectomy; SHAM, sham surgery; n.d., nondetectable.

into 5α-androstanolone *in vitro* (94). Zwain and Yen (95) established that neonatal rat astrocytes and neurons synthesize pregnenolone, DHEA, androstenedione, T, and E_2 from precursors *in vitro*. Furthermore, steroidogenesis was reduced when the steroidogenic enzymes were pharmacologically inhibited or when transcription was inhibited. In humans, adult and fetal brains are capable of metabolizing T and androstenedione *in vitro* to E_2 and T, respectively (96, 97). More recently, studies demonstrate that androgens and estrogens are synthesized *de novo* in male and female rat hippocampal slices (70, 71, 98). Steroidogenic enzyme activity, the mesocorticolimbic system, however, has not yet been examined. What is more, whether these neurally-produced steroids modulate behavior remains largely unexplored.

AAS AFFECT BEHAVIOR *VIA* ACTION ON THE MESOCORTICOLIMBIC SYSTEM

Recent studies have explored the consequences of androgen supplementation at supraphysiological (pharmacological) doses. This is relevant to the problem of AAS abuse. Importantly, when administered at pharmacological doses, AAS may act *via* different mechanisms from those under physiological conditions. AAS are performance-enhancing substances derived from T (99). The media focuses on AAS use among elite athletes and on steroid detection to ensure “fairness” in sport. In reality, use of AAS is far more widespread, and potential risks are only now becoming evident (100). As many as 3 million Americans have used AAS, which includes use in high schools, fitness centers, and “rejuvenation” clinics. A typical AAS user is a young man in his late teens or early 20s (100). Among U.S. high school students, 4–6% of boys have used AAS vs 1–2% of girls (101). This is comparable to the rates of crack cocaine or heroin use (101). It is estimated that AAS use among men in their 20s is even higher (100).

Commonly abused AAS include both aromatizable and non-aromatizable androgens (102). Elite athletes choose T because it is challenging to differentiate exogenous from endogenous sources (103). Rank-and-file users choose T because of its low cost and easy availability. Furthermore, most AAS users do not limit themselves to a single dose or type of steroid (104). Instead, users combine different steroids (“stacking”) in cycles of increasing and decreasing concentrations (“pyramiding”). AAS users take steroids orally, transdermally, or by intramuscular injection (105).

Recent research highlights a range of adverse health effects from chronic AAS abuse, including cardiovascular, hepatic, reproductive, and psychiatric dysfunction (105). However, the dangers of AAS abuse are not limited to the medical consequences of high-dose steroids themselves, but also result from risk-taking in non-social [e.g., drinking and driving (106)] and social contexts [e.g., aggression, sexual violence (107–110), and risky sex (106, 111, 112)]. Understanding the interplay of AAS and social behavior in risk-taking is particularly important in adolescents and young adults. This age group is strongly influenced by peer interactions (113, 114), exquisitely sensitive to rising levels of endogenous gonadal steroids (115), less risk-averse (116), and especially vulnerable to substance abuse (117). In part, this stems from adolescent immaturity in mPFC development (118).

Because it is not ethical to administer supraphysiological doses of AAS to normal volunteers, most of our knowledge of the behavioral effects of these drugs comes from studies of illicit users in the field and from animal studies. Furthermore, animal studies can explore consequences of AAS in an experimental context, where appearance and athletic performance are irrelevant. These studies have revealed that AAS appear to be rewarding and have potential to cause dependence. Rodents will voluntarily self-administer AAS orally (119) and by i.v. or i.c.v. injection (120). Moreover, they demonstrate tolerance, withdrawal, and fatal overdose with self-administration (121). T self-administration (i.c.v.) is blocked by the AR antagonist flutamide (121), although it appears that classical AR are not required for androgen reinforcement (122). The behavioral and physiological effects of supraphysiological doses of T resemble those of opioid overdose and are rapidly reversed by opioid antagonists (121). Likewise, many human AAS users meet DSM criteria for psychoactive substance dependence, including continued use despite negative side-effects, and withdrawal symptoms when steroids are discontinued (123).

The effects of AAS on reward and reinforcement strongly implicate involvement of the mesocorticolimbic system, since drugs of abuse act, in part, *via* DA release in NAc (124). Male rats form conditioned place preference (CPP) in response to intra-NAc infusion of T (125) or its metabolites (126), similar to the effects of DA-releasing drugs (127). Conversely, systemic or intra-NAc treatments with D_1R and D_2R antagonists block T-induced CPP (128, 129). Nonetheless, the manner in which androgens modulate DA release and signaling is still unclear. For example, acute administration of T does not induce NAc DA release (130), and in fact, AAS can reduce cocaine- or amphetamine-evoked DA release in NAc (131, 132). This latter finding is consistent with the observation that the acquisition of T self-administration is slow compared with cocaine or other addictive drugs (119). On the other hand, T upregulates the Fos protein, a marker of cellular activity, in regions of the mesolimbic DA system (133). Thus, the reinforcing effects of exogenous T may be due to its ability to modulate neural activity and DA signaling within the mesocorticolimbic circuit, but may do so without directly affecting DA release. Indeed, chronic AAS administration alters $GABA_AR$ subunit expression throughout the brain (including mesocorticolimbic regions), thus altering the physiological response to DA-independent GABAergic signaling (134, 135).

ANDROGENS MODULATE THE NEUROCHEMISTRY AND STRUCTURE OF THE MESOCORTICOLIMBIC SYSTEM

Many androgen-dependent behaviors are mediated by neurochemical changes and neuronal activity in the mesocorticolimbic system. In several mammalian species, GDX of adult males diminishes expression of copulatory behavior, which can be restored by chronic T treatment (136). Copulatory behavior, particularly ejaculation, is correlated with a T-dependent increase in DA release in the NAc (137, 138). In this section, we will discuss how androgen deprivation, AAS, and androgen synthesis influence the neurochemistry and structure of the mesocorticolimbic system.

Most studies examining T regulation of the mesocorticolimbic system have focused on DAergic transmission in the NAc and mPFC. GDX alters DA tone in the mPFC of male and female rats (139). In the mPFC, GDX decreases basal DA after 4 days but increases it after 28 days. This is likely a result of GDX increasing bursting of VTA DA neurons, altering activity of mPFC efferents to the VTA, and gradually increasing TH in the VTA (140, 141). In contrast, in the NAc, basal DA is unchanged after GDX, but the DA metabolites 3,4-dihydroxyphenylacetic acid and homovanillic acid are increased after GDX (142). This finding suggests that GDX increases DA turnover in the NAc, which might indicate faster clearance of DA from the synapse and higher rates of DA signaling at baseline. GDX also modulates evoked electrophysiological and DAergic responses in the mPFC and NAc. In superfused striatal tissue, K^+-simulated DA release was higher in GDX compared to GDX + T adult male mice (143). In the same study, reserpine, a drug that depletes DA, had the opposite effect, whereby DA release was higher in GDX + T male mice. This is in line with studies demonstrating that GDX affects storage, uptake, and/or synthesis of catecholamines in mesocorticolimbic nodes (142, 144) and helps to maintain NAc DA levels when exposed to methamphetamine (145).

Androgen-mediated structural plasticity and alterations in neurotransmitter receptor densities in the mesocorticolimbic system are other potential mechanism through which these hormones may alter cognitive/behavioral functions of this system. GDX decreases and high doses of T increase dendritic spine density in limbic regions, including the amygdala and HPC, in male rats (146, 147) and male monkeys (148). In a recent study, male rats were treated chronically with high-dose T, and brains were stained by Golgi–Cox to analyze neuronal morphology in medium spiny neurons of nucleus accumbens shell (NAcS) (149). T decreased spine density throughout the dendritic tree in the NAcS. However, T treatment did not affect total spine number, dendritic length, or arborization. Similarly, in the mPFC, GDX reduces and DHT increases dendritic spine formation in male mice (150). The effect of DHT on dendritic spine formation was reduced, but not absent, in GDX testicular feminization mutant male rats (a naturally occurring mutant with severely attenuated AR binding capacity), which suggests both androgenic and non-androgenic influence on synaptic remodeling.

Androgens can influence the function of the mesocorticolimbic nodes by their local metabolism to more potent androgens (e.g., T→DHT), further metabolism to weak androgens (e.g., T→DHT→3α-androstanediol), or metabolism to estrogens (T→E_2). 3α-androstanediol, for example, has weak androgenic effects but also acts as a robust and rapid neuromodulator *via* allosteric binding to $GABA_AR$ (66, 151). Indeed, 3α-androstanediol in the NAc facilitates CPP (a DA-dependent behavior) in rodents, likely through allosteric agonism of $GABA_AR$ in GABAergic medium spiny neurons (152). Concurrently, the aromatization of T into E_2 may also influence activity in the mesocorticolimbic system. E_2 decreases striatal DA transporter density, enhances DA synthesis and degradation (153, 154), and downregulates DA binding to D_2R in the NAc (155). In contrast, systemic treatment with the aromatase inhibitor letrozole decreases basal DA turnover in the mPFC of male and female adult rats (156). The regulation of DA turnover in the brain may be directly related to changes in phasic DA signaling. Indeed, direct pulsatile application of E_2 to striatal slices induces DA release (157) and enhances K^+-mediated DA release (158). Patch clamp analysis of ion transfer across the membrane in dissociated NAc medium spiny neurons demonstrated that there is a prompt diminution of Ca^{++} currents in response to acute E_2 (159). Taken together, these data suggest that local production of E_2 in males and females modulates DA signaling and postsynaptic neural excitability in the mesocorticolimbic system.

Few studies have examined whether neurosteroids produced in the mesocorticolimbic system influence neurochemistry. Pharmacological inhibition of Cyp17a1 regulates a DA-dependent behavior [prepulse inhibition (PPI)], but the study did not examine the direct effect on DA signaling (160). Inhibition of Cyp17a1 would decrease both androgen and estrogen signaling. DHEA, a product of Cyp17a1, is present in human, but not in laboratory rat or mouse, circulation. DHEA has a wide range of neurochemical effects, but the source of DHEA is rarely determined (161). The mesocorticolimbic system is sensitive to DHEA. For example, DHEA decreases the activity of monoamine oxidase, an enzyme necessary for the degradation of monoamines, in the NAc in male rats *in vivo* and *in vitro* (162). Pharmacological inhibition of 5αR suggests that DHT influences neurochemistry, particularly DA signaling, in the mesocorticolimbic system (163–165). Overall, these data suggest neurosteroids regulate DA turnover and DA signaling in the mesocorticolimbic system, which is important for regulating executive functions.

ANDROGENS REGULATE EXECUTIVE FUNCTION

Clinical and preclinical evidence suggest that hypogonadism and GDX have deleterious effects on executive functioning, which can often be ameliorated with androgen replacement. Furthermore, excessive androgen exposure (e.g., AAS) during adolescence and/or adulthood has detrimental effects on executive functioning. We also examine evidence that the brain compensates for a decrease in circulating androgens by increasing local androgen synthesis in the mesocorticolimbic system to mitigate deficits in executive functioning. These studies support the hypothesis that there is an optimal level of androgen signaling within the mesocorticolimbic system for proper executive functioning.

Low Androgen Signaling

Andrew and Rogers (166) were among the first to demonstrate that androgens affect executive function. In a foraging paradigm, young male chicks treated with T pecked grains of a familiar color and ignored unfamiliar, novel-colored grains, while vehicle-treated chicks demonstrated behavioral flexibility and pecked both grain colors without bias (166). The authors used the term "persistence" (also called "perseveration") to describe the inability to stop using a response strategy when it is no longer relevant or advantageous. Rogers (167) then showed that antiandrogen treatment or GDX decreased persistence in adult male chickens, whereas systemic T replacement in GDX chickens reinstated persistence. Subsequent studies in adult male rodents revealed that GDX or an antiandrogen reduced persistence, supporting the initial findings in birds (168, 169). GDX also decreases male persistence during social investigation of female conspecifics, suggesting that T increases male persistence in gaining access to potential mates (170).

T increases perseveration in operant conditioning tasks that require behavioral flexibility. Using a reversal learning task, van Hest and colleagues (171) demonstrated that GDX male rats perseverated less on the previously reinforced lever, while administration of T to GDX subjects displayed the highest rates of perseveration. Additionally, GDX male rats exposed to a conditional discrimination task in a T-maze made fewer errors during the reversal phase (i.e., decrease in perseverative errors) compared to intact subjects (172). On a delayed spatial alternation test, GDX subjects made less perseverative errors than intact subjects, but only after a delay of 6 sec or more, suggesting a concurrent deficit in working memory (173).

In men, declines in executive functioning and visuospatial ability are the most commonly reported adverse cognitive effects of androgen deprivation therapy [ADT (174)]. ADTs are administered to nearly 50% of prostate cancer patients (175) and include GnRH analogs (e.g., Histrelin), AR antagonists (e.g., flutamide), and androgenic enzyme inhibitors (e.g., abiraterone, a Cyp17a1 inhibitor) [see (176) for review]. Many ADTs decrease systemic T but might not decrease local androgen synthesis equally across tissue types (e.g., GnRH analogs). If a clinical study includes only subjects on ADTs that inhibit androgen synthesis and/or signaling in the brain, which is often not the case, then the effects of ADTs on executive function might be more clear (see below).

There is contradictory evidence on the effect of ADTs on executive functioning. For example, ADT is associated with deficits in attention and cognitive control [i.e., Trail Making B task, Stroop Interference Test (177)]. Furthermore, ADT is associated with decreases in gray matter volume in the dorsolateral and frontopolar PFC (178) and decreased neural activity and connectivity in the mPFC during tasks requiring inhibitory control (179). ADT is also associated with changes in impulsivity, emotional lability, and working memory, compared to matched non-ADT subjects (180). These findings suggest that ADT disrupts PFC function, an area particularly sensitive to androgens in males (33, 39).

However, other studies have not found an association between ADT and executive function (181–183). A recent meta-analysis of the effects of ADT on a variety of cognitive functions found that only visuospatial ability was reliably affected by ADT, whereas assays of executive functioning (e.g., Trail Making Test B, Stroop Interference Task) did not detect any significant differences (184). These findings are in line with a study in menopausal women with low T who were then treated with T and did not show changes in a range of executive functions compared to untreated subjects (185). However, the assessment tools for these studies might not be sensitive enough to detect small, yet important, changes in executive functions [e.g., (186)]. In addition, studies on ADT and executive function may lack statistical power, neglect confounding variables (183, 187), or include subjects who have not received ADT for enough time [ADT is usually administered for 2–3 years (181)]. These issues reduce the ability to detect effects of ADT on executive functioning. For example, Alibhai and colleagues (181) conducted a small study that regularly administered a battery of neuropsychological tests to ADT patients for 36 months, and ADT was not associated with deficits in cognitive flexibility or working memory. However, this study might not have utilized cognitive tests sensitive enough to detect PFC-specific deficits in executive functioning [e.g., Iowa Gambling Task (IGT)]. Moreover, 95% of ADT subjects in this study were using GnRH analogs as their sole ADT, which may not affect androgen synthesis in the brain, as would androgenic enzyme inhibitors.

High Androgen Signaling

Supraphysiological levels of androgens typically seen with AAS use also impair executive function. This has been explored in rats treated with supraphysiological levels of T and trained to work for food reward (sugar pellets) in an operant chamber (**Figures 7** and **8**). T-treated rats display deficits in different forms of cognitive flexibility, including reversal learning and extra-dimensional set-shifting (188). These rats take longer to shift their behavior when stimuli associated with rewards are reversed, or when rats must employ a novel discrimination strategy to obtain rewards. Importantly, set-shifting behavior is dependent upon D_1R in NAc (12), and AAS reduce NAc D_1R (189).

Anabolic-androgenic steroids also alter different forms of cost/benefit decision making in operant discounting tasks. In these tasks, rats choose between two retractable levers, one of which is associated with a smaller, easily obtainable reward (1 pellet) and the other with a larger reward (3 or 4 pellets) associated some cost. These costs can include effort, delay, punishment, and probability, which results in discounting of the larger reward (i.e., making it less desirable; **Figure 8**). AAS and DA have site- and task-specific effects on discounting behavior. In particular, AAS do not cause impulsivity with a consistent preference for small rewards, nor do they produce a "win-at-all-costs" strategy that always favors the large reward. Instead, there is a selective effect of AAS. Specifically, AAS-treated rats are less sensitive to effort (188), punishment (192), and delay (191), but are more sensitive to uncertainty (190). In particular, AAS may diminish sensitivity

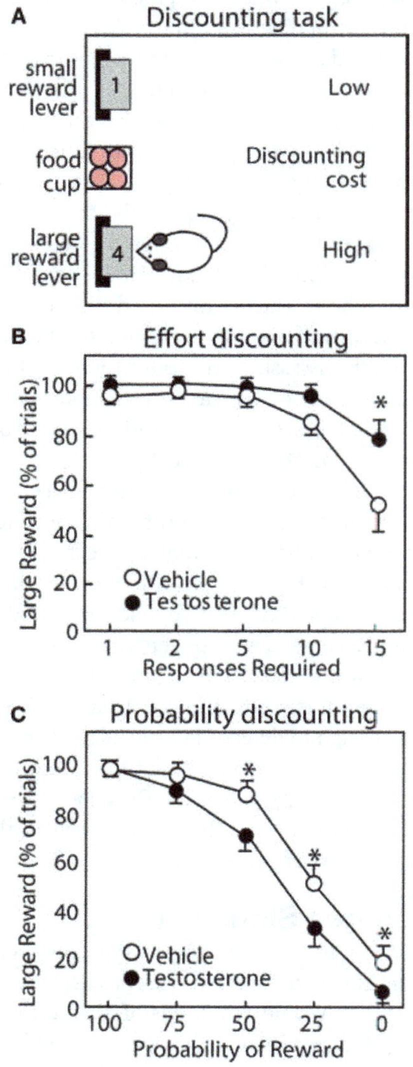

FIGURE 7 | Testosterone influences discounting behavior of male rats. **(A)** Operant task for discounting behavior. Rats choose between two levers. The small reward lever delivers 1 pellet with minimal cost. The large reward lever delivers four pellets with increasing cost throughout the session. **(B)** For effort discounting behavior, the response requirement (number of lever presses) increases. **(C)** For probability discounting, the large reward is delivered with decreasing probability. Compared with vehicle controls (open circles), testosterone (closed circles) increases preference for the large reward lever in effort discounting, but reduces preference for the large reward lever in probability discounting. Adapted with permission from Ref. (190). Values presented as mean ± SEM. $^*p \leq 0.05$.

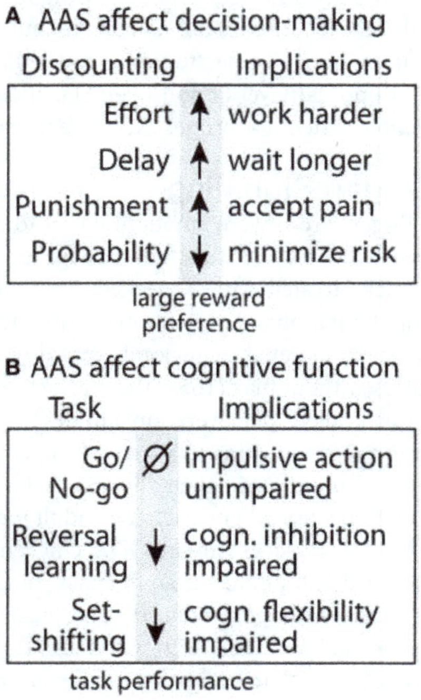

FIGURE 8 | Summary of effects of anabolic-androgenic steroids (AAS) on decision making and cognitive function. **(A)** Testosterone effects on discounting behavior for effort (190), delay (191), punishment (192), and uncertainty (190). **(B)** Testosterone effects on cognitive function and motor impulsivity in the go/no-go task (192), cognitive inhibition in the reversal learning task, and cognitive flexibility in the set-shifting task (188).

to future negative consequences, even as they render users more sensitive to unpredictable outcomes.

A wealth of studies has mapped the neurotransmitters and brain regions responsible for discounting behavior using systemic treatment with neurotransmitter receptor agonists and antagonists and selective inactivation of NAc subregions. As discussed previously, D_1R and D_2R each promote preference for the large reward in effort discounting (delivery of the large reward requires more lever presses) and probability discounting [delivery of the large reward is uncertain (193)]. Studies using inactivation of NAc subregions have revealed that effort discounting is regulated by the NAc core (NAcC), while probability discounting is regulated more prominently by the NAc shell [NAcS (194, 195)]. These findings align with modulation of D_1R and D_2R in NAc subregions by the AAS nandrolone (189) and with recent studies of effort and probability discounting in response to high-dose T (190). T reduces preference for larger reward during probability discounting (190), and AAS reduce DA receptors in NAcS (189). Conversely, T treatment increases preference for the large reward during effort discounting (190), and nandrolone increases D_2R in NAcC (189). Thus, AAS might reduce sensitivity to effort during effort discounting by increasing D_2R in NAcC.

In animal studies, it is interesting that AAS selectively alter elements of risk-taking and impulsivity. In probability discounting, risk is reflected by the potential for reward omission, and T makes rats more risk-averse, an effect that may be driven by a reduction in NAc D_1R. At the same time, they are less risk-averse in punishment discounting, whereby they risk a footshock with delivery of the large reward (190). Together, these results reveal a nuanced effect of supplemental T to increase sensitivity to reward omission and simultaneously decrease responsiveness to punishment. A similar picture emerges in assessment of how T alters different aspects of impulsivity. T has no effect on impulsive actions as measured in a go/no-go task (192), wherein rats must switch between initiating and inhibiting a response to obtain rewards. However, the same study showed that T reduces impulsive choice, assessed with a delay discounting task, in that it increases the subjects' willingness to wait for a large, delayed reward. Given the complex manner in which increasing androgen activity can influence various forms of decision making, it is unlikely that the effects of these treatments are driven by uniform increases or decreases in mesolimbic DA activity. Rather, these findings suggest that the manner in which T influences the behavioral functions depends in part on the specific costs that are being evaluated and the underlying corticostriatal circuitry that is recruited in guiding these decisions.

Studies of executive function in human AAS users are limited and restricted to male subjects. AAS abusers show impaired visuospatial working memory compared to non-users, similar to deficits seen in ADT (184), and the level of impairment is correlated with lifetime AAS use (196). A variety of evidence further implicates androgens and AAS in risk-taking behavior in humans. In a study of American high school students, AAS use was associated with risky sex, drinking and driving, carrying a weapon, and not wearing a helmet or seat belt (106). Psychological evaluations of human users have also implicated AAS in impaired decision making, which may stem from feelings of invincibility (197). Deaths among AAS users show high rates of homicide, suicide, and drug overdose (110). These possible effects of AAS abuse on risk-taking in humans might be similar to punishment discounting in rats, in that androgens increase the appetite for reward despite a risk of punishment.

Risk taking induced by AAS has a potentially dangerous social dimension as well. AAS use has been implicated in several violent murders (107–110). In surveys of current AAS users and in studies of human volunteers, increased aggression is the most consistent behavioral effect of high-dose AAS exposure in humans (103, 105). Compared with non-users, AAS users report increased sex drive (198) and increases in risky sexual behaviors [i.e., increased numbers of partners, infrequent condom usage (111)], as well as unprotected anal intercourse among HIV-positive gay men (112). Among American high school students, AAS use correlated with not using a condom and a history of sexually transmitted disease (106). Thus, a key danger of AAS abuse is the likelihood that users will engage in behaviors that harm themselves and those around them.

Individual Variation in Circulating Androgen Levels and Executive Functioning

In normal, healthy individuals, circulating levels of androgens vary dramatically, allowing for correlational analyses of androgen levels and executive function. Interestingly, perseveration and risky behavior are positively correlated with endogenous androgens in adolescence and adulthood, similar to findings from animal studies (199). For example, adolescent males that exhibit external signs of high T (e.g., hirsutism) perform better on simple repetitive tasks than those without such external signs, independent of cognitive ability (200). This early study suggested a positive correlation between endogenous androgens and persistence. Furthermore, higher androgen levels in pubertal boys correlate with a greater probability of lifetime ethanol use (201). Therefore, circulating androgens may enhance ethanol effects on behavior, potentially increasing risk-taking in one or both sexes. To address this possibility, a study compared GDX male and female rats with and without hormone replacement in the probability discounting task, to investigate the influence of ethanol and gonadal steroids on the response to uncertainty (202). At baseline, GDX + T males showed a greater preference for the large reward than GDX males. Ethanol further increased large reward preference, but only in males. These results suggest that both ethanol and T at normal physiological levels increase tolerance for a large uncertain reward.

In adults, men with higher T are more likely to choose cards from decks offering large monetary gains paired with larger, infrequent losses in the IGT, a probabilistic, risk-based decision making task (203). This result is similar to patients with damage to the OFC and ventromedial PFC (204, 205). As a result, men with higher T earned less money throughout the session, relative to men with lower T. High levels of endogenous T also correlate with economic risk-taking outside of the lab. In a study of London stock traders, morning T levels predicted risk-taking throughout the day (206). In young and menopausal women, T is not associated with changes in any measure of executive function (207–209). Taken together, such studies suggest that individual variation in systemic T levels in males, but not females, is correlated with specific aspects of executive function.

Neuroandrogens and Executive Function

In addition to acting as endocrine signals, androgens also act as intracrine, paracrine, and autocrine signals. Specific nodes within the mesocorticolimbic system might require a particular androgen concentration to function appropriately. Similarly, McEwen and Wingfield (210) posited that local glucocorticoid signaling is tightly regulated to alleviate allostatic load imposed by high circulating glucocorticoid levels. Studies utilizing extreme changes to circulating androgen concentrations, such as AAS, GDX, or ADT demonstrate the importance of systemic androgens for executive function, but they can not reveal the role of local androgen synthesis. As discussed above, local levels of T in the mesocorticolimbic system vary greatly from circulating levels and from one neural node to another. Levels of T are often two or more times higher in the mesocorticolimbic system than in the blood in intact animals, and T is still present in the mesocorticolimbic system at 6 weeks after GDX (36). These results suggest that local T synthesis is important for neural activity in the mesocorticolimbic system and executive functioning.

There are few data on how the local production of androgens in the mesocorticolimbic system influences executive functioning. Several studies report changes in T precursors or androgenic enzymes in the mesocorticolimbic system of patients with mood disorders or in animal models of depression (211–213). Depression is frequently marked by deficits in executive functions (214, 215). In fact, clinicians refer to a disorder that occurs in geriatric populations as "depression-executive dysfunction syndrome" (214, 216). Low circulating DHEA and DHEA-S levels are correlated with depression in aged human populations, and DHEA has been suggested as treatment for depression (217, 218). In a rodent model of childhood depression, DHEA levels are lower in the VTA and NAc (but not amygdala or hypothalamus), suggesting mesolimbic-specific regulation of androgens (211). Expression of several steroidogenic enzymes are altered in post-mortem analyses of depressed individuals, which include a decrease of 5α-reductase type I in the PFC (213) and Cyp17a1 in the anterior cingulate cortex [ACC (212)], and an increase in hydroxysteroid sulfotransferase 2A1 (HST, **Figure 1**) in the ACC and StAR in the dorsolateral PFC (212). Changes in the expression of these specific steroidogenic enzymes suggest active androgen synthesis and metabolism in the VTA, NAc, and PFC.

Systemic administration of steroidogenic enzyme inhibitors that cross the blood–brain barrier hint at the role of neuroandrogens in modulating executive function. Using set-shifting and reversal learning tasks, the Soma laboratory has recently found that chronic systemic administration of abiraterone (a Cyp17a1 inhibitor) enhances behavioral flexibility in intact and gonadectomized subjects [unpublished results (219)]. Furthermore, systemic administration of letrozole, an aromatase inhibitor, increases risk-taking behavior in human males (220) and improves working memory in female rats (221). In particular, the study by Goudriaan et al. (220) administered letrozole to healthy men for 1 week and tested executive function and risk-taking before and after treatment. Importantly, this treatment was used to increase circulating T, but potentially influenced steroidogenesis in the mesocorticolimbic system. Letrozole-treated subjects demonstrated an increase in risk-taking on the Balloon Analog Risk-Taking task, but not the IGT or Game of Dice, compared to their baseline and estrogen-treated subjects. These findings highlight the importance of using a variety of sensitive neurocognitive assays to detect changes in executive function. This study, along with the studies of behavioral flexibility in male rats and working memory in female rats, suggests that androgens and local androgen synthesis, and not E_2 or local androgen metabolism, have the most profound effects on executive functioning.

There have been no studies, to our knowledge, that directly (e.g., i.c.v. steroidogenic enzyme inhibitor) manipulated neural androgen synthesis and examined executive functioning. The most relevant studies examined the effects of androgenic enzyme (i.e., Cyp17a1 and 5αR) inhibitors on PPI of the acoustic startle reflex and DA signaling in the NAc (160, 163, 165). Frau and colleagues (160) administered apomorphine (a non-selective DA agonist; i.p.) to male rats to cause a deficit in PPI. The effects of apomorphine on PPI were attenuated by microinjecting (i.c.v.) the Cyp17a1 inhibitor abiraterone. Along with studies using systemic finasteride [5αR inhibitor (163, 164, 222, 223)], these results suggest that local androgen synthesis regulates DA signaling in the mesocorticolimbic system and DA-dependent behaviors. While these studies are informative, there still remains an important gap in our understanding of how neural androgen production specifically influences executive functioning.

CONCLUSION

Androgens influence a variety of behaviors and cognitive functions, which include executive functioning. Converging lines of evidence suggest that androgens can influence executive functioning *via* actions on the mesocorticolimbic system. Multiple nodes of the mesocorticolimbic system (VTA, NAc, mPFC, and OFC) contain AR and ER. Emerging evidence suggests that multiple nodes of the mesocorticolimbic system also locally synthesize androgens, estrogens, and other steroids. However, the physiological role of these neuroandrogens still remains to be determined. Reducing endogenous androgens (GDX, ADT) and administering exogenous androgens (AAS) alter the neurochemistry (e.g., DA signaling) and cytoarchitecture of the mesocorticolimbic system. In animal studies, both a reduction of endogenous androgens and pharmacological administration of exogenous androgens lead to alterations in behavioral flexibility and inhibitory control. In human studies, evidence suggests that ADT or AAS abuse can also lead to deficits in executive functioning. Future studies should investigate the roles of systemic and locally produced androgens in the mesocorticolimbic system and cognition. Taken together, such studies broaden our understanding of androgen regulation of behavior to include decision making and executive function, and also highlight neurosteroid and AAS action within the mesocorticolimbic system.

AUTHOR CONTRIBUTIONS

All authors listed have made a substantial, direct and intellectual contribution to the work and approved it for publication.

ACKNOWLEDGMENTS

The authors thank Ryan Tomm, Jordan Hamden, and Katelyn Low for comments on the manuscript.

FUNDING

This review was supported by a Bluma Tischler Postdoctoral Fellowship to DT; a grant from the National Institute on Drug Abuse of the U.S. National Institutes of Health (R01-DA029613) to RW; grants from the Natural Sciences and Engineering Research Council of Canada and the Canadian Institutes of Health Research (MOP 133579) to SF; grants from the Canadian Institutes of Health Research (MOP 133606), Canada Foundation for Innovation, and British Columbia Knowledge Development Fund to KS.

REFERENCES

1. Berthold AA. Transplantation der Hoden. *Arch Anat Physiol Wiss Med* (1849) 16:42–6.
2. Burger HG. Androgen production in women. *Fertil Steril* (2002) 77:S3–5. doi:10.1016/S0015-0282(02)02985-0
3. Werner R, Holterhus PM. Androgen action. *Endocr Dev* (2014) 27:28–40. doi:10.1159/000363610
4. Chen F, Knecht K, Birzin E, Fisher J, Wilkinson H, Mojena M, et al. Direct agonist/antagonist functions of dehydroepiandrosterone. *Endocrinology* (2005) 146:4568–76. doi:10.1210/en.2005-0368
5. Fang H, Tong W, Branham WS, Moland CL, Dial SL, Hong H, et al. Study of 202 natural, synthetic, and environmental chemicals for binding to the androgen receptor. *Chem Res Toxicol* (2003) 16:1338–58. doi:10.1021/tx030011g
6. Mo Q, Lu S, Simon NG. Dehydroepiandrosterone and its metabolites: differential effects on androgen receptor trafficking and transcriptional

activity. *J Steroid Biochem Mol Biol* (2006) 99:50–8. doi:10.1016/j.jsbmb.2005.11.011
7. Hull EM, Dominguez JM. Sexual behavior in male rodents. *Horm Behav* (2007) 52:45–55. doi:10.1016/j.yhbeh.2007.03.030
8. Soma KK, Scotti M-AL, Newman AEM, Charlier TD, Demas GE. Novel mechanisms for neuroendocrine regulation of aggression. *Front Neuroendocrinol* (2008) 29:476–89. doi:10.1016/j.yfrne.2007.12.003
9. Nelson RJ, editor. *Biology of Aggression*. New York, NY: Oxford University Press (2005).
10. Brozoski T, Brown R, Rosvold H, Goldman P. Cognitive deficit caused by regional depletion of dopamine in prefrontal cortex of rhesus monkey. *Science* (1979) 205:929–32. doi:10.1126/science.112679
11. Floresco SB. Prefrontal dopamine and behavioral flexibility: shifting from an "inverted-U" toward a family of functions. *Front Neurosci* (2013) 7:62. doi:10.3389/fnins.2013.00062
12. Haluk DM, Floresco SB. Ventral striatal dopamine modulation of different forms of behavioral flexibility. *Neuropsychopharmacology* (2009) 34:2041–52. doi:10.1038/npp.2009.21
13. Ragozzino ME. The effects of dopamine D1 receptor blockade in the prelimbic – infralimbic areas on behavioral flexibility. *Learn Mem* (2002) 9:18–28. doi:10.1101/lm.45802
14. Floresco SB, Magyar O, Ghods-Sharifi S, Vexelman C, Tse MTL. Multiple dopamine receptor subtypes in the medial prefrontal cortex of the rat regulate set-shifting. *Neuropsychopharmacology* (2006) 31:297–309. doi:10.1038/sj.npp.1300825
15. Dias R, Robbins TW, Roberts AC. Dissociable forms of inhibitory control within prefrontal cortex with an analog of the Wisconsin Card Sort Test: restriction to novel situations and independence from "on-line" processing. *J Neurosci* (1997) 17:9285–97. doi:10.1523/JNEUROSCI.17-23-09285.1997
16. McAlonan K, Brown VJ. Orbital prefrontal cortex mediates reversal learning and not attentional set shifting in the rat. *Behav Brain Res* (2003) 146:97–103. doi:10.1016/j.bbr.2003.09.019
17. Roberts AC, De Salvia MA, Wilkinson LS, Collins P, Muir JL, Everitt BJ, et al. 6-Hydroxydopamine lesions of the prefrontal cortex in monkeys enhance performance on an analog of the Wisconsin Card Sort Test: possible interactions with subcortical dopamine. *J Neurosci* (1994) 14:2531–44. doi:10.1523/JNEUROSCI.14-05-02531.1994
18. O'Neill M, Brown VJ. The effect of striatal dopamine depletion and the adenosine A2A antagonist KW-6002 on reversal learning in rats. *Neurobiol Learn Mem* (2007) 88:75–81. doi:10.1016/j.nlm.2007.03.003
19. Clarke HF, Hill GJ, Robbins TW, Roberts AC. Dopamine, but not serotonin, regulates reversal learning in the marmoset caudate nucleus. *J Neurosci* (2011) 31:4290–7. doi:10.1523/JNEUROSCI.5066-10.2011
20. Floresco SB, Tse MTL, Ghods-Sharifi S. Dopaminergic and glutamatergic regulation of effort- and delay-based decision making. *Neuropsychopharmacology* (2008) 33:1966–79. doi:10.1038/sj.npp.1301565
21. St. Onge JR, Floresco SB. Dopaminergic modulation of risk-based decision making. *Neuropsychopharmacology* (2009) 34:681–97. doi:10.1038/npp.2008.121
22. St. Onge JR, Chiu YC, Floresco SB. Differential effects of dopaminergic manipulations on risky choice. *Psychopharmacology (Berl)* (2010) 211: 209–21. doi:10.1007/s00213-010-1883-y
23. Stopper CM, Khayambashi S, Floresco SB. Receptor-specific modulation of risk-based decision making by nucleus accumbens dopamine. *Neuropsychopharmacology* (2013) 38:715–28. doi:10.1038/npp.2012.240
24. Nowend KL, Arizzi M, Carlson BB, Salamone JD. D1 or D2 antagonism in nucleus accumbens core or dorsomedial shell suppresses lever pressing for food but leads to compensatory increases in chow consumption. *Pharmacol Biochem Behav* (2001) 69:373–82. doi:10.1016/S0091-3057(01)00524-X
25. Schweimer J, Hauber W. Dopamine D1 receptors in the anterior cingulate cortex regulate effort-based decision making. *Learn Mem* (2006) 13:777–82. doi:10.1101/lm.409306
26. Loos M, Pattij T, Janssen MCW, Counotte DS, Schoffelmeer ANM, Smit AB, et al. Dopamine receptor D1/D5 gene expression in the medial prefrontal cortex predicts impulsive choice in rats. *Cereb Cortex* (2010) 20:1064–70. doi:10.1093/cercor/bhp167
27. St Onge JR, Abhari H, Floresco SB. Dissociable contributions by prefrontal D1 and D2 receptors to risk-based decision making. *J Neurosci* (2011) 31:8625–33. doi:10.1523/JNEUROSCI.1020-11.2011
28. Jenni NL, Larkin JD, Floresco SB. Prefrontal dopamine D1 and D2 receptors regulate dissociable aspects of decision making via distinct ventral striatal and amygdalar circuits. *J Neurosci* (2017) 37:6200–13. doi:10.1523/JNEUROSCI.0030-17.2017
29. Gao W, Bohl CE, Dalton JT. Chemistry and structural biology of androgen receptor. *Chem Rev* (2005) 105:3352–70. doi:10.1021/cr020456u
30. Griggs RC, Kingston W, Jozefowicz RF, Herr BE, Forbes G, Halliday D. Effect of testosterone on muscle mass and muscle protein synthesis. *J Appl Physiol* (1989) 66:498–503. doi:10.1152/jappl.1989.66.1.498
31. O'Connell LA, Hofmann HA. The vertebrate mesolimbic reward system and social behavior network: a comparative synthesis. *J Comp Neurol* (2011) 519:3599–639. doi:10.1002/cne.22735
32. Raskin K, de Gendt K, Duittoz A, Liere P, Verhoeven G, Tronche F, et al. Conditional inactivation of androgen receptor gene in the nervous system: effects on male behavioral and neuroendocrine responses. *J Neurosci* (2009) 29:4461–70. doi:10.1523/JNEUROSCI.0296-09.2009
33. Low KL, Ma C, Soma KK. Tyramide signal amplification permits immunohistochemical analyses of androgen receptors in the rat prefrontal cortex. *J Histochem Cytochem* (2017) 65:295–308. doi:10.1369/0022155417694870
34. Simerly RB, Chang C, Muramatsu M, Swanson LW. Distribution of androgen and estrogen receptor mRNA-containing cells in the rat brain: an in situ hybridization study. *J Comp Neurol* (1990) 294:76–95. doi:10.1002/cne.902940107
35. Kritzer MF. The distribution of immunoreactivity for intracellular androgen receptors in the cerebral cortex of hormonally intact adult male and female rats: localization in pyramidal neurons making corticocortical connections. *Cereb Cortex* (2004) 14:268–80. doi:10.1093/cercor/bhg127
36. Tobiansky DJ, Korol AM, Ma C, Hamden JE, Jalabert C, Tomm RJ, et al. Testosterone and corticosterone in the mesocorticolimbic system of male rats: effects of gonadectomy and caloric restriction. *Endocrinology* (2018) 159:450–64. doi:10.1210/en.2017-00704
37. Fuxjager MJ, Forbes-Lorman RM, Coss DJ, Auger CJ, Auger AP, Marler CA. Winning territorial disputes selectively enhances androgen sensitivity in neural pathways related to motivation and social aggression. *Proc Natl Acad Sci U S A* (2010) 107:12393–8. doi:10.1073/pnas.1001394107
38. Abdelgadir SE, Roselli CE, Choate JV, Resko JA. Distribution of aromatase cytochrome P450 messenger ribonucleic acid in adult rhesus monkey brains. *Biol Reprod* (1997) 57:772–7. doi:10.1095/biolreprod57.4.772
39. Finley SK, Kritzer MF. Immunoreactivity for intracellular androgen receptors in identified subpopulations of neurons, astrocytes and oligodendrocytes in primate prefrontal cortex. *J Neurobiol* (1999) 40:446–57. doi:10.1002/(SICI)1097-4695(19990915)40:4<446::AID-NEU3>3.0.CO;2-J
40. Hawrylycz MJ, Lein ES, Guillozet-Bongaarts AL, Shen EH, Ng L, Miller JA, et al. An anatomically comprehensive atlas of the adult human brain transcriptome. *Nature* (2012) 489:391–9. doi:10.1038/nature11405
41. DonCarlos LL, Sarkey S, Lorenz B, Azcoitia I, Garcia-Ovejero D, Huppenbauer C, et al. Novel cellular phenotypes and subcellular sites for androgen action in the forebrain. *Neuroscience* (2006) 138:801–7. doi:10.1016/j.neuroscience.2005.06.020
42. Aubele T, Kritzer MF. Androgen influence on prefrontal dopamine systems in adult male rats: localization of cognate intracellular receptors in medial prefrontal projections to the ventral tegmental area and effects of gonadectomy and hormone replacement on glutamate-stimulated. *Cereb Cortex* (2012) 22:1799–812. doi:10.1093/cercor/bhr258
43. Creutz LM, Kritzer MF. Mesostriatal and mesolimbic projections of midbrain neurons immunoreactive for estrogen receptor beta or androgen receptors in rats. *J Comp Neurol* (2004) 476:348–62. doi:10.1002/cne.20229
44. Kritzer MF, Creutz LM. Region and sex differences in constituent dopamine neurons and immunoreactivity for intracellular estrogen and androgen receptors in mesocortical projections in rats. *J Neurosci* (2008) 28:9525–35. doi:10.1523/JNEUROSCI.2637-08.2008
45. Low KL. *Effects of Age on Mesocorticolimbic Testosterone Levels and Androgen Receptors in Male Rats*. Vancouver: The University of British Columbia (2016). Available from: https://open.library.ubc.ca/cIRcle/collections/ubctheses/24/items/1.0300233
46. Stanić D, Dubois S, Chua HK, Tonge B, Rinehart N, Horne MK, et al. Characterization of aromatase expression in the adult male and female mouse brain. I. Coexistence with oestrogen receptors α and β, and androgen receptors. *PLoS One* (2014) 9:e90451. doi:10.1371/journal.pone.0090451

47. Roselli CE, Resko JA. Sex differences in androgen-regulated expression of cytochrome P450 aromatase in the rat brain. *J Steroid Biochem Mol Biol* (1997) 61:365–74. doi:10.1016/S0960-0760(97)80034-9
48. Pérez SE, Chen E-Y, Mufson EJ. Distribution of estrogen receptor alpha and beta immunoreactive profiles in the postnatal rat brain. *Brain Res Rev* (2003) 145:117–39. doi:10.1016/S0165-3806(03)00223-2
49. Österlund M. Differential distribution and regulation of estrogen receptor-α and -β mRNA within the female rat brain. *Mol Brain Res* (1998) 54:175–80. doi:10.1016/S0169-328X(97)00351-3
50. DonCarlos LL, Monroy E, Morrell JI. Distribution of estrogen receptor-immunoreactive cells in the forebrain of the female guinea pig. *J Comp Neurol* (1991) 305:591–612. doi:10.1002/cne.903050406
51. Mitra SW, Hoskin E, Yudkovitz J, Pear L, Wilkinson HA, Hayashi S, et al. Immunolocalization of estrogen receptor beta in the mouse brain: comparison with estrogen receptor alpha. *Endocrinology* (2003) 144:2055–67. doi:10.1210/en.2002-221069
52. Tobiansky DJ, Roma PG, Hattori T, Will RG, Nutsch VL, Dominguez JM. The medial preoptic area modulates cocaine-induced activity in female rats. *Behav Neurosci* (2013) 127:293–302. doi:10.1037/a0031949
53. Tobiansky DJ, Will RG, Lominac KD, Turner JM, Hattori T, Krishnan K, et al. Estradiol in the preoptic area regulates the dopaminergic response to cocaine in the nucleus accumbens. *Neuropsychopharmacology* (2016) 41:1897–906. doi:10.1038/npp.2015.360
54. McHenry JA, Otis JM, Rossi MA, Robinson JE, Kosyk O, Miller NW, et al. Hormonal gain control of a medial preoptic area social reward circuit. *Nat Neurosci* (2017) 20:449–58. doi:10.1038/nn.4487
55. Thomas P, Converse A, Berg HA. ZIP9, a novel membrane androgen receptor and zinc transporter protein. *Gen Comp Endocrinol* (2018) 257:130–6. doi:10.1016/j.ygcen.2017.04.016
56. Pi M, Parrill AL, Quarles LD. GPRC6A mediates the non-genomic effects of steroids. *J Biol Chem* (2010) 285:39953–64. doi:10.1074/jbc.M110.158063
57. Berg AH, Rice CD, Rahman MS, Dong J, Thomas P. Identification and characterization of membrane androgen receptors in the ZIP9 zinc transporter subfamily: I. Discovery in female Atlantic croaker and evidence ZIP9 mediates testosterone-induced apoptosis of ovarian follicle cells. *Endocrinology* (2014) 155:4237–49. doi:10.1210/en.2014-1198
58. Luo J, Liu Z, Liu J, Eugene CY. Distribution pattern of GPRC6A mRNA in mouse tissue by in situ hybridization. *Zhong Nan Da Xue Xue Bao Yi Xue Ban* (2010) 35:1–10. doi:10.3969/j.issn.1672-7347.2010.01.001
59. Lein ES, Hawrylycz MJ, Ao N, Ayres M, Bensinger A, Bernard A, et al. Genome-wide atlas of gene expression in the adult mouse brain. *Nature* (2007) 445:168–76. doi:10.1038/nature05453
60. Garza-Contreras J, Duong P, Snyder BD, Schreihofer DA, Cunningham RL. Presence of androgen receptor variant in neuronal lipid rafts. *eNeuro* (2017) 4:ENEURO.109–17. doi:10.1523/ENEURO.0109-17.2017
61. Brailoiu E, Dun SL, Brailoiu GC, Mizuo K, Sklar LA, Oprea TI, et al. Distribution and characterization of estrogen receptor G protein-coupled receptor 30 in the rat central nervous system. *J Endocrinol* (2007) 193:311–21. doi:10.1677/JOE-07-0017
62. O'Dowd BF, Nguyen T, Marchese A, Cheng R, Lynch KR, Heng HH, et al. Discovery of three novel G-protein-coupled receptor genes. *Genomics* (1998) 47:310–3. doi:10.1006/geno.1998.5095
63. Almey A, Milner TA, Brake WG. Estrogen receptors in the central nervous system and their implication for dopamine-dependent cognition in females. *Horm Behav* (2015) 74:125–38. doi:10.1016/j.yhbeh.2015.06.010
64. Zorumski CF, Paul SM, Izumi Y, Covey DF, Mennerick S. Neurosteroids, stress and depression: potential therapeutic opportunities. *Neurosci Biobehav Rev* (2013) 37:109–22. doi:10.1016/j.neubiorev.2012.10.005
65. Prough RA, Clark BJ, Klinge CM. Novel mechanisms for DHEA action. *J Mol Endocrinol* (2016) 56:R139–55. doi:10.1530/JME-16-0013
66. Reddy DS, Estes WA. Clinical potential of neurosteroids for CNS disorders. *Trends Pharmacol Sci* (2016) 37:543–61. doi:10.1016/j.tips.2016.04.003
67. Corpéchot C, Robel P, Axelson M, Sjövall J, Baulieu EE. Characterization and measurement of dehydroepiandrosterone sulfate in rat brain. *Proc Natl Acad Sci U S A* (1981) 78:4704–7. doi:10.1073/pnas.78.8.4704
68. Corpéchot C, Synguelakis M, Talha S, Axelson M, Sjövall J, Vihko R, et al. Pregnenolone and its sulfate ester in the rat brain. *Brain Res* (1983) 270:119–25. doi:10.1016/0006-8993(83)90797-7
69. Liere P, Pianos A, Eychenne B, Cambourg A, Bodin K, Griffiths W, et al. Analysis of pregnenolone and dehydroepiandrosterone in rodent brain: cholesterol autoxidation is the key. *J Lipid Res* (2009) 50:2430–44. doi:10.1194/jlr.M900162-JLR200
70. Hojo Y, Hattori T-A, Enami T, Furukawa A, Suzuki K, Ishii H-T, et al. Adult male rat hippocampus synthesizes estradiol from pregnenolone by cytochromes P45017alpha and P450 aromatase localized in neurons. *Proc Natl Acad Sci U S A* (2004) 101:865–70. doi:10.1073/pnas.2630225100
71. Munetsuna E, Hojo Y, Hattori M, Ishii H, Kawato S, Ishida A, et al. Retinoic acid stimulates 17beta-estradiol and testosterone synthesis in rat hippocampal slice cultures. *Endocrinology* (2009) 150:4260–9. doi:10.1210/en.2008-1644
72. Remage-Healey L, Dong SM, Chao A, Schlinger BA. Sex-specific, rapid neuroestrogen fluctuations and neurophysiological actions in the songbird auditory forebrain. *J Neurophysiol* (2012) 107:1621–31. doi:10.1152/jn.00749.2011
73. Saldanha CJ, Remage-Healey L, Schlinger BA. Synaptocrine signaling: steroid synthesis and action at the synapse. *Endocr Rev* (2011) 32:532–49. doi:10.1210/er.2011-0004
74. Kristensen DM, Desdoits-Lethimonier C, Mackey AL, Dalgaard MD, De Masi F, Munkbøl CH, et al. Ibuprofen alters human testicular physiology to produce a state of compensated hypogonadism. *Proc Natl Acad Sci U S A* (2018) 115:E715–24. doi:10.1073/pnas.1715035115
75. Le Goascogne C, Sananes N, Gouezou M, Takemori S, Kominami S, Baulieu EE, et al. Immunoreactive cytochrome P-45017alpha in rat and guinea-pig gonads, adrenal glands and brain. *J Reprod Fertl* (1991) 93:609–22. doi:10.1530/jrf.0.0930609
76. Sanne JL, Krueger KE. Aberrant splicing of rat steroid 17α-hydroxylase transcripts. *Gene* (1995) 165:327–8. doi:10.1016/0378-1119(95)00536-F
77. Compagnone NA, Bulfone A, Rubenstein JLR, Mellon SH. Steroidogenic enzyme p450c17 is expressed in the embryonic central nervous system. *Endocrinology* (1995) 136:5212–23. doi:10.1210/endo.136.6.7750493
78. Strömstedt M, Waterman MR. Messenger RNAs encoding steroidogenic enzymes are expressed in rodent brain. *Brain Res Mol Brain Res* (1995) 34:75–88. doi:10.1016/0169-328X(95)00140-N
79. Mellon SH, Deschepper CF. Neurosteroid biosynthesis: genes for adrenal steroidogenic enzymes are expressed in the brain. *Brain Res* (1993) 629: 283–92. doi:10.1016/0006-8993(93)91332-M
80. Guennoun R, Fiddes RJ, Gouézou M, Lombès M, Baulieu EE. A key enzyme in the biosynthesis of neurosteroids, 3β-hydroxysteroid dehydrogenase/Δ5-Δ4-isomerase (3β-HSD), is expressed in rat brain. *Brain Res Mol Brain Res* (1995) 30:287–300. doi:10.1016/0169-328X(95)00016-L
81. Kimoto T, Ishii H, Higo S, Hojo Y, Kawato S. Semicomprehensive analysis of the postnatal age-related changes in the mRNA expression of sex steroidogenic enzymes and sex steroid receptors in the male rat hippocampus. *Endocrinology* (2010) 151:5795–806. doi:10.1210/en.2010-0581
82. Hojo Y, Okamoto M, Kato A, Higo S, Sakai F, Soya H, et al. Neurosteroid synthesis in adult female rat hippocampus, including androgens and allopregnanolone. *J Steroids Horm Sci* (2014) S4:2. doi:10.4172/2157-7536.S4-002
83. Munetomo A, Hojo Y, Higo S, Kato A, Yoshida K, Shirasawa T, et al. Aging-induced changes in sex-steroidogenic enzymes and sex-steroid receptors in the cortex, hypothalamus and cerebellum. *J Physiol Sci* (2015) 65:253–63. doi:10.1007/s12576-015-0363-x
84. Furukawa A, Miyatake A, Ohnishi T, Ichikawa Y. Steroidogenic acute regulatory protein (StAR) transcripts constitutively expressed in the adult rat central nervous system: colocalization of StAR, cytochrome P-450SCC (CYP XIA1), and 3beta-hydroxysteroid dehydrogenase in the rat brain. *J Neurochem* (1998) 71:2231–8. doi:10.1046/j.1471-4159.1998.71062231.x
85. Stoffel-Wagner B. Neurosteroid biosynthesis in the human brain and its clinical implications. *Ann N Y Acad Sci* (2003) 1007:64–78. doi:10.1196/annals.1286.007
86. Stoffel-Wagner B. Neurosteroid metabolism in the human brain. *Eur J Endocrinol* (2001) 145:669–79. doi:10.1530/eje.0.1450669
87. Wagner CK, Morrell JI. Neuroanatomical distribution of aromatase mRNA in the rat brain: indications of regional regulation. *J Steroid Biochem Mol Biol* (1997) 61:307–14. doi:10.1016/S0960-0760(97)80028-3
88. Hatanaka Y, Hojo Y, Mukai H, Murakami G, Komatsuzaki Y, Kim J, et al. Rapid increase of spines by dihydrotestosterone and testosterone in hippocampal neurons: dependence on synaptic androgen receptor and kinase

networks. *Brain Res* (2015) 1621:121–32. doi:10.1016/j.brainres.2014.12.011

89. Matsunaga M, Ukena K, Tsutsui K. Androgen biosynthesis in the quail brain. *Brain Res* (2002) 948:180–5. doi:10.1016/S0006-8993(02)03147-5
90. Shen P, Schlinger BA, Campagnoni AT, Arnold AP. An atlas of aromatase mRNA expression in the zebra finch brain. *J Comp Neurol* (1995) 360:172–84. doi:10.1002/cne.903600113
91. Raab H, Beyer C, Wozniak A, Hutchison JB, Pilgrim C, Reisert I. Ontogeny of aromatase messenger ribonucleic acid and aromatase activity in the rat midbrain. *Brain Res Mol Brain Res* (1995) 34:333–6. doi:10.1016/0169-328X(95)00196-Y
92. Cook JB, Werner DF, Maldonado-Devincci AM, Leonard MN, Fisher KR, O'Buckley TK, et al. Overexpression of the steroidogenic enzyme cytochrome P450 side chain cleavage in the ventral tegmental area increases 3α,5α-THP and reduces long-term operant ethanol self-administration. *J Neurosci* (2014) 34:5824–34. doi:10.1523/JNEUROSCI.4733-13.2014
93. Agís-Balboa RC, Pinna G, Zhubi A, Maloku E, Veldic M, Costa E, et al. Characterization of brain neurons that express enzymes mediating neurosteroid biosynthesis. *Proc Natl Acad Sci U S A* (2006) 103:14602–7. doi:10.1073/pnas.0606544103
94. Snipes CA, Shore LS. Metabolism of testosterone in vitro by hypothalamus and other areas of rat brain. *Andrologia* (1982) 14:81–5. doi:10.1111/j.1439-0272.1982.tb03101.x
95. Zwain IH, Yen SS. Neurosteroidogenesis in astrocytes, oligodendrocytes, and neurons of cerebral cortex of rat brain. *Endocrinology* (1999) 140:3843–52. doi:10.1210/endo.140.8.6907
96. Schindler AE. Metabolism of androstenedione and testosterone in human fetal brain. *Prog Brain Res* (1975) 42:330. doi:10.1016/S0079-6123(08)63689-4
97. Jenkins JS, Hall CJ. Metabolism of [14C]testosterone by human foetal and adult brain tissue. *J Endocrinol* (1977) 74:425–9. doi:10.1677/joe.0.0740425
98. Hojo Y, Higo S, Ishii H, Ooishi Y, Mukai H, Murakami G, et al. Comparison between hippocampus-synthesized and circulation-derived sex steroids in the hippocampus. *Endocrinology* (2009) 150:5106–12. doi:10.1210/en.2009-0305
99. Kicman AT. Pharmacology of anabolic steroids. *Br J Pharmacol* (2008) 154:502–21. doi:10.1038/bjp.2008.165
100. Pope HG, Kanayama G, Athey A, Ryan E, Hudson JI, Baggish A. The lifetime prevalence of anabolic-androgenic steroid use and dependence in Americans: current best estimates. *Am J Addict* (2014) 23:371–7. doi:10.1111/j.1521-0391.2013.12118.x
101. Johnston L, O'Malley P, Miech R, Bachman J, Schulenberg J. *Monitoring the Future: National Survey Results on Drug Use: 1975-2014. Overview, Key Findings on Adolescent Drug Use*. Ann Arbor: Institute for Social Research, The University of Michigan (2014). p. 1–98.
102. World Anti-Doping Agency. 2014 anti-doping testing figures report. *Lab Rep* (2014) 16:202. Available from: https://www.wada-ama.org/en/resources/laboratories/anti-doping-testing-figures
103. Wood RI, Stanton SJ. Testosterone and sport: current perspectives. *Horm Behav* (2012) 61:147–55. doi:10.1016/j.yhbeh.2011.09.010
104. Gallaway S. *The Steroid Bible*. Honolulu: Belle Intl (1997).
105. Pope HG, Wood RI, Rogol A, Nyberg F, Bowers L, Bhasin S. Adverse health consequences of performance-enhancing drugs: an endocrine society scientific statement. *Endocr Rev* (2014) 35:341–75. doi:10.1210/er.2013-1058
106. Middleman AB, Faulkner AH, Woods ER, Emans SJ, DuRant RH. High-risk behaviors among high school students in Massachusetts who use anabolic steroids. *Pediatrics* (1995) 96:268–72.
107. Pope HG, Kouri EM, Powell KF, Campbell C, Katz DL. Anabolic-androgenic steroid use among 133 prisoners. *Compr Psychiatry* (1996) 37:322–7. doi:10.1016/S0010-440X(96)90013-9
108. Conacher GN, Workman DG. Violent crime possibly associated with anabolic steroid use. *Am J Psychiatry* (1989) 146:679. doi:10.1176/ajp.146.5.679b
109. Schulte HM, Hall MJ, Boyer M. Domestic violence associated with anabolic steroid abuse. *Am J Psychiatry* (1993) 150:348. doi:10.1176/ajp.150.2.348a
110. Thiblin I, Lindquist O, Rajs J. Cause and manner of death among users of anabolic androgenic steroids. *J Forensic Sci* (2000) 45:16–23. doi:10.1520/JFS14635J
111. Midgley SJ, Heather N, Best D, Henderson D, McCarthy S, Davies JB. Risk behaviours for HIV and hepatitis infection among anabolic-androgenic steroid users. *AIDS Care* (2000) 12:163–70. doi:10.1080/09540120050001832
112. Bolding G, Sherr L, Elford J. Use of anabolic steroids and associated health risks among gay men attending London gyms. *Addiction* (2002) 97:195–203. doi:10.1046/j.1360-0443.2002.00031.x
113. Sherman AM, de Vries B, Lansford JE. Friendship in childhood and adulthood: lessons across the life span. *Int J Aging Hum Dev* (2000) 51:31–51. doi:10.2190/4QFV-D52D-TPYP-RLM6
114. Sumter SR, Bokhorst CL, Steinberg L, Westenberg PM. The developmental pattern of resistance to peer influence in adolescence: will the teenager ever be able to resist? *J Adolesc* (2009) 32:1009–21. doi:10.1016/j.adolescence.2008.08.010
115. Sato SM, Schulz KM, Sisk CL, Wood RI. Adolescents and androgens, receptors and rewards. *Horm Behav* (2008) 53:647–58. doi:10.1016/j.yhbeh.2008.01.010
116. Kuntsche E, Gmel G. Alcohol consumption in late adolescence and early adulthood – where is the problem? *Swiss Med Wkly* (2013) 143:w13826. doi:10.4414/smw.2013.13826
117. Martin CA, Mainous AG, Curry T, Martin D. Alcohol use in adolescent females: correlates with estradiol and testosterone. *Am J Addict* (1999) 8:9–14. doi:10.1080/105504999306036
118. Spear LP. Consequences of adolescent use of alcohol and other drugs: studies using rodent models. *Neurosci Biobehav Rev* (2016) 70:228–43. doi:10.1016/j.neubiorev.2016.07.026
119. Johnson LR, Wood RI. Oral testosterone self-administration in male hamsters. *Neuroendocrinology* (2001) 73:285–92. doi:10.1159/000054645
120. Wood RI. Reinforcing aspects of androgens. *Physiol Behav* (2004) 83:279–89. doi:10.1016/j.physbeh.2004.08.012
121. Peters KD, Wood RI. Androgen dependence in hamsters: overdose, tolerance, and potential opioidergic mechanisms. *Neuroscience* (2005) 130:971–81. doi:10.1016/j.neuroscience.2004.09.063
122. Sato SM, Johansen JA, Jordan CL, Wood RI. Membrane androgen receptors may mediate androgen reinforcement. *Psychoneuroendocrinology* (2010) 35:1063–73. doi:10.1016/j.psyneuen.2010.01.007
123. Brower KJ, Blow FC, Young JP, Hill EM. Symptoms and correlates of anabolic-androgenic steroid dependence. *Br J Addict* (1991) 86:759–68. doi:10.1111/j.1360-0443.1991.tb03101.x
124. Volkow ND, Morales M. The brain on drugs: from reward to addiction. *Cell* (2015) 162:712–25. doi:10.1016/j.cell.2015.07.046
125. Packard MG, Cornell AH, Alexander GM. Rewarding affective properties of intra-nucleus accumbens injections of testosterone. *Behav Neurosci* (1997) 111:219–24. doi:10.1037/0735-7044.111.1.219
126. Frye CA, Rhodes ME, Rosellini R, Svare B. The nucleus accumbens as a site of action for rewarding properties of testosterone and its 5alpha-reduced metabolites. *Pharmacol Biochem Behav* (2002) 74:119–27. doi:10.1016/S0091-3057(02)00968-1
127. White NM, Packard MG, Hiroi N. Place conditioning with dopamine D1 and D2 agonists injected peripherally or into nucleus accumbens. *Psychopharmacology (Berl)* (1991) 103:271–6. doi:10.1007/BF02244216
128. Packard MG, Schroeder JP, Alexander GM. Expression of testosterone conditioned place preference is blocked by peripheral or intra-accumbens injection of α-flupenthixol. *Horm Behav* (1998) 34:39–47. doi:10.1006/hbeh.1998.1461
129. Schroeder JP, Packard MG. Role of dopamine receptor subtypes in the acquisition of a testosterone conditioned place preference in rats. *Neurosci Lett* (2000) 282:17–20. doi:10.1016/S0304-3940(00)00839-9
130. Triemstra JL, Sato SM, Wood RI. Testosterone and nucleus accumbens dopamine in the male Syrian hamster. *Psychoneuroendocrinology* (2008) 33:386–94. doi:10.1016/j.psyneuen.2007.12.006
131. Kailanto S, Kankaanpää A, Seppälä T. Subchronic steroid administration induces long lasting changes in neurochemical and behavioral response to cocaine in rats. *Steroids* (2011) 76:1310–6. doi:10.1016/j.steroids.2011.06.011
132. Kurling S, Kankaanpää A, Seppälä T. Sub-chronic nandrolone treatment modifies neurochemical and behavioral effects of amphetamine and 3,4-methylenedioxymethamphetamine (MDMA) in rats. *Behav Brain Res* (2008) 189:191–201. doi:10.1016/j.bbr.2007.12.021
133. Dimeo AN, Wood RI. Self-administration of estrogen and dihydrotestosterone in male hamsters. *Horm Behav* (2006) 49:519–26. doi:10.1016/j.yhbeh.2005.11.003
134. Henderson LP, Penatti CAA, Jones BL, Yang P, Clark AS. Anabolic androgenic steroids and forebrain GABAergic transmission. *Neuroscience* (2006) 138:793–9. doi:10.1016/j.neuroscience.2005.08.039

135. McIntyre KL, Porter DM, Henderson LP. Anabolic androgenic steroids induce age-, sex-, and dose-dependent changes in receptor subunit mRNAs in the mouse forebrain. *Neuropharmacology* (2002) 43:634–45. doi:10.1016/S0028-3908(02)00154-5
136. Beach FA, Pauker RS. Effects of castration and subsequent androgen administration upon mating behavior in the male hamster (*Cricetus auratus*). *Endocrinology* (1949) 45:211–21. doi:10.1210/endo-45-3-211
137. Pfaus JG, Damsma G, Nomikos GG, Wenkstern DG, Blaha CD, Phillips AG, et al. Sexual behavior enhances central dopamine transmission in the male rat. *Brain Res* (1990) 530:345–8. doi:10.1016/0006-8993(90)91309-5
138. van Erp AM, Miczek KA. Aggressive behavior, increased accumbal dopamine, and decreased cortical serotonin in rats. *J Neurosci* (2000) 20:9320–5. doi:10.1523/JNEUROSCI.20-24-09320.2000
139. Aubele T, Kritzer MF. Gonadectomy and hormone replacement affects in vivo basal extracellular dopamine levels in the prefrontal cortex but not motor cortex of adult male rats. *Cereb Cortex* (2011) 21:222–32. doi:10.1093/cercor/bhq083
140. Adler A, Vescovo P, Robinson JK, Kritzer MF. Gonadectomy in adult life increases tyrosine hydroxylase immunoreactivity in the prefrontal cortex and decreases open field activity in male rats. *Neuroscience* (1999) 89:939–54. doi:10.1016/S0306-4522(98)00341-8
141. Locklear MN, Michealos M, Collins WF, Kritzer MF. Gonadectomy but not biological sex affects burst-firing in dopamine neurons of the ventral tegmental area and in prefrontal cortical neurons projecting to the ventral tegmentum in adult rats. *Eur J Neurosci* (2016) 45:1–15. doi:10.1111/ejn.13380
142. Bitar MS, Ota M, Linnoila M, Shapiro BH. Modification of gonadectomy-induced increases in brain monoamine metabolism by steroid hormones in male and female rats. *Psychoneuroendocrinology* (1991) 16:547–57. doi:10.1016/0306-4530(91)90038-U
143. Shemisa K, Kunnathur V, Liu B, Salvaterra TJ, Dluzen DE. Testosterone modulation of striatal dopamine output in orchidectomized mice. *Synapse* (2006) 60:347–53. doi:10.1002/syn.20309
144. Meyers B, Kritzer MF. In vitro binding assays using 3H nisoxetine and 3H WIN 35,428 reveal selective effects of gonadectomy and hormone replacement in adult male rats on norepinephrine but not dopamine transporter sites in the cerebral cortex. *Neuroscience* (2009) 159:271–82. doi:10.1016/j.neuroscience.2008.12.010
145. Lewis C, Dluzen DE. Testosterone enhances dopamine depletion by methamphetamine in male, but not female, mice. *Neurosci Lett* (2008) 448:130–3. doi:10.1016/j.neulet.2008.10.011
146. Leranth C, Petnehazy O, MacLusky NJ. Gonadal hormones affect spine synaptic density in the CA1 hippocampal subfield of male rats. *J Neurosci* (2003) 23:1588–92. doi:10.1523/JNEUROSCI.23-05-01588.2003
147. de Castilhos J, Forti CD, Achaval M, Rasia-Filho AA. Dendritic spine density of posterodorsal medial amygdala neurons can be affected by gonadectomy and sex steroid manipulations in adult rats: a Golgi study. *Brain Res* (2008) 1240:73–81. doi:10.1016/j.brainres.2008.09.002
148. Hajszan T, MacLusky NJ, Leranth C. Role of androgens and the androgen receptor in remodeling of spine synapses in limbic brain areas. *Horm Behav* (2008) 53:638–46. doi:10.1016/j.yhbeh.2007.12.007
149. Wallin-Miller K, Li G, Kelishani D, Wood RI. Anabolic-androgenic steroids decrease dendritic spine density in the nucleus accumbens of male rats. *Neuroscience* (2016) 330:72–8. doi:10.1016/j.neuroscience.2016.05.045
150. Hajszan T, MacLusky NJ, Johansen JA, Jordan CL, Leranth C. Effects of androgens and estradiol on spine synapse formation in the prefrontal cortex of normal and testicular feminization mutant male rats. *Endocrinology* (2007) 148:1963–7. doi:10.1210/en.2006-1626
151. Reddy DS, Jian K. The testosterone-derived neurosteroid androstanediol is a positive allosteric modulator of GABAA receptors. *J Pharmacol Exp Ther* (2010) 334:1031–41. doi:10.1124/jpet.110.169854
152. Frye CA. Some rewarding effects of androgens may be mediated by actions of its 5alpha-reduced metabolite 3alpha-androstanediol. *Pharmacol Biochem Behav* (2007) 86:354–67. doi:10.1016/j.pbb.2006.10.003
153. McArthur S, McHale E, Gillies GE. The size and distribution of midbrain dopaminergic populations are permanently altered by perinatal glucocorticoid exposure in a sex- region- and time-specific manner. *Neuropsychopharmacology* (2007) 32:1462–76. doi:10.1038/sj.npp.1301277
154. Pasqualini C, Olivier V, Guibert B, Frain O, Leviel V. Acute stimulatory effect of estradiol on striatal dopamine synthesis. *J Neurochem* (2002) 65:1651–7. doi:10.1046/j.1471-4159.1995.65041651.x
155. Bazzett TJ, Becker JB. Sex differences in the rapid and acute effects of estrogen on striatal D2 dopamine receptor binding. *Brain Res* (1994) 637:163–72. doi:10.1016/0006-8993(94)91229-7
156. Kokras N, Pastromas N, Papasava D, de Bournonville C, Cornil CA, Dalla C. Sex differences in behavioral and neurochemical effects of gonadectomy and aromatase inhibition in rats. *Psychoneuroendocrinology* (2018) 87:93–107. doi:10.1016/j.psyneuen.2017.10.007
157. Becker JB. Estrogen rapidly potentiates amphetamine-induced striatal dopamine release and rotational behavior during microdialysis. *Neurosci Lett* (1990) 118:169–71. doi:10.1016/0304-3940(90)90618-J
158. Thompson TL, Moss RL. Estrogen regulation of dopamine release in the nucleus accumbens: genomic- and nongenomic-mediated effects. *J Neurochem* (1994) 62:1750–6. doi:10.1046/j.1471-4159.1994.62051750.x
159. Mermelstein PG, Becker JB. Increased extracellular dopamine in the nucleus accumbens and striatum of the female rat during paced copulatory behavior. *Behav Neurosci* (1995) 109:354–65. doi:10.1037/0735-7044.109.2.354
160. Frau R, Bini V, Pes R, Pillolla G, Saba P, Devoto P, et al. Inhibition of 17α-hydroxylase/C17,20 lyase reduces gating deficits consequent to dopaminergic activation. *Psychoneuroendocrinology* (2014) 39:204–13. doi:10.1016/j.psyneuen.2013.09.014
161. Kibaly C, Patte-Mensah C, Mensah-Nyagan AG. Molecular and neurochemical evidence for the biosynthesis of dehydroepiandrosterone in the adult rat spinal cord. *J Neurochem* (2005) 93:1220–30. doi:10.1111/j.1471-4159.2005.03113.x
162. Pérez-Neri I, Montes S, Ríos C. Inhibitory effect of dehydroepiandrosterone on brain monoamine oxidase activity: in vivo and in vitro studies. *Life Sci* (2009) 85:652–6. doi:10.1016/j.lfs.2009.09.008
163. Devoto P, Frau R, Bini V, Pillolla G, Saba P, Flore G, et al. Inhibition of 5α-reductase in the nucleus accumbens counters sensorimotor gating deficits induced by dopaminergic activation. *Psychoneuroendocrinology* (2012) 37:1630–45. doi:10.1016/j.psyneuen.2011.09.018
164. Soggiu A, Piras C, Greco V, Devoto P, Urbani A, Calzetta L, et al. Exploring the neural mechanisms of finasteride: a proteomic analysis in the nucleus accumbens. *Psychoneuroendocrinology* (2016) 74:387–96. doi:10.1016/j.psyneuen.2016.10.001
165. Frau R, Abbiati F, Bini V, Casti A, Caruso D, Devoto P, et al. Targeting neurosteroid synthesis as a therapy for schizophrenia-related alterations induced by early psychosocial stress. *Schizophr Res* (2015) 168:640–8. doi:10.1016/j.schres.2015.04.044
166. Andrew RJ, Rogers LJ. Testosterone, search behaviour and persistence. *Nature* (1972) 237:343–6. doi:10.1038/237343a0
167. Rogers LJ. Persistence and search influenced by natural levels of androgens in young and adult chickens. *Physiol Behav* (1974) 12:197–204. doi:10.1016/0031-9384(74)90173-5
168. Thompson WR, Wright JS. "Persistence" in rats: effects of testosterone. *Physiol Psychol* (1979) 7:291–4. doi:10.3758/BF03326643
169. Archer J. Testosterone and persistence in mice. *Anim Behav* (1977) 25:479–88. doi:10.1016/0003-3472(77)90023-9
170. Thor DH. Testosterone and persistence of social investigation in laboratory rats. *J Comp Physiol Psychol* (1980) 94:970–6. doi:10.1037/h0077831
171. van Hest A, van Haaren F, van de Poll NE. Perseverative responding in male and female Wistar rats: effects of gonadal hormones. *Horm Behav* (1989) 23:57–67. doi:10.1016/0018-506X(89)90074-3
172. Guillamón A, Valencia A, Calés J, Segovia S. Effects of early postnatal gonadal steroids on the successive conditional discrimination reversal learning in the rat. *Physiol Behav* (1986) 38:845–9. doi:10.1016/0031-9384(86)90052-1
173. Neese SL, Schantz SL. Testosterone impairs the acquisition of an operant delayed alternation task in male rats. *Horm Behav* (2012) 61:57–66. doi:10.1016/j.yhbeh.2011.10.003
174. Nelson CJ, Lee JS, Gamboa MC, Roth AJ. Cognitive effects of hormone therapy in men with prostate cancer. *Cancer* (2008) 113:1097–106. doi:10.1002/cncr.23658
175. Shahinian VB, Kuo Y, Freeman JL, Orihuela E, Goodwin JS. Increasing use of gonadotropin-releasing hormone agonists for the treatment of localized prostate carcinoma. *Cancer* (2005) 103:1615–24. doi:10.1002/cncr.20955

176. Fokidis HB, Adomat HH, Kharmate G, Hosseini-Beheshti E, Guns ES, Soma KK. Regulation of local steroidogenesis in the brain and in prostate cancer: lessons learned from interdisciplinary collaboration. *Front Neuroendocrinol* (2015) 36:108–29. doi:10.1016/j.yfrne.2014.08.005
177. Yang J, Zhong F, Qiu J, Cheng H, Wang K. Dissociation of event-based prospective memory and time-based prospective memory in patients with prostate cancer receiving androgen-deprivation therapy: a neuropsychological study. *Eur J Cancer Care (Engl)* (2015) 24:198–204. doi:10.1111/ecc.12299
178. Chao HH, Hu S, Ide JS, Uchio E, Zhang S, Rose M, et al. Effects of androgen deprivation on cerebral morphometry in prostate cancer patients – an exploratory study. *PLoS One* (2013) 8:e72032. doi:10.1371/journal.pone.0072032
179. Chao HH, Uchio E, Zhang S, Hu S, Bednarski SR, Luo X, et al. Effects of androgen deprivation on brain function in prostate cancer patients – a prospective observational cohort analysis. *BMC Cancer* (2012) 12:1. doi:10.1186/1471-2407-12-371
180. Wu LM, Tanenbaum ML, Dijkers MPJM, Amidi A, Hall SJ, Penedo FJ, et al. Cognitive and neurobehavioral symptoms in patients with non-metastatic prostate cancer treated with androgen deprivation therapy or observation: a mixed methods study. *Soc Sci Med* (2016) 156:80–9. doi:10.1016/j.socscimed.2016.03.016
181. Alibhai SMH, Timilshina N, Duff-Canning S, Breunis H, Tannock IF, Naglie G, et al. Effects of long-term androgen deprivation therapy on cognitive function over 36 months in men with prostate cancer. *Cancer* (2017) 123:237–44. doi:10.1002/cncr.30320
182. Alibhai SMH, Breunis H, Timilshina N, Marzouk S, Stewart D, Tannock I, et al. Impact of androgen-deprivation therapy on cognitive function in men with nonmetastatic prostate cancer. *J Clin Oncol* (2010) 28:5030–7. doi:10.1200/JCO.2010.30.8742
183. Morote J, Tabernero J, Álvarez-Ossorio JL, Ciria JP, Domínguez-Escrig JL, Vázquez F, et al. Cognitive function in patients on androgen suppression: a prospective, multicentric study. *Actas Urol Esp* (2018) 42(2):114–20. doi:10.1016/j.acuro.2017.04.007
184. McGinty HL, Phillips KM, Jim HSL, Cessna JM, Asvat Y, Cases MG, et al. Cognitive functioning in men receiving androgen deprivation therapy for prostate cancer a systematic review and meta-analysis. *Support Care Cancer* (2014) 22:2271–80. doi:10.1007/s00520-014-2285-1
185. Huang G, Wharton W, Travison TG, Ho MH, Gleason C, Asthana S, et al. Effects of testosterone administration on cognitive function in hysterectomized women with low testosterone levels: a dose-response randomized trial. *J Endocrinol Invest* (2015) 38:455–61. doi:10.1007/s40618-014-0213-3
186. Donovan KA, Walker LM, Wassersug RJ, Thompson LMA, Robinson JW. Psychological effects of androgen-deprivation therapy on men with prostate cancer and their partners. *Cancer* (2015) 121:4286–99. doi:10.1002/cncr.29672
187. Wu LM, Amidi A, Tanenbaum ML, Winkel G, Gordon WA, Hall SJ, et al. Computerized cognitive training in prostate cancer patients on androgen deprivation therapy: a pilot study. *Support Care Cancer* (2018) 26(6):1917–26. doi:10.1007/s00520-017-4026-8
188. Wallin KG, Wood RI. Anabolic–androgenic steroids impair set-shifting and reversal learning in male rats. *Eur Neuropsychopharmacol* (2015) 25:583–90. doi:10.1016/j.euroneuro.2015.01.002
189. Kindlundh AMS, Lindblom J, Bergström L, Wikberg JES, Nyberg F. The anabolic-androgenic steroid nandrolone decanoate affects the density of dopamine receptors in the male rat brain. *Eur J Neurosci* (2001) 13:291–6. doi:10.1046/j.0953-816X.2000.01402.x
190. Wallin KG, Alves JM, Wood RI. Anabolic-androgenic steroids and decision making: probability and effort discounting in male rats. *Psychoneuroendocrinology* (2015) 57:84–92. doi:10.1016/j.psyneuen.2015.03.023
191. Wood RI, Armstrong A, Fridkin V, Shah V, Najafi A, Jakowec M. Roid rage in rats? Testosterone effects on aggressive motivation, impulsivity and tyrosine hydroxylase. *Physiol Behav* (2013) 11(0–111):6–12. doi:10.1016/j.physbeh.2012.12.005
192. Cooper SE, Goings SP, Kim JY, Wood RI. Testosterone enhances risk tolerance without altering motor impulsivity in male rats. *Psychoneuroendocrinology* (2014) 40:201–12. doi:10.1016/j.psyneuen.2013.11.017
193. Winstanley CA, Floresco SB. Deciphering decision making: variation in animal models of effort- and uncertainty-based choice reveals distinct neural circuitries underlying core cognitive processes. *J Neurosci* (2016) 36:12069–79. doi:10.1523/JNEUROSCI.1713-16.2016
194. Ghods-Sharifi S, Floresco SB. Differential effects on effort discounting induced by inactivations of the nucleus accumbens core or shell. *Behav Neurosci* (2010) 124:179–91. doi:10.1037/a0018932
195. Stopper CM, Floresco SB. Contributions of the nucleus accumbens and its subregions to different aspects of risk-based decision making. *Cogn Affect Behav Neurosci* (2011) 11:97–112. doi:10.3758/s13415-010-0015-9
196. Kanayama G, Kean J, Hudson JI, Pope HG. Cognitive deficits in long-term anabolic-androgenic steroid users. *Drug Alcohol Depend* (2013) 130:208–14. doi:10.1016/j.drugalcdep.2012.11.008
197. Pope HG, Katz DL. Homicide and near-homicide by anabolic steroid users. *J Clin Psychiatry* (1990) 51:28–31.
198. Moss HB, Panzak GL, Tarter RE. Sexual functioning of male anabolic steroid abusers. *Arch Sex Behav* (1993) 22:1–12. doi:10.1007/BF01552908
199. Welker KM, Carré JM. Individual differences in testosterone predict persistence in men. *Eur J Pers* (2015) 29:83–9. doi:10.1002/per.1958
200. Broverman DM, Broverman IK, Vogel W, Palmer RD, Klaiber EL. The automatization cognitive style and physical development. *Child Dev* (1964) 35:1343. doi:10.1111/j.1467-8624.1964.tb05272.x
201. de Water E, Braams BR, Crone EA, Peper JS. Pubertal maturation and sex steroids are related to alcohol use in adolescents. *Horm Behav* (2013) 63:392–7. doi:10.1016/j.yhbeh.2012.11.018
202. Wallin-Miller KG, Chesley J, Castrillon J, Wood RI. Sex differences and hormonal modulation of ethanol-enhanced risk taking in rats. *Drug Alcohol Depend* (2017) 174:137–44. doi:10.1016/j.drugalcdep.2017.01.023
203. Stanton SJ, Liening SH, Schultheiss OC. Testosterone is positively associated with risk taking in the Iowa Gambling Task. *Horm Behav* (2011) 59:252–6. doi:10.1016/j.yhbeh.2010.12.003
204. Bechara A, Tranel D, Damasio H. Characterization of the decision-making deficit of patients with ventromedial prefrontal cortex lesions. *Brain* (2000) 123:2189–202. doi:10.1093/brain/123.11.2189
205. Bechara A, Damasio H, Damasio AR. Emotion, decision making and the orbitofrontal cortex. *Cereb Cortex* (2000) 10:295–307. doi:10.1093/cercor/10.3.295
206. Coates JM, Herbert J. Endogenous steroids and financial risk taking on a London trading floor. *Proc Natl Acad Sci U S A* (2008) 105:6167–72. doi:10.1073/pnas.0704025105
207. Castanho TC, Moreira PS, Portugal-Nunes C, Novais A, Costa PS, Palha JA, et al. The role of sex and sex-related hormones in cognition, mood and well-being in older men and women. *Biol Psychol* (2014) 103:158–66. doi:10.1016/j.biopsycho.2014.08.015
208. Henderson VW, St John JA, Hodis HN, Mccleary CA, Stanczyk FZ, Karim R, et al. Cognition, mood, and physiological concentrations of sex hormones in the early and late postmenopause. *Proc Natl Acad Sci U S A* (2013) 110:20290–5. doi:10.1073/pnas.1312353110
209. Bove RM, Brick DJ, Healy BC, Mancuso SM, Gerweck AV, Bredella MA, et al. Metabolic and endocrine correlates of cognitive function in healthy young women. *Obesity (Silver Spring)* (2013) 21:1343–9. doi:10.1002/oby.20212
210. McEwen BS, Wingfield JC. The concept of allostasis in biology and biomedicine. *Horm Behav* (2003) 43:2–15. doi:10.1016/S0018-506X(02)00024-7
211. Malkesman O, Braw Y, Ram E, Maayan R, Weizman A, Kinor N, et al. Dehydroepiandrosterone and monoamines in the limbic system of a genetic animal model of childhood depression. *Eur Neuropsychopharmacol* (2008) 18:255–61. doi:10.1016/j.euroneuro.2007.06.007
212. Qi X-R, Luchetti S, Verwer RWH, Sluiter AA, Mason MRJ, Zhou J-N, et al. Alterations in the steroid biosynthetic pathways in the human prefrontal cortex in mood disorders: a postmortem study. *Brain Pathol* (2017) 1–12. doi:10.1111/bpa.12548
213. Agis-Balboa RC, Guidotti A, Pinna G. 5α-reductase type I expression is downregulated in the prefrontal cortex/Brodmann's area 9 (BA9) of depressed patients. *Psychopharmacology (Berl)* (2014) 231:3569–80. doi:10.1007/s00213-014-3567-5
214. Alexopoulos GS. Role of executive function in late-life depression. *J Clin Psychiatry* (2003) 64(Suppl 1):18–23.
215. McDermott LM, Ebmeier KP. A meta-analysis of depression severity and cognitive function. *J Affect Disord* (2009) 119:1–8. doi:10.1016/j.jad.2009.04.022
216. Alexopoulos GS. "The depression-executive dysfunction syndrome of late life": a specific target for D3 agonists? *Am J Geriatr Psychiatry* (2001) 9:22–9. doi:10.1176/appi.ajgp.9.1.22

217. Souza-Teodoro LH, de Oliveira C, Walters K, Carvalho LA. Higher serum dehydroepiandrosterone sulfate protects against the onset of depression in the elderly: findings from the English Longitudinal Study of Aging (ELSA). *Psychoneuroendocrinology* (2016) 64:40–6. doi:10.1016/j.psyneuen.2015.11.005
218. Veronese N, De Rui M, Bolzetta F, Zambon S, Corti MC, Baggio G, et al. Serum dehydroepiandrosterone sulfate and incident depression in the elderly: the Pro.V.A. study. *Am J Geriatr Psychiatry* (2015) 23:863–71. doi:10.1016/j.jagp.2014.10.009
219. Tomm RJ, Schweitzer HR, Tobiansky DJ, Kachkovski GV, Ma CQ, Adomat HH, et al. *Local Androgen Synthesis in the Male Rat Brain and its Modulation of Behavioral Flexibility*. Washington D.C: Society for Neuroscience Conference (2017).
220. Goudriaan AE, Lapauw B, Ruige J, Feyen E, Kaufman JM, Brand M, et al. The influence of high-normal testosterone levels on risk-taking in healthy males in a 1-week letrozole administration study. *Psychoneuroendocrinology* (2010) 35:1416–21. doi:10.1016/j.psyneuen.2010.04.005
221. Taylor GT, Manzella FM, Huffman J, Cabrera OH, Hoffman J. Hormones and behavior cognition in female rats after blocking conversion of androgens to estrogens. *Horm Behav* (2017) 90:84–9. doi:10.1016/j.yhbeh.2017.02.011
222. Li L, Kang Y-X, Ji X-M, Li Y-K, Li S-C, Zhang X-J, et al. Finasteride inhibited brain dopaminergic system and open-field behaviors in adolescent male rats. *CNS Neurosci Ther* (2018) 24:115–25. doi:10.1111/cns.12781
223. Traish AM, Melcangi RC, Bortolato M, Garcia-Segura LM, Zitzmann M. Adverse effects of 5α-reductase inhibitors: what do we know, don't know, and need to know? *Rev Endocr Metab Disord* (2015) 16(3):177–98. doi:10.1007/s11154-015-9319-y

12

Clinical Features, Treatment and Outcomes Among Chinese Children with Anti-methyl-D-aspartate Receptor (Anti-NMDAR) Encephalitis

Min Zhang[1†], Wenhui Li[1†], Shuizhen Zhou[1], Yuanfeng Zhou[1], Haowei Yang[2], Lifei Yu[1], Ji Wang[1], Yi Wang[1] and Linmei Zhang[1*]*

[1] Department of Neurology, Children's Hospital of Fudan University, Shanghai, China,

[2] Department of Radiology, Children's Hospital of Fudan University, Shanghai, China

***Correspondence:**
Yi Wang
yiwang@shmu.edu.cn
Linmei Zhang
linmeizhang@outlook.com

† These authors have contributed equally to this work

Objective: Anti-N-methyl-D-aspartate receptor (anti-NMDAR) encephalitis is the most common form of autoimmune encephalitis in pediatric patients. In this study, we aimed to investigate the clinical features and long-term outcomes of pediatric patients with anti-NMDAR encephalitis in China.

Methods: We conducted a retrospective study of children (age range: 0–18 years) with anti-NMDAR encephalitis treated at Children's Hospital of Fudan University between July 2015 and November 2018. Demographic characteristics, clinical features, treatment, and outcomes were reviewed.

Results: Thirty-four patients with anti-NMDAR encephalitis were enrolled (age range: 5 months to 14 years; median age: 7 years; female: 18). The median follow- up duration was 20 months (range: 6–39 months). Eighteen (52.9%) patients initially presented with seizures and 10 (29.4%) with abnormal (psychiatric) behaviors or cognitive dysfunction. Thirty (88.2%) patients exhibited more than two symptoms during the disease course. No neoplasms were detected. Twelve (35.2%) patients had abnormal cerebrospinal fluid (CSF) findings, including leukocytosis, and increased protein concentration. Eighteen (52.9%) patients exhibited normal brain MRI findings. Electroencephalography revealed abnormal background activity in 27 (79.4%) patients, and epileptiform discharges in 16 (47.0%) patients prior to immunotherapy. All patients received first-line immunotherapy, with 30 (88.2%) and four (11.8%) patients achieving good (Modified Rankin Scale [mRS] score of 0–2) and poor outcomes (mRS score of 3–5), respectively. Initial mRS scores differed significantly between the good and poor outcome groups. Fourteen out of 18 patients (77.7%) with seizures accepted anti-epileptic drug (AED) administration, and seizure freedom was achieved in 12 out of 14 (85.7%) patients at the last follow-up. Ten of these 12 (83.3%) patients withdrew from AED treatment within 1 year.

Conclusions: Most patients achieved seizure freedom, so long-term use of AEDs may not be necessary for pediatric patients with anti-NMDAR encephalitis. Among our patients, 83.3% were sensitive to first-line immunotherapy and achieved good outcomes. Higher mRS scores before immunotherapy predicted poor outcomes, highlighting the need for a comprehensive assessment of patients with anti-NMDAR encephalitis.

Keywords: anti-NMDAR encephalitis, autoimmune encephalitis, anti-N-methyl-D-aspartate receptor, children, immunotherapy

INTRODUCTION

Anti-N-methyl-D-aspartate receptor (anti-NMDAR) encephalitis is a recently recognized autoimmune disorder in which auto-antibodies mainly target the NR1 subunit of the NMDA receptor, leading to a series of complex neuropsychiatric symptoms (1, 2). Reports of anti-NMDAR encephalitis have become more frequent over recent years, shedding light on the clinical characteristics of the disease. Anti-NMDAR encephalitis is a form of autoimmune encephalitis. Patients typically present with psychiatric symptoms, behavioral dysfunction, seizures, speech impairment, cognitive impairment, movement disorders, decreased consciousness, autonomic instability, and central hypoventilation. The disease is observed in patients of different ages and genders and may or may not be accompanied by ovarian teratomas or other tumors. Increased clinical recognition of this disease has led to an increase in the number of patients diagnosed with anti-NMDAR encephalitis.

Some research groups have summarized the clinical features of autoimmune encephalitis, providing a practical clinical approach to early diagnosis of the disease, rather than completely relying on the detection of autoantibodies (3, 4). Moreover, a meta-analysis found that earlier treatment of anti-NMDAR encephalitis leads to better outcomes among children (5). However, the clinical symptoms of anti-NMDAR encephalitis are complex, especially in younger pediatric patients, and many clinicians cannot promptly distinguish them from those of other diseases such as viral encephalitis or psychological conditions. Therefore, this study aimed to summarize the demographic characteristics, clinical features, ancillary examination results, treatments, and outcomes of Chinese children with anti-NMDAR encephalitis.

MATERIALS AND METHODS

This retrospective study included 34 pediatric patients with anti-NMDAR encephalitis, who were diagnosed at the Department of Neurology at Children's Hospital of Fudan University (Shanghai, China) between July 2015 and November 2018. The study was approved by the Ethics Committee of the Children's Hospital of Fudan University, which waived the requirement for informed consent owing to the retrospective nature of the study.

All patients met the following inclusion criteria: (a) met the diagnostic criteria for definite anti-NMDA receptor encephalitis (3); (b) treatment with first-line immunotherapy during the acute phase, including methylprednisolone and/or immunoglobulin and/or plasma exchange; (c) age between 0 and 18 years; and (d) duration of follow-up exceeding 6 months, with complete medical records. We excluded patients with other possible etiologies such as viral encephalitis or psychological conditions.

Medical information was collected from medical records or via telephone interviews and follow-up was continued until the patient died or was lost to follow-up. We reviewed patients' clinical data, including age, gender, age at disease onset, follow-up duration, initial symptoms, duration between symptom onset and diagnosis, duration between symptom onset and immunotherapy, CSF examination results, brain magnetic resonance imaging (MRI) results, results of screenings for systemic neoplasms, electroencephalography (EEG) findings, and treatment strategies. Serum and CSF samples from each patient were sent to Oumeng Biotechnology Corporation (Shanghai, China) to screen for antibodies against the NMDA receptor. All samples were evaluated for anti-NMDAR IgG antibodies via indirect immunofluorescence using EU 90 cells transfected with the NMDAR1 subunit (NR1) of the NMDAR complex and immobilized on BIOCHIPs (Euroimmun AG, Lubek, Germany). CSF leukocytosis was defined as white cell count $>5/mm^3$ while elevated CSF proteins 450 >mg/L. Tumor screening (MRI and/or CT and/or ultrasound of the chest, abdomen, and pelvic cavity) was performed once each patient was diagnosed with anti-NMDAR encephalitis. All patients were screened for tumors regularly after discharge, including MRI of the chest, abdomen, and pelvic cavity (once a year for children >12 years and biennial for children <12 years of age).

Digital-video EEG records were obtained at least once before immunotherapy, three to 6 months after immunotherapy, and at the last available follow-up. EEG data were recorded for at least 30 min. All EEG recordings were retrospectively evaluated by a pediatric epileptologist familiar with the patient's age and diagnosis, but not with his/her clinical state, symptoms, or signs. EEG data were categorized as follows: background activity (normal, generalized slowing, focal slowing, and extreme delta brushes [EDB]); interictal epileptic paroxysms such as sharp waves, spike waves, polyspike waves, or generalized discharges; focal discharges; and multifocal interictal epilepticdischarges.

Brain MRI findings were obtained from all patients before immunotherapy. Abnormal brain MRI findings were defined as hyper intensities on T2-weighted images (T2WI), fluid-attenuated inversion recovery (FLAIR) images and/or hypo intensities on T2-weighted images (T1WI). The same pediatric neurologist reviewed all the brain MRI results.

Outcomes were evaluated based on mRS scores. After discharge, outcome evaluations were performed during clinical

TABLE 1 | Patients' demographic and clinical characteristics.

Item	All patients (%)	Age under 12 (%)	Age under 6 (%)
Number	34	30	14
Female: male	18:16	16:14	8:6
Median age, range(months)	86 (5–171)	81 (5–136)	32 (5–67)
INITIAL SYMPTOMS			
Psychiatric/behavior	8 (23.5%)	8 (26.7%)	4 (28.6%)
Seizure	16 (47.1%)	13 (43.3%)	10 (71.4%)
Others	10 (29.4%)	9 (30%)	0

visits to the neurologist or via telephone follow-up. The evaluation standards were as follows: full recovery, mRS score of 0; mild deficits, mRS scores of 1–2; severe deficits, mRS scores of 3–5; or death, mRS score of 6.

We used SPSS version 19.0 for all statistical analyses (SPSS Inc., Chicago, IL, USA). Continuous variables such as age, the interval from symptom onset to definitive diagnosis, and the interval from symptom onset to immunotherapy were analyzed using independent t-tests. Categorical variables were analyzed using Fisher's exact test, and ordinal variables were analyzed using Fisher–Freeman–Halton tests. $P < 0.05$ (two-sided) were considered significant.

RESULTS

Clinical Characteristics

Clinical characteristics of the 34 included patients are presented in **Table 1**. Patients' ages ranged from 5 months to 14 years (median age: 20 months), and 18 were female (52.9%; a female-to-male ratio of 1.125). Thirty patients (88.2%) were younger than 12 years of age, and 14 patients (41.2%) were younger than 6 years of age at symptom onset. The median follow-up duration was 20 months, ranging from 6 to 39 months. The initial presentation included seizures in 18 patients (52.9%), abnormal (psychiatric) behaviors or cognitive dysfunction in 10 patients (29.4%), a movement disorder in 3 patients (8.8%), and a decreased level of consciousness in 3 patients (8.8%). Thirty patients (88.2%) developed at least two of the six symptom categories over the course of their disease. Three patients (8.8%) were hospitalized in intensive care unit (ICU) due to central hypoventilation, coma, or refractory seizures, respectively. Each of the 18 patients who experienced seizures had onset during the acute phase of anti-NMDAR encephalitis, which was defined as <3 months after symptom onset. Seizure types included repetitive seizures (16/18, 88.8%), single seizures (2/18, 11.1%), and status epileptics (9/18, 50%) **(Figure 1)**. Generalized and focal seizures were noted in 5 (27.7%) and 11(61.1%) of 18 patients, respectively **(Figure 2)**. Only two (11.1%) patients reported seizures at the last follow-up. No patients developed tumors or died during follow-up.

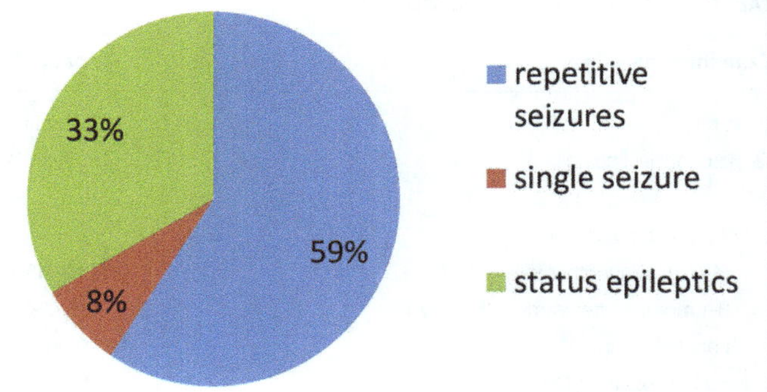

FIGURE 1 | Percentage of patients with repetitive seizures, single seizure, and status epilepticus (SE).

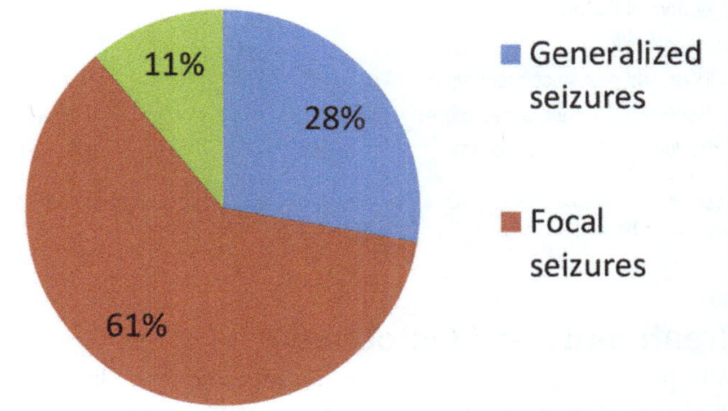

FIGURE 2 | Percentage of patients with focal, generalized, and both focal and generalized seizures epilepticus (SE).

Ancillary Examination Results

Initial CSF findings before immunotherapy are shown in **Table 2**. Eleven patients (32.4%) had CSF pleocytosis, seven (20.6%) had increased protein concentrations only, and six (17.6%) had both. Anti-NMDAR antibodies were identified in CSF obtained from 9 patients (26.5%) and both serum and CSF of 25 patients (73.5%). No patients were positive for anti-NMDAR antibodies in serum only. Brain MRI findings were normal in 19 (55.9%) of 34 patients. The remaining 15 patients (44.1%) exhibited abnormalities that included increased signal on T2WI or FLAIR images ($n = 14$, two in the temporal lobes, one in the frontal cortex, three in the thalamus, one in the parietal lobe, seven in the cerebral cortex/gray matter) and encephalomalacia ($n = 1$).

The first available EEG findings detected before immunotherapy included generalized slowing in 25/34 (73.5%) patients and focal slowing in 2/34 (5.9%). Normal background activity was observed in only 7/34 (20.6%) patients, and in 32/34 (94.1%) patients 3 months post-immunotherapy, and in all patients 9 months post-immunotherapy. Sixteen of 34 (47.1%) patients reported interictal epileptic paroxysms during the acute stage of anti-NMDAR encephalitis. This rate decreased to 14.7% ($n = 5$) 3-6 months after immunotherapy and 2.9% ($n = 1$) at the last follow-up. EDB patterns were recorded in 2/34 (5.9%) patients (**Figure 3**) and disappeared 6 months after immunotherapy **(Figure 4)**.

TABLE 2 | Results of ancillary examinations.

Examinations	All patients
Brain MRI	Numbers (%)
Total abnormal findings	18 (52.9%)
EEG	
Abnormal background	
Before immunotherapy	27(79.4%)
3–6months after immunotherapy	2(5.9%)
Last follow up	0(0%)
Interictal Epileptiform Discharge	
Before immunotherapy	16 (47.0%)
3–6months after immunotherapy	5 (14.7%)
Last follow up	2 (5.8%)
EDB	2 (5.8%)
CSF Results	
Abnormal findings	12 (35.3%)
Pleocytosis	11 (32.4%)
Increased protein concentration	7 (20.6%)
Pleocytosis and increased protein concentration	6 (17.6%)
Positive OB(Total number 11)	1 (9.1%)

EEG, electroencephalogram; EDB, extreme delta brush; CSF, cerebrospinal fluid; OB, Oligoclonal band.

Treatments and Outcomes

All patients received first-line immunotherapy, including intravenous methylprednisolone, intravenous immunoglobulin, plasma exchange, or an arbitrary combination of these treatments. The median interval between symptom onset and the start of immunotherapy treatment was 23.9 days, ranged from 7 to 42 days. The median duration of follow-up was 20 months, with a range of 6 to 39 months. Twenty-five of the 34 (73.5%) patients were treated within 30 days of first symptom appearance. Three patients (8.8%) were exclusively treated with intravenous methylprednisolone (15–30 mg/kg per day for 3–5 days), 29 patients (85.3%) with both intravenous methylprednisolone and intravenous immunoglobulin (IVIG, 0.4 g/kg per day for 5 days or 1 g/kg per day for 2 days), and two patients (5.9%) with a combination of intravenous methylprednisolone, IVIG, and plasma exchange. The median mRS score before immunotherapy was 5, which decreased to zero following 3–6 months of initial immunotherapy (**Figure 5**). By the last follow-up, 29 patients (85.2%) had fully recovered, one patient (2.9%) exhibited mild deficits (weakness on one side of the body), and four patients (11.8%) exhibited severe deficits (one with speech disturbances and memory deficits, one with dyskinesia, and two with intractable epilepsy). No deaths were noted at the last follow-up.

Comparison Between the Good and Poor Outcome Groups

Table 3 shows between-group comparisons of the good and poor outcome groups. The initial median mRS score was significantly higher in the poor outcome group than in the good outcome group ($p = 0.014$). Initial symptoms, CSF findings, the median age at the appearance of initial symptoms, the median interval between onset and diagnosis, the median interval between onset and immunotherapy, MRI findings, EEG findings, and ICU admission showed no significant between-group differences.

Comparison Between Patients Younger and Older Than 6 Years old

Table 4 shows the comparison between patients younger than 6 years old and older than 6 years. We observed no significant between-group differences for initial symptoms, CSF findings, median initial mRS score, the median interval between onset and diagnosis (d), the median interval between onset and immunotherapy (d), MRI findings, interictal epileptic discharges, or ICU admission.

DISCUSSION

Previous research has demonstrated that there are more cases of anti-NMDAR encephalitis than other kinds of autoimmune encephalitis, and that early diagnosis and aggressive medical management decrease the likelihood of morbidity and mortality (6–9). Therefore, if anti-NMDAR encephalitis is suspected and other diseases can be ruled out, treatment should begin as early as possible (10). However, there are significant differences in clinical features between pediatric and adult patients. Here we retrospectively analyzed the clinical characteristics, ancillary examination results, and outcomes of Chinese pediatric patients with anti-NMDAR encephalitis.

We observed no significant differences in sex in the present study. These findings correspond to the findings of a previous study that focused on pediatric patients with anti-NMDAR encephalitis in south-central China (11). In children, psychiatric syndromes can present as abnormal behaviors or cognitive dysfunction. This is particular true for preschool-aged children, because it is difficult for them to describe their symptoms and emotional states. Therefore, we could not make objective judgments regarding cognitive function, including the presence of memory deficits, which are independently associated with poorer outcomes (12). Instead, we attributed psychiatric symptoms and abnormal behaviors or cognitive dysfunction to a single category of symptoms. Eighteen of the 34 included patients (52.9%) initially presented with seizures, while 10 (29.4%) presented with abnormal (psychiatric) behaviors or cognitive dysfunction. We concluded that seizures and abnormal (psychiatric) behaviors and cognitive dysfunction are the most common symptoms of pediatric anti-NMDAR encephalitis, in agreement with previous findings (13–16).

Armangue et al. (9, 14) reported that younger children with anti-NMDAR encephalitis typically presented with neurologic symptoms, whereas adolescents more often presented with psychiatric symptoms. However, in our study, 75% (3/4) of adolescents presented with seizures as their initial symptom, and there was no significant difference in initial symptoms between older and younger patients (**Table 4**). This difference may be attributed to the relatively small sample of adolescents in our

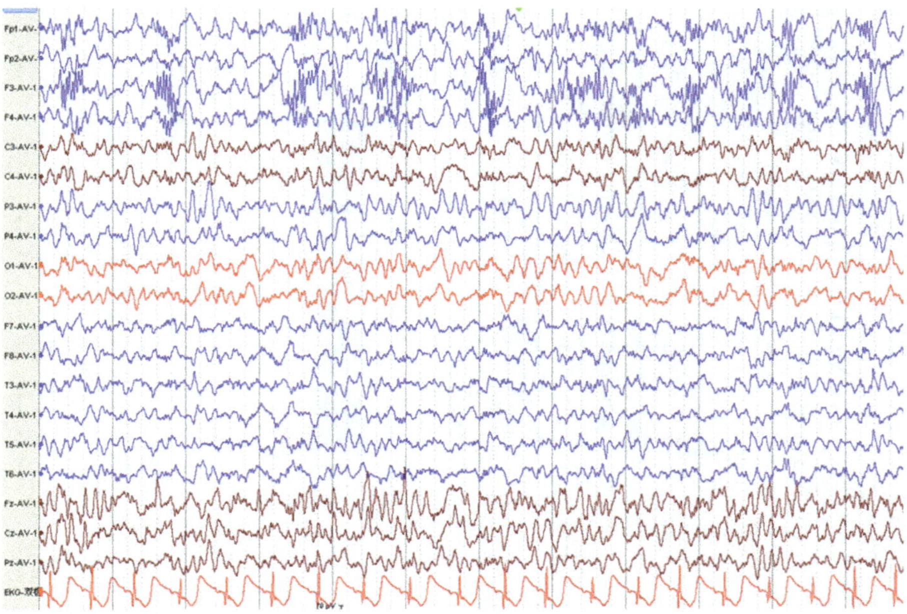

FIGURE 3 | Electroencephalography pattern of a 4-year and 5-month-old female child with anti-N-methyl-D-aspartate receptor encephalitis (Case 8), who presented with clonic seizures of her right limbs as her initial symptom. EEG was recorded 43 days after symptom onset and before immunotherapy. EEG shows bilateral frontal-predominant fast activity at 20–30 Hz riding on the generalized rhythmic delta activity (EDB).

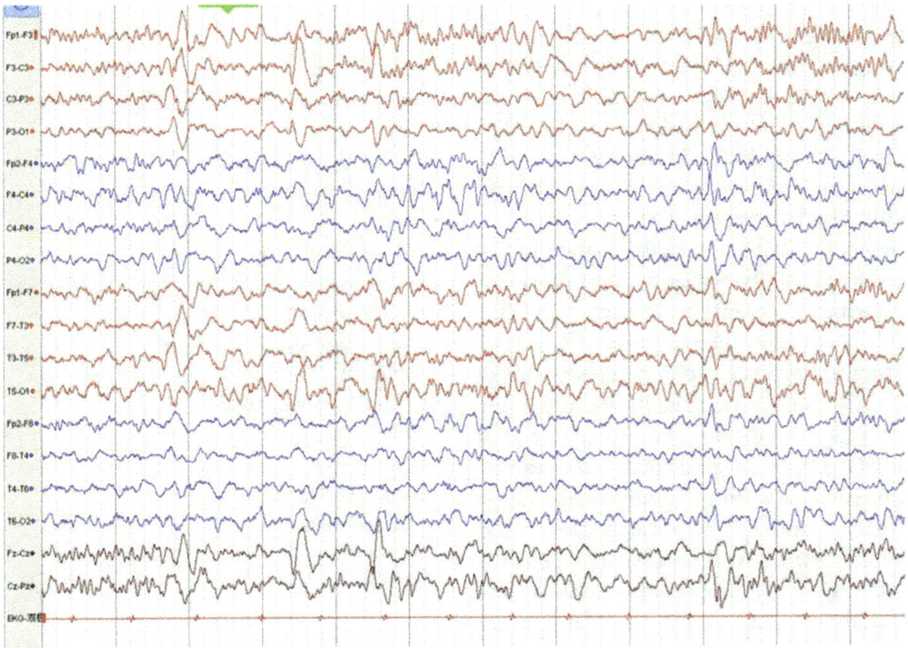

FIGURE 4 | Normal EEG was recorded six months after immunotherapy (Case 8).

study. According to the literature, adult patients more frequently present with focal seizures, while children more frequently present with generalized seizures that develop into the dominant seizure type over the course of the disease (17). In a recent study of 17 pediatric patients with anti-NMDAR encephalitis, generalized seizures were reported in 5/16 patients (31%), while focal seizures were reported in 4/16 (25%) patients, another 7/16 (44%) patients had both generalized, and focal seizures (16). In our study, among 18 patients experienced seizures, 11 (61.1%) presented with focal seizures, five (27.7%) with generalized

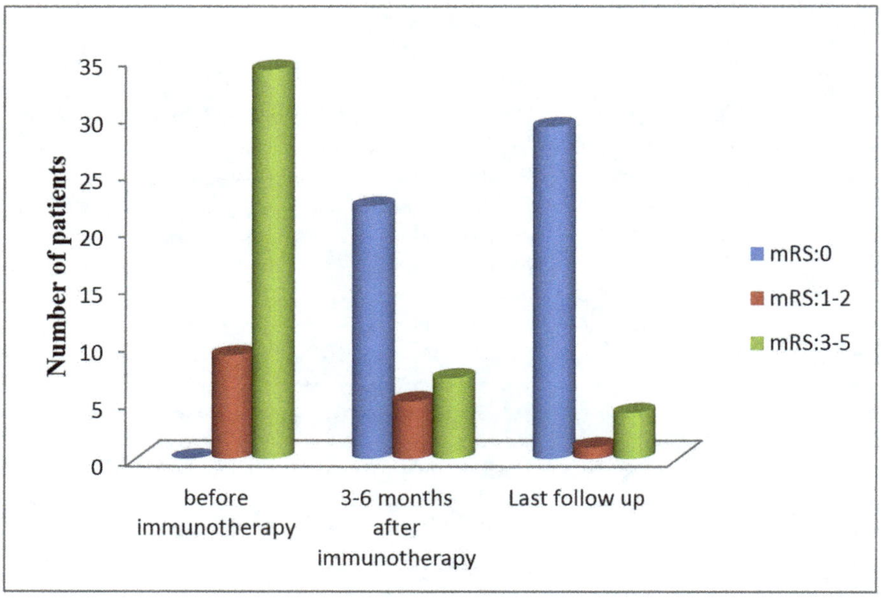

FIGURE 5 | Patients' mRS scores during the follow-up period.

seizures, and two (11.1%) with both types. Age-related differences in patients' constitutions and the use of video-EEG to determine seizure type may explain these differences.

Of the 14 patients treated with AEDs, 12 (85.7%) got seizure free during the acute stage of anti-NMDAR encephalitis, and 10 patients (71.4%) were able to withdraw from AEDs within 1 year. At the final follow-up, only two patients (14.3%) with ongoing epilepsy were treated with AEDs, indicating that long-term use of AEDs may not be necessary for pediatric patients with anti-NMDAR encephalitis. Similar results have been reported in previous studies involving both adult and pediatric patients (18). No tumors were detected in our study, which demonstrates that younger age is associated with a lower rate of teratomas (2, 11).

Although not generally helpful in diagnosing anti-NMDAR encephalitis, imaging studies play a key role in the workup of patients with suspected anti-NMDAR encephalitis because these modalities can rule out other conditions that could create a similar neurologic picture (19). A recent study demonstrated that anti-NMDA encephalitis is an autoimmune-mediated disease without specific brain MRI features. The authors categorized the brain MRI findings of patients with anti-NMDA receptor encephalitis into four types. Of these, hippocampal lesions were the most common brain abnormalities and were identified as risk factors contributing to poor prognosis (20), consistent with previous reports (21, 22). However, as with our results, some research has indicated that abnormal MRI findings do not affect prognosis as indicated by mRS scores (23). In our study, 55.9% of patients had normal brain MRI findings, and none exhibited hioppocampal lesions. This discrepancy may be due to differences between pediatric and adult patients, or to the relatively small sample size of our study. Therefore, future studies with larger samples are needed to compare brain MRI features between pediatric and adult patients.

TABLE 3 | Comparison of the good and poor outcome groups.

Item	Good outcome	Poor outcome	*P*-value
Patient number	30	4	/
Initial syndrome			/
Seizure	15	3	0.9467
Abnormal (psychiatric) behavior or cognitive dysfunction	9	1	0.7723
Others	6	0	0.5289
Abnormal CSF finding	12	2	0.8219
Median age(m)	99	24	0.1772
Median initial mRS	5	5	0.0141
Median interval between onset and diagnosis(d)	22	30	1.0000
Median interval between onset and immunotherapy(d)	20	29	0.6721
Abnormal MRI findings	12	3	0.3891
Abnormal EEG background	25	2	1.0000
Abnormal interictal epileptic discharges	14	2	0.5671
ICU stay	3	0	0.9290

Previous studies have indicated that the parietal aEEG bandwidth may separate patients with favorable and poor long-term outcomes in the early disease stages (24). In our study, the first available EEG findings that obtained before immunotherapy showed generalized slowing in 14/18 patients (77.7%), focal slowing in 2/18 patients (11.1%), and no abnormalities in 2/18 patients (11.1%), consistent with the findings of previous reports (25, 26). No patients exhibited abnormal background activity

TABLE 4 | Comparison of patients younger than 6 years old with those older than 6 years old.

Item	Age under 6 y	Age older than 6 y	*P*-value
Patient number	14	20	/
Initial syndrome			/
Seizure	10	8	0.6835
abnormal (psychiatric) behavior or cognitive dysfunction	4	6	1.0000
Others	0	6	0.0717
Abnormal CSF finding	4	8	0.7477
Median age(m)	36.5	110	0.0000
Median initial mRS	5	5	0.9830
Median interval between onset and diagnosis(d)	29.5	19	0.1010
Median interval between onset and immunotherapy(c)	27.5	17	0.0980
Abnormal MRI findings	7	8	0.8204
Abnormal EEG background	11	16	1.0000
Abnormal interictal epileptic discharges	9	7	0.1820
ICU stay	2	1	0.7450

at the final follow-up. These findings suggest that generalized slowing of EEG background activity is an important clue to diagnosing anti-NMDAR encephalitis during the acute stage, but it is not specific to anti-NMDAR encephalitis. Recent studies have demonstrated that the presence of EDB patterns is a marker of more severe disease among patients with anti-NMDAR encephalitis and corresponding with worse outcomes (27). Past researchers observed EDB patterns on EEG in 33% of patients with anti-NMDAR encephalitis (28). However, in our study, EDB patterns were detected in only 2/18 (11.1%) patients, likely due to differences in the time of EEG recording and individual differences in patients within the various study groups. Since prompt diagnosis is crucial (29), we recommend use of video-EEG monitoring for all patients with suspected anti-NMDAR encephalitis (30). Nonetheless, a recent study suggested that EDB is also not unique to anti-NMDAR encephalitis and can occur (albeit rarely) in patients with mesial temporal lobe epilepsy. While the presence of EDB should prompt suspicion of anti-NMDAR encephalitis, other possible etiologies should not be ignored (31).

Some previous studies have suggested that the prognosis is poor among patients with severe anti-NMDAR encephalitis (2, 32), but the long-term prognosis of anti-NMDAR encephalitis is good (33, 34), even in patients whose diagnoses were missed or in those with prolonged diagnostic delays who eventually recovered or substantially improved (35). Predictors of poor outcomes included younger age, decreased consciousness, memory deficits, ICU admission, treatment delay >4 weeks, lack of clinical improvement within 4 weeks, abnormal MRI, and CSF white blood cell count >20 cells/μL, etc. (2, 36–38). In our study, higher initial mRS scores predicted poor outcomes, in accordance with Anastasia Zekeridou et al. (39). However, our sample size was relatively small and further studies involving larger sample sizes are required to determine the risk factors for poor prognosis in this patient population.

According to our experience, most patients with anti-NMDAR encephalitis continue to improve within 2 years or longer, even when treated with first-line immunotherapy alone. For patients with slow clinical improvement, first-line immunotherapy can be re administered. In this study, some caretakers refused second-line immunotherapy because of cost concerns or concerns over clinical side effects, so all our patients were treated with first-line immunotherapy. Although no patients attained mRS scores of 0–2 (0%) before immunotherapy, 83.3% of them attained such scores at the final follow-up. This result indicated that first-line immunotherapy is an effective measure for pediatric patients with anti-NMDAR encephalitis. Besides, our patients' good outcomes may be associated with admission to the less intensive care unit and prompt immunotherapy after diagnosis with anti-NMDAR encephalitis.

In a recent study involving 111 patients with anti-NMDAR encephalitis, 39 (35.1%) patients were included in the severe group. Even patients with the most severe forms of anti-NMDAR encephalitis can eventually achieve good long-term outcomes after receiving early, positive, and unremitting combined immunotherapy and life support (25). Another study (40) involving 19 children with anti-NMDAR encephalitis in Thailand revealed that IVIG treatment, was associated with greater improvements in mRS scores. These findings underscore the benefits of IVIG treatment for this condition. Zhang et al. (13) analyzed the individual outcomes associated with three first-line immunotherapies and combinations of any two immunotherapies. Their findings revealed that patients treated with a combination of corticosteroids and IVIG plus second-line immunotherapy more frequently achieved full recovery than patients treated with a combination of corticosteroids and IVIG. Second-line immunotherapy with rituximab, cyclophosphamide, or both significantly improved outcomes in patients who did not respond to first-line therapy and decreased the frequency of relapses (2). Therefore, second-line immunotherapy may be necessary when patients do not achieve full recovery with first-line immunotherapy only.

Nonetheless, some recent studies have reported substantial deficits across multiple cognitive domains and behavioral problems in both adult and pediatric patients (41–44). These findings indicate that, even when good outcomes are achieved, full recovery may not be possible. Alternatively, while mRS scores are effective tools for assessing disability in patients with stroke, these scores may not be the most suitable tool for evaluating outcomes in patients with anti-NMDAR encephalitis who present with seizures and abnormal (psychiatric) behaviors or cognitive dysfunction. This is particularly true for infants who cannot walk or express their emotions. Future studies should seek to determine the most appropriate method for comprehensively assessing cognitive and social functions in patients with anti-NMDAR encephalitis at different ages.

Our study had several limitations. The functional status assessment may be susceptible to recall bias given the retrospective nature of the study. Our cohort only included patients diagnosed and treated at the Children's Hospital of Fudan University in Shanghai, which may also have introduced a selection bias. All patients were treated with first-line immunotherapy so we could not assess differences in the effects between first-line immunotherapy and other immunotherapy measures. The relationship between anti-NMDAR antibody titers and clinical symptom severity or outcomes was not examined and should be a focus of future studies.

CONCLUSION

In our study, seizure freedom was typically achieved by the final follow-up, indicating that long-term use of AEDs may not be necessary for patients with anti-NMDAR encephalitis. More than half of the patients exhibited normal brain MRI findings. Our results further indicated that generalized slowing of EEG background activity is the main characteristic of pediatric anti-NMDAR encephalitis during the acute stage. In addition, 83.3% of our patients were sensitive to first-line immunotherapy and achieved good outcomes. Higher mRS scores before immunotherapy predicted poor outcomes among pediatric patients with anti-NMDAR encephalitis. Future studies should aim to determine the most appropriate methods for comprehensively assessing cognitive and social functions in patients with anti-NMDAR encephalitis, particularly infants.

ETHICS STATEMENT

This study was approved by the Ethics Committee of Children's Hospital of Fudan University, who waived the requirement for informed consent due to the retrospective nature of the study.

AUTHOR CONTRIBUTIONS

MZ and WL wrote the initial draft of the paper. JW and LY acquired patients' demographic and clinical data through medical records and telephone interviews. YZ guided the analysis of EEG signals. HY guided the analysis of MRI and CT results, SZ guided the study design, and LZ and YW made critical revisions to the manuscript.

REFERENCES

1. Gleichman AJ, Spruce LA, Dalmau J, Seeholzer SH, Lynch DR. Anti-NMDA receptor encephalitis antibody binding is dependent on amino acid identity of a small region within the GluN1 amino terminal domain. *J Neurosci.* (2012) 32:11082–94. doi: 10.1523/JNEUROSCI.0064-12.2012
2. Titulaer MJ, McCracken L, Gabilondo I, Armangue T, Glaser C, Iizuka T, et al. Treatment and prognostic factors for long-term outcome in patients with anti-NMDA receptor encephalitis: an observational cohort study. *Lancet Neurol.* (2013) 12:157–65. doi: 10.1016/S1474-4422(12)70310-1
3. Graus F, Titulaer MJ, Balu R, Benseler S, Bien CG, Cellucci T, et al. A clinical approach to diagnosis of autoimmune encephalitis. *Lancet Neurol.* (2016) 15:391–404. doi: 10.1016/S1474-4422(15)00401-9
4. Irani SR, Gelfand JM, Al-Diwani A, Vincent A. Cell-surface central nervous system autoantibodies: clinical relevance and emerging paradigms. *Ann Neurol.* (2014) 76:168–84. doi: 10.1002/ana.24200
5. Byrne S, Walsh C, Hacohen Y, Muscal E, Jankovic J, Stocco A, et al. Earlier treatment of NMDAR antibody encephalitis in children results in a better outcome. *Neurol Neuroimmunol Neuroinflamm.* (2015) 2:e130. doi: 10.1212/NXI.0000000000000130.
6. Byrne S, McCoy B, Lych B, Webb B, King MD. Does early treatment improve outcomes in N-methyl-D-aspartate receptor encephalitis? *Dev Med Child Neurol.* (2014) 56:794–6. doi: 10.1111/dmcn.12411
7. Nijmeijer S, Bontemps S, Naeije L, Coutinho J. Anti-N-methyl- D-aspartate receptor encephalitis in a pre-teenage girl: a case report. *Eur J Pediatr.* (2014) 173:681–3. doi: 10.1007/s00431-013-2042-3
8. Salvucci A, Devine IM, Hammond D, Sheth RD. Pediatric anti-NMDA. (N-methyl D-Aspartate) receptor encephalitis. *Pediatric Neurol.* (2014) 50:507–10. doi: 10.1016/j.pediatrneurol.2014.01.012
9. Sartori S, Nosadini M, Cesaroni E, Falsaperla R, Capovilla, Beccaria F, et al. Paediatric anti-N-methyl- D-aspartate receptor encephalitis: the first Italian multicenter case series. *Eur J Paediatr Neurol.* (2015) 19:453–63. doi: 10.1016/j.ejpn.2015.02.006
10. Hong S, Klein-Gitelman M, Wainwright MS. Recognition and treatment of N-methyl- D- aspartate receptor encephalitis. *Clini Pediatric Emerg Med.* (2015) 16:3–10. doi: 10.1016/j.cpem.2015.02.003
11. Wang Y, Zhang W, Yin J, Lu Q, Yin F, He F, et al. Anti-N-methyl-d-aspartate receptor encephalitis in children of Central South China: clinical features, treatment, influencing factors, and outcomes. *J Neuroimmunol.* (2017) 312:59–65. doi: 10.1016/j.jneuroim.2017.09.005
12. Wang W, Li JM, Hu FY, Wang, R., Hong, Z, He L, Zhou D. Anti-NMDA receptor encephalitis: clinical characteristics, predictors of outcome and the knowledge gap in southwest China. *Eur. J. Neurol.* (2016) 23:621–9. doi: 10.1111/ene.12911
13. Zhang L, Wu MQ, Hao ZL, Chiang SM, Shuang K, Lin MT, et al. Clinical characteristics, treatments, and outcomes of patients with anti-N-methyl-d-aspartate receptor encephalitis: a systematic review of reported cases. *Epilepsy Behav.* (2017) 68:57–65. doi: 10.1016/j.yebeh.2016.12.019
14. Armangue T, Titulaer MJ, Malaga I, Bataller L, Gabilondo I, Graus F. Pediatric anti-NMDAR encephalitis: clinical analysis and novel findings in a series of 20 patients. *J Pediatrics.* (2013) 162:850–6. doi: 10.1016/j.jpeds.2012.10.011
15. Haberlandt E, Ensslen M, Gruber-Sedlmayr U, Plecko B, Brunner-Krainz M, Schimmel M, et al. Epileptic phenotypes, electroclinical features, and clinical characteristics in 17 children with anti-NMDAR encephalitis. *Eur J Paediatr Neurol.* (2017) 21:457–64. doi: 10.1016/j.ejpn.2016.11.016
16. Brenton JN, Goodkin HP. Antibody-mediated autoimmune encephalitis in childhood. *Pediatr Neurol.* (2016) 60:13–23. doi: 10.1016/j.pediatrneurol.2016.04.004
17. Irani SR, Bera K, Waters P, Zuliani L, Maxwell S, Zandi MS, et al. N-methyl-D-aspartate antibody encephalitis: temporal progression of clinical and paraclinical observations in a predominantly non-paraneoplastic disorder of both sexes. *Brain.* (2010) 133:1655–67. doi: 10.1093/brain/awq113
18. Liu X, Yan B, Wang R, Li C, Chen C, Zhou D, et al. Seizure outcomes in patients with anti-NMDAR encephalitis: a follow-up study. *Epilepsia.* (2017) 58:2104–11. doi: 10.1111/epi.13929
19. Zaborowski MP, Spaczynski M, Nowak-Markwitz E, Michalak S. Paraneoplastic neurological syndromes associated with ovarian tumors. *J Cancer Res Clini Oncol.* (2015) 141:99–108. doi: 10.1007/s00432-014-1745-9
20. Zhang T, Duan Y, Ye J, Xu W, Shu N, Wang C, et al. Brain MRI characteristics of patients with Anti-N-Methyl-D-aspartate receptor encephalitis and their associations with 2-year clinical outcome. *AJNR Am J Neuroradiol.* (2018) 39:824–29. doi: 10.3174/ajnr.A5593
21. Dalmau J, Lancaster E, Martinez-Hernandez E, Rosenfeld MR, Balice-Gordon R. Clinical experience and laboratory investigations in patients with anti-NMDAR encephalitis. *Lancet Neurol.* (2011) 10:63–74. doi: 10.1016/S1474-4422(10)70253-2
22. GÜnther A, Brodoehl S, Witte OW, Freesmeyer M, Dalmau JO, Redecker C. Atypical posthypoxic MRI changes in hypermetabolic regions in anti-NMDA-receptor encephalitis. *Neurology.* (2012) 79:720–21. doi: 10.1212/WNL.0b013e3182648bdc

23. Wang R, Lai XH, Liu X, Li YJ, Chen C, Li C, et al. Brain magnetic resonance-imaging findings of anti-N-methyl-D-aspartate receptor encephalitis: a cohort follow-up study in Chinese patients. *J Neurol.* (2018) 265:362–9. doi: 10.1007/s00415-017-8707-5
24. Jiang N, Guan H, Lu Q, Ren H, Peng B. Features and prognostic value of quantitative electroencephalogram changes in critically ill and non-critically Ill Anti-NMDAR encephalitis patients: a pilot study. *Front Neurol.* (2018) 9:833. doi: 10.3389/fneur.2018.00833
25. Zhang Y, Liu G, Jiang M, Chen W, He Y, Su Y. Clinical characteristics and prognosis of severe anti-N-methyl-d-aspartate receptor encephalitis patients. *Neurocrit Care.* (2018) 29:264–72. doi: 10.1007/s12028-018-0536-6
26. da Silve-Junior FP, Castro LH, Andrade JQ, Bastos CG, Moreira CH, Valerio RM, et al. Serial and prolonged EEG monitoring in anti-N-methyl-d-aspartate receptor encephalitis. *Clin Neurophysiol.* (2014) 125:1541–4. doi: 10.1016/j.clinph.2014.01.001
27. Schmitt SE, Pargeon K, Frechette ES, Hirsch LJ, Dalmau J, Friedman D, et al. Extreme delta brush: a unique EEG pattern in adults with anti-NMDA receptor encephalitis. *Neurology.* (2012) 79:1094–100. doi: 10.1212/WNL.0b013e3182698cd8
28. Huang Q, Wu Y Qin R, Wei X, Ma M. Clinical characteristics and outcomes between children and adults with anti-N-methyl-D receptor encephalitis. *J Neurol.* (2016) 263:2446–55. doi: 10.1007/s00415-016-8282-1
29. Sulentic V, Petelin Gadze Z, Derke F, Santini M, Bazadona D, Nankovic S. The effect of delayed anti-NMDAR encephalitis recognition on disease outcome. *J NeuroVirol.* (2018) 24:638–41. doi: 10.1007/s13365-018-0648-y
30. Di Capua D, García-Ptacek S, García-García ME, Abarrategui B, Porta-Etessam J, García-Morales I. Extreme delta brush in a patient with anti-NMDAR encephalitis. *Epileptic Disord.* (2013) 15:461–4. doi: 10.1684/epd.2013.0622
31. Baykan B, Gungor Tuncer O, Vanli-Yavuz EN, Baysal Kirac L, Gundogdu G, Bebek N, et al. Delta brush pattern is not unique to NMDAR encephalitis: evaluation of two independent long-term EEG cohorts. *Clin EEG Neurosci.* (2018) 49:278–84. doi: 10.1177/1550059417693168
32. Chi X, Wang W, Huang C, Wu M, Zhang L, Li J., et al. Risk factors for mortality in patients with anti-NMDA receptor encephalitis. *Acta Neurol Scand.* (2017) 136:298–304. doi: 10.1111/ane.12723
33. Mittal MK, Rabinstein AA, Hocker SE, Pittock SJ, Wijdicks EF, McKeon A. Autoimmune encephalitis in the ICU: analysis of phenotypes, serologic findings, and outcomes. *Neurocrit Care.* (2016) 24:240–50. doi: 10.1007/s12028-015-0196-8
34. Harutyunyan G, Hauer L, Dünser MW, Moser T, Pikija S, Leitinger M, et al. Risk factors for intensive care unit admission in patients with autoimmune encephalitis. *Front Immunol.* (2017) 8:835. doi: 10.3389/fimmu.2017.00835
35. Iizuka T, Sakai F, Ide T, Monzen T, Yoshii S, Iigaya M, et al. Anti-NMDA receptor encephalitis in Japan: long-term outcome without tumor removal. *Neurology.* (2008) 70:504–11. doi: 10.1212/01.wnl.0000278388.90370.c3
36. Lim JA, Lee ST, Jung KH, Kim S, Shin JW, Moon J, et al. Anti-N-methyl-D-aspartate receptor encephalitis in Korea: clinical features, treatment, and outcome. *J Clin Neurol.* (2014) 10:157–61. doi: 10.3988/jcn.2014.10.2.157
37. Balu R, McCracken L, Lancaster E, Graus F, Dalmau J, Titulaer MJ. A score that predicts 1-year functional status in patients with anti-NMDA receptor encephalitis. *Neurology.* (2019) 92:e244–52. doi: 10.1212/WNL.0000000000006783
38. Sai Y, Zhang X, Feng M, Tang J, Liau H, Tan L. Clinical diagnosis and treatment of pediatric anti-N-methyl-D-aspartate receptor encephalitis: a single-center retrospective study. *Ex Ther Med.* (2018) 16: 1442–8. doi: 10.3892/etm.2018.6329
39. Zekeridou A, Karantoni E, Viaccoz A, Ducray F, Gitiaux C, Villega F, et al. Treatment and outcome of children and adolescents with N-methyl-D-aspartate receptor encephalitis. *J Neurol.* (2015) 262:18592:185. doi: 10.1007/s00415-015-7781-9
40. Sakpichaisakul K, Patibat L, Wechapinan T, Sri-Udomkajrorn S, Apiwattanakul M, Suwannachote S. Heterogenous treatment for anti-NMDAR encephalitis in children leads to different outcomes 6–12 months after diagnosis. *J Neuroimmunol.* (2018) 324:119–25. doi: 10.1016/j.jneuroim.2018.09.007
41. de Bruijn MAAM, Aarsen FK, van Oosterhout MP, van der Knoop MM, Catsman-Berrevoets CE, Schreurs MWJ, et al. Long-term neuropsychological outcome following pediatric anti-NMDAR encephalitis. *Neurology.* (2018) 90:e1997–2005. doi: 10.1212/WNL.0000000000005605
42. Matricardi S, Patrini M, Freri E, Ragona F, Andreetta F, Narcoddi N, et al. Cognitive and neuropsychological evolution in children with anti-NMDAR encephalitis. *J Neurol.* (2016) 263:765–71. doi: 10.1007/s00415-016-8056-9
43. McKeon GL, Robinson GA, Ryan AE, Blum S, Gillis D, Finke C, et al. Cognitive outcomes following anti-N-methyl- D-aspartate receptor encephalitis: a systematic review. *J Clin Exp Neuropsychol.* (2018) 40:234–52. doi: 10.1080/13803395.2017.1329408
44. McKeon GL, Scott JG, Spooner DM, Ryan AE, Blum S, Gillis D. Cognitive and social functioning deficits after anti-N-methyl-D-aspartate receptor encephalitis: an exploratory case series. *J Int Neuropsychol Soc.* (2016) 22:828–38. doi: 10.1017/S1355617716000679

13

Childhood Emotional Abuse Moderates Associations Among Corticomotor White Matter Structure and Stress Neuromodulators in Women with and without Depression

*Carlton P. Frost[1], M. Elizabeth Meyerand[2,3], Rasmus M. Birn[1,2], Roxanne M. Hoks[1], Erin C. Walsh[4] and Heather C. Abercrombie[1]**

[1] Department of Psychiatry, University of Wisconsin-Madison, Madison, WI, United States, [2] Department of Medical Physics, University of Wisconsin-Madison, Madison, WI, United States, [3] Department of Biomedical Engineering, University of Wisconsin-Madison, Madison, WI, United States, [4] Department of Psychiatry, University of North Carolina at Chapel Hill, Chapel Hill, NC, United States

Correspondence:
Heather C. Abercrombie
heather.abercrombie@wisc.edu

Adverse caregiving during development can produce long-lasting changes to neural, endocrine, and behavioral responses to stress, and is strongly related to elevated risk of adult psychopathology. While prior experience of adversity is associated with altered sympathetic nervous system (SNS) and hypothalamic-pituitary-adrenal (HPA) axis activity, the underlying neural pathways are not completely understood. In a double-blind crossover study, we used diffusion tensor imaging (DTI) to examine whether variation in white matter structure predicts differences in HPA-SNS interactions as a function of early adversity. Participants included 74 women who exhibited a wide range of depression severity and/or childhood emotional abuse (EA). Participants attended two experimental sessions during which they were administered 20 mg cortisol (CORT) or placebo and after 90 min, viewed emotionally laden pictures while undergoing MRI scanning. Immediately after emotional picture-viewing, we collected salivary alpha-amylase (sAA) to index SNS activation. We tested whether EA moderated the relation between fractional anisotropy (FA), a measure of white matter fiber structure, and sAA. In the placebo condition, for participants with minimal history of EA, higher FA in corticomotor projections was negatively correlated with sAA, whereas in participants with severe EA, the correlation was trending in the opposite direction. Following CORT administration, FA and sAA were not related, suggesting that SNS tone during acute cortisol elevation may depend on neural pathways other than corticomotor projections. The results suggest that at baseline—though not during cortisol elevation—increased FA in these tracts is associated with lower levels of SNS activity in women with minimal EA, but not in women with severe EA. These findings provide evidence that corticomotor projections may be a key component of altered neural circuitry in adults with history of maltreatment, and may be related to alterations in stress neuromodulators in psychopathology.

Keywords: cortisol, sympathetic nervous system, hypothalamic pituitary adrenal axis, corticomotor system, emotional abuse, depression, diffusion tensor imaging, tract-based spatial statistics

INTRODUCTION

Experience of adverse caregiving in childhood is a risk factor for a variety of psychopathologies in adulthood, including major depressive disorder (MDD) and posttraumatic stress disorder (PTSD). Studies in both humans and animals show that responses to acute stress are shaped by the history of the organism (Pavlides et al., 2002; Alfarez et al., 2003; Ellis et al., 2005; Joëls and Krugers, 2007; Meewisse et al., 2007; Ehring et al., 2008). Prior adversity is at times associated with high sympathetic nervous system (SNS) response (featuring the systemic release of the catecholamine epinephrine in the medulla of the adrenal gland; Otte et al., 2005), and low hypothalamic-pituitary-adrenal (HPA) response (featuring systemic release of glucocorticoids [GCs], primarily cortisol in primates or corticosterone in rodents) to acute stress (Resnick et al., 1995; McFarlane et al., 1997; Walsh et al., 2013; Drury et al., 2016). Furthermore, it has been hypothesized that the balance between SNS and HPA responses to acute stressors is altered in individuals previously exposed to chronic and/or severe stress, so that cortisol signaling does not sufficiently contain the SNS response (Yehuda et al., 1998). The neural pathways supporting such alterations in peripheral stress physiology in individuals previously exposed to adversity are unknown.

Functional activity in a variety of brain regions and circuits, such as hippocampus, amygdala, and fronto-limbic circuitry, regulates and is modulated by stress neuromodulators such as catecholamines and GCs (Roozendaal et al., 2009; Ulrich-Lai and Herman, 2009; Hermans et al., 2014; Vogel et al., 2016). More recent research (Dum et al., 2016; Abercrombie et al., 2018) in humans and nonhuman primates has indicated a possible role for cortical premotor areas including supplementary motor area (SMA), cingulate motor areas (CMAs), and premotor cortex (PMC) in neural response to and control of stress neuromodulators. For instance, anatomical tracing in Cebus monkeys shows these areas project densely to spinal circuits innervating sympathetic preganglionic cells, which terminate in adrenal medulla, likely modulating peripheral SNS activation (Dum et al., 2016).

In addition, dorsomedial frontal cortical areas, which share substantial overlap with these premotor regions, are known substrates for GC modulation of neural activation and HPA tone (McEwen et al., 1986; Diorio et al., 1993; Radley et al., 2006). Such a pathway could constitute a potential interface by which trauma and adversity may give rise to altered HPA/SNS relationships. Indeed, numerous studies have found that patterns of dorsomedial prefrontal activation and connectivity during emotion regulation differ in individuals with history of maltreatment (McLaughlin et al., 2015; McCrory et al., 2017) and may also distinguish between individuals resilient to or at risk of psychopathology related to early adversity (Herringa, 2017).

To further elucidate the neural pathways by which adversity relates to alterations in stress response systems, we tested relations between measures of structural connectivity and SNS activation in a sample of women with varying history of childhood emotional abuse (EA) and psychopathology. We further tested how exogenous cortisol altered these relationships. The use of exogenous cortisol permits inferences about the effects of cortisol *per se*, rather than the effects of elevations in endogenous cortisol elicited by a potent, social-evaluative stressor (Dickerson and Kemeny, 2004). We pharmacologically manipulated cortisol (CORT) vs. placebo before participants viewed emotionally evocative pictures, and measured salivary alpha-amylase (sAA) following the task to index SNS activation. Alpha-amylase is an enzyme whose salivary concentration can be used as an index of SNS activity, such as when detecting autonomic dysregulation or treatment response (Nater and Rohleder, 2009). Brain structure was assessed using T1- and diffusion-weighted magnetic resonance imaging. Using functional magnetic resonance imaging (fMRI) in this sample, we previously reported that childhood EA moderated the effects of CORT on activation in SMA and adjacent premotor cortical areas, and that this activation was related to sAA, an index of sympathetic adrenal-medullary output. Because descending tracts such as corticospinal tract (CST) likely carry corticomotor axons en route to sympathetic preganglionic cells (Dum et al., 2016), we therefore hypothesized that CORT's effects on sAA would be related to their white matter structure, and that this relationship would be moderated by history of childhood EA.

MATERIALS AND METHODS

Participants

Participants were women aged 18–45 with varying depression severity and history of childhood EA. We did not specifically recruit women with anxiety disorders or PTSD, but these were not exclusionary (**Table 1**; full eligibility criteria in Supplementary Materials). Of 85 eligible participants, 80 completed the study and full data were available for 75. Data was lost to experimenter error (1 participant), scanner malfunction (1 participant), poor image quality (2 participants), and a medical condition (1 participant), and 1 participant was excluded as an extreme outlier during data analysis (see next section), bringing the final N to 74. The study protocol was approved by the University of Wisconsin Health Sciences IRB. Participants provided written informed consent and were paid for participation.

Measuring Childhood EA and Depression Severity

Childhood EA was retrospectively assessed using the Emotional Abuse subscale of the Childhood Trauma Questionnaire (CTQ), a well-validated instrument that can be used to measure aversive caregiving continuously or by categorizing participants into groups using standard cut scores (Bernstein et al., 2003). In the final sample, 14 women experienced moderate-to-extreme ("severe"), 14 experienced low-to-moderate ("moderate"), and 46 experienced none-to-minimal ("minimal") childhood EA. Timing of EA was assessed using a life history calendar (Caspi et al., 1996), which confirmed that all women endorsing EA experienced abuse prior to menarche, and many experienced ongoing EA from early childhood through adolescence.

Consistent with the NIMH Research Doman Criteria (RDoC) framework (Insel, 2014), which emphasizes the continuous nature of psychiatric disorders, we recruited women with a range of depression, anxiety, and PTSD severity. Psychopathology was assessed using the SCID-I/P for DSM-IV-TR with additional questions to assess DSM-5 criteria (First et al., 2002). Some participants experienced clinically significant anxiety (36%) and PTSD (12%); these disorders were comorbid with depression, for which we specifically recruited and which was more prevalent in our sample (61% lifetime, 43% current; **Table 1**). Depression severity was indexed using the average of Beck Depression Inventory-II (BDI-II) scores across two experimental sessions (Beck et al., 1996). A square-root transformation was applied to reduce negative skew and undue influence of extreme BDI-II scores as in prior research (van Minnen et al., 2005; Roelofs et al., 2013). In scatter plots, scores are back-transformed to preserve initial range.

Although we sought to recruit a sample in which EA and depressive symptoms were not entirely overlapping (**Table 1**), EA was nevertheless strongly associated with adult depression: the correlation in this sample is $r_{(73)} = 0.45$, $p < 0.01$. One participant's scores on the BDI-II and EA subscale of the CTQ were 0 and 25, which are respectively the lowest and highest possible scores. These values exerted extreme and anomalous influence on results: standardized residuals > 2, Cook's distance > 4 times mean, leverage >> $2p/n$, thus meeting criteria for outlier identification proposed by Rawlings et al. (1998). This was the only participant in the sample who concurrently reported extreme EA and no depressive symptomatology. Thus, this participant skewed statistical distributions and was ultimately classified as an outlier and excluded from analysis. For discussion, see Limitations Section.

TABLE 1 | Demographic and clinical characteristics.

Characteristics	CTQ emotional abuse groups		
	Minimal ($n = 46$)	Moderate ($n = 14$)	Severe ($n = 14$)
Age, years[a]	26.1 ± 6.4	31.4 ± 7.1	28.1 ± 8.0
Lifetime depressive disorder	23 (50.0)	9 (64.3)	13 (92.9)
Current depressive disorder	12 (26.1)	7 (50.0)	13 (92.9)
Current anxiety disorder	12 (26.1)	6 (42.9)	9 (64.3)
Current PTSD	0	3 (21.4)	6 (42.9)
Race[b,c]			
White	34 (73.9)	9 (64.3)	12 (85.7)
Asian	8 (17.4)	3 (21.4)	2 (14.2)
African American	3 (6.5)	1 (7.1)	0
Unknown	1 (2.2)	1 (7.1)	0
Ethnicity[b]			
Hispanic/Latina	4 (8.7)	2 (14.3)	0
Not Hispanic/Latina	42 (91.3)	11 (78.6)	14 (100)
Unknown	0	1 (7.1)	0
Education level[d]	4.4 ± 1.4	5.2 ± 1.1	4.9 ± 1.3
Childhood caregivers' education level[d]	4.5 ± 1.7	4.9 ± 1.2	5.1 ± 1.7

Values are mean ± SD, or n (groupwise %). CTQ, Childhood Trauma Questionnaire; PTSD, posttraumatic stress disorder.

[a]*There was a small but significant group difference in age, $F_{(2,73)} = 3.25$, $p = 0.04$.*

[b]*Chi-squared tests confirmed the CTQ Emotional Abuse groups did not significantly differ by racial or ethnic composition, p's > 0.34.*

[c]*Because of rounding, percentages may not total 100.*

[d]*Education categories: 1, Less than high school; 2, High school diploma or equivalent (i.e., GED); 3, Some college, no degree; 4, Associate's degree; 5, Bachelor's degree; 6, Master's degree; 7, Doctoral degree.*

Procedure

Cortisol levels were manipulated by administering 20 mg oral hydrocortisone (i.e., exogenous cortisol; CORT). In a separate experimental session, participants were given an identically appearing placebo capsule. The CORT and placebo sessions were conducted in the late afternoon into the evening (beginning at 4:15 PM) and were typically separated by 1 week (minimum of 5 days). The order of drug administration was randomized and double-blinded. Neuroimaging (diffusion tensor imaging [DTI] and fMRI) was conducted during both visits. fMRI data are described elsewhere (Abercrombie et al., 2018).

SNS Activation During CORT vs. Placebo

To index SNS activation in the context of an emotionally evocative experience, sAA was measured immediately after participants completed an emotional picture viewing task, which occurred 90 min after drug administration during fMRI (**Figure 1**). Participants viewed one of two sets of psychometrically matched pictures from the International Affective Picture System (IAPS; Lang et al., 2008) during each session.

For measurement of sAA and salivary cortisol levels, saliva samples were collected from participants throughout each session with Salivettes (Sarstedt, Nümbrecht, Germany), according to previously-described guidelines (Rohleder and Nater, 2009).

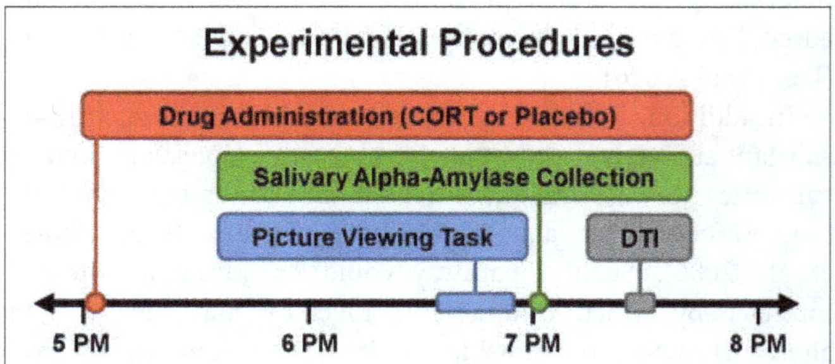

FIGURE 1 | Timing of experimental procedures. Study participation entailed two experimental sessions, which were typically separated by 1 week (minimum of 5 days). All experimental sessions were conducted late in the day (beginning at 4:15 PM) when endogenous cortisol levels are relatively low. Drug (20 mg oral hydrocortisone [CORT] or placebo) was administered slightly after 5PM. Order of drug administration across the two sessions was randomized and double-blinded. Approximately 90 min after drug administration, participants viewed emotional pictures during fMRI (described elsewhere; Abercrombie et al., 2018). Salivary alpha-amylase (sAA) was collected immediately after the emotional picture viewing task to index sympathetic nervous system (SNS) activity during CORT vs. placebo. Diffusion tensor imaging (DTI) was conducted to assess white matter structure.

sAA concentrations were assayed with an enzyme kinetic method (e.g., Bosch et al., 2003). Intra- and inter-assay coefficients of variation were below 11%. Cortisol concentrations were measured with a high sensitivity chemiluminescence immunoassay (IBL International, Hamburg, Germany; intra- and inter-assay coefficients of variation below 8%) to confirm that post-drug administration cortisol levels did not vary by group (see **Table 2**). Log-transformation was used to normalize distributions for sAA and salivary cortisol (Rohleder and Nater, 2009).

Image Collection and Preprocessing

Brain images were collected using a 3T General Electric MRI scanner (Discovery MR750; GE Medical Systems, Waukesha, WI) equipped with an 8 channel RF coil (GE Healthcare, Waukesha, WI). Structural data were acquired using a T1-weighted BRAVO pulse sequence (TI:450 ms, TR/TE/flip:8.16 ms/3.2 ms/12°, matrix:256 × 256 × 160, FOV:215.6 mm, slice thickness:1 mm). Diffusion-weighted data were acquired using a 2D echo planar imaging (EPI) sequence with ASSET parallel imaging at a geometric reduction factor of 2 in order to correct magnetic field inhomogeneities (TR/TE/flip:8,000 ms/66.2 ms/90°, matrix:128 × 128 × 76, FOV:256 mm, slice thickness:2 mm). Each axial slice was encoded with 48 directions, $b = 1,000$ s/mm^2, and eight b0 images. Field maps to correct for magnetic field distortions were also collected. Images were corrected for eddy current and fieldmap distortions, and skull-stripped (FMRIB Software Library, FSL; Smith et al., 2004). Images from the first scan session were used for analysis. Tensors were fitted with nonlinear optimization, constrained to be positive semi-definite using Camino (camino.cs.ucl.ac.uk; Cook et al., 2006). Tensor images were normalized, and scalar maps for fractional anisotropy (FA) and axial, radial, and mean diffusivity were calculated, using Diffusion Tensor Imaging ToolKit (DTI-TK, dti-tk.sourceforge.net).

To create seed regions with which to virtually dissect tracts of interest, T1 images were processed using FreeSurfer's automatic recon-all pipeline including preprocessing steps (motion correction, intensity normalization, affine registration to Talairach atlas, brain extraction), linear registration to a Gaussian classifier array for automatic subcortical segmentation (v5.3, https://surfer.nmr.mgh.harvard.edu; Fischl et al., 2002), and estimation and parcellation of cortical surfaces into functional and anatomical compartments (Desikan et al., 2006; Destrieux et al., 2010).

TABLE 2 | Salivary analytes by childhood emotional abuse (EA) severity and drug.

Measure	CTQ emotional abuse groups		
	Minima ($n = 46$)	Moderate ($n = 14$)	Severe ($n = 14$)
sAA LEVELS, U/mL			
Placebo	191.8 ± 155.9	172.9 ± 155.6	236.6 ± 193.8
CORT	166.0 ± 115.1	221.7 ± 225.9	187.4 ± 134.1
SALIVARY CORTISOL LEVELS, nmol/L			
Placebo	1.3 ± 1.6	1.7 ± 2.1	1.3 ± 0.7
CORT	55.4 ± 33.6	54.2 ± 32.7	50.6 ± 41.9

Values are mean ± SD. CORT, cortisol administration; CTQ, Childhood Trauma Questionnaire; sAA, salivary alpha-amylase.
Raw values for sAA and cortisol are shown in the table. Log-transformed values were used for analyses to normalize distributions. Neither sAA nor cortisol showed main effects or interaction for Drug (Placebo vs. CORT) or CTQ Emotional Abuse (EA), p's > 0.33.

Data Analysis

CORT's Effects on SNS Activation in Relation to EA

Proc GLM in SAS (SAS version 9.4, Cary, NC) was used to test (1) whether there was a main effect of Drug (CORT vs. Placebo) on sAA, and (2) whether effects of Drug on sAA differed with respect to EA. Analyses were conducted on log-transformed (i.e., normalized) values of sAA.

DTI

Tract-based spatial statistics (TBSS).

Individual subject maps were co-registered to a bootstrapped group template, and warps to that template were computed, by implementing DTI-TK (Zhang et al., 2007) using a custom tool (Diffusion Image Processing and Analysis, DIPA; github.com/pegasus-isi/dipa-workflow) implemented through Condor, developed by the Center for High Throughput Computing at the University of Wisconsin-Madison & Wisconsin Institutes for Discovery (chtc.cs.wisc.edu). Whole-brain, voxelwise statistical analysis of white matter structure was carried out using the TBSS method in FSL, which entails the creation of a white matter skeleton along which each subject's projected data are then analyzed (Smith et al., 2006).

To elucidate the relationship of childhood EA and adult white matter structure, general linear models were constructed accounting for age as a nuisance regressor and for depression severity, and were entered into FSL's Randomize program. Randomize performs nonparametric permutation to allow inference on data whose null distribution is not known (Winkler et al., 2014). Family-wise error rates were corrected using threshold-free cluster enhancement, which assigns voxel-wise values based on cluster-like local spatial agreement (Smith and Nichols, 2009). Next, we tested whether EA moderated the relationship between white matter structure (FA) and effects of CORT (vs. Placebo) on sAA. The difference in sAA between the CORT and Placebo days ($sAA_{CORT-Placebo}$) therefore represented our experimental variable, and an interaction term specified whether EA moderated these effects. To confirm that depression severity did not also moderate the relationship between $sAA_{CORT-Placebo}$ and FA, a model correcting for age and including terms for BDI, $sAA_{CORT-Placebo}$, and their interaction was also entered into Randomize.

Once clusters of interest were identified, they were warped from template space to participant space and mean FA values over the cluster were extracted from corresponding regions in each participant. For *post hoc* analyses, these FA values were entered into ANCOVA using SAS to characterize the relations between FA and sAA, and differences in these relations across EA groups.

Deterministic tractography

TBSS-derived clusters often include fiber bundles from multiple tracts of interest, which may be disambiguated to aid in interpreting their functional significance. To anatomically validate the affected tracts, deterministic tractography was performed in subjects' native space using Camino and visualized in TrackVis (trackvis.org; Wang et al., 2007). Significant voxels were used as seeds for streamline tractography using the fiber assignment by continuous tracking (FACT) algorithm. Streamlines were terminated at voxels with FA values less than 0.1 or when local curvature exceeded 60°. Among streamlines passing through the significant white matter clusters, tract membership was determined using anatomical landmarks and subject-specific segmentation-derived seed regions from FreeSurfer, as described in the Results. In general, when referring to "clusters," we mean voxels found significant in the TBSS model; by "tracts" we mean those a priori, anatomically-identifiable tracts whose streamlines were found to pass through the clusters of interest.

RESULTS

Participants Could Not Distinguish Between Drug Conditions

Consistent with prior research (Abercrombie et al., 2005, 2011; Wirth et al., 2011), participants did not perform above chance in distinguishing between CORT and Placebo conditions: when asked on each of the first and second visits what they thought had been administered, 60 and 67% of participants said they did not know, respectively, and of those that guessed, accuracies were 52 and 38%, *p*'s > 0.05.

Effects of CORT on SNS Activation

No main effect of Drug (CORT vs. Placebo) on sAA was observed, $F_{(1,74)} = 0.09$, $p = 0.76$ (**Table 2**). In addition, sAA level was not related to EA in either the Placebo or CORT condition or its interaction with Drug, *p*'s > 0.18. sAA was also not related to depression or its interaction with Drug, *p*'s > 0.59.

SNS Activation and White Matter Structure

TBSS-derived clusters of interest shown in **Figures 2** and **3**, and **Table 3** represent regions in which FA was significantly associated with EA, $sAA_{CORT-Placebo}$, or their interaction. Clusters associated with the interaction were centered in bilateral white matter tracts ventral to motor and premotor cortices at the level of the centrum semiovale (**Figure 3A**), at the intersection of the CST, corpus callosum (CC), thalamic radiations/corona radiata (CR), and inferior fronto-occipital fasciculus (IFOF). Corticomotor projections were identified as intersecting at least one of precentral, paracentral, caudal middle frontal, superior frontal, posterior cingulate or caudal anterior cingulate gyri, and reaching spinal cord. In addition, we adapted landmarks from prior studies (e.g., Bleyenheuft et al., 2007) to identify fibers belonging to CST proper (Figure S1). IFOF fibers terminated anteriorly in precentral, inferior or middle frontal gyri and posteriorly in parietal or superior temporal areas. CR terminated in thalamus.

The relation between tractographic "streamline" count and anatomical fiber count is highly conditional, and should be understood as a qualitative rather than quantitative tool (Jones et al., 2013b), but may offer a very coarse measure of comparative connectivity. In all participants examined, a large quantity of streamlines belonging to CST and other motor cortical projections to spinal cord were readily identified, of which the overwhelming majority traversed the cluster of interest. Approximately half or fewer of those streamlines belonging to IFOF did so, and those that did were generally limited to the tract's superior extent (i.e., terminating in superior parietal areas). CR terminating in thalamus varied in cluster membership.

Posthoc analyses were conducted to disentangle the significant TBSS interaction. Using mean cluster FA, we found that the correlation between $sAA_{CORT-Placebo}$ and FA differed across EA groups, $F_{(6, 74)} = 3.90$, $p < 0.01$, $R^2 = 0.26$. This effect was driven by Placebo-day differences in slope, $F_{(6, 74)} = 3.02$, $p = 0.01$, $R^2 = 0.21$ (**Figure 3C**), such that for women with minimal childhood EA, post-task sAA levels were negatively associated with higher cluster FA ($r = -0.30$, $p = 0.02$), but for women with history of severe EA the association was positive though did not reach significance ($r = 0.37$, $p = 0.20$). Cluster FA was unrelated to CORT-day sAA and its interaction with EA, *p*'s > 0.19 (**Table 3**). Further investigation showed that effects were mainly driven by opposing group-wise relations between sAA and radial diffusivity; axial and mean diffusivity were unrelated to sAA and EA.

FA was associated with depression severity in a cluster localized to the anterior CC (Table S1, Figure S2), but was not associated with sAA or the interaction between depression severity and sAA.

DISCUSSION

Consistent with our hypothesis, we found that the structural properties of bilateral corticomotor projections were related to SNS activation following exposure to emotional stimuli. Specifically, we found that the relation of corticomotor FA to SNS activation differed among women with history of severe childhood emotional abuse vs. those without, and CORT administration eliminated these differences. Depression severity did not moderate these effects. These findings provide evidence that these corticomotor projections may constitute an important pathway underlying alterations in stress neuromodulators in individuals with a history of abuse.

Differences in FA Are Likely Driven by Corticomotor Projections

Streamlines belonging to a variety of tracts traversed the clusters extracted from the TBSS analysis. Although tractography cannot definitively confirm or exclude the contribution of individual tracts to detectable FA effects, it can aid in interpreting likely drivers. In all participants examined, the most reliable corticofugal projections linked brainstem and spinal cord to

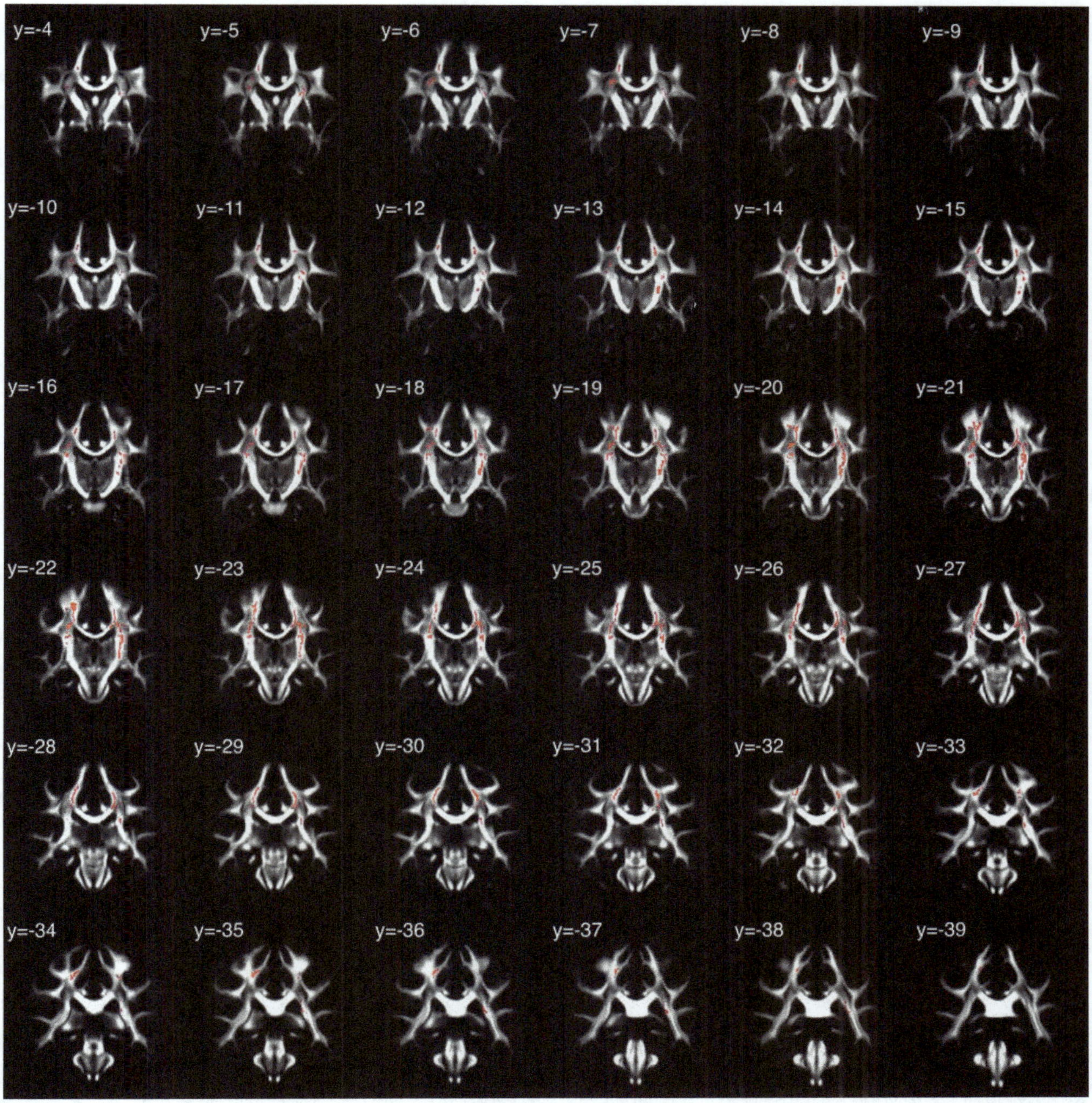

FIGURE 2 | Clusters in which the relation between fractional anisotropy (FA) and salivary alpha-amylase (sAA) was moderated by childhood emotional abuse (EA). Coronal slices are presented in montage, beginning with $y = -4$ in MNI space, radiological orientation (i.e., participants' right is on viewer's left).

sensorimotor areas (Figure S3). Using anatomical landmarks to positively identify its descending course, CST streamlines were identified as traversing the clusters of interest more reliably and in greater proportion than other tracts: of streamlines belonging to CST, over 90% were identified in multiple participants. Most such streamlines appeared to terminate on the dorsal surface of precentral and superior frontal gyri, although precise departures of fibers from a larger tract can be difficult to resolve (e.g., Jones et al., 2013a). Other premotor and sensorimotor projections reaching spinal cord showed similarly high rates of capture by our clusters.

Although a majority of streamlines of the mid-to-posterior CC traversed the clusters, the structure's interhemispheric extent—one of the most robust and undiluted white matter tracts in the brain—did not reach significance, and bilaterally the significant clusters extend well inferior to the main CC projections. This suggests that interhemispheric connectivity, while possibly involved, likely is not the principal driver our effects.

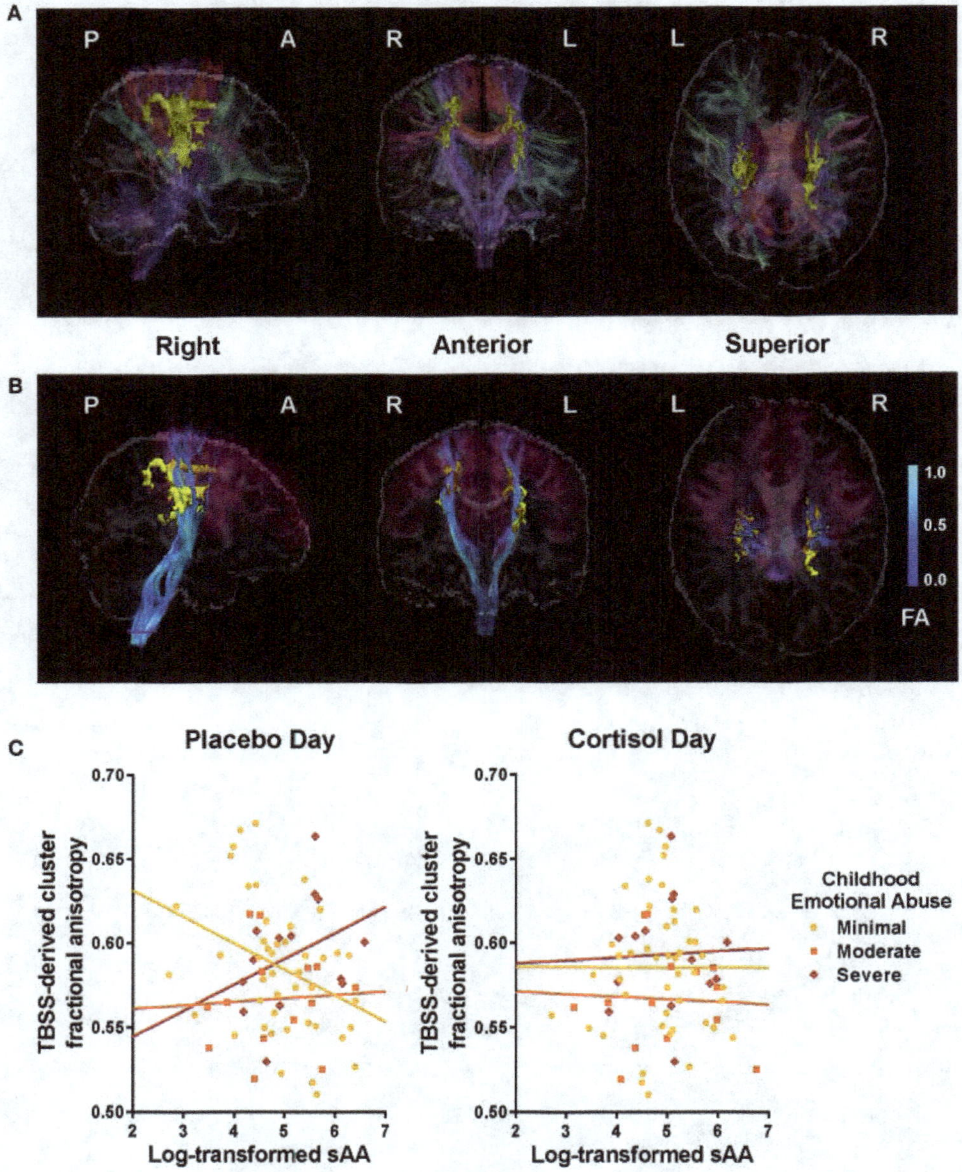

FIGURE 3 | Clusters and tracts in which the relation between fractional anisotropy (FA) and salivary alpha-amylase (sAA) was moderated by childhood emotional abuse (EA). **(A)** Tract-based spatial statistics (TBSS)-derived clusters (yellow) significantly associated with EA × $sAA_{CORT-Placebo}$ interaction, illustrated with a representative participant, and fiber tracts intersecting clusters (color indicates direction at fiber midpoint: red fibers run primarily left-right, green anterior-posterior, blue superior-inferior). See **Table 3** for listing of significant clusters. **(B)** Projection fibers (blue) originating from corticomotor regions (magenta, derived from FreeSurfer segmentation: precentral gyrus, paracentral gyrus, posterior & caudal anterior cingulate gyrus & sulcus, superior frontal gyrus, and caudal middle frontal gyrus), passing through TBSS-derived cluster (yellow), and reaching spinal cord (purple) after virtual dissection using FreeSurfer segmentation. Brighter blue indicates higher FA. **(C)** Scatter plots for sAA and cluster FA, plotted by EA. At left, Placebo-day correlations; at right, CORT-day correlations. EA moderated the association between cluster FA and sAA levels during placebo administration but not during CORT, $F_{(6,74)} = 3.90$, $p < 0.01$.

A variable proportion, typically half or fewer, of IFOF streamlines intersected the clusters, and those generally in dorsal parietal areas, in contrast to more ventral tracts such as those identified in Rodrigo et al. (2016). However, future research can aid in disentangling the possibility of crossing-fiber effects; see following section.

From a theoretical standpoint, corticomotor projections were a hypothesized structure of interest. As described in Abercrombie et al. (2018), CORT increased activation in SMA/PMC and rescued depression-related deficits in memory formation for positive stimuli in severely maltreated women. On CORT day both sAA and rescue effects were significantly related to activation in these areas. No cortical regions innervated by IFOF fibers showed this group x drug interaction. And insofar as corticomotor and adrenal activity are related, projections via CST and other descending circuits would represent a parsimonious route.

TABLE 3 | Childhood emotional abuse (EA), salivary alpha-amylase (sAA), and fractional anisotropy (FA).

Cluster	Volume (voxels)	Coordinate (peak)	Coordinate (CM)	T-Stat (peak)	P-value (corrected)
EA					
None	–	–	–	–	–
$sAA_{CORT-Placebo}$					
Left corticofugal tracts	2,373	(−28,−3,4)	(−23,−4,13)	3.74	0.01
Right corticofugal tracts	2,136	(20,−3,34)	(22,−4,15)	4.14	0.01
Left mid superior CC	114	(−18,20,27)	(−17,22,16)	3.33	0.05
Left centrum semiovale	17	(−27,4,27)	(−27,4,27)	3.71	0.05
Left superior CR	13	(−24,21,16)	(−24,21,16)	3.34	0.05
EA * $sAA_{CORT-Placebo}$					
Left corticomotor tracts	1,341	(−28,−3,4)	(−25,−4,17)	3.56	0.02
Right corticomotor tracts	1,307	(18,−3,34)	(21,−5,24)	4.22	0.03

CM, center of mass; CC, corpus callosum; CR, corona radiata; EA, Emotional Abuse subscale of the Childhood Trauma Questionnaire; $sAA_{CORT-Placebo}$, the difference in salivary alpha-amylase between the CORT and Placebo days.
Significant clusters associated with model factors.

Possible Sources of Biological Variation in Corticomotor Projection Tract Structure

Although the precise changes in axonal microstructure or fiber architecture cannot be resolved by FA (Jones et al., 2013b), interpretation depends at least in part on whether effects represent disrupted signaling or some other change in circuit function. Recently-published research (Mortazavi et al., 2018) suggests a possible, if highly speculative, mechanism to explain these effects. Histology of macaque CST found that, contrary to following smooth contours, many axons at the level of the centrum semiovale executed "microscopically sharp axonal turns and/or branches (radii $\leq$ 15 mm) into 2 sharply defined orientations, mediolateral and dorsoventral." Further, high-angle diffusion MRI, which is capable of resolving crossing fiber orientation, was unable to distinguish between crossing fibers and sharp axonal turns.

The influence of intra-voxel discrepancy in fiber orientation on FA is thought to be large, relative to that of axonal physiology (Jones et al., 2013b). It is therefore conceivable that small variations in the proportion of descending fibers deflecting to mediolateral targets in this span of CST could yield statistically detectable changes in FA, even if restricted to a small population of axons bound for spinal circuits innervating sympathetic preganglionic cells. This would also be consistent with the fact that our FA effects were driven by changes in radial, rather than axial, diffusivity. Given the novelty of the above findings, further studies in animal models—which offer the additional advantage of well-characterized adverse caregiving paradigms—may serve to test the generalizability of our results, and fully elucidate any biological source of our structural findings.

EA Moderated Associations Between Cluster FA and sAA

Under placebo, i.e., during basal levels of cortisol, the relation between SNS activation and bilateral corticomotor tract FA depended on severity of EA. Among participants with minimal history of childhood EA, FA was negatively associated with sAA, indicating that women with greater corticomotor white matter FA showed relatively lower SNS activation. For individuals with severe EA, however, results trended in the opposite direction such that higher white matter FA was weakly associated with relatively higher SNS activation.

These findings at baseline are interesting in light of recent nonhuman primate tracing studies indicating that spinal circuits influencing adrenal medulla are likely innervated by fibers from cortical motor areas (Dum et al., 2016). SMA was already known to be robustly associated with SNS tone and autonomic function (Medford and Critchley, 2010), consistent with its classical role preparing for strenuous action involving core musculature (Graziano, 2006); spinal projections therefore constitute a previously unknown, but logical, pathway with respect to modulation of peripheral stress-related activation. Previous analyses from this sample (Abercrombie et al., 2018), as well as other studies, have found functional alterations to SMA and adjacent premotor areas in individuals with history of maltreatment, especially in paradigms related to emotion regulation and executive control (for review, cf. McCrory et al., 2017). These alterations may also distinguish between individuals resilient to or at risk of psychopathology related to early adversity (Herringa, 2017). Taken together, one speculative interpretation might hold that history of exposure to EA alters the function of these areas and their projections to the SNS.

SMA and adjacent premotor areas, including dorsal cingulate, are known to integrate cognitive and affective inputs in motor planning (Picard and Strick, 2001; Shackman et al., 2011) along a continuous functional and physiological gradient: from anterior to posterior, cognitive processing converges on motor planning, and density of spinal cord-bound projections to adrenal medulla increase (Nakamura et al., 1998; Dum and Strick, 2002; Morecraft and Tanji, 2009). These systems appear to coordinate response selection and inhibition under complex, uncertain, and/or emotionally salient conditions (Nachev et al., 2008; McRae et al., 2010). However, despite their documentation in research concerning motor and some cognitive function, nomenclature for these areas varies in the emotion research discipline—perhaps due in part to limitations on spatial fidelity and resolution in functional imaging, or to challenges specific to more commonly-studied prefrontal association cortices. Study coordinates or clusters that overlap with preSMA, SMA, anterior PMC and other areas may be described using only directional or topographic terms: dorsomedial prefrontal cortex, superior frontal gyrus, dorsal anterior- or mid-cingulate, etc., whose boundaries may be defined differently across studies (see reviews: Ray and Zald, 2012; McCrory et al., 2017). It is possible that they may therefore play an under-recognized role linking emotion to behavior, particularly in the context of stress.

Furthermore, SMA in particular appears to facilitate voluntary emotion regulation (Buhle et al., 2014), alterations to which are considered a link between EA and risk of psychopathology (O'Mahen et al., 2015). Animal evidence for the role of these premotor circuits in inhibiting automatic and enabling intentional responses includes microstimulation of preSMA neurons (Isoda and Hikosaka, 2007), and macrostimulation in humans produces similar effects (Swann et al., 2012). A rodent paradigm found altered connectivity patterns in prefrontal and motor areas in female rats subjected to chronic social stress as pups (Nephew et al., 2017, 2018). Silvers et al. (2017) found that as typically-developing children reach adulthood, reactivity to aversive relative to neutral stimuli shifted from ventromedial (vmPFC) to dorsomedial prefrontal cortex (dmPFC), including preSMA, whereas Herringa and colleagues (Keding and Herringa, 2016; Wolf and Herringa, 2016) found a reverse profile of activation and limbic connectivity in children suffering from PTSD. In addition to SMA function, there is some independent evidence that CST structure is itself related to strategic aspects of emotional intelligence (Pisner et al., 2017).

That these systems should vary by exposure to early life adversity may represent divergent calibration of the neural circuitry supporting emotion regulation for vastly different environmental demands. Indeed, in a review of studies in EA populations, McCrory et al. (2017) found maltreatment-related effects on emotion regulation may persist in the absence of overt psychopathology, and suggest neural responses that are adaptive in an adverse caregiving environment confer "latent vulnerability" in adulthood. Other authors have converged on similar frameworks (e.g., Del Giudice et al., 2011; Blair and Raver, 2012; Teicher and Samson, 2013).

CORT Eliminated Effects of EA on Relations Between Cluster FA and sAA

While EA moderated the relation of corticomotor tract FA and SNS activation under baseline conditions, CORT administration eliminated these associations. Following acute cortisol elevation SNS tone may depend on neural pathways other than corticomotor projections. There is a relative dearth of studies directly examining effects of GCs on neural control of SNS; however, GCs affect a variety of structures that regulate SNS output, including the hypothalamus, amygdala, and bed nucleus of the stria terminalis (Ulrich-Lai and Herman, 2009). Research in rodents implicates amydalofugal pathways during GC elevation: whereas GCs exert negative feedback on the HPA axis in hypothalamus and cortical areas, they increase CRH in the amygdala. This affects fear-related behaviors associated with SNS activity, such as startle (Erickson et al., 2003). Indeed, a study (Song et al., 2014) specifically examining FA in tracts connecting to brainstem nuclei found depression-related alterations not in CST, but in the solitary tract, which is known to reciprocally connect to amygdala; however, they did not report on alterations due to EA. Future research is needed to determine the neural circuitry through which GCs interact with SNS function, and how circuits are affected by EA. This is relevant as evidence suggests that in some disorders, such as PTSD, there are alterations in the relation between GCs and SNS (Yehuda et al., 1998).

Implications for Etiology and Treatment of Stress-Related Psychopathology

Our findings lend further evidence to a large body of literature showing that history of maltreatment is an important etiological factor in depression and other forms of psychopathology, which has bearing on treatment selection (Nemeroff et al., 2003; Williams et al., 2016). Furthermore, early adversity alters stress response systems, and alterations in cortisol signaling and HPA regulation are more often observed in depressed adults with vs. without history of childhood adversity (Heim et al., 2008; Abercrombie et al., 2018). The current findings extend upon these literatures by implicating corticomotor projections as part of a stress responsive neural circuit whose functioning is associated with variation in early caregiving.

These premotor areas and their influence on SNS function may represent an important target for clinical intervention. In addition to their involvement in emotion regulation—an important buffer to psychopathology, as discussed in the section above, "EA moderated associations between cluster FA and sAA"—recruitment in medial premotor areas may play a compensatory role in individuals with maltreatment and/or psychiatric disorders according to several lines of evidence, including a meta-analysis (Herringa et al., 2016; McTeague et al., 2017). Corticomotor projections influencing SNS could comprise a neural circuit important for psychotherapeutic benefit in individuals with history of adverse caregiving.

This circuit may therefore be an important target for behavioral, pharmacological, or neuromodulatory interventions. It could play a role in effective treatments such as behavioral activation (Dimidjian et al., 2011; Ekers et al., 2014), aerobic exercise (Rebar et al., 2015; Schuch et al., 2016), or yoga (Pascoe and Bauer, 2015; Cramer et al., 2017). Our prior research may also suggest that interventions targeting cortisol signaling could operate in part through activation of SMA and PMC (Abercrombie et al., 2018). Repetitive Transcranial Magnetic Stimulation (rTMS) to dmPFC reduced depression severity (Downar et al., 2014), although this was applied to an area anterior to preSMA, was effective specifically in patients with lower anhedonia symptomatology, and initial replication efforts have not been successful (Bakker et al., 2015). Gutman et al. (2009) performed probabilistic structural connectivity for a target of deep brain stimulation (DBS) previously found effective in treating depression, located in the anterior limb of the internal capsule (IC), and its connectivity patterns bear some superficial resemblance to those of our TBSS-derived cluster, although of course anterior to our cluster intersecting the posterior limb of IC. Though evidence is mixed, cortical motor circuits may represent targets for psychiatric treatment with neuromodulation, possibly in combination with context-specific cognitive therapy related to emotion regulation. Based on findings suggesting that functioning within these circuits is related to early experience, effectiveness of such treatments may vary based on history of childhood adversity.

As mentioned previously, a "mismatch" may arise between phenotype—which developed in response to a stressful early environment—and post-developmental context, that increases risk of depression or other psychopathology. Progress in understanding how to re-align phenotype and environmental demands may improve the specificity of treatments beyond that achieved by accounting for early experience alone.

Limitations

As this is a cross-sectional study, we are unable to draw firm conclusions as to how childhood EA altered developmental trajectories leading to adult differences in brain structure and stress neuromodulator function. In both the current analyses and in fMRI analyses in the same sample (Abercrombie et al., 2018), we found that EA but not depression severity was associated with neural alterations. However, due to the relatively low rate of PTSD in this sample, we are unable to examine neural correlates related to PTSD.

Another limitation of our study is that we were not able to recruit a sample of adults who experienced extreme EA but who do not exhibit psychopathology, and for statistical reasons we needed to exclude a single participant who presented with extreme EA but no depressive symptoms. Future research should endeavor to include such participants with targeted recruiting to allow investigation of the role of EA in stress-related physiology along a full range of severity of psychopathology.

In addition, emerging methods for disambiguating crossing fibers may aid in establishing the exact contributions of each tract captured by our clusters of interest. Further study comparing these methods against histological studies are vital for interpretation. Finally, the present study investigates the effects of exogenous cortisol; future research must also elucidate the impact of naturalistic environmental stressors on relations among white matter structure, cortisol, and SNS activation.

CONCLUSION

We found that history of emotional abuse—but not severity of depression—moderated relations among corticomotor white matter structure and SNS activation in a sample of women with levels of depression along a broad continuum of severity. The findings may suggest that such pathways supporting neural influence on SNS activity vary based on prior experience of adverse caregiving. Furthermore, cortisol administration abolished these associations, consistent with evidence that cortisol acutely alters neural systems supporting the regulation of peripheral stress physiology.

Functional systems-based approaches to the etiology of mental disorders (Insel, 2014) offer insights into biological mechanisms that may be affected by life history, and which can be targeted for clinical applications. Disruptions to both SNS and HPA responses to stress are candidate systems in stress-related disorders such as depression and PTSD. Cortical motor systems and their efferent fibers, whose outputs appear to ultimately modulate adrenal medulla (Dum et al., 2016), may represent a neural circuit affecting alterations in stress response systems. Future studies should further characterize the action of this pathway under different neural, endocrine, and cognitive conditions, and test whether such action differs according to exposure to adverse caregiving and other forms of early life adversity.

AUTHOR CONTRIBUTIONS

HA designed the study and obtained funding. HA, EW, RH, and RB refined the design and implemented the study. EW and RH programmed the picture viewing task. EW and RB programmed scan parameters. EW, RH, CF, and HA collected data. EW and RH organized and cleaned data. EW, CF, and HA analyzed data. CF processed and analyzed neuroimaging data in consultation with RB, MM, and HA. CF wrote the first draft of the manuscript in consultation with MM and HA. HA wrote sections of the manuscript. CF, RH, and HA composed figures and tables. All authors read and approved the manuscript.

FUNDING

This research was funded by grants to HA from the National Institute of Mental Health (R01MH094478) and the University of Wisconsin-Madison Office of the Vice Chancellor for Research and Graduate Education with funding from the Wisconsin Alumni Research Foundation; a Training Program in Emotion Research grant (5T32MH018931-25, PI: Richard J. Davidson) and a Dissertation Completion Fellowship to CF; and a NCCIH grant (T32AT003378) to EW. Data were collected with the assistance of the ICTR Mobile Research Team, which is supported by the Clinical and Translational Science Award (CTSA) program through the NIH National Center for Advancing Translational Sciences (NCATS), grant UL1TR000427. The content is solely the responsibility of the authors and does not necessarily represent the official views of the NIH. The NIH had no further role in study design; in the collection, analysis, and interpretation of the data; in the writing of the report; or in the decision to submit the article for publication.

ACKNOWLEDGMENTS

We thank all of the volunteers who participated in this study, as well as A. Blumenfeld, C. Siwik, M. Dennison, A. Ehlers, C. Ernstoff, S. Goldberg, M. Kalambokidis, A. Lang, J. Nelson,

E. Osterbauer, R. Svoboda, R. Vohnoutka, A. Winter, Lane Neuroimaging Laboratory staff, and ICTR Mobile Research Team for assistance with data collection. We thank Stacey M. Schaefer, Christine Heim, Marilyn J. Essex, Ned H. Kalin, and Richard J. Davidson for consultation and advice. We thank Clemens Kirschbaum's laboratory for conducting salivary cortisol and alpha-amylase assays. We thank Do Tromp, Nagesh Adluru, Andrew Pohl, and Lea Ziskind-Conhaim for consultation on data analysis. Diffusion Image Processing and Analysis (DIPA) software package was conceived and developed primarily by Andrew J. Schoen (schoen.andrewj@gmail.com) and Nagesh Adluru (nagesh.adluru@gmail.com). Please visit https://github.com/pegasus-isi/dipa-workflow for more details. This research was supported by the computing resources and assistance of the UW-Madison Center for High Throughput Computing (CHTC) in the Department of Computer Sciences.

REFERENCES

1. Abercrombie, H. C., Frost, C. P., Walsh, E. C., Hoks, R. M., Cornejo, M. D., Sampe, M. C., et al. (2018). Neural signaling of cortisol, childhood emotional abuse, and depression-related memory bias. *Biol. Psychiatry* 3, 274–284. doi:10.1016/j.bpsc.2017.11.005
2. Abercrombie, H. C., Jahn, A. L., Davidson, R. J., Kern, S., Kirschbaum, C., and Halverson, J. (2011). Cortisol's effects on hippocampal activation in depressed patients are related to alterati ons in memory formation. *J. Psychiatr. Res.* 45, 15–23. doi:10.1016/j.jpsychires.2010.10.005
3. Abercrombie, H. C., Kalin, N. H., and Davidson, R. J. (2005). Acute cortisol elevations cause heightened arousal ratings of objectively nonarousing stimuli. *Emotion* 5, 354–359. doi:10.1037/1528-3542.5.3.354
4. Alfarez, D. N., Joëls, M., and Krugers, H. J. (2003). Chronic unpredictable stress impairs long-term potentiation in rat hippocampal CA1 area and dentate gyrus *in vitro*. *Eur. J. Neurosci.* 17, 1928–1934. doi: 10.1046 /j.1460-9568.2003.02622.x
5. Bakker, N., Shahab, S., Giacobbe, P., Blumberger, D. M., Daskalakis, Z. J., Kennedy, S. H., et al. (2015). rTMS of the dorsomedial prefrontal cortex for major depression: safety, tolerability, effectiveness, and outcome predictors for 10 Hz versus intermittent theta-burst stimulation. *Brain Stimul.* 8, 208–215. doi:10.1016/j.brs.2014.11.002
6. Beck, A. T., Steer, R. A., Ball, R., and Ranieri, W. F. (1996). Comparison of beck depression inventories -IA and -II in psychiatric outpatients. *J. Pers. Assess.* 67, 588–597. doi:10.1207/s15327 752jpa6703_13
7. Bernstein, D. P., Stein, J. A., Newcomb, M. D., Walker, E., Pogge, D., Ahluvalia, T., et al. (2003). Development and validation of a brief screening version of the childhood trauma questionnaire. *Child Abuse Negl.* 27, 169–190. doi:10.1016/S0145-2134(02)00541-0
8. Blair, C., and Raver, C. C. (2012). Child development in the context of adversity: experiential canalization of brain and behavior. *Am. Psychol.* 67, 309–318. doi:10.1037/a0027493
9. Bleyenheuft, Y., Grandin, C. B., Cosnard, G., Olivier, E., and Thonnard, J. L. (2007). Corticospinal dysgenesis and upper-limb deficits in congenital hemiplegia: a diffusion tensor imaging study. *Pediatrics* 120, e1502–e1511. doi:10.1542/peds.2007-0394
10. Bosch, J. A., de Geus, E. J. C., Veerman, E. C. I., Hoogstraten, J., and Nieuw Amerongen, A. V. (2003). Innate secretory immunity in response to laboratory stressors that evoke distinct patterns of cardiac autonomic activity. *Psychosom. Med.* 65, 245–258. doi:10.1097/01.PSY.0000058376.50240.2D
11. Buhle, J. T., Silvers, J. A., Wager, T. D., Lopez, R., Onyemekwu, C., Kober, H., et al. (2014). Cognitive reappraisal of emotion: a meta-analysis of human neuroimaging studies. *Cereb. Cortex* 24, 2981–2990. doi: 10.1093/cercor/bht154 Caspi, A., Moffitt, T. E., Thornton, A., Freedman, D., Amell, J. W., Harrington, H., et al. (1996). The life history calendar: a research and clinical assessment method for collecting retrospective event-history data. *Int. J. Methods Psychiatr. Res.* 6, 101–114. doi: 10.1002/(SICI)1234-988X(199607)6:2<101::AID-MPR156>3.3.CO;2-E Cook, P. A., Bai, Y., Nedjati-Gilani, S., Seunarine, K. K., Hall, M. G., Parker, G. J., et al. (2006). "Camino: open-source diffusion-mri reconstruction and processing," in *14th Scientific Meeting of the International Society for Magnetic Resonance in Medicine* (Seattle, DC), 2759.
12. Cramer, H., Anheyer, D., Lauche, R., and Dobos, G. (2017). A systematic review of yoga for major depressive disorder. *J. Affect. Disord.* 213, 70–77. doi:10.1016/j.jad.2017.02.006
13. Del Giudice, M., Ellis, B. J., and Shirtcliff, E. A. (2011). The adaptive calibration model of stress responsivity. *Neurosci. Biobehav. Rev.* 35, 1562–1592. doi:10.1016/j.neubiorev.2010.11.007
14. Desikan, R. S., Segonne, F., Fischl, B., Quinn, B. T., Dickerson, B. C., Blacker, D., et al. (2006). An automated labeling system for subdividing the human cerebral cortex on MRI scans into gyral based regions of interest. *Neuroimage* 31, 968–980. doi: 10.1016/j.neuroimage.2006.01.021
15. Destrieux, C., Fischl, B., Dale, A., and Halgren, E. (2010). Automatic parcellation of human cortical gyri and sulci using standard anatomical nomenclature. *Neuroimage* 53, 1–15. doi: 10.1016/j .neuroimage.2010.06.010
16. Dickerson, S. S., and Kemeny, M. E. (2004). Acute stressors and cortisol responses: a theoretical integration and synthesis of laboratory research. *Psychol. Bull.* 130, 355–391. doi: 10.1037/0033-2909.130.3.355
17. Dimidjian, S., Barrera, M., Martell, C., Muñoz, R. F., and Lewinsohn, P.
18. M. (2011). The origins and current status of behavioral activation treatments for depression. *Annu. Rev. Clin. Psychol.* 7, 1–38. doi: 10.1146/annurev-clinpsy-032210-104535
19. Diorio, D., Viau, V., and Meaney, M. J. (1993). The role of the medial prefrontal cortex (cingulate gyrus) in the regulation of hypothalamic-pituitary-adrenal responses to stress. *J. Neurosci.* 13, 3839–3847. doi: 10.1523/JNEUROSCI.13-09-03839.1993
20. Downar, J., Geraci, J., Salomons, T. V., Dunlop, K., Wheeler, S., McAndrews, M. P., et al. (2014). Anhedonia and reward-circuit connectivity distinguish nonresponders from responders to dorsomedial prefrontal repetitive transcranial magnetic stimulation in major depression. *Biol. Psychiatry* 76, 176–185. doi: 10.1016/j.biopsych.2013.10.026
21. Drury, S. S., Sánchez, M. M., and Gonzalez, A. (2016). When mothering goes awry: challenges and opportunities for utilizing evidence across rodent, nonhuman primate and human studies to better define the biological consequences of negative early caregiving. *Horm. Behav.* 77, 182–192. doi:10.1016/j.yhbeh.2015.10.007
22. Dum, R. P., and Strick, P. L. (2002). Motor areas in the frontal lobe of the primate. *Physiol. Behav.* 77, 677–682. doi: 10.1016/S0031-9384(02)00 929-0
23. Dum, R. P., Levinthal, D. J., and Strick, P. L. (2016). Motor, cognitive, and affective areas of the cerebral cortex influence the adrenal medulla. *Proc. Natl. Acad. Sci. U.S.A.* 113, 9922–9927. doi: 10.1073/pnas.1605044113
24. Ehring, T., Ehlers, A., Cleare, A. J., and Glucksman, E. (2008). Do acute psychological and psychobiological responses to trauma predict subsequent symptom severities of PTSD and depression? *Psychiatry Res.* 161, 67–75. doi:10.1016/j.psychres.2007.08.014
25. Ekers, D., Webster, L., Van Straten, A., Cuijpers, P., Richards, D., and Gilbody, S. (2014). Behavioural activation for depression; an update of meta-analysis of effectiveness and sub group analysis. *PLoS ONE* 9:e100100. doi:10.1371/journal.pone.0100100
26. Ellis, B. J., Essex, M. J., and Boyce, W. T. (2005). Biological sensitivity to context: II. empirical explorations of an evolutionary-developmental theory. *Dev. Psychopathol.* 17, 303–328. doi: 10.1017/S0954579405050157
27. Erickson, K., Drevets, W., and Schulkin, J. (2003). Glucocorticoid regulation of diverse cognitive functions in normal and pathological emotional states. *Neurosci. Biobehav. Rev.* 27, 233–246. doi: 10.1016/S0149-7634(03)00033-2
28. First, M. B., Spitzer, R. L., Gibbon, M., and Williams, J. B. W. (2002). *Structured clinical interview for DSM-IV-TR axis I disorders.* New York, NY: Biometrics Research, New York State Psychiatric Institute.
29. Fischl, B., Salat, D. H., Busa, E., Albert, M., Dieterich, M., Haselgrove, C., et al. (2002). Whole brain segmentation: automated labeling of neuroanatomical structures in the human brain. *Neuron* 33, 341–355. doi:10.1016/S0896-6273(02)00569-X
30. Graziano, M. (2006). The organization of behavioral repertoire in motor cortex. *Annu. Rev. Neurosci.* 29, 105–134. doi: 10.1146/annurev.neuro.29.051605.112924

31. Gutman, D. A., Holtzheimer, P. E., Behrens, T. E., Johansen-Berg, H., and Mayberg, H. S. (2009). A tractography analysis of two deep brain stimulation white matter targets for depression. *Biol. Psychiatry* 65, 276–282. doi:10.1016/j.biopsych.2008.09.021
32. Heim, C., Newport, D. J., Mletzko, T., Miller, A. H., and Nemeroff, C. (2008). The link between childhood trauma and depression: insights from HPA axis studies in humans. *Psychoneuroendocrinology* 33, 693–710. doi:10.1016/j.psyneuen.2008.03.008
33. Hermans, E. J., Henckens, M. J., Joëls, M., and Fernández, G. (2014). Dynamic adaptation of large-scale brain networks in response to acute stressors. *Trends Neurosci.* 37, 304–314. doi: 10.1016/j.tins.2014.03.006
34. Herringa, R. J. (2017). Trauma, PTSD, and the developing brain. *Curr. Psychiatry Rep.* 19, 69. doi: 10.1007/s11920-017-0825-3
35. Herringa, R. J., Burghy, C. A., Stodola, D. E., Fox, M. E., Davidson, R. J., and Essex, M. J. (2016). Enhanced prefrontal-amygdala connectivity following childhood adversity as a protective mechanism against internalizing in adolescence. *Biol. Psychiatry Cogn. Neurosci. Neuroimaging* 1, 326–334. doi:10.1016/j.bpsc.2016.03.003
36. Insel, T. R. (2014). The NIMH research domain criteria (RDoC) project: precision medicine for psychiatry. *Am. J. Psychiatry* 171, 395–397. doi:10.1176/appi.ajp.2014.14020138
37. Isoda, M., and Hikosaka, O. (2007). Switching from automatic to controlled action by monkey medial frontal cortex. *Nat. Neurosci.* 10, 240–248. doi: 10.1038/nn1830
38. Joëls, M., and Krugers, H. J. (2007). LTP after stress: up or down? *Neural Plast.* 2007, 93202. doi: 10.1155/2007/93202
39. Jones, D. K., Christiansen, K. F., Chapman, R. J., and Aggleton, J. P. (2013a). Distinct subdivisions of the cingulum bundle revealed by diffusion MRI fibre tracking: Implications for neuropsychological investigations. *Neuropsychologia* 51, 67–78. doi: 10.1016/j.neuropsychologia.2012.11.018
40. Jones, D. K., Knosche, T. R., and Turner, R. (2013b). White matter integrity, fiber count, and other fallacies: the do's and don'ts of diffusion MRI. *Neuroimage* 73, 239–254. doi: 10.1016/j.neuroimage.2012.06.081
41. Keding, T. J., and Herringa, R. J. (2016). Paradoxical prefrontal-amygdala recruitment to angry and happy expressions in pediatric posttraumatic stress disorder. *Neuropsychopharmacology* 41, 2903–2912. doi: 10.1038/npp.2016.104
Lang, P. J., Bradley, M. M., and Cuthbert, B. N. (2008). *International Affective Picture System (IAPS): Affective Ratings of Pictures and Instruction Manual. Technical Report A-8.* Gainesville, FL: University of Florida.
42. McCrory, E. J., Gerin, M. I., and Viding, E. (2017). Annual research review: childhood maltreatment, latent vulnerability and the shift to preventative psychiatry - the contribution of functional brain imaging. *J. Child Psychol. Psychiatry* 58, 338–357. doi: 10.1111/jcpp.12713
43. McEwen, B. S., De Kloet, E. R., and Rostene, W. (1986). Adrenal steroid receptors and actions in the nervous system. *Physiol. Rev.* 66, 1121–1188. doi:10.1152/physrev.1986.66.4.1121
44. McFarlane, A. C., Atchison, M., and Yehuda, R. (1997). The acute stress response following motor vehicle accidents and its relation to PTSD. *Ann. N. Y. Acad. Sci.* 821, 437–441. doi: 10.1111/j.1749-6632.1997.tb48299.x
45. McLaughlin, K. A., Peverill, M., Gold, A. L., Alves, S., and Sheridan, M. A. (2015). Child maltreatment and neural systems underlying emotion regulation. *J. Am. Acad. Child Adolesc. Psychiatry* 54, 753–762. doi: 10.1016/j.jaac.2015.06.010
46. McRae, K., Hughes, B., Chopra, S., Gabrieli, J. D., Gross, J. J., and Ochsner, K. N. (2010). The neural bases of distraction and reappraisal. *J. Cogn. Neurosci.* 22, 248–262. doi: 10.1162/jocn.2009.21243
47. McTeague, L. M., Huemer, J., Carreon, D. M., Jiang, Y., Eickhoff, S. B., and Etkin, A. (2017). Identification of common neural circuit disruptions in cognitive control across psychiatric disorders. *Am. J. Psychiatry* 174, 676–685. doi:10.1176/appi.ajp.2017.16040400
48. Medford, N., and Critchley, H. D. (2010). Conjoint activity of anterior insular and anterior cingulate cortex: awareness and response. *Brain Struct. Funct.* 214, 535–549. doi: 10.1007/s00429-010-0265-x
49. Meewisse, M. L., Reitsma, J. B., de Vries, G. J., Gersons, B. P. R., and Olff, M. (2007). Cortisol and post-traumatic stress disorder in adults: systematic review and meta-analysis. *Br. J. Psychiatry* 191, 387–392. doi: 10.1192/bjp.bp.106.024877
50. Morecraft, R. J., and Tanji, J. (2009). "Cingulofrontal interactions and the cingulate motor areas," in *Cingulate Neurobiology and Disease*, ed B. Vogt (Oxford: Oxford University Press), 113–144.
51. Mortazavi, F., Oblak, A. L., Morrison, W. Z., Schmahmann, J. D., Stanley, H. E., Wedeen, V. J., et al. (2018). Geometric navigation of axons in a cerebral pathway: comparing dmri with tract tracing and immunohistochemistry. *Cereb. Cortex* 28, 1219–1232. doi: 10.1093/cercor/bhx034
52. Nachev, P., Kennard, C., and Husain, M. (2008). Functional role of the supplementary and pre-supplementary motor areas. *Nat. Rev. Neurosci.* 9, 856–869. doi: 10.1038/nrn2478
53. Nakamura, K., Sakai, K., and Hikosaka, O. (1998). Neuronal activity in medial frontal cortex during learning of sequential procedures. *J. Neurophysiol.* 80, 2671–2687. doi: 10.1152/jn.1998.80.5.2671
54. Nater, U. M., and Rohleder, N. (2009). Salivary alph a-amylase as a non-invasive biomarker for the sympathetic nervous system: current state of research. *Psychoneuroendocrinology* 34, 486–496. doi: 10.1016/j.psyneuen.2009.01.014
55. Nemeroff, C. B., Heim, C. M., Thase, M. E., Klein, D. N., Rush, A. J., Schatzberg, A. F., et al. (2003). Differential responses to psychotherapy versus pharmacotherapy in patients with chronic forms of major depression and childhood trauma. *Proc. Natl. Ac ad. Sci. U.S.A.* 100, 14293–14296. doi:10.1073/pnas.2336126100
56. Nephew, B. C., Febo, M., Huang, W., Colon-Perez, L. M., Payne, L., Poirier, G. L., et al. (2018). Early life social stress and resting state functional connectivity in postpartum rat anterior cingulate circuits. *J. Affect. Disord.* 229, 213–223. doi: 10.1016/j.jad.2017.12.089
57. Nephew, B. C., Huang, W., Poirier, G. L., Payne, L., and King, J. A. (2017). Altered neural connectivity in adult female rats exposed to early life social stress. *Behav. Brain Res.* 316, 225–233. doi: 10.1016/j.bbr.2016.08.051
58. O'Mahen, H. A., Karl, A., Moberly, N., and Fedock, G. (2015). The association between childhood maltreatment and emotion regulation: two different mechanisms contributing to depression? *J. Affect. Disord.* 174, 287–295. doi:10.1016/j.jad.2014.11.028
59. Otte, C., Neylan, T. C., Pole, N., Metzler, T., Best, S., Henn-Haase, C., et al. (2005). Association between childhood trauma and catecholamine response to psychological stress in police academy recruits. *Biol. Psychiatry* 57, 27–32. doi:10.1016/j.biopsych.2004.10.009
60. Pascoe, M. C., and Bauer, I. E. (2015). A systematic review of randomised control trials on the effects of yoga on stress measures and mood. *J. Psychiatr. Res.* 68, 270–282. doi: 10.1016/j.jpsychires.2015.07.013
61. Pavlides, C., Nivon, L. G., and McEwen, B. S. (2002). Effects of chronic stress on hippocampal long-term potentiation. *Hippocampus* 12, 245–257. doi:10.1002/hipo.1116
62. Picard, N., and Strick, P. L. (2001). Imaging the premotor areas. *Curr. Opin. Neurobiol.* 11, 663–672. doi: 10.1016/S0959-4388(01)00266-5
63. Pisner, D. A., Smith, R., Alkozei, A., Klimova, A., and Killgore, W. D. (2017). Highways of the emotional intellect: white matter microstructural correlates of an ability-based measure of emotional intelligence. *Soc. Neurosci.* 12, 253–267. doi:10.1080/17470919.2016.1176600
64. Radley, J. J., Arias, C. M., and Sawchenko, P. E. (2006). Regional differentiation of the medial prefrontal cortex in regulating adaptive responses to acute emotional stress. *J. Neurosci.* 26, 12967–12976. doi: 10.1523/JNEUROSCI.4297-06.2006
65. Rawlings, J., Pantula, S., and Dickey, D. (1998). *Applied Regression Analysis: A Research Tool.* New York, NY: Springer.
66. Ray, R. D., and Zald, D. H. (2012). Anatomical insights into the interaction of emotion and cognition in the prefrontal cortex. *Neurosci. Biobehav. Rev.* 36, 479–501. doi: 10.1016/j.neubiorev.2011.08.005
67. Rebar, A. L., Stanton, R., Geard, D., Short, C., Duncan, M. J., and Vandelanotte, (2015). A meta-meta-analysis of the effect of physical activity on depressi on and anxiety in non-clinical adult populations. *Health Psychol. Rev.* 9, 366–378. doi:10.1080/17437199.2015.1022901
68. Resnick, H. S., Yehuda, R., Pitman, R. K., and Foy, D. W. (1995). Effect of previous trauma on acute plasma cortisol level following rape. *Am. J. Psychiatry* 152, 1675–1677. doi: 10.1176/ajp.152.11.1675
69. Rodrigo, M. J., Leon, I., Gongora, D., Hernandez-Cabrera, J. A., Byrne, S., and Bobes, M. A. (2016). Inferior fronto-temporo-occipital connectivity: amissing link between maltreated girls and neglectful mothers. *Soc. Cogn. Affect. Neurosci.* 11, 1658–1665. doi: 10.1093/scan/nsw080
70. Roelofs, J., van Breukelen, G., de Graaf, L. E., Beck, A. T., Arntz, A., and Huibers, M. J. H. (2013). Norms for the beck depression inventory (BDI-II) in a large Dutch community sample. *J. Psychopathol. Behav. Assess.* 35, 93–98. doi:10.1007/s10862-012-9309-2
71. Rohleder, N., and Nater, U. M. (2009). Determinants of salivary alpha-amylase in humans and methodological considerations. *Psychoneuroendocrinology* 34, 469–485. doi: 10.1016/j.psyneuen.2008.12.004
72. Roozendaal, B., McEwen, B. S., and Chattarji, S. (2009). Stress, memory and the amygdala. *Nat. Rev. Neurosci.* 10, 423–433. doi: 10.1038/nrn2651
73. Schuch, F. B., Vancampfort, D., Richards, J., Rosenbaum, S., Ward, P. B., and Stubbs, B. (2016).

74. Exercise as a treatment for depression: a meta-analysis adjusting for publication bias. *J. Psychiatr. Res.* 77, 42–51. doi: 10.1016/j.jpsychires.2016.02.023
75. Shackman, A. J., Salomons, T. V., Slagter, H. A., Fox, A. S., Winter, J. J., and Davidson, R. J. (2011). The integration of negative affect, pain and cognitive control in the cingulate cortex. *Nat. Rev. Neurosci.* 12, 154–167. doi: 10.1038/nrn2994
76. Silvers, J. A., Insel, C., Powers, A., Franz, P., Helion, C., Martin, R., et al. (2017). The transition from childhood to adolescence is marked by a general decrease in amygdala reactivity and an affect-specific ventral-to-dorsal shift in medial prefrontal recruitment. *Dev. Cogn. Neurosci.* 25, 128–137. doi: 10.1016/j.dcn.2016.06.005
77. Smith, S. M., and Nichols, T. E. (2009). Threshold-free cluster enhancement: addressing problems of smoothing, threshold dependence and localisation in cluster inference. *Neuroimage* 44, 83–98. doi: 10.1016/j.neuroimage.2008.03.061
78. Smith, S. M., Jenkinson, M., Johansen-Berg, H., Rueckert, D., Nichols, T. E., Mackay, C. E., et al. (2006). Tract-based spatial statistics: voxelwise analysis of multi-subject diffusion data. *Neuroimage* 31, 1487–1505. doi: 10.1016/j.neuroimage.2006.02.024
79. Smith, S. M., Jenkinson, M., Woolrich, M. W., Beckmann, C. F., Behrens, T. E., Johansen-Berg, H., et al. (2004). Advances in functional and structural MR image analysis and implementation as FSL. *Neuroimage* 23(Suppl. 1), S208–S219. doi: 10.1016/j.neuroimage.2004.07.051
80. Song, Y. J., Korgaonkar, M. S., Armstrong, L. V., Eagles, S., Williams, L. M., and Grieve, S. M. (2014). Tractography of the brainstem in major depressive disorder using diffusiontensor imaging. *PLoS ONE* 9:e84825. doi: 10.1371/journal.pone.0084825
81. Swann, N. C., Cai, W., Conner, C. R., Pieters, T. A., Claffey, M. P., George, J. S., et al. (2012). Roles for the pre-supplementary motor area and the right inferior frontal gyrus in stopping action: electrophysiological responses and functional and structural connectivity. *Neuroimage* 59, 2860–2870. doi: 10.1016/j.neuroimage.2011.09.049
82. Teicher, M. H., and Samson, J. A. (2013). Childhood Maltreatment and psychopathology: a case for ecophenotypic variants as clinically and
83. neurobiologically distinct subtypes. *Am. J. Psychiatry* 170, 1114–1133. doi: 10.1176/appi.ajp.2013.12070957
84. Ulrich-Lai, Y. M., and Herman, J. P. (2009). Neural regulation of endocrine and autonomic stress responses. *Nat. Rev. Neurosci.* 10, 397–409. doi: 10.1038/nrn2647
85. van Minnen, A., Wessel, I., Verhaak, C., and Smeenk, J. (2005). The relationship between autobiographical memory specificity and depressed mood following a stressful life event: a prospective study. *Br. J. Clin. Psychol.* 44(Pt 3), 405–415. doi: 10.1348/014466505X29648
86. Vogel, S., Fernández, G., Joëls, M., and Schwabe, L. (2016). Cognitive adaptation under stress: a case for the mineralocorticoid receptor. *Trends Cogn. Sci.* 20, 192–203. doi: 10.1016/j.tics.2015.12.003
87. Walsh, K., Nugent, N. R., Kotte, A., Amstadter, A. B., Wang, S., Guille, C., et al. (2013). Cortisol at the emergency room rape visit as a predictor of PTSD and depression symptoms over time. *Psychoneuroendocrinology* 38, 2520–2528. doi: 10.1016/j.psyneuen.2013.05.017
88. Wang, R., Benner, T., Sorensen, A. G., and Wedeen, V. J. (2007). "Diffusion toolkit, a software package for diffusion imaging data processing and tractography," in *Proceedings of the International Society for Magnetic Resonance Medicine* (Berlin), 15.
89. Williams, L. M., Debattista, C., Duchemin, A. M., Schatzberg, A. F., and Nemeroff, C. B. (2016). Childhood trauma predicts antidepressant response in adults with major depression: data from the randomized international study to predict optimized treatment for depression. *Transl. Psychiatry* 6, 1–7. doi: 10.1038/tp.2016.61
90. Winkler, A. M., Ridgway, G. R., Webster, M. A., Smith, S. M., and Nichols, T. E. (2014). Permutation inference for the general linear model. *Neuroimage* 92, 381–397. doi: 10.1016/j.neuroimage.2014.01.060
91. Wirth, M. M., Scherer, S. M., Hoks, R. M., and Abercrombie, H. C. (2011). The effect of cortisol on emotional responses depends on order of cortisol and placebo administration in a within-subject design. *Psychoneuroendocrinology* 36, 945–954. doi: 10.1016/j.psyneuen.2010.11.010
92. Wolf, R. C., and Herringa, R. J. (2016). Prefrontal-amygdala dysregulation to threat in pediatric posttraumatic stress disorder. *Neuropsychopharmacology* 41, 822–831. doi: 10.1038/npp.2015.209
93. Yehuda, R., McFarlane, A. C., and Shalev, A. Y. (1998). Predicting the development of posttraumatic stress disorder from the acute response to a traumatic event. *Biol. Psychiatry* 44, 1305–1313. doi: 10.1016/S0006-3223(98)00276-5
94. Zhang, H., Paul, A., Rueckert, D., and Gee, J. (2007). "Unbiased white matter atlas construction using diffusion tensor images," in *Medical Image Computing and Computer-Assisted Intervention – MICCAI 2007*, eds N. Ayache, S. Ourselin and A. Maeder (Berlin; Heidelberg: Springer), 211–218.

14

Neurological Involvement in Primary Systemic Vasculitis

Shanshan Zhang[1], Dongli Yuan[2] and Ge Tan[1]*

[1] *Department of Neurology, The First Affiliated Hospital of Chongqing Medical University, Chongqing, China,*

[2] *The Institute of Medical Information, Chongqing Medical University, Chongqing, China*

Correspondence:
Ge Tan
titot@sina.com

Primary systemic vasculitis can affect every structure in both the central and peripheral nervous system, causing varied neurological manifestations of neurological dysfunction. Early recognition of the underlying causes of the neurological symptoms can facilitate timely treatment and improve the prognosis. This review highlights the clinical manifestations of primary systemic vasculitis in the nervous system.

Keywords: primary systemic vasculitis, central nervous system, peripheral nervous system, neurological involvement, clinical manifestation

INTRODUCTION

Primary systemic vasculitis (PSV) can be defined as a heterogeneous group of uncommon diseases characterized by blood vessel inflammation and necrosis. Unlike secondary systemic vasculitis, which usually results from infections, connective tissue diseases, neoplasms, and drugs, PSV is considered to occur with no identified etiology (1). Nevertheless, recent researches have demonstrated that PSV might be associated with farming (2), silica exposure (2, 3), solvent exposure and hydrocarbons (2, 4, 5), allergy and family history of atopy (2, 6). Despite of unknown causes, two mechanisms, deposition of immune complexes and cell-mediated immunity, were found to possibly participate in the pathophysiology of PSV by causing immunological inflammation and necrosis of the vessel wall (7). And according to the classification criteria revised in 1990 by The American College of Rheumatology (8) and in 1994 and 2012 by the Chapel Hill Consensus Conferences (9, 10), the classification of PSV is based primarily on the major size of the affected vessels, although these disease-affected arteries may have overlaps in diameter.

Many neurologists have limited knowledge of PSV because most of these patients are treated by rheumatologists. However, both the central nervous system (CNS) and peripheral nervous system (PNS) are major targets in PSV and may become involved in the earliest stages; thus, patients may be referred to a neurologist first. Since the clinical manifestations of PSV are often non-specific, the differential diagnosis may be challenging.

CNS damage was reported to occur in 24% of cases with PSV, commonly due to antineutrophil cytoplasmic antibody (ANCA)-associated vasculitis and polyarteritis nodosa. The range of clinical expressions of PSV's CNS damage is relatively wide, including cerebrovascular manifestations such as hemorrhagic and ischemic stroke caused by intra/extra-cerebral vascular stenosis, aneurysm, and sinus venous thrombosis, meningeal and brain parenchymal involvement resulted from granulomatosis and perivasculitis, and encephalopathy due to cytokine damage.

Compared with the frequency of central vasculitic involvement, vasculitic peripheral neuropathies are more common and have been reported to occur in 37% of patients with PSV (11), and 25% of patients experience symptoms of peripheral neuropathy at initial presentation (12). Generally, vasculitic peripheral neuropathies result from the inflammation of precapillary arteries in the nerves, such as eosinophilic granulomatosis with polyangiitis (60–80% of patients), polyarteritis nodosa (50–100% of patients), granulomatosis with polyangiitis (Wegener's granulomatosis, 13–26.6% of cases), cryoglobulinemia (70% of cases), and microscopic polyangiitis (6–18% of cases), usually presenting in a uniform pattern such as multiplex mononeuropathy (accounting for 59–85% of cases) and symmetric polyneuropathy (41% of cases) (11–13). Nerve conduction studies have revealed a much higher frequency of peripheral neurological involvement than that in clinical case series and studies. Asymptomatic vasculitic neuropathy was detected in 21 of 270 cases (7.8%) of biopsy-proven vasculitis (14).

In addition, the introduction of nerve sonography, single-photon emission computed tomography (SPECT), magnetic resonance imaging (MRI), magnetic resonance angiography (MRA), magnetic resonance spectroscopy (MRS), and apparent diffusion coefficient (ADC) have greatly improved the diagnostic rate and accuracy of vasculitic neuropathy.

SEARCH STRATEGY

We performed an advanced literature search in PubMed and EMBASE for the period January 1, 1990, through September 1, 2017, using as a search query "systemic vasculitis" "nervous system." Eligible studies were included according to the following criteria. Only human studies that were written in English were considered. All patients included in the studies were diagnosed according to the classification criteria defined by the American College of Rheumatology or the Chapel Hill Consensus Conference. Retrospective and prospective studies were included to determine the frequency of neurological manifestations. Case reports and case series were added in the reference list only when unusual features were described. Pediatric studies were excluded because the clinical features of children and newborns are different.

LARGE-VESSEL VASCULITIS

Large vessels were defined as the aorta, vena cava, and their major branches. Large-vessel vasculitis is composed of Takayasu arteritis and giant cell arteritis.

Takayasu Arteritis

Takayasu arteritis (TA) is a rare type of primary chronic inflammatory disease, causing stenosis, occlusion and aneurysm of arteries. TA mainly affects large-caliber arteries such as the aorta and its major branches in patients younger than 40 years old (more than 90% of patients are younger than 40), with a female predominance (female to male ratio is 10:1), and is more common in Asians (1). Studies have shown that more than half of patients with TA show neurological manifestations (15, 16) that range from dizziness/headaches to ischemic or hemorrhagic stroke.

Dizziness and headache are the most common complaints in patients with TA with neurological complications, accounting for ~78.1% (214/274) and 25.5% (70/274), respectively (16). However, headache and dizziness do not necessarily indicate CNS involvement. Visual disturbances affect 4.6–59.3% of patients, and 4–21.9% of TA patients with neurological manifestations were found to have syncope as the main manifestation.

Cerebrovascular complications have always been the focus of researchers. Transient ischemic attack accounts for 3–22.2% of the nervous system manifestations caused by TA. Stroke, as the most severe complication of TA, was found to occur in 10–20% of cases (16–18). Due to lack of knowledgement, the median and average delay between symptom onset and the diagnosis of TA are 2 years (19) and 52.4 months (16), respectively, which delays the treatment of vasculitis. The majority of the strokes caused by TA are ischemic strokes, mostly due to multiple and severe stenosis or occlusive lesions in the aortic arch and its major branches. Couture and colleagues (19) evaluated the impact of stroke on the prognosis of TA patients, and after a median of seven years of follow-up, 59% of the patients had neurological deficits, 35% suffered from stroke recurrence and 24% had epilepsy. However, cerebral aneurysms and subarachnoid hemorrhage are rarely observed in TA patients. The incidence of aneurysm in TA patients is no higher than that in the general population. However, when such incidents occur, aneurysms in TA patients have a high rate of multiplicity and commonly occur in the vertebrobasilar arterial system (20). Posterior reversible encephalopathy syndrome (PRES) is an uncommon neurological complication in TA patients, mainly affecting women under the age of 30, presenting as headache, epilepsy, and neurological deficits in most patients. The pathophysiological mechanism has been suggested to be both endothelial injury and hypertension caused by TA, and the use of immunosuppressants such as cyclosporine and tacrolimus may also be a factor in the development of PRES since they can also induce endothelial dysfunction (21).

In addition, rare complications such as Horner's syndrome and intracranial granulomatosis have been reported as initial manifestations of TA. Other unusual neurological manifestations of TA that have been reported include brachial plexus palsy due to axillary artery aneurysm, unilateral sensorineural hearing loss, subclavian stealing syndrome, Moya-Moya syndrome, multiple cranial nerve palsies, cavernous sinus syndrome, and hypertrophic pachymeningitis.

Giant Cell Arteritis

Giant cell arteritis (GCA) is the most common large vasculitis in Western countries and mainly affects extracranial branches of the carotid artery and/or the aorta and its large arterial branches, usually affecting people over the age of 50 (22).

Neuro-ophthalmological manifestation is the most frequent and serious event among neurological complications of GCA, accounting for 20–28.8% of affected patients (23, 24), with 15% of them suffering from permanent visual loss (25). Visual symptoms may be caused by ischemic optic neuropathy and retinal ischemia, among which anterior ischemic optic neuropathy accounts for the largest proportion.

Cerebrovascular disease is another severe neurological manifestation, occurring in ~5% of all GCA-related neurological complications. According to recent studies, the risk ratio of cerebrovascular accident in patients with GCA vs. non-GCA comparators was 1.40 (26), and the risk of cerebrovascular complications was higher during the first year (or month) after GCA diagnosis (27, 28), which means that cerebrovascular events often occur during the active period of the disease. Epidemiological study shows that stroke is observed in 1–3% of patients (25), among which cerebral infarction is the most common (58%), followed by subarachnoid hemorrhage (24%), and cerebral hemorrhage (18%) (29). The main reasons are considered to be, on the one hand, ischemia or occlusion caused by direct involvement of carotid and vertebrobasilar arteries and, on the other hand, atherosclerotic changes of the vessels caused by chronic inflammation. The incidence of vertebrobasilar artery vascular accident in patients with GCA (35%) has been shown to be higher than that of the general population (which is usually <15%) (27, 28), and one study showed that audiovestibular dysfunction is not uncommon in GCA patients (30). It is interesting to note that in a retrospective study (25), researchers found that most GCA patients who experienced a vertebrobasilar stroke had neurological symptom onset after the start of corticosteroid treatment. However, it is still being debated whether this situation is due to a direct effect of vasculitis or vascular occlusion promoted by the effects of corticosteroids.

Peripheral nervous system involvement was found in 1–14% of GCA patients, presenting as cranial neuropathies, multiple mononeuropathy, or polyneuropathies (24); existing case reports include multiple cranial nerve palsy, trigeminal autonomic cephalalgia, occipital neuralgia, Horner syndrome, peroneal nerve palsy, cervical radiculopathy, brachial plexopathy, hypertrophic pachymeningitis, and cavernous sinus syndrome.

MEDIUM-VESSEL VASCULITIS

Medium vessels refer to the main visceral arteries and veins and their initial branches. Medium-vessel vasculitis consists of polyarteritis nodosa and Kawasaki disease.

Polyarteritis Nodosa

Polyarteritis nodosa (PAN) is a rare systemic necrotizing vasculitis mainly involving medium and small vessels, causing microaneurysm, stenosis, and thrombosis, therefore leading to ischemia or hemorrhage of the supplied tissues. PAN affects women more often than men, usually with an onset between 40 and 50 years of age (31). The condition may affect any organ; however, the most frequently affected organs are the peripheral nerves, followed by muscles, joints, kidneys, skin, gastrointestinal tract, and heart (32).

Involvement of the CNS has been reported to exist in 20–40% of PAN cases (33) and mainly occurs at late stages (2–3 years) (34). CNS involvement has been recognized as a sign of a poor prognosis, and the expected mortality rate at 5 years is 26% (35, 36). The most common manifestation of CNS involvement includes diffuse encephalopathy and a deficit of focal neurological function. Diffuse encephalopathy may present as new onset seizure and headache, reduced level of consciousness or altered vision, among which some of the cases also suffer from reversible encephalopathy syndrome (37–39). The main manifestations of focal CNS involvement include cerebral infarction (which occurs in 13–17% of PAN patients), hemorrhage, multifocal encephalopathy and episodes of neurological dysfunction that mimic multiple sclerosis (33, 40). Intracranial hemorrhage is a rare complication of PAN, and subarachnoid hemorrhage and intracerebral hemorrhage caused by aneurysms have been reported in PAN cases. The features of these aneurysms were found to be multiple, small in size, and equally located in the infratentorial and supratentorial arteries (41).

Reichart et al. (33) investigated early lacunar strokes complicating PAN and revealed that 33.3% (5/15) of strokes occurred within 1 month after the onset of PAN and 15% (2/13) shortly after the initiation of corticosteroids; ischemic strokes occurred during corticosteroid treatment in 77% (10/13) of the patients, 80% (8/10) of which occurred within 6 months after corticosteroid initiation and 50% (5/10) within 3 weeks. Combined with the results of prior studies showing that all strokes occurred while the patients were under adequate corticosteroid treatment, it was suggested that the promoting effect of corticosteroids in stroke might work by two mechanisms (33). For one thing, corticosteroids promote platelet aggregation in cerebral medium-sized arteries by increasing thromboxane A2, quickly causing a lacunar stroke. Lacunar strokes appearing 1 or more months after initiation of corticosteroids can be explained by the promoting effect of corticosteroids on thrombotic microangiopathies.

PNS involvement is the most common complication of PAN and occurs in 60–70% of cases; it has an onset early in the course of the disease, mostly within a few months of diagnosis (42). The common patterns of PNS involvement include mononeuropathy, polyneuropathy and mononeuritis multiplex, the pathophysiology of which has been recognized as vasculitis of the vasa nervorum. Sudden onset asymmetrical sensorimotor mononeuritis multiplex, which mainly affects the lower extremities, and insidious symmetrical peripheral neuropathy are typical and common in PAN (31). In addition, patients with PAN may also develop pachymeningitis (43) and present with headache or cranial nerve palsy. Sudden bilateral hearing loss (44) and visual alterations caused by optic neuropathy (45) have also been reported.

Kawasaki Disease

Kawasaki disease (KD) is a systemic vasculitis that mainly affects medium-sized vessels, occurring predominately in children under 5 years of age. Neurological complications of KD have been described in children, such as encephalopathy, seizures, cerebral infarction, intracranial hemorrhage, ataxia, and cranial nerve palsy (46). However, although rare cases of first onset have also been reported in adult patients, most reported cases are in young adults and the manifestations are due to late-onset sequelae instead of new-onset active disease. We found one case (47) describing a 20-year-old young adult with a history of KD suffering from subarachnoid hemorrhage due to an intracranial aneurysm with a stalk-like narrow neck, located at the trunk of the middle cerebral artery. As the researchers mentioned, coronary aneurysms in KD also arise in places where no branch exists. Therefore, non-bifurcation intracranial aneurysm might be related to KD and might cause intracranial hemorrhage in young adults as a late sequela.

Small-Vessel Vasculitis

Small-vessel vasculitis refers to necrotizing inflammation in the wall of small intraparenchymal arteries, arterioles, capillaries, and venules, and to a secondary degree in medium-size arteries. Vascular and perivascular inflammation leads to fibrinoid necrosis and consequently vascular necrosis, occlusion and thrombosis (10). The disease consists of two major groups, ANCA-associated vasculitis and immune complex small-vessel vasculitis.

ANCA-Associated Vasculitis

ANCA-associated vasculitis is defined as necrotizing small-vessel vasculitis with few or no immune deposits, mostly associated with myeloperoxidase (MPO) ANCA or proteinase 3 (PR3) ANCA (10). Among the cases of ANCA-associated vasculitis, CNS involvement is more common in granulomatosis with polyangiitis (GPA) and microscopic polyangiitis (MPA) than it is in eosinophilic granulomatosis with polyangiitis (EGPA) (48). Nevertheless, peripheral nerve involvement is more prevalent in EGPA than are MPA and GPA (49).

Granulomatosis With Polyangiitis (Wegener's)

Granulomatosis with polyangiitis (GPA) is characterized by necrotizing granulomatous inflammation usually associated with antibodies against PR3 and most commonly involves the upper and lower respiratory tract, and sinonasal inflammation and necrotizing glomerulonephritis are frequently present (10). Neurological complications have been shown to be present in 29–50% of all cases (50–52).

CNS involvement occurs in 7–11% of GPA patients (50, 53, 54), and when isolated cranial nerve palsies are included, the rate is 8–28% (51, 54). Since GPA can commonly involve sinonasal structures and cause granulomatous inflammation, which is capable of invading neighboring structures, the orbit, mastoid, optic nerve, chiasma, cranial nerves, meninges, and pituitary gland might be compromised, presenting as oculomotor dysfunction, mastoiditis, visual disturbances, cranial nerve palsy, headache, and endocrine dysfunction. In addition, small and medium arteries in the cranium can be involved, causing ischemia, or hemorrhage in different vascular territories (55). Cranial nerve palsy was reported to occur in 4.7–6% of GPA patients, among which the most commonly affected cranial nerves are II, VI, and VII (50, 51). The pituitary has been reported to be affected in 1.1–1.3% of GPA patients (56, 57). Meningeal pachymeningitis usually occurs i4n the early stages of GPA, with lower incidences of accompanying systemic symptoms (58), which is perhaps due to granulomatous erosion of the skull base in the early phase and may lead to a delay of diagnosis (52). The most common symptom is headache, followed by cranial nerve palsy and symptoms due to venous sinus occlusion. Vasculitis involvement can cause ischemic and hemorrhagic complications of the brain and spinal cord (58). Dysfunction of intracranial arteries may cause PRES, presenting as various symptoms (59–62). Hypophysitis has been widely reported as one of the CNS complications of GPA, and its clinical manifestations vary according to the specific sites involved. Panhypopituitarism might occur as a consequence of granulomatous inflammation of both the anterior and posterior pituitary (56). Anterior pituitary involvement may influence the release of antidiuretic hormone and present as diabetes insipidus, which was shown to occur in 47 of 58 GPA patients (81%) with sellar involvement, according to an analysis of cases performed by Peters et al. (63). Posterior pituitary inflammation may cause diminished secretion of many hormones, leading to secondary hypogonadism (occurred in 32 out of 58 sellar involved GPA patients, 55%), secondary hypothyroidism (20 out of 58 sellar involved GPA patients, 34.5%), secondary adrenal insufficiency, secondary growth hormone deficiency (19 of 58 sellar involved GPA patients, 32.8%). Compression of the pituitary stalk can result in hyperprolactinemia (5 of 58 sellar involved GPA patients, 8.6%) and galactorrhea, and visual alteration may occur if the optic chiasm is compressed (56, 57).

PNS complications have been reported to occur in 11–44% of GPA patients (54), which occurs milder and later in the course of the disease than in other ANCA-associated vasculitis (64), presenting mainly as recurrent mononeuropathies, mononeuritis multiplex, or symmetric polyneuropathy due to ischemia caused by vasculitic inflammation of the vasa nervorum. As the most frequent manifestation, distal symmetrical sensory neuropathy was reported in 7–10% of cases, followed by motor mononeuritis multiplex in 2–12% (51, 53). Commonly, peroneal (90–95%), tibial (38–55%), ulnar (35–45%), and median (26–36%) nerves are involved (29, 51).

Eosinophilic Granulomatosis With Polyangiitis (Churg-Strauss)

The characteristics of eosinophilic granulomatosis with polyangiitis (EGPA) is an eosinophil-rich and granulomatous inflammation that often involves the respiratory tract and is associated with asthma and eosinophilia (10).

Neurological involvement is common in EGPA, accounting for up to 60% of cases and usually manifesting as peripheral neuropathy that tends to present before visceral involvement (29). Therefore, early detection of peripheral nerve involvement is fundamental for early diagnosis and treatment of EGPA. The most common peripheral neurological manifestation is multiple mononeuropathy (accounting for 68% of cases with peripheral neuropathy), followed by distal symmetric polyneuropathy (28%) and asymmetric polyneuropathy (4%) (65). Since mononeuritis multiplex is typical in acute systemic vasculitis, the initial symptoms commonly present as dysesthesia, paresthesia, and edema in distal limbs, especially the lower limbs. The condition will gradually progress into asymmetrical polyneuropathy and may affect motor nerves, leading to muscle atrophy. Electrophysiological studies have shown decreases in the amplitude of sensory nerve action potentials and compound muscle action potentials, indicating the presence of axonal injury (66).

CNS involvement in EGPA is rather rare, accounting for only 6–10% of all cases (67). Cerebral infarctions and intracerebral hemorrhage resulting from intracranial vasculitis are the most common CNS presentations of EGPA. In addition, rarer manifestations have been noted, such as subarachnoid hemorrhage, cranial nerve palsy, encephalopathy, epilepsy, hydrocephalus, headache, sinus venous thrombosis, spinal hemorrhage, meningeal involvement, and optic neuropathy.

Microscopic Polyangiitis

Microscopic polyangiitis (MPA) presents with non-granulomatous inflammation with few or no immune deposits in the walls of the affected vessels, mainly associated with antibodies against MPO. Necrotizing glomerulonephritis and alveolar hemorrhage are common complications (10). Peripheral neurological involvement occurs in 55 to 79% of cases with MPA, with no special manifestations compared with those of other ANCA-associated types of vasculitis (mainly presenting as polyneuropathy and mononeuropathy); (64). CNS involvement in MPA is rare and was reported to be able to manifest as intracerebral infarction or hemorrhage, subarachnoid hemorrhage, hypertrophic pachymeningitis, PRES or spinal cord involvement (68).

Immune Complex Small-Vessel Vasculitis

Immune complex small-vessel vasculitis is characterized by moderate to marked deposits of immunoglobulin and/or complement components in the small vessel walls.

Antiglomerular Basement Membrane Disease

Antiglomerular basement membrane (anti-GBM) disease, also called Goodpasture syndrome, is a vasculitis affecting glomerular capillaries and/or pulmonary capillaries with deposition of anti-GBM autoantibodies on GBM, accounting for 5% of adult patients with glomerulonephritis and leading to acute renal failure in approximately half of the patients. Lung involvement results in pulmonary hemorrhage, and renal involvement leads to glomerulonephritis with necrosis and crescents, which are the classic presentations of anti-GBM disease (10, 69). Neurological involvement is uncommon. According to the rare cases reported (69–73), PRES is the most frequent neurological complication. All patients reported are younger than 40 and they all manifested as hypertension, renal failure, and seizures. Destruction of the blood-brain barrier resulting from inflammatory endothelial injury and increased capillary filtration due to hypertension are important factors in the pathophysiology of PRES in GBM patients.

Cryoglobulinemic Vasculitis

Cryoglobulinemic vasculitis (CV) is defined as vasculitis with cryoglobulin immune deposits affecting small vessels (predominantly capillaries, venules, or arterioles) caused by chronic inflammation, autoimmune disorders, and lymphoproliferative disorders, frequently involving skin, glomeruli, and peripheral nerves (10). Most cases of cryoglobulinemic vasculitis result from infection, B-cell lymphoproliferative disorders and autoimmune diseases, among which hepatitis C virus infection is the cause in ~80% of cases (74). In a study of 242 cases with non-infectious mixed cryoglobulinemia vasculitis (75), 117 patients (48%) were found to have no identified causal factor, also defined as idiopathic. However, no study has evaluated the neurological involvement of idiopathic cryoglobulinemia vasculitis alone. For patients with mixed CV, PNS involvement is not uncommon and typically starts with polyneuropathy that affects the sensory nerves initially and later the motor nerves, predominantly involving the lower limbs. CNS involvement is rare, and studies have shown that mixed CV may cause cerebrovascular events, PRES, hydrocephalus and intracranial hypertension (29, 76).

IgA Vasculitis (Henoch-Schönlein Purpura)

IgA vasculitis (IgAV) is characterized by IgA1-dominant immune deposits affecting small vessels, often involving the skin and gastrointestinal tract and frequently causing arthritis (10). The majority (75%) of cases occur in young people no more than 20 years of age (77), and CNS involvement has been reported to manifest as headache, decreased consciousness, seizures, focal neurological deficits, and visual and verbal abnormalities. However, PNS involvement has been documented as neuropathies of the brachial plexus and facial, peroneal, femoral and ulnar nerve, and in addition, Guillain-Barre syndrome and mononeuritis multiplex (78). Rare cases of IgAV-induced neurological manifestations have been reported in adult patients as ischemic stroke, axonal sensorimotor polyneuropathy (79, 80), mononeuritis multiplex (81, 82), acoustic neuritis, facial nerve palsy (83), intracerebral hemorrhage (84), anterior ischemic optic neuropathy (85), focal seizures (86), and encephalopathy (87).

Hypocomplementemic Urticarial Vasculitis (anti-C1q Vasculitis)

Hypocomplementemic urticarial vasculitis (HUV) is a kind of vasculitis accompanied by urticaria and hypocomplementemia affecting cutaneous small vessels and is associated with anti-C1q antibodies, commonly causing urticaria and multiorgan involvement such as glomerulonephritis, arthritis, obstructive pulmonary disease, and ocular inflammation (10). HUV may be induced by connective tissue diseases, infections (such as hepatitis B, hepatitis C and infectious mononucleosis), neoplasms and drugs; however, most cases of HUV are idiopathic (88). Neurological involvement has been occasionally reported as pseudotumor cerebri (89), lower cranial nerve (VIII, IX, and X) palsies (90) and peripheral nerve involvement such as asymmetrical multifocal axonal sensory neuropathy.

VARIABLE-VESSEL VASCULITIS

Variable-vessel vasculitis refers to vasculitis with no predominant type of vessel involved that can affect vessels of any size (small, medium, and large) and type (arteries, veins, and capillaries) (10).

Behçet's Syndrome

Behçet's syndrome is a vasculitis occurring in patients with Behçet's disease (BD) and can affect arteries or veins and lead to a relapsing inflammatory disorder in almost any tissue, with oral and genital ulcerations and uveitis as its most typical symptoms

(41). Neurological manifestations of BD, which are called neuro-BD (NBD), occur in 1.3–59% of all cases and usually affect patients aged between 20 and 40 years, with a male predominance (the male to female ratio is 2.8:1) (91–95). NBD commonly appears 3–6 years after other systemic involvement (92, 96, 97) and is considered to be caused by perivasculitis.

The manifestations of neurological involvement can be caused by either CNS parenchymal inflammation or vascular complications in the nervous system, with a reported prevalence of 67–76 vs. 12–20% in all NBD cases (93, 98). The former is considered to be caused by small vasculitis, leading to axonal damage and gliosis, frequently affecting the brain stem (occurs in 25–50% of all parenchymal NBD cases) (92, 93, 99, 100), thalamus and basal ganglia, and, only rarely, the white matter and spinal cord. The main clinical manifestations are subacute cranial neuropathy, ophthalmoparesis, meningoencephalitis, and alteration of cerebellar, pyramidal and extrapyramidal function. Uncommon symptoms such as subcortical dementia, stroke and transverse myelitis have also been reported (91, 101). Vascular complications mainly result from cerebral venous thrombosis (CVT) due to large vessels endothelial cell activation, and rarely, aneurysms due to perivasculitis to the vasa nervorum (91). CVT in BD mainly causes focal neurological deficits and seizures in young men (102). However, not all epileptic seizures in NBD patients result from CVT, and brainstem lesions may also lead to complex partial seizures (103).

In addition, perivasculitis to the vasa nervorum may also cause PNS involvement. However, this condition is extremely rare and was found in merely 8 out of 1,031 cases (0.8%); thus, its relationship with BD is still doubtful (91).

Cogan Syndrome

Cogan syndrome (CS) is a sequence of clinical manifestations due to a chronic immunological inflammatory multisystem disease of unknown origin, characterized by recurrent episodes of keratitis, vestibuloauditory dysfunction, and systemic vasculitis, frequently leading to visual loss, vertigo, sensorineural hearing loss, tinnitus and systemic manifestations (10). The syndrome mainly affects children and young adults with an average age at onset of 38 years (SD, 15.1 years; range, 9–70 years) (104).

It is worth noting that complications of the eyes and ears do not always occur at the same time (sometimes up to 9 years apart) (105) and in 20% of cases, vestibuloauditory symptoms can be the only presentation (104). Therefore, although the vestibuloauditory involvement in Cogan syndrome is mainly due to inflammation of inner ear structures rather than neurological involvement (105), its manifestations can be easily misdiagnosed as central acute vestibular syndrome of vascular origin, Ménière's disease or vestibular migraine, which are common in neurological out-patients. According to a study that enrolled 60 cases of CS at Mayo Clinic (104), all cases suffered from hearing loss, 90% of the cases experienced vertigo, and tinnitus (80%), ataxia (53%), and oscillopsia (25%) were also common during the course of the disease. Hearing loss is typically sudden, mainly involves bilateral high frequencies, and the decline in hearing fluctuates and progresses gradually. Vestibular function is commonly damaged bilaterally (accounting for 74% of cases that underwent a caloric test) and vestibular symptoms may last for days to weeks (sometimes indefinitely) with no resolution (104, 106). The vestibuloauditory symptoms listed above may recur in 1–13 years after onset (occurs in 22% of patients) (107).

TABLE 1 | Common CNS and PNS involvements of primary systemic vasculitis.

PSV	CNS involvement	PNS involvement
Takayasu arteritis	Dizziness (78.1%), headache (25.5%); visual disturbances (4.6–59.3%); syncope (4–21.9%); stroke (10–20%);	Rare
Giant cell arteritis	Neuro-ophthalmological damage (20–28.8%), stroke (1–3%), vertebrobasilar artery vascular accident (35%);	1–14% of cases; cranial neuropathies, multiple mononeuropathy, polyneuropathies;
Polyarteritis nodosa	20–40% of cases; Diffuse encephalopathy, cerebral infarction (13–17%);	60–70% of cases; Mononeuropathy, polyneuropathy, mononeuritis multiplex;
Granulomatosis with polyangiitis	8–28% of cases; Cranial nerve palsy (4.7–6%, mainly II, VI, and VII), pituitary damage (1.1–1.3%), meningeal pachymeningitis, ischemic, and hemorrhagic complications of brain and spinal cord, PRES	11–44% of cases; Recurrent mononeuropathies, mononeuritis multiplex, symmetric polyneuropathy
Eosinophilic granulomatosis with polyangiitis	6–10% of all cases; Cerebral infarctions and intracerebral hemorrhage	~60% of cases; Multiple mononeuropathy (68% of PNS cases), distal symmetric polyneuropathy (28%) and asymmetric polyneuropathy (4%)
Microscopic polyangiitis	Rare	55–79% of cases; polyneuropathy, mononeuropathy
Behçet's syndrome	CNS parenchymal inflammation (67–76% of all NBD cases): subacute cranial neuropathy, ophthalmoparesis, meningoencephalitis, alteration of cerebellar, pyramidal, and extrapyramidal function; Vascular complications in the nervous system (12–20% of all NBD cases): cerebral venous thrombosis, aneurysms	Extremely rare: 0.8% of BD cases
Cogan syndrome	Ischemic stroke (2.5–3%), encephalitis (5–6%), meningitis (5–22%), encephalopathy, myelopathy, optic nerve disorders, aneurysm, and cerebral venous thrombosis	Peripheral neuropathy (1–12.5%), cranial neuropathy (1–10%, mainly II, V, VI, and VII) and myopathy

Neurological involvement was reported in 29–56% of cases and usually occurs after eye and ear manifestations (106, 108). CNS involvement may manifest as ischemic stroke (accounting for 2.5–3% of cases reported), encephalitis (5–6%), meningitis (5–22%), encephalopathy, myelopathy, optic nerve disorders, aneurysm, and cerebral venous thrombosis. PNS conditions in Cogan syndrome patients have been reported as peripheral neuropathy (1–12.5%, frequently mononeuritis multiplex), cranial neuropathy (1–10%, mainly cranial nerve II, V, VI, and VII) and myopathy (106).

CONCLUSION

Neurological involvement is a common complication of PSV (**Table 1**), and neurologists play an important role in the identification and diagnosis of PSV patients with otherwise unexplained neurological symptoms as their chief complaint. This article summarizes the neurological manifestations of PSV and hopes to improve neuroscientists' understanding of this broad range of diseases.

AUTHOR CONTRIBUTIONS

SZ conceived the article and wrote the manuscript. DY and GT reviewed and edited the manuscript. All authors read and approved the manuscript.

ACKNOWLEDGMENTS

The authors are grateful to the Chongqing Science and Technology Commission, Chongqing Education Commission and the Chongqing Health and Family Planning Commission for funding this project.

REFERENCES

1. Gonzalez-Gay M, Garcia-Porrua C. Epidemiology of the vasculitides. *Rheum Dis Clin North Am.* (2001) 27:729–49. doi: 10.1016/S0889-857X(05)70232-5
2. Lane SE, Watts RA, Graham B, Innes NJ, Scott DGI. Are environmental factors important in primary systemic vasculitis? A case-control study. *Arthritis Rheum.* (2014) 48:814–23. doi: 10.1002/art.10830
3. Mulloy KB. Silica exposure and systemic vasculitis. *Environ Health Perspect.* (2003) 111:1933–8. doi: 10.1289/ehp.6400
4. Nuyts GD, Van VE, De VA, Daelemans RA, Rorive G, Elseviers MM, et al. Wegener granulomatosis is associated to exposure to silicon compounds: a case-control study. *Nephrol Dial Transpl.* (1995) 10:1162–5. doi: 10.1093/ndt/10.7.1162
5. Steenland NK, Thun MJ, Ferguson CW, Port FK. Occupational and other exposures associated with male end-stage renal disease: a case/control study. *Am J Public Health.* (1990) 80:153. doi: 10.2105/AJPH.80.2.153
6. Cuadrado MJ, D'Cruz D, Lloyd M, Mujic F, Khamashta MA, Hughes GRV. Allergic disorders in systemic vasculitis: a case-control study. *Br J Rheum.* (1994) 33:749. doi: 10.1093/rheumatology/33.8.749
7. Sampaio L, Silva LG, Terroso G, Nadais G, Mariz E, Ventura F. Vasculitic neuropathy. *Acta Reumatol Port.* (2011) 36:102–9.
8. Bloch DA, Michel BA, Hunder GG, McShane DJ, Arend WP, Calabrese LH, et al. The American College of Rheumatology 1990 criteria for the classification of vasculitis. Patients and methods. *Arthritis Rheum.* (1990) 33:1068–73. doi: 10.1002/art.1780330803
9. Jennette JC, Falk RJ, Andrassy K, Bacon PA, Churg J, Gross WL, et al. Nomenclature of systemic vasculitides. Proposal of an international consensus conference. *Arthritis Rheum.* (1994) 37:187–92. doi: 10.1002/art.1780370206
10. Rasmussen N. The 2012 revised international chapel hill consensus conference nomenclature of the vasculitides. *Ann Rheum Dis.* (2013) 71:16. doi: 10.1136/annrheumdis-2012-eular.1540
11. Pena CE, Pera M, Marcos J, Salas A, Testi A, Garcia MA. Peripheral neurological involvement in primary systemic vasculitis. *Ann Rheum Dis.* (2015) 74:295–6. doi: 10.1136/annrheumdis-2015-eular.2855
12. Wolf J, Schmitt V, Palm F, Grau AJ, Bergner R. Peripheral neuropathy as initial manifestation of primary systemic vasculitides. *J Neurol.* (2013) 260:1061–70. doi: 10.1007/s00415-012-6760-7
13. Finsterer J. Systemic and non-systemic vasculitis affecting the peripheral nerves. *Acta Neurologica Belgica.* (2009) 109:100–13.
14. Kurt S, Alsharabati M, Lu L, Claussen GC, Oh SJ. Asymptomatic vasculitic neuropathy. *Muscle Nerve.* (2015) 52:34–8. doi: 10.1002/mus.24494
15. Kim HJ, Suh DC, Kim JK, Kim SJ, Lee JH, Choi CG, et al. Correlation of neurological manifestations of Takayasu's arteritis with cerebral angiographic findings. *Clin Imaging.* (2005) 29:79–85. doi: 10.1016/j.clinimag.2004.04.026
16. Yang L, Zhang H, Jiang X, Song L, Qin F, Zou Y, et al. Clinical features and outcomes of Takayasu arteritis with neurological symptoms in China: a retrospective study. *J Rheum.* (2015) 42:1846–52. doi: 10.3899/jrheum.150097
17. Duarte MM, Geraldes R, Sousa R, Alarcão J, Costa J. Stroke and transient ischemic attack in takayasu's arteritis: a systematic review and meta-analysis. *J Stroke Cerebrovasc Dis.* (2016) 25:781–91. doi: 10.1016/j.jstrokecerebrovasdis.2015.12.005
18. Park MC, Lee SW, Park YB, Chung NS, Lee SK. Clinical characteristics and outcomes of Takayasu's arteritis: analysis of 108 patients using standardized criteria for diagnosis, activity assessment, and angiographic classification. *Scand J Rheumatol.* (2005) 34:284. doi: 10.1080/03009740510026526
19. Couture P, Chazal T, Rosso C, Haroche J, Léger A, Hervier B, et al. Cerebrovascular events in Takayasu arteritis: a multicenter case-controlled study. *J Neurol.* (2018) 265:757–63. doi: 10.1007/s00415-018-8744-8
20. Takayama K, Nakagawa H, Iwasaki S, Taoka T, Myouchin K, Wada T, et al. Multiple cerebral aneurysms associated with Takayasu arteritis successfully treated with coil embolization. *Rad Med Med Imaging Rad Oncol.* (2008) 26:33–8. doi: 10.1007/s11604-007-0184-9
21. Camara-Lemarroy CR, Lara-Campos JG, Perez-Contreras E, Rodriguez-Gutierrez R, Galarza-Delgado DA. Takayasu's arteritis and posterior reversible encephalopathy syndrome: a case-based review. *Clin Rheumatol.* (2013) 32:409–15. doi: 10.1007/s10067-012-2151-9
22. Buttgereit F, Dejaco C, Matteson EL, Dasgupta B. Polymyalgia rheumatica and giant cell arteritis: a systematic review. *JAMA.* (2016) 315:2442–58. doi: 10.1001/jama.2016.5444
23. Salvarani C, Cimino L, Macchioni P, Consonni D, Cantini F, Bajocchi G, et al. Risk factors for visual loss in an Italian population-based cohort of patients with giant cell arteritis. *Arthritis Rheum.* (2005) 53:293–7. doi: 10.1002/art.21075
24. Pfadenhauer K, Roesler A, Golling A. The involvement of the peripheral nervous system in biopsy proven active giant cell arteritis. *J Neurol.* (2007) 254:751–5. doi: 10.1007/s00415-006-0428-0
25. Gonzalez-Gay MA, Vazquez-Rodriguez TR, Gomez-Acebo I, Pego-Reigosa R, Lopez-Diaz MJ, Vazquez-Tri-anes MC, et al. Strokes at time of disease diagnosis in a series of 287 patients with biopsy-proven giant cell arteritis. *Medicine.* (2009) 88:227. doi: 10.1097/MD.0b013e3181af4518

26. Ungprasert P, Wijarnpreecha K, Koster MJ, Thongprayoon C, Warrington KJ. Cerebrovascular accident in patients with giant cell arteritis: a systematic review and meta-analysis of cohort studies. *Semi Arthritis Rheum.* (2016) 46:361–6. doi: 10.1016/j.semarthrit.2016.07.005
27. Chazal T, Couture P, Rosso C, Haroche J, Léger A, Hervier B, et al. Cerebrovascular events are associated with lower survival in giant cell arteritis: a case-controlled multicenter study. *Joint Bone Spine.* (2018) 85:383–5. doi: 10.1016/j.jbspin.2017.05.017
28. Pego-Reigosa R, Garcia-Porrua C, Piã±Eiro A, Dierssen T, Llorca J, Gonzalez-Gay MA. Predictors of cerebrovascular accidents in giant cell arteritis in a defined population. *Clini Exp Rheumatol.* (2004) 22:13–7.
29. Rossi CM, Di Comite G. The clinical spectrum of the neurological involvement in vasculitides. *J Neurol Sci.* (2009) 285:13–21. doi: 10.1016/j.jns.2009.05.017
30. Amordorado JC, Llorca J, Garciaporrua C, Costa C, Perezfernandez N, Gonzalezgay MA. Audiovestibular manifestations in giant cell arteritis: a prospective study. *Medicine.* (2003) 82:13–26. doi: 10.1097/00005792-200301000-00002
31. Minagar A, Fowler M, Harris MK, Jaffe SL. Neurologic presentations of systemic vasculitides. *Neurol Clin.* (2010) 28:171–84. doi: 10.1016/j.ncl.2009.09.015
32. Lhote F, Cohen P, Guillevin L. Polyarteritis nodosa, microscopic polyangiitis and Churg-Strauss syndrome. *Semin Respir Crit Care Med.* (1998) 19:27–45. doi: 10.1055/s-2007-1009380
33. Reichart MD, Bogousslavsky J, Janzer RC. Early lacunar strokes complicating polyarteritis nodosa: thrombotic microangiopathy. *Neurology.* (2000) 54:883–9. doi: 10.1212/WNL.54.4.883
34. Moore PM, Cupps TR. Neurological complications of vasculitis. *Ann Neurol.* (2010) 14:155–67. doi: 10.1002/ana.410140202
35. Gomes V, Capela C, Rodrigues C, Gonc,alves F. Polyarteritis nodosa with central and peripheral neurological involvement. *Eur J Intern Med.* (2013) 24:e118. doi: 10.1016/j.ejim.2013.08.300
36. Guillevin L, Lhote F, Gayraud M, Cohen P, Jarrousse B, Lortholary O, et al. Prognostic factors in polyarteritis nodosa and Churg-Strauss syndrome. A prospective study in 342 patients. *Medicine.* (1996) 75:17–28. doi: 10.1097/00005792-199601000-00003
37. Arai M, Shigeno K, Wada M. [A reversible posterior leukoencephalopathy syndrome in a patient with classical polyarteritis nodosa]. *Rinsho shinkeigaku.* (1997) 37:64–6.
38. Navinan MR, Subasinghe CJ, Kandeepan T, Kulatunga A. Polyarteritis nodosa complicated by posterior reversible encephalopathy syndrome: a case report. *BMC Res Notes.* (2014) 7:89. doi: 10.1186/1756-0500-7-89
39. Stanzani L, Fusi L, Gomitoni A, Roncoroni M, Villa P, Grampa G. A case of posterior reversible encephalopathy during polyarteritis nodosa vasculitis. *Neurol Sci.* (2008) 29:163–7. doi: 10.1007/s10072-008-0929-y
40. Ueno KI, Matsushima A, Hineno A, Fukushima K, Tazawa KI, Matsuda M, et al. Polyarteritis nodosa with central nervous system involvement mimicking relapsingremitting multiple sclerosis. *Modern Rheumatol.* (2014) 24:525–8. doi: 10.3109/14397595.2013.852849
41. Oomura M, Yamawaki T, Naritomi H, Terai T, Shigeno K. Polyarteritis nodosa in association with subarachnoid hemorrhage. *Intern Med.* (2006) 45:655–8. doi: 10.2169/internalmedicine.45.1632
42. Ribi C, Cohen P, Pagnoux C, Mahr A, Arène JP, Puéchal X, et al. Treatment of polyarteritis nodosa and microscopic polyangiitis without poor-prognosis factors: a prospective randomized study of one hundred twenty-four patients. *Arthritis Rheum.* (2010) 62:1186–97. doi: 10.1002/art.27340
43. Song JS, Lim MK, Park BH, Park W. Acute pachymeningitis mimicking subdural hematoma in a patient with polyarteritis nodosa. *Rheumatol Int.* (2005) 25:637–40. doi: 10.1007/s00296-005-0615-9
44. Rubin F, Tran Khai Hoan N, Bonfils P. Sudden bilateral hearing loss revealing polyarteritis nodosa. *Eur Ann Otorhinol Head Neck Dis.* (2014) 131:265–6. doi: 10.1016/j.anorl.2014.03.003
45. Vazquez-Romo KA, Rodriguez-Hernandez A, Paczka JA, Nu-o-Suarez MA, Rocha-Mu-oz AD, Zavala-Cerna MG. Optic neuropathy secondary to polyarteritis nodosa, case report, and diagnostic challenges. *Front Neurol.* (2017) 8:490. doi: 10.3389/fneur.2017.00490
46. Alves NR, Magalhaes CM, Almeida Rde F, Santos RC, Gandolfi L, Pratesi R. Prospective study of Kawasaki disease complications: review of 115 cases. *Rev Assoc Med Bras.* (1992) 57:295–300.
47. Ishida A, Matsuo S, Kawamura S, Nishikawa T. Subarachnoid hemorrhage due to nonbranching aneurysm of the middle cerebral artery in a young adult with a history of Kawasaki disease. *Surg Neurol Int.* (2014) 5:5. doi: 10.4103/2152-7806.125285
48. Graf J. Central nervous system disease in antineutrophil cytoplasmic antibodies-associated vasculitis. *Rheum Dis Clini North Am.* (2017) 43:573–8. doi: 10.1016/j.rdc.2017.06.006
49. Imboden JB. Involvement of the peripheral nervous system in polyarteritis nodosa and antineutrophil cytoplasmic antibodies-associated vasculitis. *Rheum Dis Clini North Am.* (2017) 43:633–9. doi: 10.1016/j.rdc.2017.06.011
50. De Groot K, Schmidt DK, Arlt AC, Gross WL, Reinhold-Keller E. Standardized neurologic evaluations of 128 patients with Wegener granulomatosis. *Arch Neurol.* (2001) 58:1215–21. doi: 10.1001/archneur.58.8.1215
51. Nishino H, Rubino FA, DeRemee RA, Swanson JW, Parisi JE. Neurological involvement in Wegener's granulomatosis: an analysis of 324 consecutive patients at the Mayo Clinic. *Ann Neurol.* (1993) 33:4–9. doi: 10.1002/ana.410330103
52. Choi HA, Lee MJ, Chung CS. Characteristics of hypertrophic pachymeningitis in patients with granulomatosis with polyangiitis. *Cephalalgia.* (2016) 36:169–70. doi: 10.1177/0333102416670318
53. Stone JH. Limited versus severe Wegener's granulomatosis: baseline data on patients in the Wegener's granulomatosis etanercept trial. *Arthritis Rheum.* (2003) 48:2299. doi: 10.1002/art.11075
54. Reinholdkeller E, Beuge N, Latza U, De GK, Rudert H, Nölle B, et al. An interdisciplinary approach to the care of patients with Wegener's granulomatosis: long-term outcome in 155 patients. *Arthritis Rheum.* (2000) 43:1021–32. doi: 10.1002/1529--0131(200005)43:5<1021::AID-ANR10>3.0.CO;2-J
55. Seror R, Mahr A, Ramanoelina J, Pagnoux C, Cohen P, Guillevin L. Central nervous system involvement in wegener granulomatosis. *Medicine.* (2006) 85:54–65. doi: 10.1097/01.md.0000200166.90373.41
56. Kapoor E, Cartin-Ceba R, Specks U, Leavitt J, Erickson B, Erickson D. Pituitary dysfunction in granulomatosis with polyangiitis: the mayo clinic experience. *J Clini Endocrinol Metabol.* (2014) 99:3988–94. doi: 10.1210/jc.2014-1962
57. De Parisot A, Puechal X, Langrand C, Raverot G, Gil H, Perard L, et al. Pituitary involvement in granulomatosis with polyangiitis: report of 9 patients and review of the literature. *Medicine.* (2015) 94:e748. doi: 10.1097/MD.0000000000000748
58. De Luna G, Terrier B, Kaminsky P, Le Quellec A, Maurier F, Solans R, et al. Central nervous system involvement of granulomatosis with polyangiitis: clinical-radiological presentation distinguishes different outcomes. *Rheumatology.* (2015) 54:424–32. doi: 10.1093/rheumatology/keu336
59. Arteaga-Müller G, Camara-Lemarroy CR, Rizo-Topete L, Guerrero-González E, Sánchez-Martinez C, Cruz-Valdez J. Granulomatosis with polyangiitis and posterior reversible encephalopathy syndrome. *J Neurol Sci.* (2016) 362:204–5. doi: 10.1016/j.jns.2016.01.048
60. Zabihiyeganeh MO, Jahed AD, Poormoghim HA. Reversible posterior leukoencephalopathy and splenic infarction in a patient with Wegener granulomatosis. *Int J Rheum Dis.* (2010) 13:232. doi: 10.1111/j.1756-185X.2010.01524.x
61. Ohta T, Sakano T, Shiotsu M, Furue T, Ohtani H, Kinoshita Y, et al. Reversible posterior leukoencephalopathy in a patient with Wegener granulomatosis. *Pediatr Nephrol.* (2004) 19:442–4. doi: 10.1007/s00467-003-1286-y
62. Pugnet G, Pagnoux C, Bézanahary H, Ly KH, Vidal E, Guillevin L. Progressive multifocal encephalopathy after cyclophosphamide in granulomatosis with polyangiitis (wegener) patients: case report and review of the literature. *Clini Exp Rheumatol.* (2013) 31(Suppl. 75):S62–4.

63. Peters JE, Gupta V, Saeed IT, Offiah C, Jawad ASM. Severe localised granulomatosis with polyangiitis (Wegener's granulomatosis) manifesting with extensive cranial nerve palsies and cranial diabetes insipidus: a case report and literature review. *BMC Neurol.* (2018) 18:59. doi: 10.1186/s12883-018-1058-8
64. Cattaneo L, Chierici E, Pavone L, Grasselli C, Manganelli P, Buzio C, et al. Peripheral neuropathy in Wegener's granulomatosis, Churg-Strauss syndrome and microscopic polyangiitis. *J Neurol Neurosurg Psychiatr.* (2007) 78:1119–23. doi: 10.1136/jnnp.2006.111013
65. Sehgal M, Swanson JW, DeRemee RA, Colby TV. Neurologic manifestations of Churg-Strauss syndrome. *Mayo Clini Proc.* (1995) 70:337–41. doi: 10.4065/70.4.337
66. Hattori N, Ichimura M, Nagamatsu M, Li M, Yamamoto K, Kumazawa K, et al. Clinicopathological features of Churg-Strauss syndrome-associated neuropathy. *Brain.* (1999) 122(Pt 3):427–39. doi: 10.1093/brain/122.3.427
67. Guillevin L, Cohen P, Gayraud M, Lhote F, Jarrousse B, Casassus P. Churg-Strauss syndrome. Clinical study and long-term follow-up of 96 patients. *Medicine.* (1999) 78:26–37. doi: 10.1097/00005792-199901000-00003
68. Decker ML, Emery DJ, Smyth PS, Lu JQ, Lacson A, Yacyshyn E. Microscopic polyangiitis with spinal cord involvement: a case report and review of the literature. *J Stroke Cerebrovasc Dis.* (2016) 25:1696–704. doi: 10.1016/j.jstrokecerebrovasdis.2016.01.034
69. Camara-Lemarroy CR, Cruz-Moreno MA, Gamboa-Sarquis RN, Gonzalez-Padilla KA, Tamez-Perez HE, Galarza-Delgado DA. Goodpasture syndrome and posterior reversible encephalopathy syndrome. *J Neurol Sci.* (2015) 354:135–7. doi: 10.1016/j.jns.2015.05.002
70. Lahmer T, Kuchle C, Schirmer L, Heemann U, Lutz J, Thurmel K. Kidney transplant after preexisting posterior reversible encephalopathy syndrome induced by Goodpasture's syndrome. *Exp Clini Transplant.* (2012) 10:299–301. doi: 10.6002/ect.2011.0177
71. Ozkok A, Elcioglu OC, Bakan A, Atilgan KG, Alisir S, Odabas AR. Reversible posterior leukoencephalopathy in the course of Goodpasture syndrome. *Renal Failure.* (2012) 34:254–6. doi: 10.3109/0886022X.2011.647211
72. Cha B, Kim DY, Jang H, Hwang SD, Choi HJ, Kim MJ. Unusual case of posterior reversible encephalopathy syndrome in a patient with anti-glomerular basement membrane antibody glomerulonephritis: a case report and review of the literature. *Electrolyte Blood Pressure.* (2017) 15:12–6. doi: 10.5049/EBP.2017.15.1.12
73. Gutiérrez-Sánchez MJ, Petkov-Stoyanov V, Martín-Navarro JA. Reversible posterior leukoencephalopathy syndrome in Goodpasture syndrome. *Nefrologia.* (2012) 32:540–3. doi: 10.3265/Nefrologia.pre2012.Mar.11427
74. Terrier B, Cacoub P. Cryoglobulinemia vasculitis: an update. *Curr Opinion Rheumatol.* (2013) 25:10–8. doi: 10.1097/BOR.0b013e32835b15f7
75. Terrier B, Krastinova E, Marie I, Launay D, Lacraz A, Belenotti P, et al. Management of noninfectious mixed cryoglobulinemia vasculitis: data from 242 cases included in the CryoVas survey. *Blood.* (2012) 119:5996–6004. doi: 10.1182/blood-2011-12-396028
76. Ferri C, La Civita L, Cirafisi C, Siciliano G, Longombardo G, Bombardieri S, et al. Peripheral neuropathy in mixed cryoglobulinemia: clinical and electrophysiologic investigations. *J Rheumatol.* (1992) 19:889–95.
77. Ortiz-Sanjuán F, Calvo- Río V, Loricera J, Mata C, Penagos LM, Alvarez L, et al. Henoch-schönlein purpura: clinical spectrum of the disease in 417 patients from a single center. *Arthritis Rheum.* (2013) 65:S1122. doi: 10.1002/art.38216
78. Garzoni L, Vanoni F, Rizzi M, Simonetti GD, Simonetti BG, Ramelli GP, et al. Nervous system dysfunction in Henoch-Schönlein syndrome: systematic review of the literature. *Rheumatology.* (2009) 48:1524–9. doi: 10.1093/rheumatology/kep282
79. Soydemir Ö, Dotan Ak P, Aktan Z, Gözke E. Peripheral neuropathy: rare manifestation in Henoch-Schönlein purpura. *Eur J Neurol.* (2014) 21:711.
80. De Luna G, Vasco PG, Terrier B, Calleja JL, Fraile G. Henoch Schönlein purpura at diagnosis in 3 adult patients: acute onset with peripheral nervous system dysfunction. *Eur J Intern Med.* (2013) 24:e116. doi: 10.1016/j.ejim.2013.08.294
81. Fukushima K. Severe intestinal lesions and neuropathy associated with henoch-schonlein purpura. *Intern Med.* (2013) 52:2009–10. doi: 10.2169/internalmedicine.52.0616
82. Campbell SB, Hawley CM, Staples C. Mononeuritis multiplex complicating Henoch-Schonlein purpura. *Aust N Z J Med.* (1994) 24:580. doi: 10.1111/j.1445-5994.1994.tb01767.x
83. Fiaux E, Benhamou Y, Cailleux N, Levesque H. A rare case of Henoch-Schönlein purpura with neurological involvement. *Intern Med J.* (2010) 40:795–6. doi: 10.1111/j.1445-5994.2010.02298.x
84. Karamadoukis L, Ludeman L, Williams AJ. Henoch-Schönlein purpura with intracerebral haemorrhage in an adult patient: a case report. *J Med Case Rep.* (2008) 2:200. doi: 10.1186/1752-1947-2-200
85. Chuah J, Meaney T. Anterior ischaemic optic neuropathy secondary to Henoch-Schönlein Purpura. *Eye.* (2005) 19:1028. doi: 10.1038/sj.eye.6701764
86. Fielding RE, Hawkins CP, Hand MF, Heath PD, Davies SJ. Seizures complicating adult Henoch-Schonlein purpura. *Nephrol Dialysis Transplant.* (1998) 13:761–2. doi: 10.1093/ndt/13.3.759
87. Perez C, Maravi E, Olier J, Guarch R. MR imaging of encephalopathy in adult Henoch-Shonlein purpura. *Am J Roentgenol.* (2000) 175:922–3. doi: 10.2214/ajr.175.3.1750922a
88. Filosto M, Cavallaro T, Pasolini G, Broglio L, Tentorio M, Cotelli M, et al. Idiopathic hypocomplementemic urticarial vasculitis-linked neuropathy. *J Neurol Sci.* (2009) 284:179–81. doi: 10.1016/j.jns.2009.03.027
89. Lieberman J, Gephardt G, Calabrese LH. Urticaria, nephritis, and pseudotumor cerebri. *Cleve Clin J Med.* (1990) 57:197–210. doi: 10.3949/ccjm.57.2.197
90. Koul PA, Wahid A, Shah SU, Koul AN, Saleem SM. Hypocomplementemic urticarial vasculitis and lower cranial nerve palsies. *J Assoc Physicians India.* (2000) 48:536–7.
91. Al-Araji A, Kidd DP. Neuro-Behçet's disease: epidemiology, clinical characteristics, and management. *Lancet Neurol.* (2009) 8:192–204. doi: 10.1016/S1474-4422(09)70015-8
92. Akman-Demir G, Serdaroglu P, Tasçi B. Clinical patterns of neurological involvement in Behcet's disease: evaluation of 200 patients. *Brain.* (1999) 122:2171–81. doi: 10.1093/brain/122.11.2171
93. Siva A, Kantarci OH, Saip S, Altintas A, Hamuryudan V, Islak C, et al. Behçet's disease: diagnostic and prognostic aspects of neurological involvement. *J Neurol.* (2001) 248:95–103. doi: 10.1007/s004150170242
94. Farah S, Al-Shubaili A, Montaser A, Hussein JM, Malaviya AN, Mukhtar M, et al. Behcet's syndrome: a report of 41 patients with emphasis on neurological manifestations. *J Neurol Neurosurg Psychiatr.* (1998) 64:382–4. doi: 10.1136/jnnp.64.3.382
95. Davatchi F, Chams-Davatchi C, Shams H, Nadji A, Faezi T, Akhlaghi M, et al. Adult Behcet's disease in Iran: analysis of 6075 patients. *Int J Rheum Dis.* (2016) 19:95–103. doi: 10.1111/1756-185X.12691
96. Kidd DP. Neurological complications of Behcet's syndrome. *J Neurol.* (2017) 264:2178–83. doi: 10.1007/s00415-017-8436-9
97. Siva A, Saip S. The spectrum of nervous system involvement in Behçet's syndrome and its differential diagnosis. *J Neurol.* (2009) 256:513–29. doi: 10.1007/s00415-009-0145-6
98. Kurtuncu M, Aydin BN, Gunduz T, Ala S, Akman-Demir G. Neuro-Behcet's disease: analysis of 430 patients. *J Neurol Sci.* (2017) 381:121–2. doi: 10.1016/j.jns.2017.08.376
99. Al-Fahad SA, Al-Araji AH. Neuro-Behcet's disease in Iraq: a study of 40 patients. *J Neurol Sci.* (1999) 170:105–11. doi: 10.1016/S0022-510X(99)00165-3
100. Kidd D, Steuer A, Denman AM, Rudge P. Neurological complications in Behçet's syndrome. *Brain.* (1999) 122:2183–94. doi: 10.1093/brain/122.11.2183
101. Hirohata S. Histopathology of central nervous system lesions in Behcet's disease. *J Neurol Sci.* (2008) 267:41–7. doi: 10.1016/j.jns.2007.09.041
102. Kurt EA, Kocer N, Ozguler Y, Ucar D, Uygunoglu U, Islak C, et al. An outcome survey of 100 patients with cerebral venous sinus thrombosis due to Behcet's syndrome followed up at a single, dedicated center. *Arthritis Rheumatol.* (2016) 68:3966–7. doi: 10.1002/art.39977
103. Kutlu G, Semercioglu S, Ucler S, Erdal A, Inan LE. Epileptic seizures in Neuro-Behcet disease: why some patients develop seizure and others not? *Seizure.* (2015) 26:32–5. doi: 10.1016/j.seizure.2015.01.013

104. Gluth MB, Baratz KH, Matteson EL, Driscoll CL. Cogan syndrome: a retrospective review of 60 patients throughout a half century. *Mayo Clin Proc.* (2006) 81:483–8. doi: 10.4065/81.4.483

105. Van DS, Mccoll G, Walter M, Jennens I, Bhathal P, Wicks IP. Prolonged prodrome, systemic vasculitis, and deafness in cogan's syndrome. *Ann Rheum Dis.* (2001) 60:69–71. doi: 10.1136/ard.60.1.69

106. Antonios N, Silliman S. Cogan syndrome: an analysis of reported neurological manifestations. *Neurologist.* (2012) 18:55–63. doi: 10.1097/NRL.0b013e31823fa3a0

107. Grasland A, Pouchot J, Hachulla E, Blétry O, Papo T, Vinceneux P. Typical and atypical Cogan's syndrome: 32 cases and review of the literature. *Rheumatology.* (2004) 43:1007. doi: 10.1093/rheumatology/keh228

108. Bicknell JM, Holland JV. Neurologic manifestations of Cogan syndrome. *Neurology.* (1978) 28:278–81. doi: 10.1212/WNL.28.3.278

15

Application of Plasma Exchange in Steroid-Responsive Encephalopathy

Yuting Jiang [1†], Xin Tian [1†], Yixue Gu [1], Feng Li [1] and Xuefeng Wang [1,2]*

[1] *Chongqing Key Laboratory of Neurology, Department of Neurology, the First Affiliated Hospital of Chongqing Medical University, Chongqing, China,*
[2] *Center of Epilepsy, Beijing Institute for Brain Disorders, Beijing, China*

***Correspondence:**
Xuefeng Wang
xfyp@163.com*

† These author have contributed equally to this work and share first authorship

Plasma exchange has been widely used in autoimmune neurological diseases and is the standard treatment for myasthenia gravis crisis and Guillain-Barre syndrome. A growing body of research suggests that, in the clinical application of steroid-responsive encephalopathy, such as for Hashimoto's encephalopathy, limbic encephalitis, systemic lupus erythematosus encephalopathy, ANCA-associated vasculitis encephalopathy, and acute disseminated encephalomyelitis, plasma exchange is a safe, and effective option when steroids or other immunosuppressive therapies are ineffective in the short term or when contraindications are present. Additionally, plasma exchange can also be used alone or in combination with steroids, immunoglobulins, or other immunosuppressive agents to treat steroid-responsive encephalopathy. This paper reviews the clinical application of plasma exchange in steroid-responsive encephalopathy, including its indications, onset time, course, curative effects, and side effects.

Keywords: plasma exchange, steroid, clinical practice, course, onset time, side effects

INTRODUCTION

Plasma exchange is also known as therapeutic plasma exchange (1). The seventh special issue of the Therapeutic Apheresis in Clinical Practice treatment guidelines, published in 2016 by the American Society for Apheresis, defines plasma exchange as a therapeutic procedure in which the patient's blood is separated into plasma and other blood components by medical devices, and then the plasma is removed and replaced by a replacement solution such as a colloidal solution (albumin and/or plasma) or a combination of crystal/colloidal solutions, thus eliminating or reducing unwanted substances (2). Castillo et al. (3) considered encephalopathy to be accompanied by cognitive impairment and one or more of the following: (i) neuropsychiatric symptoms (hallucinations or delusions and paranoia); (ii) myoclonus; (iii) seizure; and/or (iv) focal neurologic deficits. Steroid responsiveness refers to the complete or nearly complete return to normal neurological baseline status after steroid treatment, while steroid unresponsiveness refers to lack of improvement after at least 4–6 weeks of a sufficient dose of steroids (4). In this paper, steroid-responsive encephalopathy is a general term used to describe diseases characterized by diffuse brain injury and their responsiveness to steroids. These diseases include Hashimoto's encephalopathy, limbic encephalitis, systemic lupus erythematosus encephalopathy, ANCA-associated vasculitis encephalopathy, and acute disseminated encephalomyelitis. Plasma exchange is a rapid-onset, safe, and effective option for patients with steroid-responsive encephalopathy who fail to respond to steroids in the short term or for patients who are unable to tolerate the side effects of steroid therapies. It can also be used as an initial treatment (see **Table 1**).

HISTORY OF PLASMA EXCHANGE

Plasma exchange dates back to 1914. Able et al. (18) described the separation of cell components and plasma from the blood of dogs with uremia. The separated components were mixed with replacement solution and then returned to the subject. Regular plasma exchange began to be used in humans in 1952. Researchers found that repeated plasma exchange reduced the amount of pathological proteins in patients with multiple myeloma (19). In 1960, Schwab and Fahey (20) reported that plasma exchange in Waldenstrom's macroglobulin and hyperviscosity syndrome achieved good therapeutic effects. Therefore, plasma exchange became the standard treatment for Waldenstrom's macroglobulin. In the 1980s, studies reported that plasma exchange was an effective treatment for systemic lupus erythematosus encephalopathy and acute disseminated encephalomyelitis; thereafter, plasma exchange began to be used as a treatment for steroid-responsive encephalopathy (4, 21).

UNKNOWN MECHANISMS OF PLASMA EXCHANGE OR POTENTIALLY INVOLVED MECHANISMS UNDER EXPLORATION

Clearing Pathogenic Antibodies From Plasma

The mechanism of plasma exchange for treating systemic lupus erythematosus encephalopathy is the rapid removal of pathogenic autoantibodies such as anti-nuclear antibodies from the blood (22). Anti-neutrophil cytoplasmic antibodies (ANCAs) play an important role in the pathogenesis of ANCA-related vasculitis encephalopathy, and the clearance of pathogenic antibodies from blood by plasma exchange can improve the therapeutic effects (2). Plasma exchange can also effectively remove pathogenic antibodies and can be combined with immunotherapy to suppress the production of autoantibodies and effectively treat limbic encephalitis (23). The mechanism of plasma exchange for treating acute disseminated encephalomyelitis is the removal of autoantibodies (antibodies against myelin oligodendrocyte glycoprotein) as well as complement components and cytokines (4).

Increasing the Susceptibility of Antibody-Producing Cells to Immunosuppressant and Chemotherapeutic Drugs

Plasma exchange can also induce proliferation of antibody-producing cells and increase the synthetic ability of antibodies as well as the susceptibility of antibody-producing cells to immunosuppressive or chemotherapy drugs (23). Studies have reported that plasma exchange can increase the synthetic activity of B cells and increase the susceptibility of antibody-producing cells to immunosuppressive agents (24).

Removing Immune Complexes From Plasma and Enhancing the Function of Macrophages and Monocytes

Plasma exchange can not only directly promote the removal of immune complexes from patients with systemic lupus erythematosus (22) but also upregulate red blood cell (RBC) complement receptors and increase the binding of RBC and immune complexes to remove immune complexes from the circulation. Steven et al. (25) studied the effect of plasma exchange on monocyte function and found that monocytes significantly increased their bactericidal effect by increasing the level of proteolytic enzymes in immune-complex-mediated diseases.

Removing Pathogenic Cytokines and Adhesion Molecules From Plasma

The concentration of soluble adhesion molecules ICAM-1 and VCAM-1 may be decreased after plasma exchange in patients with ANCA-associated vasculitis (26). Yeh et al. (27) found that double-filtration plasmapheresis can effectively remove IL-2, IL-4, IL-5, tumor necrosis factor alpha, and interferon gamma from the serum of patients.

CLINICAL APPLICATION OF PLASMA EXCHANGE IN STEROID-RESPONSIVE ENCEPHALOPATHY

Indications of Plasma Exchange for the Treatment of Steroid-Responsive Encephalopathy

Therapeutic plasma exchange is an established treatment method for known or suspected immune-mediated diseases (28). In 2016, the American Society for Apheresis published treatment guidelines for plasma exchange based on evidence-based medical research and proposed that Hashimoto's encephalopathy is a category II indication for plasma exchange and that the recommended level is 2C. Anti-N-methyl-D-aspartate receptor encephalitis is a category I indication, and the recommended level is 1C. Plasma exchange for the treatment of severe systemic lupus erythematosus, including systemic lupus erythematosus encephalopathy, is a category II indication, and the recommended level is 2C (2). Plasma exchange for the treatment of acute disseminated encephalomyelitis is a class II indication, and the recommended level is 2C (2) (See **Tables 2, 3**).

Volume, Interval Time, and Frequency of Plasma Exchange for the Treatment of Steroid-Responsive Encephalopathy

The efficacy of plasma exchange is often related to the volume of plasma exchanged, which is dependent on the estimated plasma volume of the patient. The formula for estimating the plasma volume of the patient uses the patient's weight and hematocrit: $EPV=[0.065 \times wt\ (kg)] \times [1-Hct]$. This formula provides a reliable prediction of the therapeutic effect in clinical

TABLE 1 | Case reports of plasma exchange for steroid-responsive encephalopathy.

References	Diagnosis	Number	Clinical feature	Failed treatments	Process of plasma exchange	Side effects	Therapeutic effect
Nagpal and Pande (5)	Hashimoto's encephalopathy	One	52-year-old female, aphasia, memory loss, and tremor	Corticosteroids, thyroxine	Three plasma exchange procecures; the volume of Plasma exchanged per procedure was 1.8 L.	Not mentioned	After the third plasma exchange, all neuropsychiatric symptoms improved.
Gul et al. (6)	Hashimoto's encephalopathy	Two	Case 1: 8-year-old female, status epilepticus	Antiepileptic drugs, immunoglobulin, steroids	Five sessions	Not mentioned	Status epilepticus was controlled after plasma exchange.
			Case 2: 17-year-old female, status epilepticus	Immunoglobulin, Antiepileptic drugs, steroids	Five sessions	Not mentioned	After plasma exchange, epilepsy was controlled without recurrence.
Simmons and Staley (7)	Hashimoto's encephalopathy	Two	Case 1: 55-year-old female, gait ataxia, memory loss, mood change	Mycophenolate, mofetil	Five sessions; the volume of plasma exchanged per session was one times the plasma volume.	Slight citrate toxicity	Three months after plasma exchange, the patient's gait ataxia improved without obvious changes in daily activities.
			Case 2: 49-year-old female, insomnia, altered state of consciousness, mental symptoms	Steroids, immunoglobulin	Two course courses no. 1 (one times the plasma volume/session for five sessions), the second and third course were all (one times the plasma volume/session for three sessions	Transient hypotension, headache	After the first plasma exchange, orientation and daily activity improved, and the anti-thyroid peroxidase antibody was reduced from >1,000 units before plasma exchange to 286 units. The anti-thyroid peroxidase antibody was 538 units at 1 month after the first course of plasma exchange, the psychiatric symptoms were improved after the second and third courses, and the anti-thyroid peroxidase antibody was <63 units after the third course of plasma exchange.
Endres et al. (8)	Hashimoto's encephalopathy	One	55-year-old female, rapid progressive dementia, stupor, silence	Antidepressants, antipsychotics, steroids	Five sessions	Not mentioned	After plasma exchange, all symptoms were significantly improved, but verbal fluency was still lacking.
Tran et al. (9)	Hashimoto's encephalopathy	One	72-year-old female, cerebellar ataxia, cognitive dysfunction	Steroids, mycophenolate, immunoglobulin	Induction period: Two sessions/week for 6 weeks and then one procedure/week (1.5 times the plasma volume for 6 weeks, followed by 2 sessions/week (one times the plasma volume) and then 1 procedure/week. After 9.5 months, readjust to two sessions/week	Citrate toxicity somnolence lower limb spasm	Clinical symptoms were alleviated after the induction of plasma exchange, the patient could walk normally, and memory was restored. Anti-thyroid peroxidase antibody levels decreased, but when the plasma exchange sessions were reduced to one procedure/week, and the patient experienced recurrence. Therefore, plasma exchange was administered at the rate of 2 sessions/week, and the patient's gait was improved (stable and lively).

(Continued)

TABLE 1 | Continued

References	Diagnosis	Number	Clinical feature	Failed treatments	Process of plasma exchange	Side effects	Therapeutic effect
Batra et al. (10)	Anti-NMDA receptor limbic encephalitis	One	34-year-old female, abnormal mental behavior,	Acyclovir, immunoglobulin	1.2 times the plasma volume/ procedure for five sessions, once every other day, with 5% albumin as the replacement fluid	Not mentioned	Symptoms improved significantly after 1 month, and antibody tests were negative. Symptoms were significantly relieved.
Mazzi et al. (11)	Nonparaneoplastic limbic encephalitis associated with the anti-GAD antibody	One	21-year-old female, intractable epilepsy, memory loss	Antiepileptics, steroids, immunoglobulin	Sixteen sessions with 1.4 times the plasma volume replaced during each procedure	Not mentioned	Seizures were significantly reduced after the third plasma exchange session.
Martin et al. (12)	Anti-VGKC antibody-positive limbic encephalitis	One	69-year-old male, memory loss, Abnormal mental behavior	Steroids, immunoglobulin, mycophenolate, mofetil	One time the plasma volume/session (2 sessions/week) for 6 weeks	Not mentioned	Anti-VGKC antibody levels decreased, and clinical symptoms were well controlled.
Özkale et al. (13)	Two cases of anti-NMDA receptor encephalitis One case of serologic negative Autoimmune Limbic encephalitis One case of paraneoplastic limbic Encephalitis	Four	Headache, Status epilepticus psychiatric symptom	Steroid, immunoglobulin	Six sessions on average	Not mentioned	The neurological symptoms of all patients improved after plasma exchange.
Hussein et al. (14)	Systemic lupus erythematosus encephalopathy	One	17-year-old female headache, double vision, facial paralysis	Cyclosporin	Six sessions	Not mentioned	Cyclophosphamide and methylprednisolone (1 g/d for 3 days) combined with six plasma exchange resulted in significant improvement in clinical symptoms.
Bartolucci et al. (15)	Systemic lupus erythematosus encephalopathy	Ten	Average age: 30 Female: 8, male: 2 psychiatric symptoms, aseptic meningitis, cognitive decline	Not mentioned	Three sessions/week for three weeks and then two or three sessions/week, according to the clinical outcome	Not mentioned	After plasma exchange, 54% (7/13) had complete remission, and 46% (6/13) had partial remission. The European consensus lupus activity score (ECLAM) and systematic lupus activity index (SLEDAI) decreased to 1.2 and 3.9 respectively from 6.9 and 30.7.Disappeared upon head MRI examination, and consciousness level and mental state began to recover. The PR3-ANCA antibody decreased from 164 U/ml to 15.7 U/ml.
Shinozaki et al. (16)	Acute disseminated encephalomyelitis	One	Headache, confused and delirious state, no eyelash, corneal or light reflexes	Intravenous methylprednisolone (1,000 mg per day for 5 days)	Plasma exchange (PE) plus continuous hemodiafiltration using 1.5 times the circulating plasma volume, daily PE with CHDF for 3 days	Not mentioned	On the day after initiation of SPE + CHDF, the patient's corneal and bilateral light reflexes were dramatically recovered.
Balestri et al. (17)	Acute disseminated encephalomyelitis	One	An eight-year-old female, comatose and generalized tonic-clonic seizures, unable to raise her head, walk, or speak, and facial paresis	Methylprednisolone, immunoglobulin, and Interferon beta-1b	Six courses with 1,400 cc of plasma exchanged once every 2 days)	Not mentioned	Dramatic recovery was observed over the next 2 weeks, and the patient was able to walk, speak, and raise her left forearm.

TABLE 2 | Category of recommendation for plasma exchange (2).

Category for plasma exchange	Detailed description
I	Plasma exchange is used as first-line treatment alone or in conjunction with other treatments.
II	Plasma exchange is used as second-line treatment alone or in conjunction with other treatments.
III	The optimal role of plasma exchange has not been determined, and decisions should be personalized.
IV	Published evidence confirms or suggests that plasma exchange is ineffective or even harmful and that IRB approval is required if it is to be used in these circumstances.

applications. In general, macromolecular substances (immune globulin, lipoprotein cholesterol, cold globulin, etc.) inside and outside of blood vessels become slowly redistributed, achieving a gradual balance. Thus, clearance during a single treatment is limited. One is the concentration of substances in the blood vessels, while the other is the volume of plasma exchanged. Based on these two factors, the percentage of the decrease in pathogenic substances after treatment compared with the pretreatment level can be determined as follows: $X_1 = X_{0e}\text{-}V_e/\mathrm{EPV}$, where X_1 is the final plasma concentration, X_{0e} is the initial plasma concentration, V_e is the volume of plasma exchange, and EPV is the estimated plasma volume of patients. If the volume of plasma exchange is equal to the patient's EPV, pretreatment values will drop by 63%, and if the volume of plasma exchange is equal to 1.4 times the EPV, pretreatment values will drop by 75%. However, in the process of a single exchange, the volume of plasma exchanged is further increased. As a result, the pretreatment level decreases less, and thus, the exchange volume would increase, subsequently increasing the duration of treatment and associated costs. For most indications of plasma exchange (including Hashimoto's encephalopathy, limbic encephalitis, systemic lupus erythematosus encephalopathy, ANCA-associated vasculitis encephalopathy, acute disseminated encephalomyelitis, etc.), the volume of plasma exchanged per treatment is 1–1.5 times the plasma volume (30). For a single plasma exchange treatment, this volume will not cause reductions in the overall load of the serum levels caused by partial rebound. Several consecutive plasma exchange sessions, separated by 24–48 h, can remove a substantial percentage of the total body burden. In general, if the rate of production is moderate, then at least five sessions within 7–10 days are required to remove 90% of the patient's initial overall load, and additional sessions will be needed if the production is rapid (30).

Curative Effects

Cook et al. (31) retrospectively analyzed plasma exchange for the treatment of 10 Hashimoto's encephalopathy cases and showed that 90% of the symptoms of Hashimoto's encephalopathy significantly improved after plasma exchange. Neuwelt (32) reported the use of plasma exchange in eight systemic lupus erythematosus encephalopathy patients who failed to respond to

TABLE 3 | Recommended levels for plasma exchange (2, 29).

Recommendation	Grade 1A	Grade 1B	Grade 1C	Grade 2A	Grade 2B	Grade 2C
The quality of evidence	RCT without significant limitation or overwhelming evidence from observational studies.	RCT has important limitations (inconsistent results, methodological defects) or exceptionally strong evidence from observational studies.	Case series or observational studies.	RCT without significant limitation or overwhelming evidence from observational studies.	RCT has important limitations (inconsistent results, methodological defects) or exceptionally strong evidence from observational studies.	Case series or observational studies.
Detailed description	Strong recommendation, high-quality evidence.	Strong recommendation, moderate-quality evidence.	Strong recommendation, low-quality, or very low-quality evidence.	Weak recommendation, high-quality evidence.	Weak recommendation, moderate-quality evidence.	Weak recommendation, low-quality, or very low-quality evidence.

cyclophosphamide, among whom six were completely relieved of their clinical symptoms. In 2010, a non-blinded prospective study by Wong et al. (33) included nine cases of limbic encephalitis with positive anti-VGKC antibody, and each patient underwent five plasma exchange sessions combined with steroid and immunoglobulin treatment. After treatment, the VGKC antibody titer of all patients returned to normal within 1–4 months. After 1–3 months, clinical and cognitive tests showed that memory function had improved. After 6–9 months, the swelling subsided, and the signal was recovered on brain MRI.

Adverse Reactions

Plasma exchange is a relatively safe treatment, mostly with reports of only mild side effects, of which the most common are hypotension, hypocalcemia, urticaria, bleeding (due to loss of platelets or clotting factors), and arrhythmia. These adverse reactions are mainly related to anticoagulants, the replacement fluid used, and central venous catheterization. The incidence of hypocalcemia is 1.5–9% and is related to citrate. The main symptoms include paresthesia, muscle spasm, and arrhythmia. In addition, acid-base imbalance can be induced by citrate. The use of albumin as a replacement fluid may lead to the consumption of clotting factors and immunoglobulin and thus increase the risk of bleeding and infection. Fresh frozen plasma used as a replacement solution may cause HIV and hepatitis virus infection (34). Adverse reactions associated with central venous catheterization include infection, sepsis, thrombosis, and pneumothorax. Hemolysis and hypotension may occur, but the incidence of serious side effects such as severe hypotension, acute pulmonary edema, myocardial infarction, and death is 1.6–22% (35). In 2007, the world plasma exchange registry reported that the incidence of side effects from plasma exchange was 5.7% and that no death occurred in 838 patients who underwent plasma exchange; a plasma exchange team in Canada analyzed 91,000 sessions of plasma exchange and found that the incidence of serious side effects caused by plasma exchange was 0.4%. In addition, blood transfusion-related side effects are more common when plasma is used as the replacement fluid (36). Basic-Jukic et al. (34) studied the side effects of plasma exchange in the treatment of neurological diseases, including 152 patients from January 1982 to December 2003, with a total of 4,857 plasma exchanges performed. The incidence of side effects was 4.74% (231/4857), and the side effects were mostly mild to moderate. In summary, a few studies have reported on the side effects of plasma exchange for steroid-responsive encephalopathy, the results indicate that plasma exchange may be a safe treatment for steroid-responsive encephalopathy.

APPLICATION OF PLASMA EXCHANGE IN DIFFERENT TYPES OF STEROID-RESPONSIVE ENCEPHALOPATHY

Application of Plasma Exchange in Hashimoto's Encephalopathy

Hashimoto's encephalopathy (also known as autoimmune thyroiditis-related steroid-responsive encephalopathy) was first reported by the British scholar Brain in 1966. Hashimoto's encephalopathy is related to Hashimoto's thyroiditis, as anti-thyroid antibodies were found in serum. The patients' thyroid function can be classified as normal, hypothyroidism or hyperthyroidism (37, 38). The clinical manifestations mainly include two types: vasculitis type, mainly including recurrent stroke-like episodes, seizures, and mental abnormality, and diffuse progressive type, which manifests as cognitive dysfunction (including memory and language dysfunction) dementia, behavior change, confusion, mental derangement, and coma (5). The most common clinical manifestations are seizures, followed by psychiatric symptoms (39). Elevated levels of anti-thyroid peroxidase antibodies (anti-TPOAb) and/or anti-thyroglobulin antibodies (anti-TgAb) are important laboratory characteristics for the diagnosis of Hashimoto's encephalopathy; elevated anti-thyroid peroxidase antibody levels are most common and are observed in 86% of patients with Hashimoto's encephalopathy, while 48% of the patients with Hashimoto's encephalopathy have elevated anti-thyroglobulin antibody levels (6). Although the pathophysiological mechanism of Hashimoto's encephalopathy is still not clear, high concentrations of anti-thyroid antibodies and effective treatment with immunosuppressive agents both support the important role of autoimmune mechanisms in Hashimoto's encephalopathy (40), which is the theoretical basis of plasma exchange in the treatment of Hashimoto's encephalopathy. Although steroids are the first-line treatment for Hashimoto's encephalopathy (41), no randomized controlled trials have been performed, so the optimal dose and duration of steroids remain unclear. Steroid responsiveness is determined by the dose and administration method. Usually, intravenous methylprednisone (500–1,000 mg/d) is administered for 3–7 days, followed by oral prednisone 1–2 mg/kg/d for 6–8 weeks, and in most cases, clinical improvement is observed within the first 4–6 weeks of treatment (4). When patients are unable to tolerate the side effects of steroid or have no response to steroids in the short term, plasma exchange can be performed to improve treatment efficacy. Moreover, a few reports have demonstrated that plasma exchange can be used for the initial treatment (39).

History of Plasma Exchange as a Treatment for Hashimoto's Encephalopathy

In 2001, Boers and Colebatch (42) was the first to report that plasma exchange could effectively treat Hashimoto's encephalopathy that failed to respond to corticosteroids. The author reported a 47-year-old Uruguayan man who was treated for upper limb postural tremor and gait disorder. During hospitalization, the patient developed seizures, short-term memory impairment, visual hallucination, auditory hallucinations, and paranoid delusions. Electroencephalogram (EEG) showed diffuse slow wave activity but no epileptic discharge. Cerebrospinal fluid showed increased pressure and protein (1.06 g/l), but other cerebrospinal fluid examinations (including polymerase chain reaction of herpes simplex virus), brain magnetic resonance plain scan, and enhancement showed no abnormalities. Examinations for thyroid stimulating hormone (TSH) were normal, but the levels of microsomal antibodies and anti-thyroglobulin antibodies significantly increased, so the diagnosis of Hashimoto's encephalopathy was established after ruling out other causes. Intravenous methylprednisolone was initiated, but 4 weeks later, the patient still experienced tremor and difficulty eating and dressing himself, so four plasma exchange sessions were performed with the exchange of 1.5–2 times the estimated plasma volume per session. After the first plasma exchange, the patient's condition improved, and after the fourth plasma exchange, the patient was able to dress, eat, talk, and work independently; in addition, his antibody levels decreased. Afterward, the patient experienced two relapses, and the symptoms were relieved after plasma exchange. Multiple studies have subsequently supported this treatment (5, 6, 40, 43–45). Nieuwenhuis et al. (45) reported a 48-year-old patient with subacute Hashimoto's encephalopathy, and the main manifestations were rapid progressive dementia, visual hallucinations, and myoclonus. Plasma exchange was used as the initial treatment of Hashimoto's encephalopathy, and clinical symptoms relieved after the first plasma exchange.

Onset Time of Plasma Exchange for Hashimoto's Encephalopathy

Most of the cases in which plasma exchange used to treat Hashimoto's encephalopathy showed positive effects after the first plasma exchange. Clinical symptoms of Hashimoto's encephalopathy were found to be improved after the first plasma exchange in a report by Boers and Colebatch (42). In addition, Bektas et al. (43) reported one Hashimoto's encephalopathy in which the patient's status epilepticus was controlled after the first plasma exchange.

The Course of Plasma Exchange for Hashimoto's Encephalopathy

Most studies on plasma exchange for Hashimoto's encephalopathy lack a specific description of the number of plasma exchange sessions used. Nieuwenhuis et al. (45) used three sessions plasma exchange to treat Hashimoto's encephalopathy successfully. Bektas et al. (43) used nine sessions plasma exchange, while Nagpal and Pande (5) and Gul Mert et al. (6) reports that the number of plasma exchange sessions for the treatment of Hashimoto's encephalopathy should be five. These results are consistent with the American Society for Apheresis, which recommends a total of 3–9 sessions plasma exchange for Hashimoto's encephalopathy, with the most common number of plasma exchange being five and exchanges being performed once every other day. The volume of plasma exchanged per treatment should be 1–1.5 times the estimated plasma volume, and albumin should be used as the replacement solution (2, 5, 31, 45).

Clinical Practice of Plasma Exchange for Hashimoto's Encephalopathy

Hussain et al. (44) reported a case of 54-year-old woman with hypothyroidism who presented with progressive cognitive impairment, gait disturbance, and seizures; based on an anti-thyroid microsomal antibody titer of 1:1,600 and the presence of head abnormalities on MRI without other reasons for cognitive impairment, a definite diagnosis of Hashimoto's encephalopathy was made. The patient began oral prednisone at a dose of 60 mg/d, and her cognitive function, apraxia, and gait disorder improved, but memory impairment remained. Because the patient could not tolerate the side effects of prednisone, the dose was gradually reduced to 15 mg/d. As the patient's cognitive function and gait disorder worsened with the reduction in the dose of prednisone, plasma exchange was performed, with five sessions per course and two courses of plasma exchange at intervals of 5 months. Four weeks after the first course of treatment, the patient's cognitive function markedly improved, and anti-thyroid microsomal antibody levels were reduced to 1:400. Cognitive function began to decline a few months later, but after the patient underwent the second course of plasma exchange, cognitive function continuously improved. Pari et al. (40) reported a 19-year-old girl who had been in good health but experienced a seizure. One month later, she had difficulty finding words and understanding language, along with symptoms of confusion, and disorientation. Electroencephalogram showed a non-convulsive status epilepticus, with a slightly elevated number of cells in CSF, with normal glucose and protein levels. PCR analysis of herpes simplex virus, adenovirus and enterovirus in cerebrospinal fluid were all negative. Brain MRI was normal. An 18F-FDG PET on the left temporal lobe, insula, temporoparietal junction, the right side of the parietal lobe metabolism reduced, diagnosis of Hashimoto's encephalopathy, intravenous methylprednisolone 1 g/d for 8 days, but no obvious improvement was observed. Electroencephalogram improved after five plasma exchange sessions, antithyroglobulin antibody, and thyroid peroxidase antibody, respectively pretreatment of >1,000 IU/ml (normal <4.1 IU/ml), 519 IU/ml (normal for <5.6 IU/ml) dropped to 462 IU/ml, 30 IU/ml. Symptoms of difficulty finding words and understanding speech also improved. In most studies, steroids work within the first 4–6 weeks, while other studies have shown that the time to complete recovery may range from 4 months to 10 years (4). However, in this case, the course of steroids was shorter. If used for a longer duration, the effect may be more pronounced. The patient may be responsive to steroid treatment, but if the clinical symptoms are severe or worsen, plasma exchange can be used to quickly relieve these symptoms. Cook et al. (31) retrospectively analyzed a study on the treatment of Hashimoto's encephalopathy with plasma exchange in 10 cases and showed that 90% of patients had significantly improved symptoms after plasma exchange. Because plasma exchange alone or with other treatments have been used as the second-line treatment for Hashimoto's encephalopathy, in 2016, the American Society for Apheresis published treatment guidelines for plasma exchange and proposed that Hashimoto's encephalopathy is a category II indication of plasma exchange. Moreover, because only observational studies or case series have reported the efficacy of plasma exchange on Hashimoto's encephalopathy and randomized controlled studies are lacking, the recommended level is 2C (2). This study was supported by Simmons and Staley (the volume of plasma exchanged per treatment was 1.0 times the plasma volume) (7) and Endres et al. (8). In addition, Tran et al. (9) found that long-term plasma exchange can be used for maintenance treatment in patients with Hashimoto's encephalopathy accompanied by cerebellar ataxia.

Plasma Exchange in Combination With Other Drugs for Hashimoto's Encephalopathy

Plasma exchange is usually combined with steroid, immunoglobulin, and antiepileptic drugs as well as immunosuppressants to treat Hashimoto's encephalopathy (5, 39, 44). Bektas et al. (43) reported a 12-year-old patient with Hashimoto's encephalopathy that mainly manifested status epilepticus, but after the first plasma exchange, his status epilepticus was controlled; subsequently, prednisone combined with a total of nine sessions plasma exchange resulted in normal mental and neurological status in 2 months. Gul et al. (6) also reported two successful cases in which plasma exchange combined with steroid, intravenous immunoglobulin, and antiepileptic drugs to treat Hashimoto's encephalopathy.

However, at present, only case reports and case analyses have shown that plasma exchange is effective at treating Hashimoto's encephalopathy, and because plasma exchange was initiated after failure to respond to steroids or immunoglobulin therapy in most of the studies, we cannot completely rule out the delayed effects of steroids. Nevertheless, because of the narrow time window between clinical symptom improvement and plasma exchange, plasma exchange can be considered for the treatment of Hashimoto's encephalopathy when steroids are ineffective in the short term or when patients cannot tolerate the side effects of steroids, and a few studies have shown that plasma exchange is effective as an initial treatment for Hashimoto's encephalopathy.

Side Effects of Plasma Exchange for Hashimoto's Encephalopathy

Plasma exchange is a relatively safe and effective treatment. The application of plasma exchange for the treatment of Hashimoto's encephalopathy is rare, and few studies have evaluated the occurrence of side effects from plasma exchange in Hashimoto's encephalopathy patients. Hussain et al. (44) reported a 54-year-old patient with Hashimoto's encephalopathy treated with plasma exchange who developed a urinary tract infection.

Application of Plasma Exchange for Limbic Encephalitis

Limbic encephalitis is a neuropsychiatric disease characterized by inflammation of the limbic system, including the hippocampus, amygdala, and less frequently the frontobasal and insular regions. The clinical manifestations are subacute onset of cognitive impairment (mainly short-term memory loss), epilepsy, and mental disorder (46, 47). Radja et al. (48) reported that 97% of VGKC-associated limbic encephalitis presented with memory impairment, 85% with seizures, and 33% with emotional change. Brain MRI may present edema or inflammation that occur selectively on unilateral or bilateral limbic systems, especially in the medial temporal region (49). Electroencephalogram usually shows focal or diffuse slow waves or epileptiform discharge (50), and cerebrospinal fluid usually shows lymphocytosis, slight protein elevation, oligoclonal band positivity, and an increase in the IgG index (51, 52). Limbic encephalitis can be divided into infectious and autoimmune limbic encephalitis according to the etiology. Infectious limbic encephalitis is usually caused by the direct invasion of the brain by pathogens such as herpes simplex virus, while autoimmune limbic encephalitis is caused by an autoimmune disorder and can be divided into paraneoplastic and non-paraneoplastic limbic encephalitis (50).

In 1968, Corsellis et al. (53) used the term "limbic encephalitis" for the first time to describe six patients characterized by progressive memory loss, confusion, and seizures. Of those patients, four had tumors, and three had bronchial carcinomas. An autopsy found that the limbic gray matter in all patients' temporal lobes exhibited inflammation and degeneration, indicating that there was a link between limbic encephalitis and tumors. Gultekin et al. (52) analyzed the relationship between 50 cases of limbic encephalitis and tumors and found that limbic encephalitis commonly occurs with small cell lung cancer (52%, 68/132), testicular cancer (11%, 14/132), and thymoma (5%, 6/132).There were also reports of paraneoplastic limbic encephalitis with non-Hodgkin's lymphoma, neuroblastoma, colon cancer, ovarian cancer, breast cancer, prostate cancer, etc. Since 1988, several studies have confirmed that patients with tumors outside the central nervous system but have neuropsychiatric symptoms have antitumor and brain tissue antibodies in their serum, including anti-Hu, anti-Yo, anti-CRMP5, anti-Ri, anti-Ma2, and anti-amphiphysin antibodies. Since 2000, studies have shown that some limbic encephalitis are detected antibodies against neuronal cell-surface antigens or antibodies against neuronal ion channels, including voltage-gated potassium channels and ligand-gated ion channels and antibodies against VGKC, NMDA, and AMPA receptors, thus providing a therapeutic basis for plasma exchange (47, 50).

History of Plasma Exchange for the Treatment of Limbic Encephalitis

Buckley et al. (54) first reported that plasma exchange successfully treated a case of limbic encephalitis. The report described a 47-year-old female stylist with myasthenia gravis. Thymoma was removed 4 years after she was diagnosed with myasthenia gravis, and after her diagnosis of myasthenia gravis for 10 years, her symptoms of myasthenia gravis recurred, the following year, the patient exhibited significant short-term memory loss, irritability, disorientation, inattention, and slowed thinking. The doses of cyclophosphamide and prednisone were reduced, and the patient started using loxapine (fourth generation antipsychotic medication), but her mental status did not improve significantly. After 7 weeks, the patient was transferred to the intensive care unit due to myasthenia crisis, and the myasthenia gravis symptoms were relieved with increased immunosuppression, but her mental status still did not improve. Brain CT and MRI were normal, while cerebrospinal fluid cytology and PCR of herpes simplex virus were negative. The electroencephalogram showed nonspecific slow waves. In the first 10 years after the diagnosis of myasthenia gravis, the VGKC antibody was normal, and significantly increased (750 pM) after the onset of psychiatric symptoms, so the patient was diagnosed with anti-VGKC receptor limbic encephalitis. The myasthenia gravis symptoms and limbic system symptoms improved after six sessions of plasma exchange. Jaben and Winters (55) studied the treatment of five anti-VGKC antibody-related diseases with plasma exchange, of those, four were anti-VGKC antibody-related limbic encephalitis with the main clinical manifestations of memory impairment, seizures, and personality changes. All patients were given 1.0 times the plasma volume during each session every other day for a total of 5–6 sessions. Among these patients, three limbic encephalitis were treated with other immunosuppressive agents at the same time, and one significantly experienced symptom relief with plasma exchange alone. Although there have been a number of cases in which plasma exchange was used to treat limbic encephalitis, plasma exchange in combination with steroid and immunoglobulins have also been used to treat all types of limbic encephalitis. Steroid and immunoglobulin treatments are first-line therapy for limbic encephalitis whereas plasma exchange is not (56). Rather, it is implemented when steroid and immunoglobulin therapy has no obvious effect in the short term, alternatively, plasma exchange may be used in combination with steroid and immunoglobulin to treat limbic encephalitis.

Onset Time of Plasma Exchange for Limbic Encephalitis

At present, most studies that describe plasma exchange for limbic encephalitis lack a description of the onset time of plasma exchange. Schimme et al. (57) reported a 12-year-old girl with NMDA receptor encephalitis performed with eight sessions of plasma exchange over 13 days. The patient's clinical symptoms markedly improved after the second plasma exchange, and her ability to walk was partially recovered. This treatment schedule was consistent with the onset time of plasma exchange for anti-NMDA receptor encephalitis that was unresponsive to immunoglobulin (0.4 g/kg/d for 5 days) combined with methylprednisolone (1 g/d for 5 days) in the short term, as reported by Wang et al. (58) in 2015, consciousness was regained after the second plasma exchange. Mazzi et al. (11) reported a case of non-paraneoplastic limbic encephalitis with anti-GAD antibody, in which seizures were significantly reduced by the third plasma exchange. Rypulak et al. (59) reported a 23-year-old patient with NMDA receptor encephalitis who received plasma exchange, and after the third session, the patient's neurological symptoms significantly improved. The GCS score increased to 11 points from 6 points.

The Course of Plasma Exchange for Limbic Encephalitis

In the study of Batra et al. (10) and Jaben and Winters (55), the number of plasma exchange sessions used to treat limbic encephalitis ranged from 5 to 6. In 2016, the American Society for Apheresis recommended the use of plasma exchange once every other day to treat anti-NMDA receptor encephalitis, and the volume of plasma exchanged per session was 1–1.5 times the plasma volume. Albumin was used as the replacement fluid, and a total of 5–6 sessions were performed. For the treatment of paraneoplastic neuropathy (PNS), including paraneoplastic limbic encephalitis, plasma exchange is recommended once daily or every other day for a total of 5–6 sessions, and the volume of plasma exchanged per procedure should be 1–1.5 times the plasma volume (2).

Clinical Practice of Plasma Exchange for the Treatment of Limbic Encephalitis

Plasma exchange is initiated when steroid and immunoglobulin treatments fail to treat limbic encephalitis, alternatively, it can be combined with steroid and immunoglobulin treatments. Therefore, plasma exchange is usually not the first choice. However, at present, no randomized controlled trials have analyzed the therapeutic effect of plasma exchange on limbic encephalitis. In 2011, Markakis et al. (60) reported a case of a 48-year-old female who presented with mental disorders and disorientation 2 years before admission; the patient rapidly developed anterograde amnesia, irritability, hallucinations, refractory temporal lobe seizure, and obvious short-term memory loss in a few weeks. The enhanced T2 weighted sequence of brain MRI suggested bilateral temporal lobe swelling and revealed a high signal intensity in the medial temporal lobe. High concentrations of anti-GAD antibodies were found in serum and cerebrospinal fluid. A diagnosis of anti-GAD antibody-associated limbic encephalitis was established. After methylprednisolone (1 g/d for 5 days) failed, plasma exchange was initiated, each session involved the replacement of 1.2 times the plasma volume. After a total of seven sessions, the epilepsy was under control, but the patient's cognitive function did not improve. Subsequently, the patient underwent one plasma exchange session every 3 weeks along with oral prednisone (1 mg/kg, gradually reduced to 0.25 mg/kg, for at least 1 year). The seizures did not recur, and a simple intelligence test showed that language and visual memory improved, in addition, anti-GAD antibody levels were reduced at the 1-year follow-up. Mccarthy et al. (61) reported one case of a 32-year-old pregnant woman with anti-NMDA receptor encephalitis, in the first 2 weeks of pregnancy, a new symptom developed, continuous daily headache, and in the maternity clinic, the patient experienced a rapid onset of visual and auditory hallucinations, illusions, irritability, paranoid, delusional within 24 h. One week later, the patient lost consciousness, and seizures began to occur. Brain MRI was normal, EEG showed diffuse slow waves, and cerebrospinal fluid protein was elevated to 726 mg/l (normal is 150–450 mg/l). Steroids were initiated (methyl prednisolone 1 g/d for 5 days, then slowly reduced), but the patient became aggravated, and hence stayed in the intensive care unit. After plasma exchange (1.5 times the plasma volume per session), the patient's symptoms improved significantly, and after 8 weeks, the symptoms of encephalopathy were completely resolved. Van Ael et al. (62) used steroids to treat a 26-year-old woman with GAD antibody limbic encephalitis, but the treatment was unsuccessful. Plasma exchange was subsequently initiated, and marked improvements in clinical symptoms, including memory, seizures, and imaging findings were observed. At the 14-month follow-up, the level of GAD antibody, which was initially >7,000 IU, was decreased by plasma exchange to <1,000 IU. Moreover, several other studies have shown that plasma exchange is more effective than intravenous immunoglobulin and steroids for the treatment of limbic encephalitis, including in pregnant women (10, 12, 61, 63). Korff et al. (64) found that plasma exchange was the most effective at reducing antibody levels in limbic encephalitis.

Plasma Exchange in Combination With Other Drugs for the Treatment of Limbic Encephalitis

Plasma exchange is rarely used alone in the treatment of limbic encephalitis, but it is often used in combination with other immunomodulatory therapies such as steroids and/or immunoglobulin. Vincent et al. (65) analyzed the clinical features and treatment of 10 cases of anti-VGKC-antibody-associated limbic encephalitis. Among those cases, seven were treated with plasma exchange combined with steroids or immunoglobulin, and the results showed that four patients experienced a significant curative effect, two patients experienced a slight curative effect, and only one patient did not experience an effect. Desena et al. (66) analyzed the use of plasma exchange to treat 14 cases of anti-NMDA receptor encephalitis, including three adults, 10 patients began plasma exchange after failure to respond to steroids, and the results showed that 7/10 NMDA receptor encephalitis patients who underwent plasma exchange exhibited an average increase in the modified Rankin scale of 0.4, and 3/10 patients exhibited an average increase in the modified Rankin scale of 0.1 after treatment with steroids. The results indicated that plasma exchange combined with steroids was more effective than steroids alone for the treatment of anti-NMDA receptor encephalitis.

However, no randomized controlled trials have been performed to support the therapeutic effect of plasma exchange on limbic encephalitis, and plasma exchange is primarily initiated when the patient exhibits no response to steroid treatment in the short term (perhaps because steroid treatment requires a longer time period to elicit effects). Thus, the therapeutic effect of steroid treatment cannot be completely excluded, especially when it is combined with plasma exchange or immunoglobulin, so improvements in the patient's condition should not be attributed solely to plasma exchange. However, the patients receiving plasma exchange had better outcomes, and plasma exchange exhibited a time-dependent effect. The coincidence was small, and a few cases reported plasma exchange as the initial treatment of Hashimoto's encephalopathy. Therefore, plasma exchange may be considered when patients have contraindications to steroid treatment or slow onset time in the short term, but randomized controlled trials are needed for confirmation.

Side Effects of Plasma Exchange for Limbic Encephalitis

Suppiej et al. (67) analyzed the efficacy and side effects of plasma exchange for pediatric NMDA receptor encephalitis and showed two cases of transient hypotension that improved after rehydration therapy and blood vessel vasopressors, one case of allergic reaction and shock because of autonomic dysfunction, and one case of pulmonary embolism. Wong et al. (33) prospectively studied nine VGKC antibody-positive limbic encephalitis patients who underwent five sessions of plasma exchange with 50 ml/kg of plasma volume exchanged per session. Side effects associated with plasma exchange were observed in two patients: one had methicillin-resistant staphylococcus aureus septicemia and vertebral body inflammation, while the other had femoral artery puncture hematoma, deep vein thrombosis, and pulmonary embolism, which improved after treatment. Miyauchi et al. (68) reported an 11-year-old patient with anti-NMDA receptor encephalitis who developed hypotension shock ~1 h after plasma exchange, but the patient's condition improved after rescue. Rypulak et al. (59) reported that hemodynamic instability and coagulation dysfunction occur after treatment of anti-NMDA receptor encephalitis with plasma exchange, and a prolonged interval between plasma exchange sessions can help prevent unwanted side effects. Therefore, the vital signs of patients, especially patients with anti-NMDA receptor encephalitis, should be closely monitored.

Application of Plasma Exchange in Systemic Lupus Encephalopathy

Systemic lupus erythematosus encephalopathy, also known as neuropsychiatric systemic lupus erythematosus (NPSLE), is a common neurological complication of systemic lupus erythematosus (SLE) (69), patients with NPSLE present a variety of neuropsychological symptoms, including aseptic meningitis, cerebrovascular disease, demyelination, headaches, movement disorders, seizures, confusion, anxiety, cognitive decline, and mood disorders (70), and NPSLE is the main cause of disability and death in patients with systemic lupus erythematosus. The pathogenesis of neuropsychiatric lupus involves a variety of inflammatory factors, autoantibodies, vascular lesions caused by immune complexes, and neuronal dysfunction mediated by autoantibodies (71). For many years, steroids as the first-line drug for systemic lupus erythematosus encephalopathy, often intravenous methylprednisolone (1,000 mg for 3 d), and then oral prednisone (1 mg/kg/d) gradually tapered and stopped within 3–12 months, but long-term use of the steroid has obvious side effects. When SLE encephalopathy has contraindications to steroid, or steroid is not sufficient or ineffective in the short term, plasma exchange may be a rapid-onset, safe, and effective option (72). In 2016, the American Society for Apheresis (ASFA) recommended plasma exchange as a class II indication for severe SLE, including lupus encephalopathy, and the recommended level is 2C (2).

History of Plasma Exchange for Systemic Lupus Erythematosus Encephalopathy

In 1976, Jones et al. (71) treated eight SLE patients with plasma exchange and found that plasma exchange can reduce the level of immune complexes in SLE. In 1981, Evans et al. (21) reported a 44-year-old nurse who developed systemic lupus erythematosus encephalopathy 12 years after the diagnosis of SLE, the disease mainly manifests as schizophrenia-like psychosis, personality changes, mood changes, cognitive disorders, delusions, hallucinations, and irrational thoughts and behaviors. High doses of antipsychotic medications such as thiazine, chlorpromazine, and haloperidol combined with prednisone at 200 mg/day failed to treat the patient's mental symptoms. Immune complex levels were significantly increased in the blood and cerebrospinal fluid, and electroencephalograms showed irregular delta waves of 7–8 Hz per s, hence, four sessions of plasma exchange were performed after 35–38 days.

An obvious improvement in the patient's mental status was observed 3 days after the fourth plasma exchange. Four weeks later, the dose of prednisone was reduced to 15 mg/d, and all the antipsychotic drugs were stopped at the same time, the patient's mental function and EEG performance gradually returned to normal, and the levels of immune complex and anti-neuronal antibody decreased correspondingly, indicating that plasma exchange can effectively treat lupus encephalopathy in patients with high levels of circulating immune complexes. In 1988, Unterweger et al. (73) reported a case of a 15-year-old girl with lupus encephalopathy. Three years after diagnosis of SLE, the patient manifested a severe depressive episode accompanied by suicidal ideation, disorientation, and delusional behavior, hence, steroids were initiated. After 7 days, the patient still had clinical manifestations of encephalopathy, mainly dementia, and delusions. The symptoms still did not significantly improve within 3 weeks of continued steroids. Therefore, plasma exchange was performed once every 2 days, with a total of five sessions performed over 10 days. The levels of circulating immune complexes decreased, antibody levels decreased, and the symptoms were relieved. Two weeks after the last plasma exchange session, the patient had recovered completely, and based on the results of psychological testing, the patient's attention and memory had returned to normal. Since then, studies have reported that plasma exchange can effectively treat systemic lupus encephalopathy (15, 69, 71, 74, 75). Plasma exchange has recently been reported to successfully treat one lupus encephalopathy case with catatonia as the main manifestation, avoiding the use of electroshock treatment (76). But no randomized controlled trials have confirmed the effect of plasma exchange on systemic lupus erythematosus encephalopathy.

The Course of Plasma Exchange for Systemic Lupus Erythematosus Encephalopathy

Kato et al. (77) reported three sessions of plasma exchange for the treatment of systemic lupus erythematosus encephalopathy, and Hussein et al (44) and Perisse et al (76) successfully treated systemic lupus encephalopathy using six sessions. Most studies reporting the use of plasma exchange for lupus encephalopathy lack a specific description of their methods. According to the reports on plasma exchange, for other immune mechanisms mediated neurological diseases, and according to studies reporting the plasma exchange clearance kinetics of immunoglobulin, it should be performed once daily or every other day, with the volume of plasma exchanged per procedure at 1–1.5 times the estimated plasma volume, and a total of 3–6 sessions of plasma exchange.

Clinical Practice of Plasma Exchange for the Treatment of Systemic Lupus Erythematosus Encephalopathy

Mild SLE encephalopathy needs only symptomatic treatment, but for severe SLE encephalopathy (disturbance of consciousness, seizures, severe depression, psychotic symptoms, etc.) and lupus encephalopathy in which steroids and cyclophosphamide have contraindications, high concentrations of immune complexes, and steroids have no obvious curative effect in the short term. Plasma exchange can treat lupus encephalopathy effectively, safely, and quickly (78–80). By removing pathogenic autoantibodies, immunoglobulin, immune complexes, and toxins, plasma exchange can also increase the function of regulatory T cells (23, 78). Kato et al. (77) reported a 48-year-old male with lupus encephalopathy that manifested as organic encephalopathy syndrome, specifically exhibiting mental behavior abnormalities, disorientation, memory, and intelligence impairments. Plasma exchange was performed after steroid treatment was deemed ineffective. After the first plasma exchange, the patient's consciousness improved, and their clinical symptoms were relieved. Subsequently, the steroid treatment was continued. Three days after the first plasma exchange session, a second plasma exchange session was conducted, the patient's disorientation was immediately alleviated. Quinter-Del-Rio AI et al. (79) studied a 14-year-old girl with SLE encephalopathy presenting with seizure, after steroid treatment failed, the clinical symptoms were significantly relieved with plasma exchange (1 session/d for 4 days). Gokhale et al. (69) reported three cases of lupus encephalopathy, two of which presented with status epilepticus. Plasma exchange combined with cyclophosphamide was initiated when steroid and cyclophosphamide treatment failed, and the clinical symptoms of all three patients were significantly relieved. Some scholars believe that the combination of synchronous plasma exchange and cyclophosphamide is effective for the treatment of SLE encephalopathy. Neuwelt (32) studied 26 patients who met the 1999 American Society of Rheumatology diagnostic criteria for lupus encephalopathy and treated them with plasma exchange with or without cyclophosphamide. Symptoms were relieved in 74% of patients. Euler et al (80) used plasma exchange and cyclophosphamide to treat 14 cases of severe SLE, of which 12 had complete remission of clinical symptoms within 6 years of follow-up after cessation of treatment.

SLE encephalopathy has various clinical manifestations, and its pathogenesis and pathophysiological mechanisms are still being explored. Although plasma exchange has been shown to be effective at treating SLE encephalopathy, there is a lack of randomized controlled trials to support the efficacy of plasma exchange. Thus, clinicians must weigh the pros and cons of the risk and costs, as well as other factors, to determine whether plasma exchange should be performed. In addition, large-sample, multicenter, randomized controlled trials are still needed to confirm the therapeutic effect of plasma exchange.

Side Effects of Plasma Exchange for the Treatment of Systemic Lupus Erythematosus Encephalopathy

Although plasma exchange does have a few side effects, potential life-threatening side effects are very rare, and their incidence is <0.15% (75). Bartolucci et al. (15) analyzed the side effects of plasma exchange as adjuvant treatment for lupus encephalopathy and found five cases: one case of transient hypocalcemia, one case of venous fistula of the indwelling venous catheter, one case of allergic skin reaction to albumin, and two cases of central venous catheter infection.

Plasma Exchange for the Treatment of ANCA-associated Vasculitis Encephalopathy

ANCA-associated vasculitis includes granulomatosis with polyangiitis (GPA: formerly Wegener's granulomatosis), microscopic polyangiitis (MPA), and eosinophilic granulomatosis with polyangiitis (EGPA: formerly Churg-Strauss syndrome), which is a group of systemic vasculitis characterized by oligovascular oligoimmune necrosis inflammation. ANCAs can be detected in the serum of most patients (81). ANCA-associated vasculitis can lead to systemic organ damage, mainly renal and lung, of which renal damage is more prevalent (70%) (81). However, the manifestations that cause central nervous system damage are not common, with an incidence of ~5–15%. In addition, there is no significant difference in the incidence of each type of ANCA-related vasculitis-induced central nervous system damage. Usually, central nervous system damage is caused by cerebral or spinal vasculitis and granulomas, and the clinical manifestations are complex, ranging from headache to cognitive impairment, memory loss, epilepsy, disturbance of consciousness, paresthesia, etc. (81). Encephalopathy is not a disease, rather, it is a clinical syndrome that describes global brain dysfunction. Mental status alteration is the most typical manifestation, and changes in personality and/or behavior can indicate deterioration in cognitive functioning, a reduction in the level of consciousness, and specific localizing features of injury, such as seizures, ataxia, tremor, and other focal motor signs. There may also be systemic symptoms, such as headache, fever, vomiting, and loss of appetite. In summary, ANCA-associated vasculitis encephalopathy is a global brain dysfunction caused by ANCA-associated vasculitis (82).

Untreated ANCA-associated vasculitis usually leads to death, with a mortality rate as high as 90% in the natural course of 2 years, since the 1950s, when steroids became the basic treatment for ANCA-associated vasculitis, the five-year survival rate has increased to 48%, and after the 1980s, when steroids began to be combined with cyclophosphamide to treat ANCA-associated vasculitis, symptoms could be relieved in 80–90% of patients (83). Because ANCAs play an important role in the pathogenesis of disease, the use of plasma exchange to clear pathogenic antibodies from circulation, and increase the ability of the reticuloendothelial system to clear immune complexes can be combined with immunosuppressive agents for the treatment of severe ANCA-associated vasculitis (84), such as ANCA-associated vasculitis encephalopathy. However, due to the low incidence of ANCA-associated vasculitis encephalopathy, systematic studies on the treatment of ANCA-associated vasculitis encephalopathy by plasma exchange are lacking. There is currently no description of the specific dose and course of plasma exchange for ANCA-associated vasculitis encephalopathy. According to the reports on plasma exchange for other immune mechanisms mediating neurological diseases, it may be recommended once daily or every other day, with the volume of plasma exchanged per session at 1–1.5 times the estimated plasma volume, and a total of five sessions of plasma exchange should be performed.

Clinical Practice of Plasma Exchange for the Treatment of ANCA-associated Vasculitis Encephalopathy

The treatment of ANCA-associated vasculitic encephalopathy with plasma exchange is uncommon. In 2000, Deshpande et al. (85) reported a 15-year-old girl with renal failure who developed lethargy for 3 months and suffered from decreased appetite and vomiting in the week prior to admission. At 24 h after admission, renal biopsy showed that 29 of 43 glomeruli contained a mixture of fibrous crescents and cells. The patient was diagnosed with microscopic polyangiitis, and the patient was discharged after her condition improved. Three weeks after discharge, the patient had a severe headache and blurred vision, and blood pressure was 139/92 mmHg. Subsequently, the patient experienced three epileptic seizures, followed by a loss of consciousness, and irritability. Phenytoin and carbamazepine were used to control the seizures, and T2-weighted and T2 FLAIR sequences of brain MRI showed multiple increased signal intensities in the peripheral gray matter of the cerebral hemisphere, especially in the occipital cortex. Vasculitis caused widespread cerebral ischemia. EEG indicated changes consistent with encephalopathy. Headache, disturbance of consciousness, and blurred vision were relieved after the first plasma exchange session, the patient then underwent three sessions of plasma exchange, performed every other day, and after five consecutive plasma exchange sessions, cyclophosphamide was administered intravenously. After 2 months, the abnormal signals on brain MRI showed improvement. Nishio et al (86) reported reversible posterior leukoencephalopathy syndrome caused by vascular damage from Wegener's granulomatosis. A female with Wegener's granulomatosis presented severe headache, nausea, and seizures after severe intestinal complications. Blood pressure was 126/60 mmHg, brain CT showed low-density shadows in the bilateral posterior parietal and occipital lobes, and brain MRI showed high-intensity signals on the T2-weighted sequence in the bilateral occipital white matter, parietal lobe, and frontal lobe. Cerebrospinal fluid was normal. Thus, the diagnosis was reversible posterior white matter encephalopathy syndrome. Two courses of methylprednisolone combined with plasma exchange were administered, followed by intravenous cyclophosphamide at 400 mg/week. After 13 days, brain MRI showed that the abnormal signal had almost completely disappeared. The patient's consciousness and mental status also began to recover, and the concentration of PR3-ANCA antibodies decreased from 164 to 15.7 U/ml, and the intestinal symptoms were relieved. However, studies that treat ANCA-associated vasculitis encephalopathy with plasma exchange are very rare, so more studies are needed in the future to provide supporting evidence of the therapeutic effect of plasma exchange.

Plasma Exchange for the Treatment of Acute Demyelinating Encephalomyelitis

Acute disseminated encephalomyelitis is an immune-mediated single-phase acute inflammatory demyelinating disease of the central nervous system, which mainly affects the white matter of the brain, brainstem and spinal cord (87). It is common in children and young adults, and most cases occur after viral or bacterial infections or within 2–4 weeks of vaccination (<5%) This disease can exhibit acute or subacute onset, with clinical manifestations of encephalopathy (disturbance of consciousness and behavior change) and multifocal neurological defects. In 2007, an international pediatric multiple sclerosis research group noted that encephalopathy not explained by fever is a necessary clinical manifestation of acute disseminated encephalomyelitis (87, 88), and in the prodromal stage, upper respiratory tract infection, and gastrointestinal symptoms are usually observed. The diagnosis is mainly based on clinical manifestations and imaging examination. Typical cerebrospinal fluid changes include increased pressure, increased lymphocytes, increased protein (usually <1.0 mg/l), and normal glucose. The gamma globulin and IgG levels in cerebrospinal fluid can increase, as can myelin basic protein, with a rare oligoclonal band. Electroencephalography examination presents a slow wave on imaging and is of great value in the diagnosis of acute disseminated encephalomyelitis, especially brain MRI, which can detect multiple or extensive white matter or deep gray matter lesions (thalamus and basal ganglia) within 5–14 days after the onset of symptoms (88, 89).

The pathogenesis of acute disseminated encephalomyelitis is not very clear. Cell-mediated immune dysfunction may play a main role. Humoral factors, including antibodies, complement, immune complex, and cytokines, also play an important role (78), so priority is given to immune modulators (90). No randomized controlled trials have been performed on children or adults to determine the best treatment for ADEM. Systemic intravenous large doses of corticoids are currently considered to be first-line therapy (89). Early intravenous methylprednisolone can shorten the course of the disease. Plasma exchange has been reported to be effective in the treatment of acute disseminated encephalomyelitis when the diagnosis of acute disseminated encephalomyelitis is delayed and cannot be early except for infectious diseases where steroid cannot be used, where there are contraindications to steroid, or where the effects of steroid are not obvious in the short term (90).

History of Plasma Exchange for the Treatment of Acute Disseminated Encephalomyelitis

In 1981, Newton et al. successfully treated the first case of acute disseminated encephalomyelitis caused by acute infection through plasma exchange alone (4). Subsequently, Cotter et al. (91) reported the case of a 22-year-old male with acute disseminated encephalomyelitis caused by mycoplasma pneumoniae infection. Eight days after onset, the patient improved after plasma exchange alone. Several studies have shown that plasma exchange can effectively treat acute disseminated encephalomyelitis. However, the current therapeutic effect of plasma exchange lacks the support of randomized controlled trials.

Onset Time of Plasma Exchange for the Treatment of Acute Disseminated Encephalomyelitis

Plasma exchange for the treatment of acute disseminated encephalomyelitis usually takes effect after the first plasma exchange (88). Kanter et al. (92) reported that plasma exchange for the treatment of two cases of acute disseminated encephalomyelitis, in which one improved neurological function within a few hours during the first plasma exchange. Shah et al. (93) noted, in their study of plasma exchange for the treatment of one acute disseminated encephalomyelitis, that the neurological deficit was improved after the first plasma exchange, which was supported by findings reported in the study by Yi et al. (94).

Course of Plasma Exchange for the Treatment of Acute Disseminated Encephalomyelitis

The course of plasma exchange for the treatment of acute disseminated encephalomyelitis has not been determined. Borras-Novell et al. (90) and Stricker et al. (95), in the study of plasma exchange for treating acute fulminant disseminated encephalomyelitis, included four cases of acute disseminated encephalomyelitis. The number of plasma exchange sessions was 3–10, predominantly 5, and plasma exchange was performed once daily with the volume of plasma exchanged per procedure set at one times the plasma volume, with 5% albumin used as replacement fluid, and all patients improved. Therefore, for the treatment of acute disseminated encephalomyelitis, 3–10 sessions are recommended, typically five, performed once a day or every other day, with the volume of plasma exchanged per sessions set at one times the plasma volume and albumin used as the replacement fluid.

Clinical Practice of Plasma Exchange in Acute Disseminated Encephalomyelitis

Miyazawa et al. (96) reported an eleven-year-old patient with acute disseminated encephalomyelitis. Brain MRI revealed extensive multiple high-intensity lesions in the white matter on T2-weighted imaging. Intravenous immunoglobulin (0.125 g/kg/d for 3 days) was administered after 10 days of illness, and 11 days after onset, oral prednisone was initiated at a dose of 60 mg/d, but the patient did not improve. Twelve days after onset, intravenous methylprednisolone was administered (1,000 mg/d) for 3 days. Fourteen days after onset, the patient became comatose, and spinal magnetic resonance T2 weighted images showed cervical segmental spinal cord swelling and abnormally high signal because of the patients' neurologic deterioration. At 17–20 days after onset, three plasma exchange sessions were started using 5% albumin as the replacement fluid. She regained full consciousness, and MRI improved. Lin et al. (97) described plasma exchange for the successful treatment of two cases of acute disseminated encephalomyelitis, including a 26-year-old woman who had a history of rubella vaccination, characterized by disturbance of consciousness, speech, ataxia, and myoclonus. Brain magnetic resonance T2 weighted images revealed high-intensity signals in the brain stem, cerebellum, basal ganglia, thalamus, and white matter of the cerebral ventricles. Initially, she received intravenous methylprednisolone (1,000 mg/d for 5 days and then 500 mg/d for 2 days) and then oral prednisone. However, her neurological function began to deteriorate, and one seizure occurred after 3 days of intravenous methylprednisolone. Five sessions of plasma exchange were initiated, with one session performed every 2 days, and 5% of albumin was used as the replacement fluid. Her symptoms were alleviated after the third plasma exchange. Another a 65-year-old patient presented with acute disseminated encephalomyelitis, unconsciousness, speech disorder, emotional dissonance, and slow movement. T2-weighted images of the brain magnetic resonance showed high-intensity signals in the bilateral cerebral hemisphere, an elevated number of cells in the cerebrospinal fluid, normal glucose, and moderately elevated protein levels. She received five plasma exchange sessions (once every 2 days, with 5% albumin as the replacement fluid). After the fourth plasma exchange, her symptoms began to resolve.

Since most studies have shown that the standard dose of immunoglobulin for the treatment of acute disseminated encephalomyelitis is 0.4 g/kg/d for 5 days, steroids are usually administered intravenously at a dose of 20–30 mg/kg/d for (3–5 days), followed by oral prednisone at a dose of 1–2 mg/kg/d (87). Miyazawa and Lin et al reported that a poor response to intravenous immunoglobulin and steroids may be related to inadequate immunoglobulin and steroid dosing. Even so, the delayed effects of steroid and immunoglobulin treatments cannot be excluded as a component of symptom resolution because of the narrow time window between symptom improvement and plasma exchange, indicating that plasma exchange can effectively treat fulminant acute disseminated encephalomyelitis. In addition, Stricker et al. (95) reported four cases of acute disseminated encephalomyelitis due to delayed diagnosis and cannot exclude infection, which were significantly improved by plasma exchange alone. Keegan et al. (98) reviewed 59 cases of acute and severe central nervous system demyelination treated with plasma exchange at the Mayo clinic, including 10 patients with acute disseminated encephalomyelitis (ADEM), of whom 40% experienced symptom relief. Therefore, plasma exchange treatment for acute disseminated encephalomyelitis is effective, and few side effects have been reported. However, there is still a lack of support from randomized controlled studies.

Other types of steroid-responsive encephalopathy are very rarely reported, including hypoglycemic encephalopathy (99) and steroid-responsive encephalopathy caused by cholesterol thrombosis (100), and currently, there are no reports on the effects of plasma exchange therapy on these types.

CONCLUSION

In conclusion, plasma exchange is a widely accepted treatment method for autoimmune neurological diseases because it is safe, rapid-onset, and effective. Plasma exchange may be effective for patients with steroid-responsive encephalopathy who do not respond to treatment with steroids in the short term or those who have contraindications for steroid treatment, including patients with Hashimoto's encephalopathy, limbic encephalitis, SLE encephalopathy, ANCA-associated vasculitis encephalopathy, or acute disseminated encephalomyelitis. The main limitation of this study is the lack of systematic treatments reported in the literature. The current data are almost entirely derived from case reports and case analyses. Moreover, plasma exchange is often applied in combination with steroids and other immunosuppressive agents, hence, no high-quality evidence is available to prove the efficacy of plasma exchange on steroid-responsive encephalopathy.

AUTHOR CONTRIBUTIONS

YJ, XT, and XW provided the initial idea and outline of content for the manuscript. All authors contributed content and critically reviewed and edited the manuscript.

FUNDING

This study was supported by the National Clinical Key Specialty Construction Foundation of China and the National Natural Science Foundation of China (Nos. 81471319, 81671301).

REFERENCES

1. Schwartz J. Evidence-based guideline update: plasmapheresis in neurologic disorders. *Neurology*. (2011) 77:e105–6; author reply: e6. doi: 10.1212/WNL.0b013e318230b33f
2. Schwartz J, Padmanabhan A, Aqui N, Balogun RA, Connelly-Smith L, Delaney M, et al. Guidelines on the use of therapeutic apheresis in clinical practice-evidence-based approach from the writing committee of the american society for apheresis: the seventh special issue. *J Clin Apheresis*. (2016) 31:149–62. doi: 10.1002/jca.21470
3. Castillo P, Woodruff B, Caselli R, Vernino S, Lucchinetti C, Swanson J, et al. Steroid-responsive encephalopathy associated with autoimmune thyroiditis. *Arch Neurol*. (2006) 63:197–202. doi: 10.1001/archneur.63.2.197
4. Mocellin R, Walterfang M, Velakoulis D. Hashimoto's encephalopathy: epidemiology, pathogenesis and management. *CNS Drugs*. (2007) 21:799–811. doi: 10.2165/00023210-200721100-00002
5. Nagpal T, Pande S. Hashimoto's encephalopathy: response to plasma exchange. *Neurol. India*. (2004) 52:245–7.
6. Gul Mert G, Horoz OO, Herguner MO, Incecik F, Yildizdas RD, Onenli Mungan N, et al. Hashimoto's encephalopathy: four cases and review of literature. *Int J Neurosci*. (2014) 124:302–6. doi: 10.3109/00207454.2013.836706
7. Simmons SC, Staley EM, Dorn DP, Nails AP, Marques MB, Pham HP et al. Therapeutic plasma exchange For Hashimoto's encephalopathy. *J Clin Apher*. (2018) 33:444–6. doi: 10.1002/jca.21597
8. Endres D, Vry MS, Dykierek P, Riering AN, Lungen E, Stich O, et al. Plasmapheresis responsive rapid onset dementia with predominantly frontal dysfunction in the context of Hashimoto's encephalopathy. *Front Psychiatry*. (2017) 8:212. doi: 10.3389/fpsyt.2017.00212
9. Tran MH, Mkhikian H, Sy M, Perez-Alvarez I, Demetriou M. Long-term plasma exchange as maintenance therapy for cerebellar-type Hashimoto's encephalopathy, a case report. *Transfus Apher Sci*. (2018) 57:418–20. doi: 10.1016/j.transci.2018.05.027
10. Batra R, Pang Y, Friedman MT. Therapeutic plasma exchange in anti-N-methyl-D-aspartate-receptor (anti-NMDA-R) encephalitis associated with benign ovarian teratoma. *J Clin Apher*. (2012) 27:227–8. doi: 10.1002/jca.21212
11. Mazzi G, Roia DD, Cruciatti B, Mata S, Catapano R. Plasma exchange for anti-GAD associated non paraneoplastic limbic encephalitis. *Transfus Apher Sci*. (2008) 39:229–33. doi: 10.1016/j.transci.2008.09.005
12. Martin IW, Martin CL, Dunbar NM, Lee SL, Szczepiorkowski ZM. Therapeutic plasma exchange as a steroid-sparing therapy in a patient with limbic encephalitis due to antibodies to voltage-gated potassium channels. *J Clin Apher*. (2016) 31:63–5. doi: 10.1002/jca.21395

13. Ozkale M, Erol I, Ozkale Y, Kozanoglu I. Overview of therapeutic plasma exchange in pediatric neurology: a single-center experience. *Acta Neurol Belgica.* (2018) 118:451–8. doi: 10.1007/s13760-018-0961-5
14. Hussein M, Mooij J, Roujouleh H. Cerebral lupus in patients whilst on treatment for lupus nephritis with cyclosporine. *J Clin Neurosci.* (2003) 10:104–6. doi: 10.1016/S0967-5868(02)00260-6
15. Bartolucci P, Brechignac S, Cohen P, Le Guern V, Guillevin L. Adjunctive plasma exchanges to treat neuropsychiatric lupus: a retrospective study on 10 patients. *Lupus.* (2007) 16:817–22. doi: 10.1177/0961203307081840
16. Shinozaki K, Oda S, Sadahiro T, Nakamura M, Abe R, Nakamura S, et al. A case report of plasmapheresis in the treatment of acute disseminated encephalomyelitis. *Ther Apher Dial.* (2008) 12:401–5. doi: 10.1111/j.1744-9987.2008.00617.x
17. Balestri P, Grosso S, Acquaviva A, Bernini M. Plasmapheresis in a child affected by acute disseminated encephalomyelitis. *Brain Dev.* (2000) 22:123–6. doi: 10.1016/S0387-7604(99)00115-1
18. Abel JJ, Rowntree LG, Turner BB. Plasma removal with return of corpuscles (plasmaphaeresis). The journal of pharmacology and experimental therapeutics Vol. V. No. 6, July, 1914. *Transfusion Sci.* (1990) 11:166–77.
19. Adams WS, Blahd WH, Bassett SH. A method of human plasmapheresis. *Proc Soc Exp Biol Med.* (1952) 80:377–9. doi: 10.3181/00379727-80-19629
20. Schwab PJ, Fahey JL. Treatment of Waldenstrom's macroglobulinemia by plasmapheresis. *N Engl J Med.* (1960) 263:574–9. doi: 10.1056/NEJM196009222631202
21. Evans DT, Giles M, Horne DJ, d'Apice AJ, Riglar A, Toh BH. Cerebral lupus erythematosus responding to plasmaphaeresis. *Postgraduate Med J.* (1981) 57:247–51. doi: 10.1136/pgmj.57.666.247
22. Popescu A, Kao AH. Neuropsychiatric systemic lupus erythematosus. *Curr Neuropharmacol.* (2011) 9:449–57. doi: 10.2174/157015911796557984
23. Winters JL. Plasma exchange: concepts, mechanisms, and an overview of the American Society for Apheresis guidelines. *Hematol Am Soc Hematol Educ Program.* (2012) 2012:7–12. doi: 10.1182/asheducation-2012.1.7
24. Dau PC. Increased antibody production in peripheral blood mononuclear cells after plasma exchange therapy in multiple sclerosis. *J Neuroimmunol.* (1995) 62:197–200. doi: 10.1016/0165-5728(95)00121-4
25. Steven MM, Tanner AR, Holdstock GE, Cockerell R, Smith J, Smith DS, et al. The effect of plasma exchange on the *in vitro* monocyte function of patients with immune complex diseases. *Clin Exp Immunol.* (1981) 45:240–5.
26. Tesar V, Jelinkova E, Masek Z, Jirsa M Jr, Zabka J, Bartunkova J, et al. Influence of plasma exchange on serum levels of cytokines and adhesion molecules in ANCA-positive renal vasculitis. *Blood Purif.* (1998) 16:72–80. doi: 10.1159/000014316
27. Yeh JH, Wang SH, Chien PJ, Shih CM, Chiu HC. Changes in serum cytokine levels during plasmapheresis in patients with myasthenia gravis. *Eur J Neurol.* (2009) 16:1318–22. doi: 10.1111/j.1468-1331.2009.02729.x
28. Natarajan N, Weinstein R. Therapeutic apheresis in neurology critical care. *J Intensive Care Med.* (2005) 20:212–25. doi: 10.1177/0885066605276816
29. Guyatt GH, Oxman AD, Vist GE, Kunz R, Falck-Ytter Y, Alonso-Coello P, et al. GRADE: an emerging consensus on rating quality of evidence and strength of recommendations. *BMJ* (2008) 336:924–6. doi: 10.1136/bmj.39489.470347.AD
30. Kaplan AA. Therapeutic plasma exchange: a technical and operational review. *J Clin Apheresis.* (2013) 28:3–10. doi: 10.1002/jca.21257
31. Cook MK, Malkin M, Karafin MS. The use of plasma exchange in Hashimoto's encephalopathy: a case report and review of the literature. *J Clin Apheresis* (2015) 30:188–92. doi: 10.1002/jca.21353
32. Neuwelt CM. The role of plasmapheresis in the treatment of severe central nervous system neuropsychiatric systemic lupus erythematosus. *Ther Apher Dial.* (2003) 7:173–82. doi: 10.1046/j.1526-0968.2003.00032.x
33. Wong SH, Saunders MD, Larner AJ, Das K, Hart IK. An effective immunotherapy regimen for VGKC antibody-positive limbic encephalitis. *J Neurol Neurosurg Psychiatry.* (2010) 81:1167–9. doi: 10.1136/jnnp.2009.178293
34. Basic-Jukic N, Kes P, Glavas-Boras S, Brunetta B, Bubic-Filipi L, Puretic Z. Complications of therapeutic plasma exchange: experience with 4857 treatments. *Ther Apher Dial.* (2005) 9:391–5. doi: 10.1111/j.1744-9987.2005.00319.x
35. Kaynar L, Altuntas F, Aydogdu I, Turgut B, Kocyigit I, Hacioglu SK, et al. Therapeutic plasma exchange in patients with neurologic diseases: retrospective multicenter study. *Transfusion Apher Sci.* (2008) 38:109–15. doi: 10.1016/j.transci.2007.11.002
36. Casian A, Jayne D. Plasma exchange in the treatment of Wegener's granulomatosis, microscopic polyangiitis, Churg-Strauss syndrome and renal limited vasculitis. *Curr Opin Rheumatol.* (2011) 23:12–7. doi: 10.1097/BOR.0b013e32834120c1
37. Brain L, Jellinek EH, Ball K. Hashimoto's disease and encephalopathy. *Lancet.* (1966) 2:512–4. doi: 10.1016/S0140-6736(66)92876-5
38. Riangwiwat T, Sangtian J, Sriphrapradang C. Steroid-responsive encephalopathy: an under recognised aspect of Hashimoto's thyroiditis. *BMJ Case Rep.* (2015) 2015:bcr2014208969. doi: 10.1136/bcr-2014-208969
39. Chong JY, Rowland LP, Utiger RD. Hashimoto encephalopathy: syndrome or myth? *Arch Neurol.* (2003) 60:164–71. doi: 10.1001/archneur.60.2.164
40. Pari E, Rinaldi F, Premi E, Codella M, Rao R, Paghera B, et al. A follow-up (1)(8)F-FDG brain PET study in a case of Hashimoto's encephalopathy causing drug-resistant status epilepticus treated with plasmapheresis. *J Neurol.* (2014) 261:663–7. doi: 10.1007/s00415-013-7228-0
41. Laurent C, Capron J, Quillerou B, Thomas G, Alamowitch S, Fain O, et al. Steroid-responsive encephalopathy associated with autoimmune thyroiditis (SREAT): characteristics, treatment and outcome in 251 cases from the literature. *Autoimmun Rev.* (2016) 15:1129–33. doi: 10.1016/j.autrev.2016.09.008
42. Boers PM, Colebatch JG. Hashimoto's encephalopathy responding to plasmapheresis. *J Neurol Neurosurg Psychiatry.* (2001) 70:132. doi: 10.1136/jnnp.70.1.132
43. Bektas O, Yilmaz A, Kendirli T, Siklar Z, Deda G. Hashimoto encephalopathy causing drug-resistant status epilepticus treated with plasmapheresis. *Pediatr Neurol.* (2012) 46:132–5. doi: 10.1016/j.pediatrneurol.2011.11.009
44. Hussain NS, Rumbaugh J, Kerr D, Nath A, Hillis AE. Effects of prednisone and plasma exchange on cognitive impairment in Hashimoto encephalopathy. *Neurology.* (2005) 64:165–6. doi: 10.1212/01.WNL.0000148580.98997.C5
45. Nieuwenhuis L, Santens P, Vanwalleghem P, Boon P. Subacute Hashimoto's encephalopathy, treated with plasmapheresis. *Acta Neurolog Belgica.* (2004) 104:80–3.
46. Mori M, Kuwabara S, Yoshiyama M, Kanesaka T, Ogata T, Hattori T. Successful immune treatment for non-paraneoplastic limbic encephalitis. *J Neurol Sci.* (2002) 201:85–8. doi: 10.1016/S0022-510X(02)00188-0
47. Honnorat J. Autoimmune limbic encephalitis: an expanding concept. *Lancet Neurol.* (2010) 9:24–5. doi: 10.1016/S1474-4422(09)70333-3
48. Radja GK, Cavanna AE. Treatment of VGKC complex antibody-associated limbic encephalitis: a systematic review. *J Neuropsychiatry Clin Neurosci.* (2013) 25:264–71. doi: 10.1176/appi.neuropsych.13020022
49. Dirr LY, Elster AD, Donofrio PD, Smith M. Evolution of brain MRI abnormalities in limbic encephalitis. *Neurology.* (1990) 40:1304–6. doi: 10.1212/WNL.40.8.1304
50. Vedeler CA, Storstein A. Autoimmune limbic encephalitis. *Acta Neurol Scand Suppl.* (2009) 120:63–7. doi: 10.1111/j.1600-0404.2009.01204.x
51. Lawn ND, Westmoreland BF, Kiely MJ, Lennon VA, Vernino S. Clinical, magnetic resonance imaging, and electroencephalographic findings in paraneoplastic limbic encephalitis. *Mayo Clin Proceed.* (2003) 78:1363–8. doi: 10.4065/78.11.1363
52. Gultekin SH, Rosenfeld MR, Voltz R, Eichen J, Posner JB, Dalmau J. Paraneoplastic limbic encephalitis: neurological symptoms, immunological findings and tumour association in 50 patients. *Brain.* (2000) 123 (Pt 7):1481–94. doi: 10.1093/brain/123.7.1481
53. Corsellis JA, Goldberg GJ, Norton AR. "Limbic encephalitis" and its association with carcinoma. *Brain.* (1968) 91:481–96. doi: 10.1093/brain/91.3.481
54. Buckley C, Oger J, Clover L, Tuzun E, Carpenter K, Jackson M, et al. Potassium channel antibodies in two patients with reversible limbic encephalitis. *Ann Neurol.* (2001) 50:73–8. doi: 10.1002/ana.1097
55. Jaben EA, Winters JL. Plasma exchange as a therapeutic option in patients with neurologic symptoms due to antibodies to voltage-gated potassium

channels: a report of five cases and review of the literature. *J Clin Apher.* (2012) 27:267–73. doi: 10.1002/jca.21233
56. Gastaldi M, Thouin A, Vincent A. Antibody-mediated autoimmune encephalopathies and immunotherapies. *Neurotherapeutics.* (2016) 13:147–62. doi: 10.1007/s13311-015-0410-6
57. Schimmel M, Bien CG, Vincent A, Schenk W, Penzien J. Successful treatment of anti-N-methyl-D-aspartate receptor encephalitis presenting with catatonia. *Arch Dis Childhood.* (2009) 94:314–6. doi: 10.1136/adc.2008.149021
58. Wang RJ, Chen BD, Qi D. Anti-N-methyl-D-aspartate receptor encephalitis concomitant with multifocal subcortical white matter lesions on magnetic resonance imaging: a case report and review of the literature. *BMC Neurol.* (2015) 15:107. doi: 10.1186/s12883-015-0366-5
59. Rypulak E, Borys M, Piwowarczyk P, Fijalkowska M, Potrec B, Sysiak J, et al. Successful treatment of anti-NMDA receptor encephalitis with a prompt ovarian tumour removal and prolonged course of plasmapheresis: a case report. *Mol Clin Oncol.* (2016) 5:845–9. doi: 10.3892/mco.2016.1054
60. Markakis I, Alexopoulos H, Poulopoulou C, Akrivou S, Papathanasiou A, Katsiva V, et al. Immunotherapy-responsive limbic encephalitis with antibodies to glutamic acid decarboxylase. *J Neurol Sci.* (2014) 343:192–4. doi: 10.1016/j.jns.2014.05.032
61. McCarthy A, Dineen J, McKenna P, Keogan M, Sheehan J, Lynch T, et al. Anti-NMDA receptor encephalitis with associated catatonia during pregnancy. *J Neurol.* (2012) 259:2632–5. doi: 10.1007/s00415-012-6561-z
62. Van Ael Y, Amir R, Cras P. Anti-GAD antibodies, a rare cause of limbic encephalitis: a case report. *Acta Neurol Belgica.* (2016) 116:105–7. doi: 10.1007/s13760-015-0493-1
63. Shahani L. Steroid unresponsive anti-NMDA receptor encephalitis during pregnancy successfully treated with plasmapheresis. *BMJ Case Rep.* (2015) 2015:bcr2014208823. doi: 10.1136/bcr-2014-208823
64. Korff CM, Parvex P, Cimasoni L, Wilhelm-Bals A, Hampe CS, Schwitzgebel VM, et al. Encephalitis associated with glutamic acid decarboxylase autoantibodies in a child: a treatable condition? *Arch Neurol.* (2011) 68:1065–8. doi: 10.1001/archneurol.2011.177
65. Vincent A, Buckley C, Schott JM, Baker I, Dewar BK, Detert N, et al. Potassium channel antibody-associated encephalopathy: a potentially immunotherapy-responsive form of limbic encephalitis. *Brain.* (2004) 127 (Pt 3):701–12. doi: 10.1093/brain/awh077
66. DeSena AD, Noland DK, Matevosyan K, King K, Phillips L, Qureshi SS, et al. Intravenous methylprednisolone versus therapeutic plasma exchange for treatment of anti-N-methyl-D-aspartate receptor antibody encephalitis: a retrospective reiview. *J Clin Apher.* (2015) 30:212–6. doi: 10.1002/jca.21363
67. Suppiej A, Nosadini M, Zuliani L, Pelizza MF, Toldo I, Bertossi C, et al. Plasma exchange in pediatric anti-NMDAR encephalitis: a systematic review. *Brain Dev.* (2016) 38:613–22. doi: 10.1016/j.braindev.2016.01.009
68. Miyauchi A, Monden Y, Osaka H, Takahashi Y, Yamagata T. A case of anti-NMDAR encephalitis presented hypotensive shock during plasma exchange. *Brain Dev.* (2016) 38:427–30. doi: 10.1016/j.braindev.2015.10.009
69. Gokhale YA, Bhide S, Rajadhyaksha S, Bichile LS, Hase NK. Plasmapheresis: an adjunct therapy in severe progressive neuropsychiatric lupus. *J Assoc Phys India.* (2001) 49:986–9.
70. The American College of Rheumatology nomenclature and case definitions for neuropsychiatric lupus syndromes. *Arthritis Rheum.* (1999) 42:599–608. doi: 10.1002/1529-0131(199904)42:4<599::AID-ANR2>3.0.CO;2-F
71. Jones JV, Cumming RH, Bucknall RC, Asplin CM. Plasmapheresis in the management of acute systemic lupus erythematosus? *Lancet.* (1976) 1:709–11. doi: 10.1016/S0140-6736(76)93088-9
72. Magro-Checa C, Zirkzee EJ, Huizinga TW, Steup-Beekman GM. Management of neuropsychiatric systemic lupus erythematosus: current approaches and future perspectives. *Drugs.* (2016) 76:459–83. doi: 10.1007/s40265-015-0534-3
73. Unterweger B, Klein G, Fleischhacker WW. Plasma exchange for cerebral lupus erythematosus. *Biol Psychiatry.* (1988) 24:946–7. doi: 10.1016/0006-3223(88)90233-8
74. Barath S, Soltesz P, Kiss E, Aleksza M, Zeher M, Szegedi G, et al. The severity of systemic lupus erythematosus negatively correlates with the increasing number of CD4+CD25(high)FoxP3+ regulatory T cells during repeated plasmapheresis treatments of patients. *Autoimmunity.* (2007) 40:521–8. doi: 10.1080/08916930701610028
75. Cid J, Carbasse G, Andreu B, Baltanas A, Garcia-Carulla A, Lozano M. Efficacy and safety of plasma exchange: ann 11-year single-center experience of 2730 procedures in 317 patients. *Transfus Apher Sci.* (2014) 51:209–14. doi: 10.1016/j.transci.2014.08.018
76. Perisse D, Amoura Z, Cohen D, Saintigny P, Mekhloufi F, Mazet P, et al. Case study: effectiveness of plasma exchange in an adolescent with systemic lupus erythematosus and catatonia. *J Am Acad Child Adoles Psychiatry.* (2003) 42:497–9. doi: 10.1097/01.CHI.0000046820.95464.86
77. Kato T, Shiratori K, Kobashigawa T, Hidaka Y. Systemic lupus erythematosus with organic brain syndrome: serial electroencephalograms accurately evaluate therapeutic efficacy. *Internal Med.* (2006) 45:95–9. doi: 10.2169/internalmedicine.45.1363
78. Lassmann H, Brunner C, Bradl M, Linington C. Experimental allergic encephalomyelitis: the balance between encephalitogenic T lymphocytes and demyelinating antibodies determines size and structure of demyelinated lesions. *Acta Neuropathol.* (1988) 75:566–76. doi: 10.1007/BF00686201
79. Quintero-Del-Rio AI, Van M. Neurologic symptoms in children with systemic lupus erythematosus. *J Child Neurol.* (2000) 15:803–7. doi: 10.1177/088307380001501207
80. Euler HH, Schroeder JO, Harten P, Zeuner RA, Gutschmidt HJ. Treatment-free remission in severe systemic lupus erythematosus following synchronization of plasmapheresis with subsequent pulse cyclophosphamide. *Arthritis Rheum.* (1994) 37:1784–94. doi: 10.1002/art.1780371212
81. Lally L, Spiera R. Current therapies for ANCA-associated vasculitis. *Annu Rev Med.* (2015) 66:227–40. doi: 10.1146/annurev-med-011514-023051
82. Davies E, Connolly DJ, Mordekar SR. Encephalopathy in children: an approach to assessment and management. *Arch Dis Childhood.* (2012) 97:452–8. doi: 10.1136/adc.2011.300998
83. Rubio-Agusti I, Salavert M, Bataller L. Limbic encephalitis and related cortical syndromes. *Curr Treat Options Neurol.* (2013) 15:169–84. doi: 10.1007/s11940-012-0212-7
84. Ribi C, Cohen P, Pagnoux C, Mahr A, Arene JP, Puechal X, et al. Treatment of polyarteritis nodosa and microscopic polyangiitis without poor-prognosis factors: a prospective randomized study of one hundred twenty-four patients. *Arthritis Rheum.* (2010) 62:1186–97. doi: 10.1002/art.27340
85. Deshpande PV, Gilbert R, Alton H, Milford DV. Microscopic polyarteritis with renal and cerebral involvement. *Pediatr Nephrol.* (2000) 15:134–5. doi: 10.1007/s004670000428
86. Nishio M, Yoshioka K, Yamagami K, Morikawa T, Konishi Y, Hayashi N, et al. Reversible posterior leukoencephalopathy syndrome: a possible manifestation of Wegener's granulomatosis-mediated endothelial injury. *Modern Rheumatol.* (2008) 18:309–14. doi: 10.3109/s10165-008-0052-1
87. Pohl D, Tenembaum S. Treatment of acute disseminated encephalomyelitis. *Curr Treat Options Neurol.* (2012) 14:264–75. doi: 10.1007/s11940-012-0170-0
88. Krupp LB, Tardieu M, Amato MP, Banwell B, Chitnis T, Dale RC, et al. International pediatric multiple sclerosis study group criteria for pediatric multiple sclerosis and immune-mediated central nervous system demyelinating disorders: revisions to the 2007 definitions. *Multiple Scler.* (2013) 19:1261–7. doi: 10.1177/1352458513484547
89. Gray MP, Gorelick MH. Acute disseminated encephalomyelitis. *Pediatr Emergency Care.* (2016) 32:395–400. doi: 10.1097/PEC.0000000000000825
90. Borras-Novell C, Garcia Rey E, Perez Baena LF, Jordan Garcia I, Catella Cahiz D, Cambra F. Therapeutic plasma exchange in acute disseminated encephalomyelitis in children. *J Clin Apher.* (2015) 30:335–9. doi: 10.1002/jca.21388
91. Cotter FE, Bainbridge D, Newland AC. Neurological deficit associated with *Mycoplasma pneumoniae* reversed by plasma exchange. *Br Med J.* (1983) 286:22. doi: 10.1136/bmj.286.6358.22
92. Kanter DS, Horensky D, Sperling RA, Kaplan JD, Malachowski ME, Churchill WH Jr. Plasmapheresis in fulminant acute disseminated encephalomyelitis. *Neurology.* (1995) 45:824–7. doi: 10.1212/WNL.45.4.824

93. Shah AK, Tselis A, Mason B. Acute disseminated encephalomyelitis in a pregnant woman successfully treated with plasmapheresis. *J Neurol Sci.* (2000) 174:147–51. doi: 10.1016/S0022-510X(00)00260-4
94. Yi CH, La Vega-Talbott M, Friedman MT. Treatment of acute disseminated encephalomyelitis with plasmapheresis in a 16-year-old female, a case report and literature review. *J Clin Apher.* (2014) 29:339–40. doi: 10.1002/jca.21327
95. Stricker RB, Miller RG, Kiprov DD. Role of plasmapheresis in acute disseminated (postinfectious) encephalomyelitis. *J Clin Apher.* (1992) 7:173–9. doi: 10.1002/jca.2920070403
96. Miyazawa R, Hikima A, Takano Y, Arakawa H, Tomomasa T, Morikawa A. Plasmapheresis in fulminant acute disseminated encephalomyelitis. *Brain Dev.* (2001) 23:424–6. doi: 10.1016/S0387-7604(01)00256-X
97. Lin CH, Jeng JS, Yip PK. Plasmapheresis in acute disseminated encephalomyelitis. *J Clin Apher.* (2004) 19:154–9. doi: 10.1002/jca.20022
98. Keegan M, Pineda AA, McClelland RL, Darby CH, Rodriguez M, Weinshenker BG. Plasma exchange for severe attacks of CNS demyelination: predictors of response. *Neurology.* (2002) 58:143–6. doi: 10.1212/WNL.58.1.143
99. Mathur JL, Rajabi F, Schroeder A, Becker TK. Case of steroid-responsive encephalopathy from hypoglycaemia. *BMJ Case Rep.* (2017) 2017:bcr-2017-221262. doi: 10.1136/bcr-2017-221262
100. Laloux P. Steroid-responsive leucoencephalopathy due to cholesterol embolism. *J Neurol Neurosurg Psychiatry.* (2007) 78:112. doi: 10.1136/jnnp.2006.105981

16

Sex Steroids and Adult Neurogenesis in the Ventricular-Subventricular Zone

Giovanna Ponti[1,2], Alice Farinetti[2,3], Marilena Marraudino[2,3], GianCarlo Panzica[2,3] and Stefano Gotti[2,3]*

[1] Department of Veterinary Sciences, University of Turin, Grugliasco, Turin, Italy, [2] Neuroscience Institute Cavalieri Ottolenghi (NICO), Orbassano, Turin, Italy, [3] Department of Neuroscience "Rita Levi-Montalcini", University of Turin, Turin, Italy

***Correspondence:**
Giovanna Ponti
giovanna.ponti@unito.it

The forebrain ventricular-subventricular zone (V-SVZ) continuously generates new neurons throughout life. Neural stem cells (type B1 cells) along the lateral ventricle become activated, self-renew, and give rise to proliferating precursors which progress along the neurogenic lineage from intermediate progenitors (type C cells) to neuroblasts (type A cells). Neuroblasts proliferate and migrate into the olfactory bulb and differentiate into different interneuronal types. Multiple factors regulate each step of this process. Newly generated olfactory bulb interneurons are an important relay station in the olfactory circuits, controlling social recognition, reproductive behavior, and parental care. Those behaviors are strongly sexually dimorphic and changes throughout life from puberty through aging and in the reproductive age during estrous cycle and gestation. Despite the key role of sex hormones in regulating those behaviors, their contribution in modulating adult neurogenesis in V-SVZ is underestimated. Here, we compare the literature highlighting the sexual dimorphism and the differences across the physiological phases of the animal for the different cell types and steps through the neurogenic lineage.

Keywords: ventricular-subventricular zone, sexual dimorphism, estrogens, testosterone, neural stem cells, puberty, estrous cycle, pregnancy

INTRODUCTION

The subventricular zone-olfactory bulb (V-SVZ-OB) system has fascinated scientists for over than 25 years. In fact, this region harbors, in many mammals, a huge neurogenesis persisting until aging (1). In rodents, this process involves multiple steps, each one of them representing a model for different biological and pathological processes with unique features. In fact, this neurogenic process encompasses a germinal layer located in the ventricular-subventricular zone of the forebrain (V-SVZ), along the ventricle in which neural stem cells undergo self-renewal (2) and differentiation to intermediate progenitors (type C cells), then to immature neurons (type A cells) (3–5). Newly generated, type A, cells undergo tangential migration along the rostral migratory stream (RMS) up to the OB (6, 7). There, they migrate radially to the appropriate cell layer and differentiate into interneurons (8). Neurogenesis is thus a complex process consisting in proliferation, migration, apoptosis, and differentiation occurring in each of those levels with specific features (9, 10). The proper turnover enforced by proliferation, migration as well as apoptosis in the OB, is essential for optimizing olfaction [(11); **Figure 1**]. Therefore, the study of V-SVZ is capital for many purposes: understanding unregulated cell growth in tumor formations (12, 13), preventing or replacing cell loss in aging (1, 14, 15), decreasing neurodegenerative disease risks (16–18), and improving stroke treatments (18).

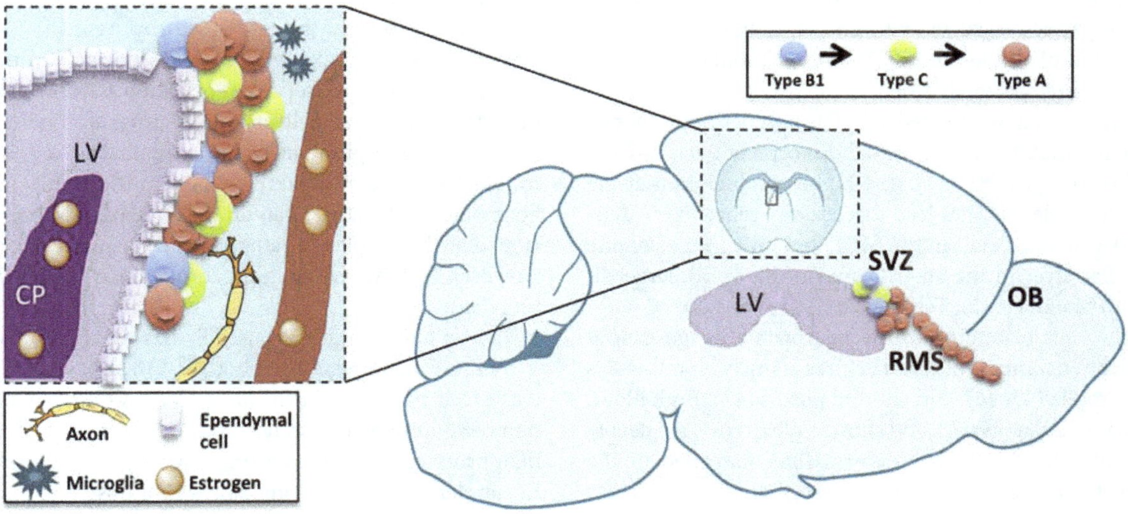

FIGURE 1 | Schematic drawing summarizing adult neurogenesis in the V-SVZ/OB system. Adult neurogenesis is a multiple-step process, occurring in three different subregions: the ventricular-subventricular zone (V-SVZ), the rostral migratory stream (RMS), and the olfactory bulb (OB). Sex hormones reaching the lateral ventricle (LV) through the choroid plexus (CP) or blood vessels (BV) modulate each of those steps either directly on neurogenic lineage or indirectly through other component of the stem-cell niche or the parenchyma.

Despite a huge interest on the endogenous and exogenous factors affecting adult neurogenesis in V-SVZ-OB system (19), few studies have focused on the role of gonadal hormones. This flaw is surprising since steroids have a key role in hippocampal neurogenesis both during development and in adulthood (20–22). Furthermore, V-SVZ-OB system is involved in social and reproductive behaviors, which are strongly regulated by sexual steroids (23, 24) and are targets for xenoestrogens (25–27). Moreover, estrogen receptors (ERs) and enzymes involved in the biosynthesis of steroids such as aromatase, the enzyme converting testosterone (T) into estradiol, are expressed in the V-SVZ (28) and in the OB of adult (29, 30) and developing (31) rats and mice (32). However, while the importance of steroids in the regulation of adult neurogenesis in the hippocampus has been widely studied, its role in the V-SVZ-OB system is more debated. Here, we want to focus on the available data in order to encourage a discussion addressing the open questions in the field.

SEXUAL DIMORPHISM IN V-SVZ-OB SYSTEM

Sexual dimorphism in the V-SVZ-OB system is an open question. Only few studies compared the two sexes and most of them are limited to a few ages. Indeed, the extent of neurogenesis in this region changes along life and it is likely to be affected by changes in the endocrine system.

Neurogenesis is more prominent in adult female mice compared with males. In 3-month-old C57/BL6J mice, females displayed higher proliferating rates in V-SVZ, RMS, and OB, and lower apoptotic cells in V-SVZ in both estrus and pregnancy (33) than males. Similarly, the number of neuronal progenitors (SOX2+) in the V-SVZ of females was higher than males in young adults but not in pups (34).

On the other hand, in other studies, the density of apoptotic cells in accessory (AOB) and main (MOB) OB was similar in the two sexes (35). Some differences affect transiently specific features of the V-SVZ-OB system. For instance, peripubertal males displayed higher rates of apoptosis (33), as well as of proliferation in the V-SVZ compared with females (35), but, in 2-month-old animals, the proliferation rate in the V-SVZ is similar in the two sexes and 1 month later there was a similar supply of newly generated cells in both the MOB and the AOB (35).

Multiple factors may explain the discrepancy among the data. From a technical point of view, the methods used to assess cell proliferation may highlight a different subset of the cycling population. In fact, while the total number of cycling cells identified with PCNA was measured by Diaz (33), the study of Nunez-Parra (35) highlighted only the cells in the S-phase, labeled by BrdU 2 h after the injection of the marker. Thus, it may reflect differences in the cell-cycle length between the two ages, or differences in the composition of the V-SVZ, e.g., a decrease in the number of type C cells, which have a longer S-phase length compared with type A cells (4, 5) or even differential sensitivities of BrdU antibodies (36), although the use of two different anti-BrdU antibodies by Nunez-Parra et al. is likely to have decreased this issue. Moreover, since different subregions in the V-SVZ give rise to different interneurons in the OB (37), it is possible that sexual dimorphism is limited to some of them. In addition to that, the extent of neurogenesis is dissimilar in different mouse strains (38) and it might be differently regulated. In fact, other reports indicate that the higher number of proliferating cells in the V-SVZ of females is limited to mature animals, i.e., 6–8 months old (39). Interestingly, this dimorphism is abolished (SJL/J) or reverted (BALB/C) in different strains (39). Accordingly, in two months old C57BL6 mice, the density of newly generated cells is higher in the AOB of males than females, while no sexual dimorphism has been reported for MOB (34). Similarly, no sexual dimorphism was observed in the number of newly generated cells in the AOB of young-adult CD1 mice, although the age of those mice was not specified (40).

In Wistar rats, males exhibited a higher number of proliferating cells than females and this sexual dimorphism was already established before puberty (41). The higher proliferation at the level of the ventricle does not lead to a sex difference in the density of newly generated cells in the MOB, but only in the volume of the granular layer in the anterior part of the AOB, larger in males than in females [(42); **Table 1**].

Beside the cells belonging to the neurogenic linage, neural stem-cell niche encompass other structures, namely blood vessels (43, 44), microglia (45, 46), and choroid plexus (47). Both blood vessels (48), microglia (49, 50), and choroid plexus (51) are deeply affected by sex steroids. These structures, thus, may mediate the effect of sex steroids on adult neurogenesis (**Figure 1**).

Moreover, V-SVZ neurogenesis may also be modulated in a trans-synaptic way by other neuronal circuits which may be sensible to sexual steroids, e.g., serotonin or dopamine system (52, 53), and cholinergic neurons (54).

In general, estrogens are neuroprotective and stimulate differentiation and proliferation while progestins and androgens stimulate differentiation and cell survival (21). However, the V-SVZ-OB system has its unique features. In conclusion, a number of factors can affect adult neurogenesis in the V-SVZ-OB system, and it is likely that some of them are sexually dimorphic and change throughout lifetime. In this picture, the endocrine system may play a key role.

HORMONAL REGULATION OF V-SVZ NEUROGENESIS IN ADULT FEMALES

Circulating hormone levels dramatically change during the life of female rodents, during both estrous cycle and pregnancy. These changes may affect neurogenesis. In particular, E_2 levels control the estrous cycle, pregnancy, and sexual behavior (32, 55).

TABLE 1 | Sexually dimorphic features in the subventricular zone-olfactory bulb (V-SVZ-OB) system.

Model	Feature	Higher in:	Where	Reference
Prepubertal Wistar rats	Proliferation rates	Males	V-SVZ	(41)
	Volume of the granule cell layer	Males	Anterior AOB	(42)
	Newly generated cells	Males	Anterior AOB	(42)
Peripubertal mice	Apoptotic cells	Males	V-SVZ	(33)
P60 C57/BL6 mice	Newly generated cells	Males	AOB	(34)
P90 C57/BL6 mice (estrous and pregnancy)	Proliferation rates	Females	V-SVZ, RMS, OB	(33)
	SOX2 + progenitors	Females	V-SVZ, RMS, OB	(34)
P180-P240 C57/BL6 mice	Proliferation rates	Females	V-SVZ, RMS, OB	(39)
P180-P240 BALB/c mice	Proliferation rates	Males	V-SVZ, RMS, OB	(39)

Since OB has a key role in mother's offspring recognition, it is not surprising that the rate of neurogenesis in V-SVZ transiently increase during pregnancy (56). Indeed, two peaks of cell proliferations were observed at gestation day 7 and at postpartum day 7, while at delivery the neurogenic rate is similar to matched aged virgin females (56). The first peak is evident also in females mated with sterile males, so it depends on maternal hormonal levels rather than on the embryo. However, this effect is mediated by prolactin rather than E_2 or progesterone (56, 57). However, E_2 may have an indirect role, since it stimulates prolactin release (58).

In the adult female mouse, E_2 has an inhibitory effect on V-SVZ-OB neurogenesis in both V-SVZ and OB. First, it decreases cell proliferation in the V-SVZ in different models. The number of proliferating cells in the V-SVZ is lower during estrus, than proestrus (39). Moreover, in ovariectomized females, acute E_2 supplementation for one day, with a dose comparable to the estrus, decreases cell proliferation in the V-SVZ (59). On the other hand, this effect was not detected by long-term treatment [3 weeks (60)] or with a lower dose of E_2 (61), comparable with diestrus (62). Differences in the effect of ovariectomy may be due to an interplay of many component of the neural stem-cell niche. In fact, ovariectomized mice express both ERα and ERβ, but E_2 supplementation selectively upregulates ERβ (51). T metabolite 5α-dihydrotestosterone (5αDHT) decreases the expression of AR in the choroid plexus of ovariectomized mice (51).

Male pheromones stimulate the production of ovarian hormones (63) as well as the neurogenesis in adult females (35, 64, 65). However, E_2 does not increase neurogenesis (66), nor cell proliferation in V-SVZ or neuroblasts density in OB, but it decreases cell survival in AOB, but not in MOB (24).

In the OB, E_2 has different effects depending on the region. In the MOB, in adulthood rather than during development, E_2 is able to impair the survival of newly generated cells (59) and MOB functionality (60). Interestingly, as demonstrated in aromatase-KO mice, developmental E_2 has the opposite effect in the AOB: the absence of E_2 during development decreases the survival of adult generated cells in the AOB. This phenotype can be reverted by adult E_2 treatment. On the contrary, the lack of estrogens during development neither alters cell proliferation in the V-SVZ, nor its response to E_2 (60).

In contrast to mice, the proliferation rate in the rat V-SVZ does not change during pregnancy, while it increases at delivery (67). As for mice, E_2 role in female rat is highly debated. Proliferation in the V-SVZ is not affected neither by ovariectomy nor by acute T or E_2 supplementation (41). No studies are available on the long-term effects of ovariectomy despite it deeply alter choroid plexus transcriptome which may indirectly affect the neural stem-cell niche (68). However, E_2 decreases the survival of newly generated cells in the AOB, but not in the MOB [(29, 30); **Figure 2; Table 2**].

The different effects of E_2 in mice and rats may be related with the lack of ERα and ERβ in the mouse V-SVZ (76) and with the presence of ERα receptor in the rat (28), although other pathways may be involved (21). For example, no information is available at the moment, concerning the expression of membrane ER (GPER) in rodent V-SVZ.

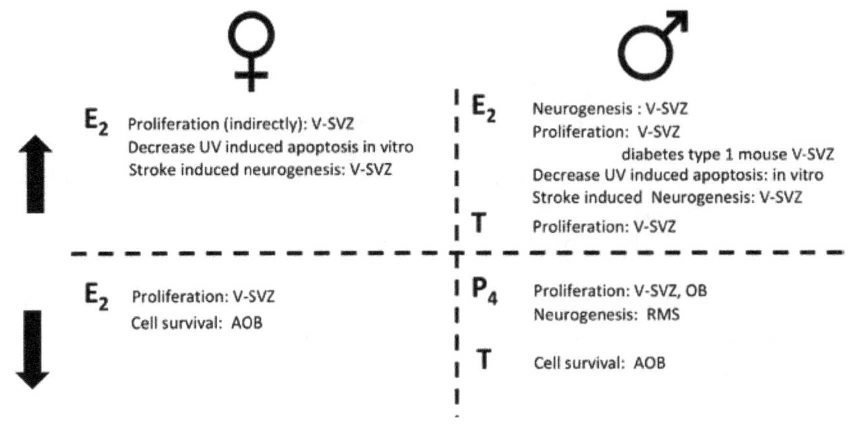

FIGURE 2 | The role of sex hormones in adult neurogenesis for females (left) and for males (right). On the top, steroid hormones induce an increase (↑) in the reported actions; on the bottom steroid hormones induce a decrease (↓) in the reported actions. Estradiol (E_2); progesterone (P_4); testosterone (T).

TABLE 2 | Summary of the hormonal regulations in the subventricular zone-olfactory bulb (V-SVZ-OB) system of adult male and female rodents.

	Hormone	Effect	Where	Reference
Hormonal regulation of V-SVZ neurogenesis in adult females				
Mouse	Estrogen	↓ Proliferation	V-SVZ	(39)
		↑ Proliferation (indirectly)	V-SVZ	(56, 57)
		↓ UV-induced apoptosis	*In vitro*	(34)
		↑ Stroke-induced neurogenesis	V-SVZ	(61, 69, 70)
		↓ Cell survival	MOB	(59)
		↓ Functionality	MOB	(60)
Mouse, rat	5α-dihydrotestosterone	↓ Expression AR	Choroid plexus	(51)
		↓ Cell survival	AOB	(29, 30, 66)
Hormonal regulation of V-SVZ neurogenesis in adult males				
Mouse	Castration	↑ Proliferation	V-SVZ	(39)
		↓ Apoptosis	V-SVZ	(39)
	Estrogen	↓ UV-induced apoptosis	*In vitro*	(34)
		↑ Stroke-induced neurogenesis	V-SVZ	(61, 69, 70)
Type 1 diabetes mouse model		↑ Proliferation	V-SVZ	(71)
		↓ Cell survival	AOB	(72)
Rat	5α-dihydrotestosterone	↓ Expression AR	Choroid plexus	(51)
	castration	↑ Expression ERβ	Choroid plexus	(51)
		↓ Proliferation	V-SVZ	(41)
	Estrogen	↑ Proliferation	V-SVZ	(41)
		↑ Stroke-induced neurogenesis	V-SVZ	(73, 74)
		↑ DCX + cells after stroke	V-SVZ	(73)
		↓ Cell death	V-SVZ	(74)
	Testosterone	↑ Proliferation	V-SVZ	(41)
	Progesterone	↓ Proliferation	V-SVZ/OB	(75)
		↓ Neurogenesis	RMS	(75)

HORMONAL REGULATION OF V-SVZ NEUROGENESIS IN ADULT MALES

The effect of sexual steroids is complex also in males. In fact, castration increased the number of proliferating cells and decreased the number of apoptotic ones in the V-SVZ of C57BL6 and SJL/J adult males, i.e., 6–8 months old (39).

Neurogenesis is influenced by pheromones related to aggressive (35) and paternal behavior (77, 78). In fact, the response to pheromones is sex specific and affected by hormonal levels. Indeed, female pheromones stimulate neurogenesis in adult males (64), although the survival of newly generated cells in the AOB in males does not change after opposite sex pheromones exposure, as in females (65). Interestingly, male pheromones as well as female ones, enhance proliferation in the V-SVZ of males (35), although it did not change the ratio of SOX2 cells among the BrdU labeled ones (64). However, low T levels feminize neurogenic response, increasing newly generated cell survival in the AOB, following male pheromone exposure, without affecting cell proliferation in RMS and V-SVZ, leading to attraction to male cues (72).

E_2 have a neuroprotective effect on V-SVZ precursors. In fact, it is able to restore proliferation in a type 1 diabetes mouse model (71). Only a few choroid plexus genes are altered by castration in rats (68): ERβ expression increased when compared with sham operated rats (51), while ARs expression decreased after 5αDHT treatment (51).

Unlike in females, T or E_2 are required for maintaining physiological neurogenic rate in the V-SVZ of peripubertal rats (41). In fact, the number of proliferating cells and the number of type C progenitors is restored by hormonal treatment in castrated rats, but this effect is restricted to the lateral wall of the V-SVZ (41).

Progesterone and its metabolites, decrease cell proliferation in the V-SVZ-OB of adult rats [2 months old (75)]. The number of newly generated cells in the final part of the RMS is decreased by progesterone metabolites. It is not clear, however, whether this effect is due to a reduction in cell proliferation, of cell survival or, less likely, in the migration rate (**Figure 2**; **Table 2**).

HORMONAL REGULATION OF V-SVZ NEUROGENESIS IN PATHOLOGICAL CONDITIONS

Beside an effect in physiological conditions, sex steroids may have a neuroprotective role after different insults. In fact, while no effect of sex steroid treatment was observed on cell death *in vitro*, E_2 prevented apoptosis after UV insults in both male- and female-derived V-SVZ cells, whereas no T effect was reported [(34); **Table 2**].

Stroke induced an increase in the number of newly generated cells, which was significantly higher in females. As for UV-induced apoptosis, E_2 enhances neurogenesis after ischemic stroke, *in vivo*, in mice of both sexes (61, 69, 79) and rats (73). This increase is present 96 h but not 24 h after stroke (61). The presence of ERα and ERβ, as well as AR is required for the stroke-induced neurogenesis in female mice, since it is abolished in transgenic mice lacking those receptors (69). Interestingly, those receptors are not directly expressed in the V-SVZ (61) suggesting that they may act indirectly through other cells.

Gonadal hormones are supposed to have a key role also in many diseases which display a different incidence and severity in the two sexes (80). V-SVZ neurogenesis may have a prominent role in some of them as: Parkinson disease (17, 81), Multiple sclerosis (82, 83), Alzheimer disease (84), autism (85), schizophrenia (86), and in psychiatric and cognitive disorders (87). However, only limited data are available on the effect of neuroactive steroids on the V-SVZ neurogenesis in those diseases. Moreover, many studies report controversial data on changes in the V-SVZ neurogenesis that may be related on the experimental model as in Parkinson disease (17).

CONCLUDING REMARKS

Despite the huge amount of studies on adult neurogenesis in the V-SVZ-OB system, still few data focus on its regulation by steroids. The role of steroids on V-SVZ-OB neurogenesis is highly complex. Generally, neurogenesis is more affected by T in males, while E_2 has a higher influence on females. However, the same hormone may determine a different effect depending on sex, age, strain, brain region, and neurogenic process. It is also possible that the different extent of V-SVZ-OB neurogenesis may reflects behavioral differences described among many strains of mice (88) as observed in other brain regions (89, 90). Those differences may be genetic (91, 92) or depend on a lack of maternal care during development (93). Profound differences exist between males and females. Some of them are actively determined by steroids levels in adults, while others are established during development. Moreover, sexual hormone's levels changes along life. Important species-specific differences exist between different rodent models. Despite some similarities, adult neurogenesis is regulated by different factors in the V-SVZ-OB system compared with the SGZ of the hippocampus. Furthermore, different cell populations, or different steps of the neurogenic lineage may be sensible to a specific hormone.

The extent of adult neurogenesis in the V-SVZ-OB changes along with each of the above mentioned parameters. However, it is not clear which features are directly or indirectly involved. It is, thus, important to consider all those parameters altogether.

AUTHOR CONTRIBUTIONS

All the authors equally contributed to the search for the sources and to the writing of the manuscript.

ACKNOWLEDGMENTS

We are grateful to the Fondazione Cavalieri Ottolenghi for hosting our laboratories in its premises.

FUNDING

We acknowledge the support from Fondazione Cavalieri Ottolenghi, the University of Torino (Ricerca locale to SG, GP, and GCP), and Fondazione CRT—RF 2015.2564 (to SG). This study was supported by Ministero dell'Istruzione, dell'Università e della Ricerca—MIUR projects "Dipartimenti di Eccellenza 2018–2022" to the Dept. of Neurosciences "Rita Levi Montalcini" and to the Dept. of Veterinary Sciences.

REFERENCES

1. Apple DM, Solano-Fonseca R, Kokovay E. Neurogenesis in the aging brain. *Biochem Pharmacol* (2017) 141:77–85. doi:10.1016/j.bcp.2017.06.116
2. Lois C, Alvarez-Buylla A. Proliferating subventricular zone cells in the adult mammalian forebrain can differentiate into neurons and Glia. *Proc Natl Acad Sci U S A* (1993) 90(5):2074–7. doi:10.1073/pnas.90.5.2074
3. Doetsch F, García-Verdugo JM, Alvarez-Buylla A. Cellular composition and three-dimensional organization of the subventricular germinal zone in the adult mammalian brain. *J Neurosci* (1997) 17(13):5046–61.
4. Ponti G, Obernier K, Guinto C, Jose L, Bonfanti L, Alvarez-Buylla A. Cell cycle and lineage progression of neural progenitors in the ventricular-subventricular zones of adult mice. *Proc Natl Acad Sci U S A* (2013) 110(11):E1045–54. doi:10.1073/pnas.1219563110

5. Ponti G, Obernier K, Alvarez-Buylla A. Lineage progression from stem cells to new neurons in the adult brain ventricular-subventricular zone. *Cell Cycle* (2013) 12(11):1649–50. doi:10.4161/cc.24984
6. Luskin MB. Restricted proliferation and migration of postnatally generated neurons derived from the forebrain subventricular zone. *Neuron* (1993) 11(1):173–89. doi:10.1016/0896-6273(93)90281-U
7. Lois C, Alvarez-Buylla A. Long-distance neuronal migration in the adult mammalian brain. *Science* (1994) 264(5162):1145–8. doi:10.1126/science.8178174
8. Gheusi G, Lepousez G, Lledo P-M. Adult-born neurons in the olfactory bulb: integration and functional consequences. *Curr Top Behav Neurosci* (2013) 15:49–72. doi:10.1007/7854_2012_228
9. Barral S, Beltramo R, Salio C, Aimar P, Lossi L, Merighi A. Phosphorylation of histone H2AX in the mouse brain from development to senescence. *Int J Mol Sci* (2014) 15(1):1554–73. doi:10.3390/ijms15011554
10. Capilla-Gonzalez V, Lavell E, Quinones-Hinojosa A, Guerrero-Cazares H. Regulation of subventricular zone-derived cells migration in the adult brain. *Adv Exp Med Biol* (2015) 853:1–21. doi:10.1007/978-3-319-16537-0_1
11. Mouret A, Lepousez G, Gras J, Gabellec MM, Lledo PM. Turnover of newborn olfactory bulb neurons optimizes olfaction. *J Neurosci* (2009) 29(39):12302–14. doi:10.1523/JNEUROSCI.3383-09.2009
12. Jackson EL, Alvarez-Buylla A. Characterization of adult neural stem cells and their relation to brain tumors. *Cells Tissues Organs* (2008) 188(1–2):212–24. doi:10.1159/000114541
13. Kusne Y, Sanai N. The SVZ and its relationship to stem cell based neurooncogenesis. *Adv Exp Med Biol* (2015) 853:23–32. doi:10.1007/978-3-319-16537-0_2
14. Luo J, Daniels SB, Lennington JB, Notti RQ, Conover JC. The aging neurogenic subventricular zone. *Aging Cell* (2006) 5(2):139–52. doi:10.1111/j.1474-9726.2006.00197.x
15. Capilla-Gonzalez V, Herranz-Perez V, Garcia-Verdugo JM. The aged brain: genesis and fate of residual progenitor cells in the subventricular zone. *Front Cell Neurosci* (2015) 9:365. doi:10.3389/fncel.2015.00365
16. Lamm O, Ganz J, Melamed E, Offen D. Harnessing neurogenesis for the possible treatment of Parkinson's disease. *J Comp Neurol* (2014) 522(12):2817–30. doi:10.1002/cne.23607
17. van den Berge SA, van Strien ME, Hol EM. Resident adult neural stem cells in Parkinson's disease—the brain's own repair system? *Eur J Pharmacol* (2013) 719(1–3):117–27. doi:10.1016/j.ejphar.2013.04.058
18. Zhang Z, Chopp M. Neural stem cells and ischemic brain. *J Stroke* (2016) 18(3):267–72. doi:10.5853/jos.2016.00206
19. Lim DA, Alvarez-Buylla A. Adult neural stem cells stake their ground. *Trends Neurosci* (2014) 37(10):563–71. doi:10.1016/j.tins.2014.08.006
20. Mahmoud R, Wainwright SR, Galea LA. Sex hormones and adult hippocampal neurogenesis: regulation, implications, and potential mechanisms. *Front Neuroendocrinol* (2016) 41:129–52. doi:10.1016/j.yfrne.2016.03.002
21. Heberden C. Sex steroids and neurogenesis. *Biochem Pharmacol* (2017) 141:56–62. doi:10.1016/j.bcp.2017.05.019
22. Galea LAM, Duarte-Guterman P. Hormones and the regulation of adult neurogenesis in the hippocampus and beyond: where are we now? Introduction to the special issue on hormonal regulation of adult neurogenesis: implications for disease. *Front Neuroendocrinol* (2016) 41:1–2. doi:10.1016/j.yfrne.2016.06.001
23. Peretto P, Paredes RG. Frontiers in neurosciencesocial cues, adult neurogenesis, and reproductive behavior. In: Mucignat-Caretta C, editor. *Neurobiology of Chemical Communication.* Boca Raton, FL: CRC Press/Taylor & Francis(c) (2014).
24. Brus M, Trouillet AC, Hellier V, Bakker J. Estradiol-induced neurogenesis in the female accessory olfactory bulb is required for the learning of the male odor. *J Neurochem* (2016) 138(3):457–68. doi:10.1111/jnc.13677
25. Rodriguez-Gomez A, Filice F, Gotti S, Panzica G. Perinatal exposure to genistein affects the normal development of anxiety and aggressive behaviors and nitric oxide system in CD1 male mice. *Physiol Behav* (2014) 133:107–14. doi:10.1016/j.physbeh.2014.05.020
26. Hicks KD, Sullivan AW, Cao J, Sluzas E, Rebuli M, Patisaul HB. Interaction of bisphenol A (BPA) and soy phytoestrogens on sexually dimorphic sociosexual behaviors in male and female rats. *Horm Behav* (2016) 84:121–6. doi:10.1016/j.yhbeh.2016.06.010
27. Ho SM, Cheong A, Adgent MA, Veevers J, Suen AA, Tam NN, et al. Environmental factors, epigenetics, and developmental origin of reproductive disorders. *Reprod Toxicol* (2017) 68:85–104. doi:10.1016/j.reprotox.2016.07.011
28. Isgor C, Watson SJ. Estrogen receptor alpha and beta mRNA expressions by proliferating and differentiating cells in the adult rat dentate gyrus and subventricular zone. *Neuroscience* (2005) 134(3):847–56. doi:10.1016/j.neuroscience.2005.05.008
29. Hoyk Z, Varga C, Parducz A. Estrogen-induced region specific decrease in the density of 5-bromo-2-deoxyuridine-labeled cells in the olfactory bulb of adult female rats. *Neuroscience* (2006) 141(4):1919–24. doi:10.1016/j.neuroscience.2006.05.053
30. Hoyk Z, Csákvári E, Gyenes A, Siklós L, Harada N, Párducz A. Aromatase and estrogen receptor beta expression in the rat olfactory bulb: neuroestrogen action in the first relay station of the olfactory pathway? *Acta Neurobiol Exp* (2014) 74(1):1–14.
31. Horvath TL, Wikler KC. Aromatase in developing sensory systems of the rat brain. *J Neuroendocrinol* (1999) 11(2):77–84. doi:10.1046/j.1365-2826.1999.00285.x
32. Bakker J, Baum MJ. Role for estradiol in female-typical brain and behavioral sexual differentiation. *Front Neuroendocrinol* (2008) 29(1):1–16. doi:10.1016/j.yfrne.2007.06.001
33. Diaz D, Valero J, Airado C, Baltanas FC, Weruaga E, Alonso JR. Sexual dimorphic stages affect both proliferation and serotonergic innervation in the adult rostral migratory stream. *Exp Neurol* (2009) 216(2):357–64. doi:10.1016/j.expneurol.2008.12.013
34. Kim JY, Casaccia-Bonnefil P. Interplay of hormones and p53 in modulating gender dimorphism of subventricular zone cell number. *J Neurosci Res* (2009) 87(15):3297–305. doi:10.1002/jnr.21940
35. Nunez-Parra A, Pugh V, Araneda RC. Regulation of adult neurogenesis by behavior and age in the accessory olfactory bulb. *Mol Cell Neurosci* (2011) 47(4):274–85. doi:10.1016/j.mcn.2011.05.003
36. Leuner B, Glasper ER, Gould E. Thymidine analog methods for studies of adult neurogenesis are not equally sensitive. *J Comp Neurol* (2009) 517(2):123–33. doi:10.1002/cne.22107
37. Merkle FT, Mirzadeh Z, Alvarez-Buylla A. Mosaic organization of neural stem cells in the adult brain. *Science* (2007) 317(5836):381–4. doi:10.1126/science.1144914
38. Li Q, Michaud M, Stewart W, Schwartz M, Madri JA. Modeling the neurovascular niche: murine strain differences mimic the range of responses to chronic hypoxia in the premature newborn. *J Neurosci Res* (2008) 86(6):1227–42. doi:10.1002/jnr.21597
39. Tatar C, Bessert D, Tse H, Skoff RP. Determinants of central nervous system adult neurogenesis are sex, hormones, mouse strain, age, and brain region. *Glia* (2013) 61(2):192–209. doi:10.1002/glia.22426
40. Oboti L, Savalli G, Giachino C, De Marchis S, Panzica GC, Fasolo A, et al. Integration and sensory experience-dependent survival of newly-generated neurons in the accessory olfactory bulb of female mice. *Eur J Neurosci* (2009) 29(4):679–92. doi:10.1111/j.1460-9568.2009.06614.x
41. Farinetti A, Tomasi S, Foglio B, Ferraris A, Ponti G, Gotti S, et al. Testosterone and estradiol differentially affect cell proliferation in the subventricular zone of young adult gonadectomized male and female rats. *Neuroscience* (2015) 286:162–70. doi:10.1016/j.neuroscience.2014.11.050
42. Peretto P, Giachino C, Panzica GC, Fasolo A. Sexually dimorphic neurogenesis is topographically matched with the anterior accessory olfactory bulb of the adult rat. *Cell Tissue Res* (2001) 306(3):385–9. doi:10.1007/s00441-001-0471-1
43. Colin-Castelan D, Ramirez-Santos J, Gutierrez-Ospina G. Differential vascular permeability along the forebrain ventricular neurogenic niche in the adult murine brain. *J Neurosci Res* (2016) 94(2):161–9. doi:10.1002/jnr.23682
44. Tavazoie M, Van der Veken L, Silva-Vargas V, Louissaint M, Colonna L, Zaidi B, et al. A specialized vascular niche for adult neural stem cells. *Cell Stem Cell* (2008) 3(3):279–88. doi:10.1016/j.stem.2008.07.025
45. Lenz KM, McCarthy MM. A starring role for microglia in brain sex differences. *Neuroscientist* (2015) 21(3):306–21. doi:10.1177/1073858414536468
46. Sato K. Effects of microglia on neurogenesis. *Glia* (2015):1394–405. doi:10.1002/glia.22858
47. Silva-Vargas V, Maldonado-Soto AR, Mizrak D, Codega P, Doetsch F. Age-dependent niche signals from the choroid plexus regulate adult neural

stem cells. *Cell Stem Cell* (2016) 19(5):643–52. doi:10.1016/j.stem.2016.06.013
48. Akishita M, Yu J. Hormonal effects on blood vessels. *Hypertens Res* (2012) 35(4):363–9. doi:10.1038/hr.2012.4
49. Habib P, Beyer C. Regulation of brain microglia by female gonadal steroids. *J Steroid Biochem Mol Biol* (2015) 146:3–14. doi:10.1016/j.jsbmb.2014.02.018
50. Rebuli ME, Gibson P, Rhodes CL, Cushing BS, Patisaul HB. Sex differences in microglial colonization and vulnerabilities to endocrine disruption in the social brain. *Gen Comp Endocrinol* (2016) 238:39–46. doi:10.1016/j.ygcen.2016.04.018
51. Santos CR, Duarte AC, Quintela T, Tomas J, Albuquerque T, Marques F, et al. The choroid plexus as a sex hormone target: functional implications. *Front Neuroendocrinol* (2017) 44:103–21. doi:10.1016/j.yfrne.2016.12.002
52. Young SZ, Taylor MM, Bordey A. Neurotransmitters couple brain activity to subventricular zone neurogenesis. *Eur J Neurosci* (2011) 33(6):1123–32. doi:10.1111/j.1460-9568.2011.07611.x
53. Tong CK, Chen J, Cebrian-Silla A, Mirzadeh Z, Obernier K, Guinto CD, et al. Axonal control of the adult neural stem cell niche. *Cell Stem Cell* (2014) 14(4):500–11. doi:10.1016/j.stem.2014.01.014
54. Paez-Gonzalez P, Asrican B, Rodriguez E, Kuo CT. Identification of distinct ChAT(+) neurons and activity-dependent control of postnatal SVZ neurogenesis. *Nat Neurosci* (2014) 17(7):934–42. doi:10.1038/nn.3734
55. Taziaux M, Keller M, Bakker J, Balthazart J. Sexual behavior activity tracks rapid changes in brain estrogen concentrations. *J Neurosci* (2007) 27(24): 6563–72. doi:10.1523/JNEUROSCI.1797-07.2007
56. Shingo T, Gregg C, Enwere E, Fujikawa H, Hassam R, Geary C, et al. Pregnancy-stimulated neurogenesis in the adult female forebrain mediated by prolactin. *Science* (2003) 299(5603):117–20. doi:10.1126/science.1076647
57. Larsen CM, Grattan DR. Prolactin, neurogenesis, and maternal behaviors. *Brain Behav Immun* (2012) 26(2):201–9. doi:10.1016/j.bbi.2011.07.233
58. Amenomori Y, Chen CL, Meites J. Serum prolactin levels in rats during different reproductive states. *Endocrinology* (1970) 86(3):506–10. doi:10.1210/endo-86-3-506
59. Brock O, Keller M, Veyrac A, Douhard Q, Bakker J. Short term treatment with estradiol decreases the rate of newly generated cells in the subventricular zone and main olfactory bulb of adult female mice. *Neuroscience* (2010) 166(2):368–76. doi:10.1016/j.neuroscience.2009.12.050
60. Veyrac A, Bakker J. Postnatal and adult exposure to estradiol differentially influences adult neurogenesis in the main and accessory olfactory bulb of female mice. *FASEB J* (2011) 25(3):1048–57. doi:10.1096/fj.10-172635
61. Suzuki S, Gerhold LM, Bottner M, Rau SW, Dela Cruz C, Yang E, et al. Estradiol enhances neurogenesis following ischemic stroke through estrogen receptors alpha and beta. *J Comp Neurol* (2007) 500(6):1064–75. doi:10.1002/cne.21240
62. Nelson JF, Felicio LS, Osterburg HH, Finch CE. Differential contributions of ovarian and extraovarian factors to age-related reductions in plasma estradiol and progesterone during the estrous cycle of C57BL/6J mice. *Endocrinology* (1992) 130(2):805–10. doi:10.1210/endo.130.2.1733727
63. Bronson FH, Maruniak JA. Differential effects of male stimuli on follicle-stimulating hormone, luteinizing hormone, and prolactin secretion in prepubertal female mice. *Endocrinology* (1976) 98(5):1101–8. doi:10.1210/endo-98-5-1101
64. Koyama S, Soini HA, Foley J, Novotny MV, Lai C. Stimulation of cell proliferation in the subventricular zone by synthetic murine pheromones. *Front Behav Neurosci* (2013) 7:101. doi:10.3389/fnbeh.2013.00101
65. Oboti L, Schellino R, Giachino C, Chamero P, Pyrski M, Leinders-Zufall T, et al. Newborn interneurons in the accessory olfactory bulb promote mate recognition in female mice. *Front Neurosci* (2011) 5:113. doi:10.3389/fnins.2011.00113
66. Oboti L, Trova S, Schellino R, Marraudino M, Harris NR, Abiona OM, et al. Activity dependent modulation of granule cell survival in the accessory olfactory bulb at puberty. *Front Neuroanat* (2017) 11:44. doi:10.3389/fnana.2017.00044
67. Furuta M, Bridges RS. Gestation-induced cell proliferation in the rat brain. *Brain Res Dev Brain Res* (2005) 156(1):61–6. doi:10.1016/j.devbrainres.2005.01.008
68. Quintela T, Marcelino H, Deery MJ, Feret R, Howard J, Lilley KS, et al. Sex-related differences in rat choroid plexus and cerebrospinal fluid: a cDNA microarray and proteomic analysis. *J Neuroendocrinol* (2016) 28(1). doi:10.1111/jne.12340
69. Li J, Siegel M, Yuan M, Zeng Z, Finnucan L, Persky R, et al. Estrogen enhances neurogenesis and behavioral recovery after stroke. *J Cereb Blood Flow Metab* (2011) 31(2):413–25. doi:10.1038/jcbfm.2010.181
70. Cheng Y, Su Q, Shao B, Cheng J, Wang H, Wang L, et al. 17Beta-estradiol attenuates poststroke depression and increases neurogenesis in female ovariectomized rats. *Biomed Res Int* (2013) 2013:392434. doi:10.1155/2013/392434
71. Saravia F, Revsin Y, Lux-Lantos V, Beauquis J, Homo-Delarche F, De Nicola AF. Oestradiol restores cell proliferation in dentate gyrus and subventricular zone of streptozotocin-diabetic mice. *J Neuroendocrinol* (2004) 16(8):704–10. doi:10.1111/j.1365-2826.2004.01223.x
72. Schellino R, Trova S, Cimino I, Farinetti A, Jongbloets BC, Pasterkamp RJ, et al. Opposite-sex attraction in male mice requires testosterone-dependent regulation of adult olfactory bulb neurogenesis. *Sci Rep* (2016) 6:36063. doi:10.1038/srep36063
73. Zheng J, Zhang P, Li X, Lei S, Li W, He X, et al. Post-stroke estradiol treatment enhances neurogenesis in the subventricular zone of rats after permanent focal cerebral ischemia. *Neuroscience* (2013) 231(Suppl C):82–90. doi:10.1016/j.neuroscience.2012.11.042
74. Brown CM, Suzuki S, Jelks KA, Wise PM. Estradiol is a potent protective, restorative, and trophic factor after brain injury. *Semin Reprod Med* (2009) 27(3):240–9. doi:10.1055/s-0029-1216277
75. Giachino C, Galbiati M, Fasolo A, Peretto P, Melcangi RC. Effects of progesterone derivatives, dihydroprogesterone and tetrahydroprogesterone, on the subependymal layer of the adult rat. *J Neurobiol* (2004) 58(4):493–502. doi:10.1002/neu.10290
76. Merchenthaler I, Lane MV, Numan S, Dellovade TL. Distribution of estrogen receptor alpha and beta in the mouse central nervous system: in vivo autoradiographic and immunocytochemical analyses. *J Comp Neurol* (2004) 473(2):270–91. doi:10.1002/cne.20128
77. Mak GK, Weiss S. Paternal recognition of adult offspring mediated by newly generated CNS neurons. *Nat Neurosci* (2010) 13(6):753–8. doi:10.1038/nn.2550
78. Feierstein CE. Linking adult olfactory neurogenesis to social behavior. *Front Neurosci* (2012) 6:173. doi:10.3389/fnins.2012.00173
79. Cheng M-F. Hypothalamic neurogenesis in the adult brain. *Front Neuroendocrinol* (2013) 34(3):167–78. doi:10.1016/j.yfrne.2013.05.001
80. Panzica G, Melcangi RC. Structural and molecular brain sexual differences: a tool to understand sex differences in health and disease. *Neurosci Biobehav Rev* (2016) 67:2–8. doi:10.1016/j.neubiorev.2016.04.017
81. He XJ, Nakayama H. Transiently impaired neurogenesis in MPTP mouse model of Parkinson's disease. *Neurotoxicology* (2015) 50:46–55. doi:10.1016/j.neuro.2015.07.007
82. Mecha M, Feliu A, Carrillo-Salinas FJ, Mestre L, Guaza C. Mobilization of progenitors in the subventricular zone to undergo oligodendrogenesis in the Theiler's virus model of multiple sclerosis: implications for remyelination at lesions sites. *Exp Neurol* (2013) 250:348–52. doi:10.1016/j.expneurol.2013.10.011
83. Akkermann R, Beyer F, Kury P. Heterogeneous populations of neural stem cells contribute to myelin repair. *Neural Regen Res* (2017) 12(4):509–17. doi:10.4103/1673-5374.204999
84. Zhang P, Xie MQ, Ding YQ, Liao M, Qi SS, Chen SX, et al. Allopregnanolone enhances the neurogenesis of midbrain dopaminergic neurons in APPswe/PSEN1 mice. *Neuroscience* (2015) 290:214–26. doi:10.1016/j.neuroscience.2015.01.019
85. Kotagiri P, Chance SA, Szele FG, Esiri MM. Subventricular zone cytoarchitecture changes in autism. *Dev Neurobiol* (2014) 74(1):25–41. doi:10.1002/dneu.22127
86. Liu YH, Lai WS, Tsay HJ, Wang TW, Yu JY. Effects of maternal immune activation on adult neurogenesis in the subventricular zone-olfactory bulb pathway and olfactory discrimination. *Schizophr Res* (2013) 151(1-3):1–11. doi:10.1016/j.schres.2013.09.007
87. Apple DM, Fonseca RS, Kokovay E. The role of adult neurogenesis in psychiatric and cognitive disorders. *Brain Res* (2017) 1655:270–6. doi:10.1016/j.brainres.2016.01.023

88. Kohl J, Autry AE, Dulac C. The neurobiology of parenting: a neural circuit perspective. *Bioessays* (2017) 39(1):1–11. doi:10.1002/bies.201600159
89. Mathieson WB, Wilkinson M, Brown RE, Bond TL, Taylor SW, Neumann PE. FOS and FOSB expression in the medial preoptic nucleus pars compacta of maternally active C57BL/6J and DBA/2J mice. *Brain Res* (2002) 952(2):170–5. doi:10.1016/S0006-8993(02)03078-0
90. Mathieson WB, Taylor SW, Marshall M, Neumann PE. Strain and sex differences in the morphology of the medial preoptic nucleus of mice. *J Comp Neurol* (2000) 428(2):254–65. doi:10.1002/1096-9861(20001211)428:2<254::AID-CNE5>3.0.CO;2-A
91. Holmes A, Wrenn CC, Harris AP, Thayer KE, Crawley JN. Behavioral profiles of inbred strains on novel olfactory, spatial and emotional tests for reference memory in mice. *Genes Brain Behav* (2002) 1(1):55–69. doi:10.1046/j.1601-1848.2001.00005.x
92. Levy F, Keller M. Olfactory mediation of maternal behavior in selected mammalian species. *Behav Brain Res* (2009) 200(2):336–45. doi:10.1016/j.bbr.2008.12.017
93. Sauce B, Goes CP, Forti I, O do Monte BG, Watanabe IM, Cunha J, et al. A link between thrifty phenotype and maternal care across two generations of intercrossed mice. *PLoS One* (2017) 12(5):e0177954. doi:10.1371/journal.pone.0177954

17

Neural Androgen Synthesis and Aggression: Insights From a Seasonally Breeding Rodent

Kathleen M. Munley, Nikki M. Rendon and Gregory E. Demas*

Program in Neuroscience, Department of Biology, Center for the Integrative Study of Animal Behavior, Indiana University, Bloomington, IN, United States

***Correspondence:**
Kathleen M. Munley
kmunley@indiana.edu

Aggression is an essential social behavior that promotes survival and reproductive fitness across animal systems. While research on the neuroendocrine mechanisms underlying this complex behavior has traditionally focused on the classic neuroendocrine model, in which circulating gonadal steroids are transported to the brain and directly mediate neural circuits relevant to aggression, recent studies have suggested that this paradigm is oversimplified. Work on seasonal mammals that exhibit territorial aggression outside of the breeding season, such as Siberian hamsters (*Phodopus sungorus*), has been particularly useful in elucidating alternate mechanisms. These animals display elevated levels of aggression during the non-breeding season, in spite of gonadal regression and reduced levels of circulating androgens. Our laboratory has provided considerable evidence that the adrenal hormone precursor dehydroepiandrosterone (DHEA) is important in maintaining aggression in both male and female Siberian hamsters during the non-breeding season, a mechanism that appears to be evolutionarily-conserved in some seasonal rodent and avian species. This review will discuss research on the neuroendocrine mechanisms of aggression in Siberian hamsters, a species that displays robust neural, physiological, and behavioral changes on a seasonal basis. Furthermore, we will address how these findings support a novel neuroendocrine pathway for territorial aggression in seasonal animals, in which adrenal DHEA likely serves as an essential precursor for neural androgen synthesis during the non-breeding season.

Keywords: aggression, androgens, brain, dehydroepiandrosterone, steroid-converting enzymes, hamster, seasonality

INTRODUCTION

Aggression is a well-studied social behavior that is universally exhibited across vertebrates in various social contexts (1, 2). Among conspecifics, aggression is typically displayed when two or more individuals compete for a critical limited resource, such as mates, territories, or food. In seasonally breeding vertebrates, elevated territorial aggression is most often exhibited during the breeding season, when individuals compete for access to resources that will increase their chances of reproductive success. A substantial body of work on male territorial aggression has shown that elevated levels of circulating androgens, including testosterone (T), are correlated with increased aggressive behaviors during the breeding season [reviewed in the studies by Cunningham et al. (3) and Fuxjager et al. (4)]. For example, studies from seasonally breeding birds [(5, 6); but see the study by Apfelbeck et al. (7)]; lizards (8, 9); and rodent species, including mice [(10); but see the study by Trainor and Marler (11)], gerbils (12, 13), and hamsters (14, 15), have demonstrated that castration decreases intermale aggression in a reproductive context, but that this reduction can be alleviated by exogenous T administration. Moreover, individuals with higher endogenous levels of T oftentimes display greater aggression toward conspecifics and may exhibit dominance over animals with lower circulating T levels (16, 17).

Interestingly, some seasonally breeding species exhibit equivalent or increased levels of territorial aggression outside of the breeding season, despite gonadal regression and reduced circulating levels of androgens [reviewed in the study by Soma et al. (18)]. A particularly remarkable example of a species that displays elevated aggression during the non-breeding season is Siberian hamsters (*Phodopus sungorus*), which exhibit robust changes in morphology, physiology, and behavior on a seasonal basis. Siberian hamsters breed during the summer months and cease breeding and undergo gonadal regression, a reduction in body mass, and changes in thermoregulation during the winter months (19). These natural seasonal adaptations can be elicited in the laboratory by housing animals in light cycles that mimic the photoperiods of the breeding and non-breeding seasons (20, 21). For example, animals exposed to short, winter-like days (i.e., >12.5 h of light/day) in the laboratory, which mimic the photoperiod conditions of the non-breeding season, exhibit gonadal regression, a reduction in body mass, and a change in pelage color from brown to white (22, 23). These characteristic changes in physiology are associated with increased levels of aggression in both male (15, 24) and female hamsters (25, 26). Thus, Siberian hamsters are an excellent model for elucidating how seasonal variations in photoperiod can alter the neuroendocrine mechanisms associated with territorial aggression.

SEASONAL SHIFTS IN NEUROENDOCRINE MECHANISMS UNDERLYING AGGRESSION

Pineal Melatonin Regulates Seasonal Changes in Aggression

Although several biotic and abiotic factors vary on a seasonal basis, photoperiod (day length) is the primary environmental cue that is used by animals to shape seasonal shifts in reproductive physiology and social behavior [reviewed in the studies by Prendergast et al. (27) and Walton et al. (28)]. These differences in physiology and behavior are produced *via* a complex neural circuit, which begins with the perception of environmental light *via* retinal ganglion cells and culminates in the transduction of information about day length into a neuroendocrine signal within the pineal gland. The pineal gland secretes melatonin, an indolamine that plays a prominent role in establishing and maintaining biological rhythms, in response to photoperiodic information. Because melatonin secretion tends to be high at night and low during the day, changes in photoperiod cause associated changes in the pattern and duration of melatonin secretion, which convey information about day length to the central nervous system [reviewed in the studies by Bartness et al. (29) and Goldman (30)].

Previous work has implicated pineal melatonin in the modulation of neuroendocrine mechanisms underlying seasonal aggression *via* direct actions on neural substrates, such as the hypothalamus and pituitary gland, and *via* peripheral actions on the adrenal glands and gonads [reviewed in the studies by Haller et al. (31) and Boringer and Nelson (32)]. In seasonally breeding vertebrates, melatonin has regulatory functions at all levels of the hypothalamic–pituitary–gonadal (HPG) and hypothalamic–pituitary–adrenal (HPA) axes and binds to melatonin-type I receptors (MT_1) located on the hypothalamus (33, 34), anterior pituitary gland (35, 36), gonads (37, 38), and adrenals (39, 40). Collectively, the presence of MT_1 at different tiers of the HPA and HPG axes suggests that melatonin alters gonadal and adrenal steroid synthesis on a seasonal basis. More specifically, long days induce a lower duration of melatonin secretion, which upregulates the HPG axis relative to the HPA axis to promote gonadal steroid secretion [reviewed in the study by Tsutsui et al. (41)]. Conversely, short days result in prolonged melatonin secretion, which upregulates the HPA axis relative to the HPG axis and elevates adrenal steroid synthesis (26, 42). The action of melatonin at the level of the adrenals is particularly intriguing, since several species of seasonally breeding animals that display year-round territorial aggression increase serum dehydroepiandrosterone (DHEA), an adrenal androgen, during the non-breeding season.

DHEA Promotes Territorial Aggression During the Non-Breeding Season

In recent years, it has become increasingly evident that DHEA is an important modulator of seasonal aggression in birds and rodents [reviewed in the study by Soma et al. (43)]. DHEA is an androgen that is secreted by the adrenal cortex in certain mammals, including hamsters and squirrels (15, 44). Although DHEA is synthesized peripherally, circulating DHEA is capable of passing through the blood–brain barrier and can be metabolized to active androgens and estrogens, such as T and estradiol (E_2), *via* a multi-step conversion in brain regions that express the appropriate steroidogenic enzymes (45, 46). Alternatively, some seasonally breeding animals are capable of steroid synthesis *de novo* from cholesterol, and these "neurosteroids" can bind directly to androgen receptor (AR) and estrogen receptors (ERα and ERβ) to regulate social behaviors (47, 48). Because DHEA has a low affinity for AR and ER, high endogenous levels of DHEA would be required to activate these receptors and induce changes in behavior (49). Therefore, it is likely that region-specific metabolism of circulating DHEA and/or neurally synthesized DHEA into active androgens and estrogens is primarily responsible for modulating the neural circuits relevant to territorial aggression during the non-breeding season, since these steroids bind with high affinity to AR and ER in neurons and glia.

Results from studies on seasonally breeding animals have illuminated a few potential neuroendocrine pathways by which androgens can act on relevant neural circuits to modulate seasonal changes in aggression (**Figure 1**). Briefly, the classical neuroendocrine model proposes that circulating gonadal steroids pass through the blood–brain barrier and act on neural circuits relevant to aggression by directly binding to

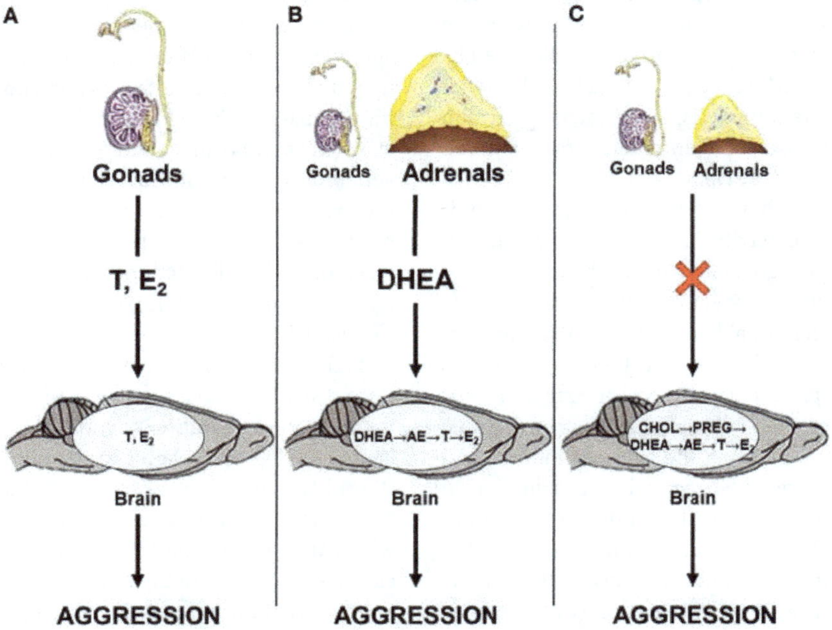

FIGURE 1 | Neuroendocrine pathways by which androgens could affect territorial aggression in seasonally breeding animals. **(A)** Gonadal steroids, such as testosterone (T) and estradiol (E_2), act directly on the brain; **(B)** adrenal dehydroepiandrosterone (DHEA) is locally converted to T and/or E_2; and **(C)** steroids are produced *de novo* in the brain from cholesterol (CHOL) *via* conversion to pregnenolone (PREG) and, subsequently, to DHEA, androstenedione (AE), T, and E_2 in the absence of steroid production from the gonads and adrenal glands.

AR or ER (**Figure 1A**). This mechanism likely predominates during the breeding season, when animals exhibit elevated levels of circulating androgens. However, outside of the breeding season, circulating gonadal steroids are low and adrenal steroids, such as DHEA, may serve as an important source of neural T and E_2. Thus, during the non-breeding season, circulating DHEA may serve as a prohormone and be converted to active androgens and estrogens in the brain after passing through the blood–brain barrier (**Figure 1B**). Alternatively, neurosteroids may be synthesized *de novo* from cholesterol (**Figure 1C**). These different neuroendocrine mechanisms culminate in region-specific binding of active steroids to AR and ER, respectively, which modulates seasonal changes in territorial aggression.

Adrenal DHEA as a Source of Neurally-Derived Androgens in Siberian Hamsters

Both male and female Siberian hamsters exhibit pronounced changes in reproductive physiology and territorial aggression across seasonal phenotypes (19). Several studies have demonstrated that male and female hamsters housed in short-day photoperiods display decreased levels of circulating gonadal steroids (23, 25), but increased levels of serum DHEA (15, 26). Furthermore, short-day males and females display elevated levels of aggression (21, 25), and similar increases in aggressive behaviors are observed in long-day animals administered short day-like levels of melatonin (24, 26). Interestingly, short-day males that receive adrenalectomies exhibit reduced levels of aggressive behaviors, yet adrenal demedullation, in which the catecholamine-secreting adrenal medulla is removed, produces no change in aggression (24). Furthermore, photoperiod has no effect on serum or adrenal cortisol content, and cortisol treatment does not affect levels of aggression in short- or long-day males (50). Collectively, these findings suggest that the neuroendocrine control of territorial aggression is dependent on seasonal changes in photoperiod and melatonin secretion, but is independent of gonadal steroids. Moreover, these data suggest that certain adrenocortical steroids may facilitate increases in aggression during the non-breeding season.

Recent studies from our group have focused on elucidating the neuroendocrine mechanisms responsible for increased territorial aggression during the non-breeding season. Specifically, we have examined the potential role of the HPA axis in modulating aggression. We have shown that male and female hamsters housed in short-day photoperiods decrease serum DHEA levels following an aggressive encounter, suggesting that short days may facilitate the conversion of circulating DHEA to T and E_2 (51, 52). Moreover, short-day female hamsters exhibit changes in adrenal morphology and have significantly higher adrenal DHEA content relative to long-day females. In addition, short- but not long-day females show elevated serum DHEA following adrenocorticotropic hormone (ACTH) challenge, in which the HPA axis is stimulated *via* exogenous administration of ACTH. Exogenous melatonin administration also stimulates adrenal DHEA release and elevates circulating DHEA and aggression in female hamsters (26). Taken together, these findings suggest that melatonin is responsible for coordinating a "seasonal switch" from gonadal to adrenal regulation of aggression by acting directly on the adrenal glands. In addition, these data suggest that DHEA peripherally regulates seasonal aggression.

We have also compared the abundance of gonadal and adrenal steroid receptors in brain regions associated with aggression or reproduction across seasonal phenotypes. We found that photoperiod does not affect glucocorticoid receptor (GR) levels in male hamsters in regions associated with aggressive behavior, including the medial amygdala (MeA) and the medial prefrontal cortex, or in the hippocampus, an area that shows changes in GR levels across photoperiods in other animals (50). In contrast, short-day female hamsters exhibit increases in ERα abundance in brain regions associated with aggression, including the periaqueductal gray (PAG), lateral septum (LS), and bed nucleus of the stria terminalis (BnST), but not in nuclei associated with reproduction, including the preoptic area (POA), arcuate nucleus (ARC), and anteroventral periventricular nucleus of the hypothalamus (53). Likewise, short-day males elevate ERα expression in brain nuclei associated with aggression, including the BnST, MeA, and central amygdala (54). While the presence of steroidogenic enzymes in these brain nuclei has yet to be confirmed, these data suggest that localized variation in neural ERα abundance may be responsible for seasonal changes in territorial aggression.

In summary, our findings provide compelling evidence that adrenal DHEA serves as a critical precursor of neurally-derived androgens in non-breeding Siberian hamsters (**Figure 2**). We have shown that short-day female hamsters display increased levels of aggression, but show no change in other social behaviors, such as investigation [**Figure 2A**; (53)]. In addition, short-day females increase serum DHEA, yet display reduced circulating levels of E_2 compared to long-day females [**Figure 2B**; (25, 53)]. Finally, female hamsters exhibit region-specific changes in ERα abundance, which may be a consequence of increased negative feedback from the HPG axis during the non-breeding season. Specifically, short-day females elevate ERα receptors in regions associated with aggression, such as the PAG, but not in nuclei associated with reproduction, such as the ARC [**Figure 2C**; (53)]. It is likely that these elevations in ERα abundance upregulate the activity of brain nuclei associated with aggressive behaviors and, consequently, increase territorial aggression during the non-breeding season.

NEURALLY-DERIVED STEROID SYNTHESIS IN OTHER SPECIES

Mice

Like Siberian hamsters, some species of deer mice (*Peromyscus sp.*) undergo seasonal changes in reproductive physiology and behavior. For example, male beach mice (*P. polionotus*) and deer mice (*P. maniculatus*) increase territorial aggression during the non-breeding season, in spite of gonadal regression and low circulating levels of androgens (55, 56). Intriguingly, California mice (*P. californicus*) do not undergo gonadal regression in response to short-day photoperiods, yet still exhibit elevated levels of aggression during the non-breeding season (57, 58). Together, these data suggest that increases in aggression during the non-breeding season are independent of circulating gonadal steroid levels and that, instead, localized neural androgen and estrogen synthesis may be responsible.

Recent work on the neuroendocrine mechanisms underlying seasonal aggression in deer mice has primarily examined neural ER abundance in brain nuclei associated with aggressive behaviors. Both short-day male beach mice and male deer mice exhibit increases in ERα abundance and expression in the BnST, yet display decreases in ERβ abundance and expression in the BnST and MeA. These changes in ERα- and ERβ-immunoreactivity are correlated with increased levels of aggression (59). Moreover, selective activation of either ERα or ERβ is associated with increased aggression in short-day male beach mice, and these increases in aggression are not correlated with changes in estrogen-dependent gene expression in the BnST and POA (60). While it is unclear whether adrenal DHEA is a source of neural estrogens in this signaling pathway, these findings suggest that ER abundance increases in a region-specific manner and primarily *via* non-genomic pathways to increase territorial aggression during the non-breeding season in *Peromyscus species* that are reproductively responsive to changes in photoperiod.

In contrast, mice that reproduce year-round or are physiologically non-responsive to changes in photoperiod do not exhibit similar changes in steroid hormone synthesis. For example, house mice (*Mus musculus*) decrease aggression in response to exogenous DHEA administration (61, 62). Furthermore, seasonally breeding male California mice, which do not undergo gonadal regression during non-breeding season, still elevate aggression and circulating E_2 levels in response to short days. However, non-breeding aggression in this species is independent of changes in ERα abundance, as short-day and long-day males show no differences in ERα and ERβ immunostaining in the LS, BnST, MeA, or POA (58, 63). Collectively, these findings indicate that some rodent species may not utilize circulating DHEA to maintain year-round territorial aggression. Additionally, these studies suggest that only seasonally breeding mice that are physiologically responsive to changes in day length alter neural ER abundance to elevate non-breeding aggression.

Birds

Most avian species have distinct breeding and non-breeding seasons, and many of these species display high levels of territorial aggression throughout the year [reviewed in the study by Soma (64)]. Like seasonally breeding rodents, birds undergo gonadal regression and exhibit pronounced reductions in plasma androgen levels during the non-breeding season, yet still exhibit levels of aggression that are often quantitatively and qualitatively similar to that displayed during the breeding season (65, 66). Moreover, castration of non-breeding male song sparrows has no effect on territorial aggression (67). Thus, while breeding season aggression is mediated by gonadal steroids, territorial aggression exhibited outside of the breeding season may be regulated by non-gonadal steroids in some male songbirds (68, 69).

Several studies have provided evidence that DHEA is an indirect source of neural androgens and estrogens in song sparrows (*Melospiza melodia*) during the non-breeding season. Male song sparrows display elevated circulating DHEA levels during the non-breeding season, which typically match seasonal changes in territorial aggression (66, 70). In addition, non-breeding male song sparrows display elevated plasma DHEA in

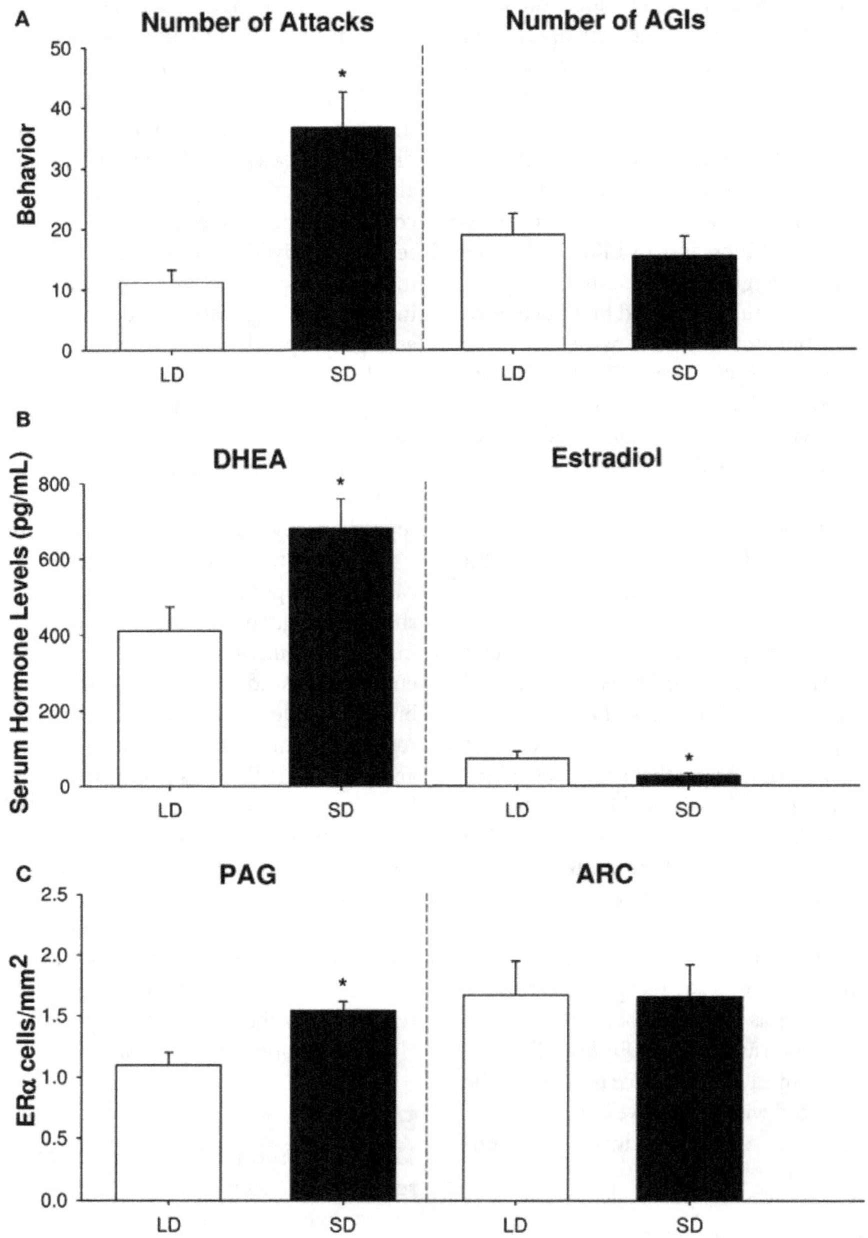

FIGURE 2 | Aggressive behavior, serum hormone profiles, and neural estrogen receptor-α (ERα) abundance differ across reproductive phenotypes of female Siberian hamsters. **(A)** Number of attacks and anogenital investigations (AGIs), **(B)** serum dehydroepiandrosterone (DHEA) and estradiol levels (in pg/mL), and **(C)** ERα cell density (in cells/mm²) in the periaqueductal gray (PAG) and arcuate nucleus of the hypothalamus (ARC) in short-day and long-day female hamsters following 10 weeks of photoperiodic treatment. Bar heights represent mean ± SEM. "*" indicates a significant difference between groups ($P < 0.05$). Data are modified and reprinted with permission from the authors (25, 53).

the jugular vein exiting the brain, but not in the peripherally-located brachial vein, following a simulated territorial intrusion [STI; (71)]. Non-breeding male song sparrows also have higher 3β-hydroxysteroid dehydrogenase (3β-HSD) activity, an enzyme that converts DHEA to the androgen precursor androstenedione, in brain regions associated with aggression, including the LS, BnST, and the taenial amygdala, the avian equivalent of the MeA (72). Furthermore, sparrows exhibit increased aromatase activity, an enzyme that converts T to E_2, and increased ERα and ERβ mRNA expression in brain nuclei that regulate aggression (73, 74). A more recent study confirmed that neural levels of DHEA, T, and E_2 are higher in brain tissue than in circulation and that a single STI event alone can induce localized changes in neural DHEA levels (75). Taken together, these data suggest that circulating DHEA is an important source of neurally-derived steroids and that DHEA metabolism in the brain stimulates territorial aggression during the non-breeding season of birds.

Interestingly, there is emerging evidence that this mechanism is evolutionarily-conserved in some tropical bird species, but not others. Non-breeding male spotted antbirds (*Hylophylax n. naevioides*) elevate plasma DHEA, reduce circulating T, and display similar aggressive behaviors compared to breeding males (76, 77). In contrast, non-breeding European nuthatches (*Sitta europaea*) do not elevate aggressive behaviors following exogenous DHEA administration (78), and non-breeding male European starlings (*Sturnus vulgaris*) exhibit lower plasma DHEA levels compared to breeding males (79), indicating that these species maintain year-round territorial aggression independently of DHEA. Intriguingly, inhibiting AR and aromatase activity reduces territorial aggression in breeding, but not non-breeding male European stonechats (*Saxicola torquatus rubicola*), suggesting that steroid hormones only regulate territorial aggression in a breeding context (80, 81). Because the neuroendocrine mechanisms underlying seasonal aggression in songbirds vary considerably across species and context, additional studies in this area of research are warranted.

CONCLUSION AND FUTURE DIRECTIONS

Several species of seasonally breeding animals maintain or elevate territorial aggression during the non-breeding season, despite reductions in circulating gonadal steroids. Although our work on Siberian hamsters suggests that non-breeding animals metabolize adrenal DHEA to locally synthesize neural androgens and induce changes in aggressive behaviors, several aspects of these mechanisms have yet to be proven experimentally. Future studies should compare peripheral and central levels of gonadal and adrenal steroids across reproductive phenotypes and investigate whether neurosteroid concentrations and AR and ERβ abundance, in addition to ERα abundance, vary seasonally in brain nuclei associated with aggression. Moreover, little is known about how photoperiod affects the activity of enzymes involved in gonadal steroid synthesis (e.g., 3β-HSD and aromatase), both in the brain and in systemic circulation. It is important that future work addresses this area of research to pinpoint the sex steroid synthesis pathway cascades that are critical in establishing seasonal differences in aggression. Ongoing and future studies in hamsters and other seasonal species will continue to provide important insights into the role of neurally-active steroid hormones in the regulation of aggression.

AUTHOR CONTRIBUTIONS

KM and GD drafted the manuscript, with editorial contributions from NR.

ACKNOWLEDGMENTS

We thank previous and current members of the Demas lab for their assistance in data collection and analysis and for their intellectual contributions to the projects discussed in this review. We also thank Wolfgang Goymann and Brian Trainor for their valuable comments on a previous version of this manuscript and Takayoshi Ubuka, Ishwar Parhar, and Vance Trudeau for the invitation to submit this review.

FUNDING

This work was supported in part by National Science Foundation grant IOB-0543798 (to GD), National Institutes of Health grant MH109942 (to GD), National Science Foundation Doctoral Dissertation Improvement Grant IOS-1406063 (to NR and GD), National Institutes of Health Training Grant T32HD049336 (to NR), and a National Science Foundation Graduate Research Fellowship (to NR).

REFERENCES

1. Simon NG. Hormonal processes in the development and expression of aggressive behavior. In: Pfaff DW, Arnold AP, Etgen AM, Fahrbach SE, Rubin RT, editors. *Hormones, Brain and Behavior*. New York: Academic Press (2002). p. 339–92.
2. Nelson RJ. *Biology of Aggression*. New York: Oxford University Press (2006).
3. Cunningham RL, Lumia AR, McGinnis MY. Androgen receptors, sex behavior, and aggression. *Neuroendocrinology* (2012) 96(2):131–40. doi:10.1159/000337663
4. Fuxjager MJ, Trainor BC, Marler CA. What can animal research tell us about the link between androgens and social competition in humans? *Horm Behav* (2017) 92:182–9. doi:10.1016/j.yhbeh.2016.11.014
5. Tsutsui K, Ishii S. Effects of sex steroids on aggressive behavior of adult male Japanese quail. *Gen Comp Endocrinol* (1981) 44(4):480–6. doi:10.1016/0016-6480(81)90336-1
6. Harding CF, Walters MJ, Collado D, Sheridan K. Hormonal specificity and activation of social behavior in male red-winged blackbirds. *Horm Behav* (1988) 22(3):402–18. doi:10.1016/0018-506X(88)90011-6
7. Apfelbeck B, Mortega KG, Kiefer S, Kipper S, Goymann W. Life-history and hormonal control of aggression in black redstarts: blocking testosterone does not decrease territorial aggression, but changes the emphasis of vocal behaviours during simulated territorial intrusions. *Front Zool* (2013) 10(1):8. doi:10.1186/1742-9994-10-8
8. Adkins E, Schlesinger L. Androgens and the social behavior of male and female lizards (*Anolis carolinensis*). *Horm Behav* (1979) 13(2):139–52. doi:10.1016/0018-506X(79)90053-9
9. Moore MC. Testosterone control of territorial behavior: tonic-release implants fully restore seasonal and short-term aggressive responses in free-living castrated lizards. *Gen Comp Endocrinol* (1988) 70(3):450–9. doi:10.1016/0016-6480(88)90121-9
10. Haug M, Brain PF, Kamis AB. A brief review comparing the effects of sex steroids on two forms of aggression in laboratory mice. *Neurosci Biobehav Rev* (1986) 10(4):463–8. doi:10.1016/0149-7634(86)90007-2
11. Trainor BC, Marler CA. Testosterone, paternal behavior, and aggression in the monogamous California mouse (*Peromyscus californicus*). *Horm Behav* (2001) 40(1):32–42. doi:10.1006/hbeh.2001.1652
12. Sayler A. The effect of anti-androgens on aggressive behavior in the gerbil. *Physiol Behav* (1970) 5(6):667–71. doi:10.1016/0031-9384(70)90228-3
13. Yahr P, Coquelin A, Martin A, Scouten CW. Effects of castration of aggression between male Mongolian gerbils. *Behav Biol* (1977) 19(2):189–205. doi:10.1016/S0091-6773(77)91482-1
14. Hume JM, Wynne-Edwards KE. Castration reduces male testosterone, estradiol, and territorial aggression, but not paternal behavior in biparental dwarf hamsters (*Phodopus campbelli*). *Horm Behav* (2005) 48(3):303–10. doi:10.1016/j.yhbeh.2005.04.001
15. Scotti MA, Belén J, Jackson JE, Demas GE. The role of androgens in the mediation of seasonal territorial aggression in male Siberian hamsters (*Phodopus sungorus*). *Physiol Behav* (2008) 95(5):633–40. doi:10.1016/j.physbeh.2008.09.009
16. Hiadlovská Z, Mikula O, Macholán M, Hamplová P, Vošlajerová Bímová B, Daniszová K. Shaking the myth: body mass, aggression, steroid hormones, and social dominance in wild house mouse. *Gen Comp Endocrinol* (2015) 223:16–26. doi:10.1016/j.ygcen.2015.09.033

17. Williamson CM, Lee W, Romeo RD, Curley JP. Social context-dependent relationships between mouse dominance rank and plasma hormone levels. *Physiol Behav* (2017) 171:110–9. doi:10.1016/j.physbeh.2016.12.038
18. Soma KK, Scotti MA, Newman AEM, Charlier TD, Demas GE. Novel mechanisms for neuroendocrine regulation of aggression. *Front Neuroendocrinol* (2008) 29(4):476–89. doi:10.1016/j.yfrne.2007.12.003
19. Heldmaier G, Steinlechner S. Seasonal control of energy requirements for thermoregulation in the Djungarian hamster (*Phodopus sungorus*), living in natural photoperiod. *J Comp Physiol* (1981) 142(4):429–37. doi:10.1007/BF00688972
20. Garrett JW, Campbell CS. Changes in social behavior of the male golden hamster accompanying photoperiodic changes in reproduction. *Horm Behav* (1980) 14(4):303–19. doi:10.1016/0018-506X(80)90020-3
21. Jasnow AM, Huhman KL, Bartness TJ, Demas GE. Short-day increases in aggression are inversely related to circulating testosterone concentrations in male Siberian hamsters (*Phodopus sungorus*). *Horm Behav* (2000) 38(2): 102–10. doi:10.1006/hbeh.2000.1604
22. Bartness TJ, Wade GN. Photoperiodic control of seasonal body weight cycles in hamsters. *Neurosci Biobehav Rev* (1985) 9(4):599–612. doi:10.1016/0149-7634(85)90006-5
23. Jasnow AM, Huhman KL, Bartness TJ, Demas GE. Short days and exogenous melatonin increase aggression of male Syrian hamsters (*Mesocricetus auratus*). *Horm Behav* (2002) 42(1):13–20. doi:10.1006/hbeh.2002.1797
24. Demas GE, Polacek KM, Durazzo A, Jasnow AM. Adrenal hormones mediate melatonin-induced increases in aggression in male Siberian hamsters (*Phodopus sungorus*). *Horm Behav* (2004) 46(5):582–91. doi:10.1016/j.yhbeh.2004.07.001
25. Scotti MA, Place NJ, Demas GE. Short-day increases in aggression are independent of circulating gonadal steroids in female Siberian hamsters (*Phodopus sungorus*). *Horm Behav* (2007) 52(2):183–90. doi:10.1016/j.yhbeh.2007.03.029
26. Rendon NM, Rudolph LM, Sengelaub DR, Demas GE. The agonistic adrenal: melatonin elicits female aggression via regulation of adrenal androgens. *Proc Biol Sci* (2015) 282(1819). doi:10.1098/rspb.2015.2080
27. Prendergast BJ, Nelson RJ, Zucker I. Mammalian seasonal rhythms: behavior and neuroendocrine substrates. In: Pfaff DW, editor. *Hormones, Brain and Behavior*. New York: Academic Press (2003). p. 93–156.
28. Walton JC, Weil ZM, Nelson RJ. Influence of photoperiod on hormones, behavior, and immune function. *Front Neuroendocrinol* (2011) 32(3):303–19. doi:10.1016/j.yfrne.2010.12.003
29. Bartness TJ, Bradley J, Hastings MH, Bittman EL, Goldman BD. The timed infusion paradigm for melatonin delivery: what has it taught us about the melatonin signal, its reception, and the photoperiodic control of seasonal responses? *J Pineal Res* (1993) 15(4):161–90. doi:10.1111/j.1600-079X.1993.tb00903.x
30. Goldman BD. Mammalian photoperiodic system: formal properties and neuroendocrine mechanisms of photoperiodic time measurement. *J Biol Rhythms* (2001) 16(4):283–301. doi:10.1177/074873001129001980
31. Haller J, Makara GB, Kruk MR. Catecholaminergic involvement in the control of aggression: hormones, the peripheral sympathetic, and central noradrenergic systems. *Neurosci Biobehav Rev* (1998) 22(1):85–97. doi:10.1016/S0149-7634(97)00023-7
32. Boringer JC, Nelson RJ. Photoperiodic regulation of behavior: *Peromyscus* as a model system. *Semin Cell Dev Biol* (2017) 61:82–91. doi:10.1016/j.semcdb.2016.06.015
33. Bae S-E, Wright IK, Wyse C, Samson-Desvignes N, Le Blanc P, Laroche S, et al. Regulation of pituitary MT1 melatonin receptor expression by gonadotrophin-releasing hormone (GnRH) and early growth response factor-1 (Egr-1): *in vivo* and *in vitro* studies. *PLoS One* (2014) 9(3):e90056. doi:10.1371/journal.pone.0090056
34. Wood S, Loudon A. Clocks for all seasons: unwinding the roles and mechanisms of circadian and interval timers in the hypothalamus and pituitary. *J Endocrinol* (2014) 222(2):R39–59. doi:10.1530/JOE-14-0141
35. Williams LM, Lincoln GA, Mercer JG, Barrett P, Morgan PJ, Clarke IJ. Melatonin receptors in the brain and pituitary gland of hypothalamo-pituitary disconnected Soay rams. *J Neuroendocrinol* (1997) 9(8):639–43. doi:10.1046/j.1365-2826.1997.00625.x
36. Chowdhury VS, Ubuka T, Tsutsui K. Review: melatonin stimulates the synthesis and release of gonadotropin-inhibitory hormone in birds. *Gen Comp Endocrinol* (2013) 181:175–8. doi:10.1016/j.ygcen.2012.08.005
37. Frungieri MB, Mayerhofer A, Zitta K, Pignataro OP, Calandra RS, Gonzalez-Calvar SI. Direct effect of melatonin on Syrian hamster testes: melatonin subtype 1a receptors inhibition of androgen production, and interaction with the local corticotropin-releasing hormone system. *Endocrinology* (2005) 146(3):1541–52. doi:10.1210/en.2004-0990
38. McGuire NL, Kangas K, Bentley GE. Effects of melatonin on peripheral reproductive function: regulation of testicular GnIH and testosterone. *Endocrinology* (2011) 152(9):3461–70. doi:10.1210/en.2011-1053
39. Skinner DC, Robinson JE. Melatonin-binding sites in the gonadotroph-enriched zona tuberalis of ewes. *J Reprod Fertil* (1995) 104(2):243–50. doi:10.1530/jrf.0.1040243
40. Richter HG, Torres-Farfan C, Garcia-Sesnich J, Abarzua-Catalan L, Henriquez MG, Alvarez-Felmer M, et al. Rhythmic expression of functional MT1 melatonin receptors in the rat adrenal gland. *Endocrinology* (2008) 149(3):995–1003. doi:10.1210/en.2007-1009
41. Tsutsui K, Ubuka T, Bentley GE, Kriegsfeld LJ. Review: regulatory mechanisms of gonadotropin-inhibitory hormone (GnIH) synthesis and release in photoperiodic animals. *Front Neurosci* (2013) 7:60. doi:10.3389/fnins.2013.00060
42. Paterson AT, Vickers C. Melatonin and the adrenal-cortex relationship to territorial aggression in mice. *Physiol Behav* (1981) 27:983–7. doi:10.1016/0031-9384(81)90358-9
43. Soma KK, Rendon NM, Boonstra R, Albers HE, Demas GE. DHEA effects on brain and behavior: insights from comparative studies of aggression. *J Steroid Biochem Mol Biol* (2015) 145:261–72. doi:10.1016/j.jsbmb.2014.05.011
44. Boonstra R, Lane JE, Boutin S, Bradley A, Desantis L, Newman AEM, et al. Plasma DHEA levels in wild, territorial red squirrels: seasonal variation and effect of ACTH. *Gen Comp Endocrinol* (2008) 158(1):61–7. doi:10.1016/j.ygcen.2008.05.004
45. Beck SG, Handa RJ. Dehydroepiandrosterone (DHEA): a misunderstood adrenal hormone and spine-tingling neurosteroid? *Endocrinology* (2004) 145(3):43–68. doi:10.1210/en.2003-1703
46. Labrie F, Luu-The V, Bélanger A, Lin SX, Simard J, Pelletier G, et al. Is dehydroepiandrosterone a hormone? *J Endocrinol* (2005) 187(2):169–96. doi:10.1677/joe.1.06264
47. Tsutsui K, Ukena K, Usui M, Sakamoto H, Takase M. Novel brain function: biosynthesis and actions of neurosteroids in neurons. *Neurosci Res* (2000) 36(4):261–73. doi:10.1016/S0168-0102(99)00132-7
48. Do Rego JL, Seong JY, Burel D, Leprince J, Vaudry D, Luu-The V, et al. Regulation of neurosteroid biosynthesis by neurotransmitters and neuropeptides. *Front Endocrinol* (2012) 3:4. doi:10.3389/fendo.2012.00004
49. Webb SJ, Geoghegan TE, Prough RA, Michael Miller KK. The biological actions of dehydroepiandrosterone involves multiple receptors. *Drug Metab Rev* (2006) 38(1–2):89–116. doi:10.1080/03602530600569877
50. Scotti MA, Rendon NM, Greives TM, Romeo RD, Demas GE. Short-day aggression is independent of changes in cortisol or glucocorticoid receptors in male Siberian hamsters (*Phodopus sungorus*). *J Exp Zoo A Ecol Genet Physiol* (2015) 323(5):331–41. doi:10.1002/jez.1922
51. Scotti MA, Schmidt KL, Newman AEM, Bonu TN, Soma KK, Demas GE. Aggressive encounters differentially affect serum dehydroepiandrosterone and testosterone concentrations in male Siberian hamsters (*Phodopus sungorus*). *Horm Behav* (2009) 56(4):376–81. doi:10.1016/j.yhbeh.2009.07.004
52. Rendon NM, Demas GE. Bi-directional actions of dehydroepiandrosterone and aggression in female Siberian hamsters. *J Exp Zoo A Ecol Genet Physiol* (2016) 325(2):116–21. doi:10.1002/jez.2001
53. Rendon NM, Amez AC, Proffitt MR, Bauserman ER, Demas GE. Aggressive behaviours track transitions in seasonal phenotypes of female Siberian hamsters. *Funct Ecol* (2017) 31(5):1071–81. doi:10.1111/1365-2435.12816
54. Kramer KM, Simmons JL, Freeman DA. Photoperiod alters central distribution of estrogen receptor α in brain regions that regulate aggression. *Horm Behav* (2008) 53(2):358–65. doi:10.1016/j.yhbeh.2007.11.002
55. Trainor BC, Kyomen HH, Marler CA. Estrogenic encounters: how interactions between aromatase and the environment modulate aggression. *Front Neuroendocrinol* (2006) 27(2):170–9. doi:10.1016/j.yfrne.2005.11.001
56. Trainor BC, Martin LB, Greiwe KM, Kulhman JR, Nelson RJ. Social and photoperiod effects on reproduction in five species of *Peromyscus*. *Gen Comp Endocrinol* (2006) 148(2):252–9. doi:10.1016/j.ygcen.2006.03.006
57. Nelson RJ, Gubernick DJ, Blom JM. Influence of photoperiod, green food, and water availability on reproduction in male California mice (*Peromyscus californicus*). *Physiol Behav* (1995) 57(6):1175–80. doi:10.1016/0031-9384(94)00380-N

58. Trainor BC, Finy MS, Nelson RJ. Rapid effects of estradiol on male aggression depend on photoperiod in reproductively non-responsive mice. *Horm Behav* (2008) 53(1):192–9. doi:10.1016/j.yhbeh.2007.09.016
59. Trainor BC, Rowland MR, Nelson RJ. Photoperiod affects estrogen receptor α, estrogen receptor β and aggressive behavior. *Eur J Neurosci* (2007) 26(1):207–18. doi:10.1111/j.1460-9568.2007.05654.x
60. Trainor BC, Lin S, Finy MS, Rowland MR, Nelson RJ. Photoperiod reverses the effects of estrogens on male aggression via genomic and nongenomic pathways. *Proc Natl Acad Sci U S A* (2007) 104(23):9840–5. doi:10.1073/pnas.0701819104
61. Schlegel ML, Spetz JF, Robel P, Haug M. Studies on the effects of dehydroepiandrosterone and its metabolites on attack by castrated mice on lactating intruders. *Physiol Behav* (1985) 34(6):867–70. doi:10.1016/0031-9384(85)90005-8
62. Perché F, Young J, Robel P, Simon NG, Haug M. Prenatal testosterone treatment potentiates the aggression-inhibiting effect of the neurosteroid dehydroepiandrosterone in female mice. *Aggress Behav* (2001) 27(2):130–8. doi:10.1002/ab.5
63. Laredo SA, Villalon Landeros R, Dooley JC, Steinman MQ, Orr V, Silva AL, et al. Nongenomic effects of estradiol on aggression under short day photoperiods. *Horm Behav* (2013) 64(3):557–65. doi:10.1016/j.yhbeh.2013.06.002
64. Soma KK. Testosterone and aggression: berthold, birds and beyond. *J Neuroendocrinol* (2006) 18(7):543–51. doi:10.1111/j.1365-2826.2006.01440.x
65. Wingfield JC, Hahn TP. Testosterone and territorial behaviour in sedentary and migratory sparrows. *Anim Behav* (1994) 47(1):77–89. doi:10.1006/anbe.1994.1009
66. Soma KK, Wingfield JC. Dehydroepiandrosterone in songbird plasma: seasonal regulation and relationship to territorial aggression. *Gen Comp Endocrinol* (2001) 123(2):144–55. doi:10.1006/gcen.2001.7657
67. Wingfield JC. Control of territorial aggression in a changing environment. *Psychoneuroendocrinology* (1994) 19(5–7):709–21. doi:10.1016/0306-4530(94)90052-3
68. Soma KK, Sullivan KA, Tramontin AD, Saldanha CJ, Schlinger BA, Wingfield JC. Acute and chronic effects of an aromatase inhibitor on territorial aggression in breeding and nonbreeding male song sparrows. *J Comp Physiol A* (2000) 186(7–8):759–69. doi:10.1007/s003590000129
69. Heimovics SA, Fokidis HB, Soma KK. Brain aromatase and territorial aggression across the seasons in male song sparrows. In: Balthazart J, Ball GF, editors. *Brain, Aromatase, Estrogens and Behavior*. Oxford: Oxford University Press (2013). p. 199–220.
70. Newman AEM, Soma KK. Corticosterone and dehydroepiandrosterone in songbird plasma and brain: effects of season and acute stress. *Eur J Neurosci* (2009) 29(9):1905–14. doi:10.1111/j.1460-9568.2009.06748.x
71. Newman AEM, Pradhan DS, Soma KK. Dehydroepiandrosterone and corticosterone are regulated by season and acute stress in a wild songbird: jugular versus brachial plasma. *Endocrinology* (2008) 149(5):2537–45. doi:10.1210/en.2007-1363
72. Pradhan DS, Newman AEM, Wacker DW, Wingfield JC, Schlinger BA, Soma KK. Aggressive interactions rapidly increase androgen synthesis in the brain during the non-breeding season. *Horm Behav* (2010) 57(4–5):381–9. doi:10.1016/j.yhbeh.2010.01.008
73. Soma KK, Schlinger BA, Wingfield JC, Saldanha CJ. Brain aromatase, 5α-reductase, and 5β-reductase change seasonally in wild male song sparrows: relationship to aggressive and sexual behavior. *J Neurobiol* (2003) 56(3):209–21. doi:10.1002/neu.10225
74. Wacker DW, Wingfield JC, Davis JE, Meddle SL. Seasonal changes in aromatase and androgen receptor, but not estrogen receptor mRNA expression in the brain of the free-living male song sparrow, *Melospiza melodia morphna*. *J Comp Neurol* (2010) 518(18):3819–35. doi:10.1002/cne.22426
75. Heimovics SA, Prior NH, Ma C, Soma KK. Rapid effects of an aggressive interaction on dehydroepiandrosterone, testosterone and oestradiol levels in the male song sparrow brain: a seasonal comparison. *J Neuroendocrinol* (2016) 28(2):12345. doi:10.1111/jne.12345
76. Hau M, Stoddard ST, Soma KK. Territorial aggression and hormones during the non-breeding season in a tropical bird. *Horm Behav* (2004) 45(1):40–9. doi:10.1016/j.yhbeh.2003.08.002
77. Hau M, Beebe K. Plastic endocrine regulation of year-round territorial aggression in tropical male spotted antbirds. *Gen Comp Endocrinol* (2011) 172(2):305–13. doi:10.1016/j.ygcen.2011.03.016
78. Landys MM, Goymann W, Soma KK, Slagsvold T. Year-round territorial aggression is independent of plasma DHEA in the European nuthatch *Sitta europaea*. *Horm Behav* (2013) 63(1):166–72. doi:10.1016/j.yhbeh.2012.10.002
79. Pintér O, Péczely P, Zsebok S, Zelena D. Seasonal changes in courtship behavior, plasma androgen levels and in hypothalamic aromatase immunoreactivity in male free-living European starlings (*Sturnus vulgaris*). *Gen Comp Endocrinol* (2011) 172(1):151–7. doi:10.1016/j.ygcen.2011.02.002
80. Canoine V, Gwinner E. Seasonal differences in the hormonal control of territorial aggression in free-living European stonechats. *Horm Behav* (2002) 41(1):1–8. doi:10.1006/hbeh.2001.1720
81. Marasco V, Fusani L, Dessì-Fulgheri F, Canoine V. Non-migratory stonechats show seasonal changes in the hormonal regulation of non-seasonal territorial aggression. *Horm Behav* (2011) 60(4):414–9. doi:10.1016/j.yhbeh.2011.07.010

18

Neurosteroids in Adult Hippocampus of Male and Female Rodents: Biosynthesis and Actions of Sex Steroids

Yasushi Hojo[1] and Suguru Kawato[2,3,4]*

[1] *Department of Biochemistry, Faculty of Medicine, Saitama Medical University, Moroyama, Saitama, Japan,* [2] *Department of Biophysics and Life Sciences, Graduate School of Arts and Sciences, The University of Tokyo, Tokyo, Japan,* [3] *Department of Urology, Graduate School of Medicine, Juntendo University, Tokyo, Japan,* [4] *Department of Cognitive Neuroscience, Faculty of Pharma-Science, Teikyo University, Tokyo, Japan*

Correspondence:
Yasushi Hojo
yhojo@saitama-med.ac.jp

The brain is not only the target of steroid hormones but also is able to locally synthesize steroids *de novo*. Evidence of the local production of steroids in the brain has been accumulating in various vertebrates, including teleost fish, amphibia, birds, rodents, non-human primates, and humans. In this review, we mainly focus on the local production of sex steroids in the hippocampal neurons of adult rodents (rats and mice), a center for learning and memory. From the data of the hippocampus of adult male rats, hippocampal principal neurons [pyramidal cells in CA1–CA3 and granule cells in dentate gyrus (DG)] have a complete system for biosynthesis of sex steroids. Liquid chromatography with tandem-mass-spectrometry (LC-MS/MS) enabled us to accurately determine the levels of hippocampal sex steroids including 17β-estradiol (17β-E2), testosterone (T), and dihydrotestosterone (DHT), which are much higher than those in blood. Next, we review the steroid synthesis in the hippocampus of female rats, since previous knowledge had been biased toward the data from males. Recently, we clarified that the levels of hippocampal steroids fluctuate in adult female rats across the estrous cycle. Accurate determination of hippocampal steroids at each stage of the estrous cycle is of importance for providing the account for the fluctuation of female hippocampal functions, including spine density, long-term potentiation (LTP) and long-term depression (LTD), and learning and memory. These functional fluctuations in female had been attributed to the level of circulation-derived steroids. LC-MS/MS analysis revealed that the dendritic spine density in CA1 of adult female hippocampus correlates with the levels of hippocampal progesterone and 17β-E2. Finally, we introduce the direct evidence of the role of hippocampus-synthesized steroids in hippocampal function including neurogenesis, LTP, and memory consolidation. Mild exercise (2 week of treadmill running) elevated synthesis of DHT in the hippocampus, but not in the testis, of male rats, resulting in enhancement of neurogenesis in DG. Concerning synaptic plasticity, hippocampus-synthesized E2 is required for LTP induction, whereas hippocampus-synthesized DHT is required for LTD induction. Furthermore, hippocampus-synthesized E2 is involved in memory consolidation tested by object recognition and object placement tasks, both of which are hippocampus-dependent.

Keywords: hippocampus, neurosteroids, estradiol, testosterone, dihydrotestosterone, estrous cycle, synaptic plasticity, neurogenesis

INTRODUCTION

Extensive evidence has been accumulated that the systems of local steroid synthesis exist in the organs other than gonads and adrenal since 1980s (1, 2). Local production of steroids in the brain has been investigated in various vertebrates, including teleost fish (3, 4), amphibia (5–7), birds (8, 9), rodents (10–14), non-human primates, and humans (15–17).

For clinical purposes, the importance of neurosteroids is increasing. Because of the limitation to invade human brain tissues, quantitative determination of steroids in cerebrospinal fluid (CSF) has been applied to detect the alteration of the allopregnanolone (Allo) level under physiological/pathological conditions, including epilepsy (18, 19), and reproductive mood disorders (20, 21).

Sex steroids including 17β-estradiol (17β-E2), testosterone (T), and dihydrotestosterone (DHT) are also synthesized in the brain. In this review, we mainly focus on the local production of sex steroids, particularly, E2, T, and DHT in the hippocampal neurons of adult rodents (rats and mice).

In addition to the genomic effects, sex steroids modulate neural functions in a rapid/non-genomic manner [reviewed in Ref. (22)]. Using the hippocampal slices of rodents, rapid effects of sex steroids have been extensively investigated. E2 modulates long-term potentiation (LTP) (23, 24) and long-term depression (LTD) (25, 26) in CA1 synapses. E2 induces LTP in CA1 under the weak theta burst stimulation (weak-TBS), which is not strong enough to induce LTP alone (27). Exogenous application of E2, T, and DHT to rat hippocampal slices, rapidly increases dendritic spines in CA1 pyramidal cells (27, 28).

Using exogenous application of steroids, these investigations demonstrated that rapid effects of sex steroids are mediated through estrogen receptors (ERα and ERβ) or androgen receptors (AR), located at the pre/post synapses (25, 28–30), followed by the activation of kinases which phosphorylate the molecules essential for synaptic plasticity. Upon LTP-induction, E2 drives src tyrosine kinase and the extracellular signal-related protein kinase/MAPK (Erk MAPK), resulting in phosphorylation of NMDA receptor (23). In case of E2-induced LTP by weak-TBS, Erk MAPK, PKA, PKC, PI3K, and CaMkII phosphorylate NR2B subunit (27). In addition to postsynaptic modulation, E2 also activates ERs in presynapses, resulting in potentiation of glutamate release (31) or disinhibition of GABAergic axon terminal (32). Concerning spinogenesis, E2, T, or DHT drives Erk MAPK, p38 MAPK, PKA, PKC, PI3K, and LIMK (27, 28), which may phosphorylate cortactin (33, 34) and cofilin (35, 36), leading to actin polymerization and spinogenesis.

Do the effects of hippocampus-synthesized E2, T and DHT share the common mechanism described above? It is difficult, however, to directly demonstrate the roles of hippocampus-synthesized E2, T, and DHT, because of the supply of E2, T, and DHT from testis or ovary. It is necessary to perform the experiment under the depletion of circulation-derived E2, T, and DHT, although the possibility is not excluded that 'peripherally produced precursors (e.g., pregnenolone and progesterone) convert into E2, T, or DHT in the hippocampus (**Figure 1A**). Several investigations are introduced in the Section "Physiological Roles of Hippocampus-Synthesized Steroids."

STEROID BIOSYNTHESIS IN THE HIPPOCAMPUS

Steroid Biosynthesis in the Hippocampus of Adult Male Rodents

Until about 15 years ago, it had not been elucidated whether adult hippocampal neurons have a complete system for synthesis of sex hormones (from cholesterol to androgens or estrogens) since P450(17α), which is required for synthesis of dehydroepiandrosterone (DHEA) from pregnenolone (PREG), had been thought to be absent in the brain of mammals. Any effort to demonstrate the existence of P450(17α) or its enzymatic activity had been unsuccessful (38–41) despite the presence of DHEA in the rodent brain even after castration (1, 2).

By using the hippocampus of adult male rats, the localization of P450(17α) in the principal neurons [pyramidal cells in CA1–CA3 and granule cells in dentate gyrus (DG)] was demonstrated (42, 43). Immunohistochemistry and *in situ* hybridization studies revealed that StAR and other enzymes, including P450scc, 3β-hydroxysteroid dehydrogenase (3β-HSD), 17β-HSD, 5α-reductase (types 1 and 2), and P450arom, are also localized in the hippocampal principal neurons of adult male rats and mice (37, 42–48). Studies with radioactive steroids directly demonstrated synthesis of PREG, DHEA, T, DHT, and E2 in slices or cultured hippocampal neurons from adult male rats in early 2000s (42, 43, 47, 49). These results suggest that complete systems for steroidogenesis exist in the hippocampal neurons of adult male rodents.

Interestingly, an electron microscopic (EM) analysis revealed synaptic localization of steroidogenic enzymes including P450 (17α), P450arom, and 3β-HSD in the hippocampus of adult male rats (42, 50), implying the synaptic synthesis of sex steroids. EM and Western immunoblot analysis revealed localization of steroid receptors including ERα, ERβ, AR, and progesterone receptor (PR) in the hippocampal synapses of rodents (25, 28–30, 51, 52).

Although these results give information about the potential to synthesize steroids in the hippocampus, it remains unclear whether hippocampus-synthesized steroids are effective enough to modulate hippocampal functions. To answer this question, it is necessary to quantitatively determine the concentration of steroids in the hippocampus. From early 2000s, quantitative determination of steroids, such as PREG, DHEA, and T in brain with mass-spectrometry (MS) began to emerge (53–58). The presence of pregnenolone sulfate (PREGS) in the brain of mammals had been a matter of debate (59).

To detect small amounts of steroids in the brain, purification of samples and selection of appropriate derivatization reagents are indispensable. Extracts from brain tissue contain various kinds of impurities (lipids and other steroids) which mask derivatization and ionization of the steroid of interest, resulting in decrease of detection efficiency of MS. Purification of the extracts by hybrid-SPE cartridges before LC–ESI-MS/MS enabled the detection of PREGS in the rat hippocampus (60). Concerning the detection of sex steroids, we removed impurities from hippocampal extracts and separated into fractions containing an individual steroid, with C18 column and normal phase HPLC before derivatization.

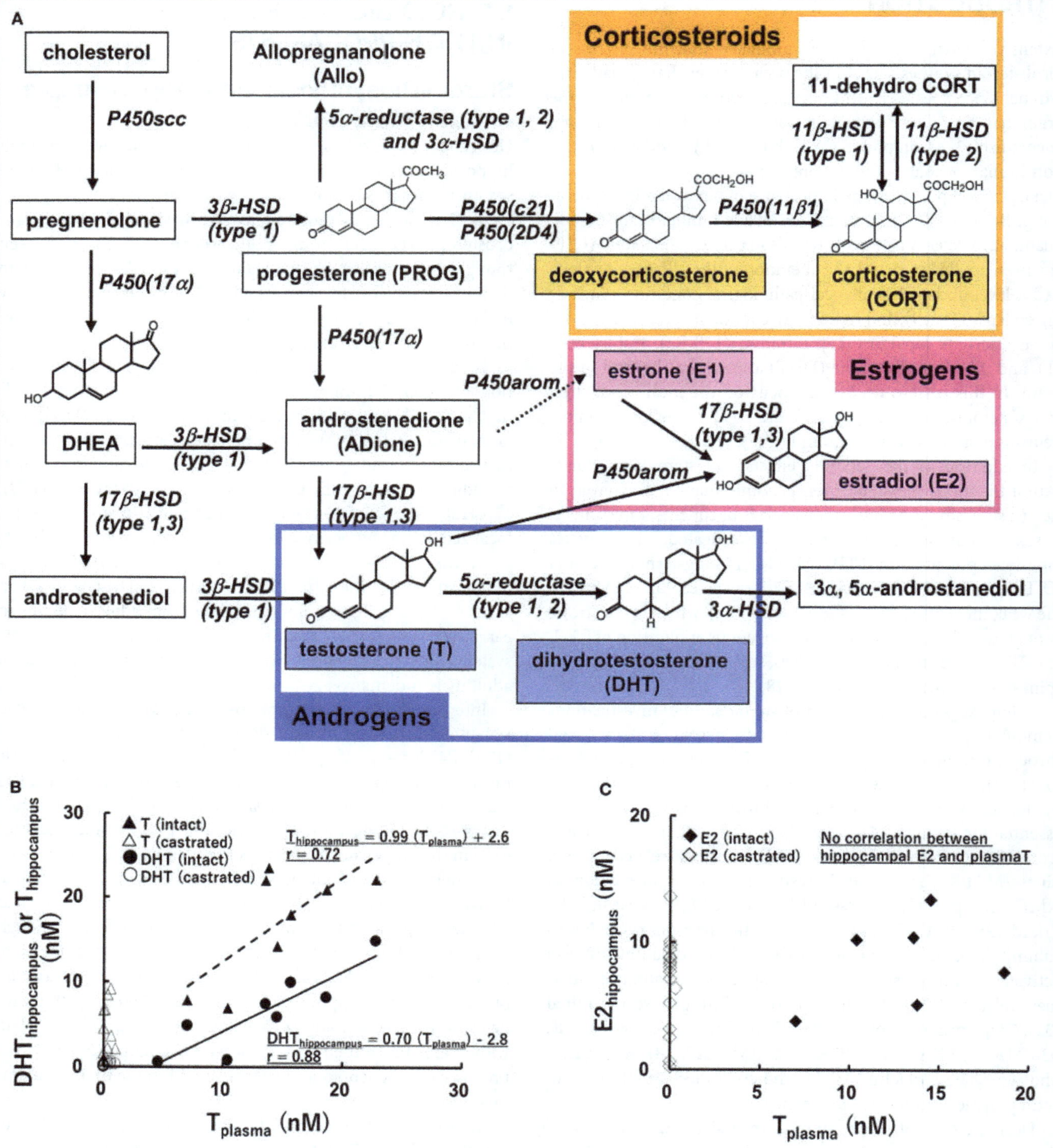

FIGURE 1 | (A) Biosynthetic pathway of steroids in rat hippocampus [modified from Ref. (11)]. Estrogens, androgens, and corticosteroids are represented with pink, blue, and orange boxes, respectively. **(B,C)** Relationship between the level of plasma T and those of hippocampal androgens [T and dihydrotestosteron (DHT)] **(A)**, or that of hippocampal E2 **(B)**. Vertical axis represents hippocampal steroids and horizontal axis represents plasma T, a precursor of DHT and E2. The regression lines and Pearson's "*r*" are indicated [modified from Ref. (37)].

Next, picolinoyl-derivatization was selected for steroids of interest (E2, T, DHT, and E1) to increase ionization efficiency (61, 62). Concerning E2, further derivatization with pentafluorobenzyl was performed to elevate volatility. In combination with these improvements, LC-MS/MS enabled us to quantitatively determine the concentration of E2, T, DHT, and E1 in the hippocampus, with high accuracy and reproducibility (37). Caruso and collaborators also determined the levels of steroids including E2, T, and DHT in rat hippocampus, with LC-MS/MS methods (63). These results support that the significant amount of sex steroids exists in the hippocampus.

Correlation between the level of hippocampal androgen (T and DHT) and that of plasma T (**Figure 1**) was observed (37, 64). Hippocampal estrogen (E2), however, did not correlate with plasma T (**Figure 1**) (37, 64). Using male and female rats, Melcangi's laboratory extensively analyzed the correlation of steroid levels among plasma, CSF and various brain regions (63). According to this work, the levels of E2, T, and DHT in the hippocampus or CSF positively correlated with those in plasma, but no significant correlation of E2 level was observed between in the hippocampus and CSF (63).

Synthesis and Fluctuation of Steroids in the Hippocampus of Adult Female Rodents

Equally important is to clarify whether local steroid production occurs in female hippocampus, because sex hormones have a great impact on functions of female hippocampus [reviewed in Ref. (65)]. The knowledge of the hippocampus-synthesized steroids, however, had been biased toward the data from males (11–13) because of the estrous cycle in female animals. In case of rats and mice, estrous cycle comprises of four stages [proestrus: Pro, estrus: Est, diestrus1 (also called metestrus): D1, and diestrus2 (also called diestrus): D2], and each stage switches in 1 day in this order (66). Hippocampal functions such as spatial memory (67–71), LTP (72, 73), and spine/synapse density (74–78), fluctuate across the estrous cycle. To investigate hippocampal steroid synthesis in female rodents, therefore, fourfold as much data as those of male must be acquired.

LC-MS/MS analysis revealed the accurate concentrations of progesterone (PROG), androstenedione (ADione), T, E1, and E2 in the hippocampus of adult female rats at each stage of estrous cycle (**Table 1**) (79). The levels of plasma steroids exhibit typical estrous cycle dependent changes, in agreement with the previous study (80). The level of hippocampal E2 highly correlates with that of plasma E2, in agreement with other study (63). Concerning the correlation of PROG level between in hippocampus and in plasma, our data exhibit highly positive correlation, whereas others have no correlation (63). It may be due to the difference of samples used for calculation of correlations, rats of both sexes (male and diestrus female) in Caruso et al. (63) and only female (all four stages of the estrous cycle) in our study (79).

Surprisingly, mRNA levels of steroidogenic enzymes, including StAR, P450(17α), 17β-HSD (types 1 and 3), 5α-reductase (types 1 and 2), and P450arom, did not fluctuate in the hippocampus across the estrous cycle (79, 81). Steroid receptors, including ERα, ERβ, AR, and PR, also kept their expression level constant. Moreover, no sex difference was observed concerning these enzymes in the hippocampus whose expression levels are approximately 1/300 ~ 1/1000 of those in gonads or adrenals(79, 81, 82).

Penetration of plasma E2 into the hippocampus, however, is not able to account for the level of hippocampal E2 because hippocampal E2 is much higher than that in plasma. There are two possibilities for explanation of hippocampal E2 fluctuation. The first is the fluctuation of blood PROG which is well known to fluctuate across the estrous cycle (80). This peripherally produced PROG may penetrate hippocampus and be converted into E2, resulting in E2 fluctuation. The other is the fluctuation of activity of kinases including MAPK, Akt, and LIMK, across the estrous cycle (72, 83, 84). The activity of P450arom

TABLE 1 | Mass spectrometric analysis of the concentration of steroids in the hippocampus and plasma of adult rats.

	Male	Female[b]				
		Proestrus	Estrus	Diestrus 1	Diestrus 2	OVX
(A) Hippocampus[a]						
17β-E2	8.4[c] (n^d = 6)	4.3 (n = 6)	1.0 (n = 4)	0.51 (n = 3)	0.67 (n = 4)	0.70 (n = 4)
T	16.9 (n = 8)	1.1 (n = 12)	2.3 (n = 4)	1.3 (n = 3)	1.2 (n = 4)	0.17 (n = 4)
Dihydrotestosteron (DHT)	6.6 (n = 8)	0.62 (n = 7)				
Progesterone (PROG)	14.6 (n = 4)	55.7 (n = 4)	40.7 (n = 4)	87.0 (n = 3)	48.0 (n = 4)	24.5 (n = 5)
Androstenedione	1.5 (n = 4)	1.6 (n = 4)	0.7 (n = 4)	1.1 (n = 4)	0.83 (n = 4)	
E1	0.015 (n = 4)	0.36 (n = 4)	0.045 (n = 4)	0.05 (n = 4)	0.10 (n = 4)	0.025 (n = 3)
Allopregnanolone	1.0 (n = 3)	16.4 (n = 3)				
(B) Plasma						
17β-E2	0.014 (n = 5)	0.111 (n = 6)	0.017 (n = 6)	0.009 (n = 5)	0.029 (n = 6)	0.005 (n = 5)
T	14.6 (n = 8)	0.10 (n = 4)	0.013 (n = 4)	0.020 (n = 3)	0.06 (n = 4)	0.005 (n = 5)
DHT	0.63 (n = 8)					
PROG	6.8 (n = 4)	20.5 (n = 4)	16.7 (n = 4)	51.6 (n = 3)	24.1 (n = 4)	10.1 (n = 5)
Androstenedione	0.61 (n = 4)	1.0 (n = 4)	0.06 (n = 4)	0.119 (n = 4)	0.33 (n = 4)	
E1	0.007 (n = 4)	0.082 (n = 4)	0.004 (n = 4)	0.009 (n = 4)	0.031 (n = 4)	0.002 (n = 4)

[a] *Hippocampus was homogenized immediately after dissection from a decapitated head. This condition reflects the basal concentration of steroids in hippocampus.*
[b] *Female samples were prepared from rats at each stage of estrous cycle (Proestrus, Estrus, Diestrus1, and Diestrus 2) and ovariectomized (OVX) rats.*
[c] *Data are expressed as mean and are represented as nanomolar. Concentration in nanomolar is calculated using the average volume of 0.14 mL for one whole hippocampus that has 0.14 ± 0.02 g wet weight (n = 86). We assume that tissue having 1 g of wet weight has an approximate volume of 1 mL, since the major part of tissue consists of water whose 1 mL weight is 1 g (47).*
[d] *Number of animals.*
Modified from Ref. (37, 79, 81).

(E2 synthase) changes upon phosphorylation (85). If the activity of kinases fluctuates, then following the fluctuation of P450arom activity may generate hippocampal E2 fluctuation, even if the mRNA levels of steroidogenic enzymes do not change across the estrous cycle.

Female hippocampus is equipped with systems for androgen synthesis from PROG [P450(17α), 17β-HSD (types 1 and 3), 5α-reductase (types 1 and 2)] and synthesizes DHT (**Table 1**) (81). In female hippocampus, a large amount of Allo is also synthesized from peripherally produced PROG because 5α-reductase is responsible for Allo synthesis (53, 63, 81).

Regulation of Local Production of Steroids in Hippocampus

A stimulation with NMDA for 30 min increases the levels of PREG and E2 in the hippocampal slices of adult male rats (42, 43, 47), suggesting that neural activity-dependent Ca^{2+} influx drives local production of PREG and E2.

Reduction of P450arom activity by phosphorylation *via* kinases (PKA and PKC) is an important mechanism which regulates E2 synthesis. Balthazart et al. demonstrated that this phosphorylation occurred in the quail brain within 15 min (85–87). In the cultured hippocampal neurons of female rats, E2 application facilitated the phosphorylation of P450arom, suggesting negative feedback mechanism (88).

As slow/genomic modulators, *cis*-retinoic acid (89) and gonadotropin-releasing hormone (GnRH) (75) were examined using hippocampal slice culture from neonatal rats. Forty-eight-hour treatment with 1 μM of 9-*cis*-retinoic acid increased the expression levels of P450(17α) and P450arom in the cultured hippocampal slices from male rats, *via* retinoid X receptor signaling (89). On the other hand, 8 days of treatment with GnRH enhanced local E2 production (75, 90). Hippocampal E2 synthesis was also increased by a stereotaxic injection of GnRH into the hippocampus of adult female rats (91).

Interestingly, behaviors, including social interaction (92, 93) and exercise (94), alter local production of steroids in the hippocampus. Social isolation (housing individually for 8 weeks) upregulated the mRNA levels of P450arom and StAR in the hippocampus of adult male rats, compared with pair housed rats (92), whereas environmental enrichment (housing in a group of nine in a large cage for 8 weeks) increased the mRNA levels of 5α-reductase type 1 and 3α-HSD (93).

PHYSIOLOGICAL ROLES OF HIPPOCAMPUS-SYNTHESIZED STEROIDS

Hippocampus-Synthesized DHT Enhances Neurogenesis in DG

Adult hippocampal neurogenesis occurs in DG throughout life in mammals (95). Sex steroids (96–99) and exercise (100, 101) enhance adult hippocampal neurogenesis of rodents, but the involvement of sex steroids in the exercise-induced neurogenesis, had been poorly understood.

Recently, Okamoto et al. revealed that mild exercise (30 min/day for 2 weeks) increased synthesis of hippocampal DHT, resulting in the neurogenesis enhancement (94). Injection of flutamide, an AR antagonist, suppressed the exercise-induced increase in neurogenesis, suggesting the involvement of androgens. However, surprisingly, castration (depletion of androgen from blood circulation) did not suppress this effect, suggesting the involvement of hippocampus-synthesized androgens. Indeed, the increase in DHT and 5α-reductase (DHT synthase) mRNA, were observed in the hippocampus of castrated rats after exercise (94). This study provides the direct evidence of the role of hippocampus-synthesized steroids in hippocampal functions.

Modulation of LTP/LTD Induced by Hippocampus-Synthesized Steroids

The physiological roles of hippocampus-synthesized sex steroids (E2 and DHT) in LTP/LTD were demonstrated *in vitro* studies using acute hippocampal slices and selective inhibitors of steroidogenic enzymes. A perfusion with letrozole, a selective inhibitor of P450arom, suppressed the magnitude of LTP in CA1–CA3 synapses of adult male rats (102), and in DG synapses of young (3- to 4-week old) male rats (103–104), within 10–20 min. ICI182,780, a selective antagonist of ERα/β, mimicked this suppressive effect (102), suggesting that hippocampus-synthesized E2 is required for full induction of LTP *via* synaptic ER. Conversely, hippocampus-synthesized DHT is required for the induction of LTD, from the data showing that low frequency stimulation (1 Hz, 15 min)-induced LTD was suppressed in the presence of finasteride, an inhibitor of 5α-reductase (105). In addition to sex steroids, the effect of hippocampus-synthesized PREG is reported, in which the application of aminoglutethimide, an inhibitor of P450scc, decreased the field excitatory postsynaptic potentials in granule cells in 20 min (103). Although the molecular mechanism underlying these effects remains unclear, a possible explanation may be provided by analogy from the data, showing that exogenous application of E2 rapidly (within 30 min) enhanced LTP by driving kinase network (Erk MAPK, PKA, PKC, PI3K, and CaMKII) in a non-genomic manner (27, 106).

Role of Hippocampus-Synthesized E2 in Hippocampus-Dependent Memory

Recently, the role of hippocampus-synthesized E2 in hippocampus-dependent memory consolidation was provided using OVX mice (107). Immediate after the training, bilateral infusion of letrozole into the dorsal hippocampus blocked the transient elevation of hippocampal E2 (within 30 min), and impaired object recognition and object placement memory consolidation (107). Under the same condition except for infusion of E2, this group previously demonstrated that E2 enhanced hippocampal memory consolidation *via* rapid activation of Erk MAPK and PI3K/Akt (108, 109), suggesting that learning experience-induced E2 elevation in the hippocampus rapidly activates kinase cascades.

CONCLUSION

Hippocampus-synthesized steroids as well as circulation-derived ones, are of importance for hippocampal functions.

A possible molecular mechanism for rapid effect of hippocampus-synthesized steroids may be kinase networks which modulate hippocampal functions, including spinogenesis (106, 110), LTP (27), learning, and memory (108, 109).

AUTHOR CONTRIBUTIONS

YH wrote the manuscript. SK brushed up the initial draft of the manuscript written by YH.

REFERENCES

1. Baulieu EE. Neurosteroids: of the nervous system, by the nervous system, for the nervous system. *Recent Prog Horm Res* (1997) 52:1–32.
2. Corpechot C, Robel P, Axelson M, Sjovall J, Baulieu EE. Characterization and measurement of dehydroepiandrosterone sulfate in rat brain. *Proc Natl Acad Sci U S A* (1981) 78:4704–7. doi:10.1073/pnas.78.8.4704
3. Diotel N, Do Rego JL, Anglade I, Vaillant C, Pellegrini E, Vaudry H, et al. The brain of teleost fish, a source, and a target of sexual steroids. *Front Neurosci* (2011) 5:137. doi:10.3389/fnins.2011.00137
4. Xing L, Goswami M, Trudeau VL. Radial glial cell: critical functions and new perspective as a steroid synthetic cell. *Gen Comp Endocrinol* (2014) 203:181–5. doi:10.1016/j.ygcen.2014.03.010
5. Tsutsui K, Haraguchi S, Fukada Y, Vaudry H. Brain and pineal 7alpha-hydroxypregnenolone stimulating locomotor activity: identification, mode of action and regulation of biosynthesis. *Front Neuroendocrinol* (2013) 34:179–89. doi:10.1016/j.yfrne.2013.05.002
6. Tsutsui K, Haraguchi S, Matsunaga M, Koyama T, Do Rego JL, Vaudry H. 7alpha-Hydroxypregnenolone, a new key regulator of amphibian locomotion: discovery, progress and prospect. *Gen Comp Endocrinol* (2012) 176:440–7. doi:10.1016/j.ygcen.2011.11.020
7. Vaudry H, Do Rego JL, Burel D, Luu-The V, Pelletier G, Vaudry D, et al. Neurosteroid biosynthesis in the brain of amphibians. *Front Endocrinol* (2011) 2:79. doi:10.3389/fendo.2011.00079
8. Heimovics SA, Prior NH, Ma C, Soma KK. Rapid effects of an aggressive interaction on dehydroepiandrosterone, testosterone and oestradiol levels in the male song sparrow brain: a seasonal comparison. *J Neuroendocrinol* (2016) 28:12345. doi:10.1111/jne.12345
9. Remage-Healey L, Saldanha CJ, Schlinger BA. Estradiol synthesis and action at the synapse: evidence for "synaptocrine" signaling. *Front Endocrinol* (2011) 2:28. doi:10.3389/fendo.2011.00028
10. Do Rego JL, Seong JY, Burel D, Leprince J, Luu-The V, Tsutsui K, et al. Neurosteroid biosynthesis: enzymatic pathways and neuroendocrine regulation by neurotransmitters and neuropeptides. *Front Neuroendocrinol* (2009) 30:259–301. doi:10.1016/j.yfrne.2009.05.006
11. Hojo Y, Higo S, Kawato S, Hatanaka Y, Ooishi Y, Muakami G, et al. Hippocampal synthesis of sex steroids and corticosteroids: essential for modulation of synaptic plasticity. *Front Endocrinol* (2011) 2:43. doi:10.3389/fendo.2011.00043
12. Mukai H, Kimoto T, Hojo Y, Kawato S, Murakami G, Higo S, et al. Modulation of synaptic plasticity by brain estrogen in the hippocampus. *Biochim Biophys Acta* (2010) 1800:1030–44. doi:10.1016/j.bbagen.2009.11.002
13. Ooishi Y, Kawato S, Hojo Y, Hatanaka Y, Higo S, Murakami G, et al. Modulation of synaptic plasticity in the hippocampus by hippocampus-derived estrogen and androgen. *J Steroid Biochem Mol Biol* (2012) 131:37–51. doi:10.1016/j.jsbmb.2011.10.004
14. Tsutsui K, Ukena K, Sakamoto H, Okuyama S, Haraguchi S. Biosynthesis, mode of action, and functional significance of neurosteroids in the purkinje cell. *Front Endocrinol* (2011) 2:61. doi:10.3389/fendo.2011.00061
15. Azcoitia I, Yague JG, Garcia-Segura LM. Estradiol synthesis within the human brain. *Neuroscience* (2011) 191:139–47. doi:10.1016/j.neuroscience.2011.02.012
16. Melcangi RC, Panzica G, Garcia-Segura LM. Neuroactive steroids: focus on human brain. *Neuroscience* (2011) 191:1–5. doi:10.1016/j.neuroscience.2011.06.024
17. Naftolin F, Horvath TL, Jakab RL, Leranth C, Harada N, Balthazart J. Aromatase immunoreactivity in axon terminals of the vertebrate brain. An immunocytochemical study on quail, rat, monkey and human tissues. *Neuroendocrinology* (1996) 63:149–55. doi:10.1159/000126951
18. Biagini G, Rustichelli C, Curia G, Vinet J, Lucchi C, Pugnaghi M, et al. Neurosteroids and epileptogenesis. *J Neuroendocrinol* (2013) 25:980–90. doi:10.1111/jne.12063
19. Meletti S, Lucchi C, Monti G, Giovannini G, Bedin R, Trenti T, et al. Decreased allopregnanolone levels in cerebrospinal fluid obtained during status epilepticus. *Epilepsia* (2017) 58:e16–20. doi:10.1111/epi.13625
20. Martinez PE, Rubinow DR, Nieman LK, Koziol DE, Morrow AL, Schiller CE, et al. 5alpha-reductase inhibition prevents the luteal phase increase in plasma allopregnanolone levels and mitigates symptoms in women with premenstrual dysphoric disorder. *Neuropsychopharmacology* (2016) 41:1093–102. doi:10.1038/npp.2015.246
21. Schiller CE, Schmidt PJ, Rubinow DR. Allopregnanolone as a mediator of affective switching in reproductive mood disorders. *Psychopharmacology* (2014) 231:3557–67. doi:10.1007/s00213-014-3599-x
22. Murakami G, Hojo Y, Kato A, Komatsuzaki Y, Horie S, Soma M, et al. Rapid nongenomic modulation by neurosteroids of dendritic spines in the hippocampus: androgen, oestrogen and corticosteroid. *J Neuroendocrinol* (2018) 30:e12561. doi:10.1111/jne.12561
23. Bi R, Broutman G, Foy MR, Thompson RF, Baudry M. The tyrosine kinase and mitogen-activated protein kinase pathways mediate multiple effects of estrogen in hippocampus. *Proc Natl Acad Sci U S A* (2000) 97:3602–7. doi:10.1073/pnas.97.7.3602
24. Foy MR, Xu J, Xie X, Brinton RD, Thompson RF, Berger TW. 17beta-estradiol enhances NMDA receptor-mediated EPSPs and long-term potentiation. *J Neurophysiol* (1999) 81:925–9. doi:10.1152/jn.1999.81.2.925
25. Mukai H, Tsurugizawa T, Murakami G, Kominami S, Ishii H, Ogiue-Ikeda M, et al. Rapid modulation of long-term depression and spinogenesis via synaptic estrogen receptors in hippocampal principal neurons. *J Neurochem* (2007) 100:950–67. doi:10.1111/j.1471-4159.2006.04264.x
26. Vouimba RM, Foy MR, Foy JG, Thompson RF. 17beta-estradiol suppresses expression of long-term depression in aged rats. *Brain Res Bull* (2000) 53:783–7. doi:10.1016/S0361-9230(00)00377-4
27. Hasegawa Y, Hojo Y, Kojima H, Ikeda M, Hotta K, Sato R, et al. Estradiol rapidly modulates synaptic plasticity of hippocampal neurons: involvement of kinase networks. *Brain Res* (2015) 1621:147–61. doi:10.1016/j.brainres.2014.12.056
28. Hatanaka Y, Hojo Y, Mukai H, Murakami G, Komatsuzaki Y, Kim J, et al. Rapid increase of spines by dihydrotestosterone and testosterone in hippocampal neurons: dependence on synaptic androgen receptor and kinase networks. *Brain Res* (2015) 1621:121–32. doi:10.1016/j.brainres.2014.12.011
29. Milner TA, Ayoola K, Drake CT, Herrick SP, Tabori NE, McEwen BS, et al. Ultrastructural localization of estrogen receptor beta immunoreactivity in the rat hippocampal formation. *J Comp Neurol* (2005) 491:81–95. doi:10.1002/cne.20724
30. Tabori NE, Stewart LS, Znamensky V, Romeo RD, Alves SE, McEwen BS, et al. Ultrastructural evidence that androgen receptors are located at extranuclear sites in the rat hippocampal formation. *Neuroscience* (2005) 130:151–63. doi:10.1016/j.neuroscience.2004.08.048
31. Smejkalova T, Woolley CS. Estradiol acutely potentiates hippocampal excitatory synaptic transmission through a presynaptic mechanism. *J Neurosci* (2010) 30:16137–48. doi:10.1523/JNEUROSCI.4161-10.2010
32. Tabatadze N, Huang G, May RM, Jain A, Woolley CS. Sex differences in molecular signaling at inhibitory synapses in the hippocampus. *J Neurosci* (2015) 35:11252–65. doi:10.1523/JNEUROSCI.1067-15.2015
33. Hering H, Sheng M. Activity-dependent redistribution and essential role of cortactin in dendritic spine morphogenesis. *J Neurosci* (2003) 23:11759–69. doi:10.1523/JNEUROSCI.23-37-11759.2003
34. Iki J, Inoue A, Bito H, Okabe S. Bi-directional regulation of postsynaptic cortactin distribution by BDNF and NMDA receptor activity. *Eur J Neurosci* (2005) 22:2985–94. doi:10.1111/j.1460-9568.2005.04510.x
35. Aizawa H, Wakatsuki S, Ishii A, Moriyama K, Sasaki Y, Ohashi K, et al. Phosphorylation of cofilin by LIM-kinase is necessary for semaphorin 3A-induced growth cone collapse. *Nat Neurosci* (2001) 4:367–73. doi:10.1038/86011

36. Liston C, Cichon JM, Jeanneteau F, Jia Z, Chao MV, Gan WB. Circadian glucocorticoid oscillations promote learning-dependent synapse formation and maintenance. *Nat Neurosci* (2013) 16:698–705. doi:10.1038/nn.3387
37. Hojo Y, Higo S, Ishii H, Ooishi Y, Mukai H, Murakami G, et al. Comparison between hippocampus-synthesized and circulation-derived sex steroids in the hippocampus. *Endocrinology* (2009) 150:5106–12. doi:10.1210/en.2009-0305
38. Compagnone NA, Mellon SH. Neurosteroids: biosynthesis and function of these novel neuromodulators. *Front Neuroendocrinol* (2000) 21:1–56. doi:10.1006/frne.1999.0188
39. Le Goascogne C, Sananès N, Gouézou M, Takemori S, Kominami S, Baulieu EE, et al. Immunoreactive cytochrome P-450(17 alpha) in rat and guinea-pig gonads, adrenal glands and brain. *J Reprod Fertil* (1991) 93:609–22. doi:10.1530/jrf.0.0930609
40. Mellon SH, Deschepper CF. Neurosteroid biosynthesis: genes for adrenal steroidogenic enzymes are expressed in the brain. *Brain Res* (1993) 629: 283–92. doi:10.1016/0006-8993(93)91332-M
41. Robel P, Bourreau E, Corpéchot C, Dang DC, Halberg F, Clarke C, et al. Neuro-steroids: 3 beta-hydroxy-delta 5-derivatives in rat and monkey brain. *J Steroid Biochem* (1987) 27:649–55. doi:10.1016/0022-4731(87)90133-6
42. Hojo Y, Hattori TA, Enami T, Furukawa A, Suzuki K, Ishii HT, et al. Adult male rat hippocampus synthesizes estradiol from pregnenolone by cytochromes P45017alpha and P450 aromatase localized in neurons. *Proc Natl Acad Sci U S A* (2004) 101:865–70. doi:10.1073/pnas.2630225100
43. Kawato S, Hojo Y, Kimoto T. Histological and metabolism analysis of P450 expression in the brain. *Methods Enzymol* (2002) 357:241–9. doi:10.1016/S0076-6879(02)57682-5
44. Agís-Balboa RC, Pinna G, Zhubi A, Maloku E, Veldic M, Costa E, et al. Characterization of brain neurons that express enzymes mediating neurosteroid biosynthesis. *Proc Natl Acad Sci U S A* (2006) 103:14602–7. doi:10.1073/pnas.0606544103
45. Castelli MP, Casti A, Casu A, Frau R, Bortolato M, Spiga S, et al. Regional distribution of 5alpha-reductase type 2 in the adult rat brain: an immunohistochemical analysis. *Psychoneuroendocrinology* (2013) 38:281–93. doi:10.1016/j.psyneuen.2012.06.008
46. Furukawa A, Miyatake A, Ohnishi T, Ichikawa Y. Steroidogenic acute regulatory protein (StAR) transcripts constitutively expressed in the adult rat central nervous system: colocalization of StAR, cytochrome P-450SCC (CYP XIA1), and 3beta-hydroxysteroid dehydrogenase in the rat brain. *J Neurochem* (1998) 71:2231–8. doi:10.1046/j.1471-4159.1998.71062231.x
47. Kimoto T, Tsurugizawa T, Ohta Y, Makino J, Tamura H, Hojo Y, et al. Neurosteroid synthesis by cytochrome p450-containing systems localized in the rat brain hippocampal neurons: N-methyl-D-aspartate and calcium-dependent synthesis. *Endocrinology* (2001) 142:3578–89. doi:10.1210/endo.142.8.8327
48. Wehrenberg U, Prange-Kiel J, Rune GM. Steroidogenic factor-1 expression in marmoset and rat hippocampus: co-localization with StAR and aromatase. *J Neurochem* (2001) 76:1879–86. doi:10.1046/j.1471-4159.2001.00207.x
49. Prange-Kiel J, Wehrenberg U, Jarry H, Rune GM. Para/autocrine regulation of estrogen receptors in hippocampal neurons. *Hippocampus* (2003) 13:226–34. doi:10.1002/hipo.10075
50. Higo S, Hojo Y, Ishii H, Komatsuzaki Y, Ooishi Y, Murakami G, et al. Endogenous synthesis of corticosteroids in the hippocampus. *PLoS One* (2011) 6:e21631. doi:10.1371/journal.pone.0021631
51. Mitterling KL, Spencer JL, Dziedzic N, Shenoy S, McCarthy K, Waters EM, et al. Cellular and subcellular localization of estrogen and progestin receptor immunoreactivities in the mouse hippocampus. *J Comp Neurol* (2010) 518:2729–43. doi:10.1002/cne.22361
52. Waters EM, Torres-Reveron A, McEwen BS, Milner TA. Ultrastructural localization of extranuclear progestin receptors in the rat hippocampal formation. *J Comp Neurol* (2008) 511:34–46. doi:10.1002/cne.21826
53. Caruso D, Pesaresi M, Maschi O, Giatti S, Garcia-Segura LM, Melcangi RC. Effect of short-and long-term gonadectomy on neuroactive steroid levels in the central and peripheral nervous system of male and female rats. *J Neuroendocrinol* (2010) 22:1137–47. doi:10.1111/j.1365-2826.2010.02064.x
54. Ebner MJ, Corol DI, Havlikova H, Honour JW, Fry JP. Identification of neuroactive steroids and their precursors and metabolites in adult male rat brain. *Endocrinology* (2006) 147:179–90. doi:10.1210/en.2005-1065
55. Higashi T, Ninomiya Y, Iwaki N, Yamauchi A, Takayama N, Shimada K. Studies on neurosteroids XVIII LC-MS analysis of changes in rat brain and serum testosterone levels induced by immobilization stress and ethanol administration. *Steroids* (2006) 71:609–17. doi:10.1016/j.steroids.2006.03.003
56. Liere P, Akwa Y, Weill-Engerer S, Eychenne B, Pianos A, Robel P, et al. Validation of an analytical procedure to measure trace amounts of neursteroids in brain tissue by gas chromatography-mass spectrometry. *J Chromatogr B Biomed Sci Appl* (2000) 739:301–12. doi:10.1016/S0378-4347(99)00563-0
57. Liu S, Sjovall J, Griffiths WJ. Neurosteroids in rat brain: extraction, isolation, and analysis by nanoscale liquid chromatography-electrospray mass spectrometry. *Anal Chem* (2003) 75:5835–46. doi:10.1021/ac0346297
58. Meffre D, Pianos A, Liere P, Eychenne B, Cambourg A, Schumacher M, et al. Steroid profiling in brain and plasma of male and pseudopregnant female rats after traumatic brain injury: analysis by gas chromatography/mass spectrometry. *Endocrinology* (2007) 148:2505–17. doi:10.1210/en.2006-1678
59. Schumacher M, Liere P, Akwa Y, Rajkowski K, Griffiths W, Bodin K, et al. Pregnenolone sulfate in the brain: a controversial neurosteroid. *Neurochem Int* (2008) 52:522–40. doi:10.1016/j.neuint.2007.08.022
60. Rustichelli C, Pinetti D, Lucchi C, Ravazzini F, Puia G. Simultaneous determination of pregnenolone sulphate, dehydroepiandrosterone and allopregnanolone in rat brain areas by liquid chromatography-electrospray tandem mass spectrometry. *J Chromatogr B Analyt Technol Biomed Life Sci* (2013) 930:62–9. doi:10.1016/j.jchromb.2013.04.035
61. Yamashita K, Kobayashi S, Tsukamoto S, Numazawa M. Synthesis of pyridine-carboxylate derivatives of hydroxysteroids for liquid chromatography-electrospray ionization-mass spectrometry. *Steroids* (2007) 72:50–9. doi:10.1016/j.steroids.2006.10.005
62. Yamashita K, Okuyama M, Watanabe Y, Honma S, Kobayashi S, Numazawa M. Highly sensitive determination of estrone and estradiol in human serum by liquid chromatography-electrospray ionization tandem mass spectrometry. *Steroids* (2007) 72:819–27. doi:10.1016/j.steroids.2007.07.003
63. Caruso D, Pesaresi M, Abbiati F, Calabrese D, Giatti S, Garcia-Segura LM, et al. Comparison of plasma and cerebrospinal fluid levels of neuroactive steroids with their brain, spinal cord and peripheral nerve levels in male and female rats. *Psychoneuroendocrinology* (2013) 38:2278–90. doi:10.1016/j.psyneuen.2013.04.016
64. Barron AM, Hojo Y, Mukai H, Higo S, Ooishi Y, Hatanaka Y, et al. Regulation of synaptic plasticity by hippocampus synthesized estradiol. *Horm Mol Biol Clin Investig* (2011) 7:361–75. doi:10.1515/HMBCI.2011.118
65. Frick KM, Kim J, Tuscher JJ, Fortress AM. Sex steroid hormones matter for learning and memory: estrogenic regulation of hippocampal function in male and female rodents. *Learn Mem* (2015) 22:472–93. doi:10.1101/lm.037267.114
66. Goldman JM, Murr AS, Cooper RL. The rodent estrous cycle: characterization of vaginal cytology and its utility in toxicological studies. *Birth Defects Res B Dev Reprod Toxicol* (2007) 80:84–97. doi:10.1002/bdrb.20106
67. Frick KM, Berger-Sweeney J. Spatial reference memory and neocortical neurochemistry vary with the estrous cycle in C57BL/6 mice. *Behav Neurosci* (2001) 115:229–37. doi:10.1037/0735-7044.115.1.229
68. Paris JJ, Frye CA. Estrous cycle, pregnancy, and parity enhance performance of rats in object recognition or object placement tasks. *Reproduction* (2008) 136:105–15. doi:10.1530/REP-07-0512
69. Pompili A, Tomaz C, Arnone B, Tavares MC, Gasbarri A. Working and reference memory across the estrous cycle of rat: a long-term study in gonadally intact females. *Behav Brain Res* (2010) 213:10–8. doi:10.1016/j.bbr.2010.04.018
70. Sutcliffe JS, Marshall KM, Neill JC. Influence of gender on working and spatial memory in the novel object recognition task in the rat. *Behav Brain Res* (2007) 177:117–25. doi:10.1016/j.bbr.2006.10.029
71. Warren SG, Juraska JM. Spatial and nonspatial learning across the rat estrous cycle. *Behav Neurosci* (1997) 111:259–66. doi:10.1037/0735-7044.111.2.259
72. Bi R, Foy MR, Vouimba RM, Thompson RF, Baudry M. Cyclic changes in estradiol regulate synaptic plasticity through the MAP kinase pathway. *Proc Natl Acad Sci U S A* (2001) 98:13391–5. doi:10.1073/pnas.241507698
73. Warren SG, Humphreys AG, Juraska JM, Greenough WT. LTP varies across the estrous cycle: enhanced synaptic plasticity in proestrus rats. *Brain Res* (1995) 703:26–30. doi:10.1016/0006-8993(95)01059-9
74. Gould E, Woolley CS, Frankfurt M, McEwen BS. Gonadal steroids regulate dendritic spine density in hippocampal pyramidal cells in adulthood. *J Neurosci* (1990) 10:1286–91. doi:10.1523/JNEUROSCI.10-04-01286.1990

75. Prange-Kiel J, Jarry H, Schoen M, Kohlmann P, Lohse C, Zhou L, et al. Gonadotropin-releasing hormone regulates spine density via its regulatory role in hippocampal estrogen synthesis. *J Cell Biol* (2008) 180:417–26. doi:10.1083/jcb.200707043
76. Woolley CS, Gould E, Frankfurt M, McEwen BS. Naturally occurring fluctuation in dendritic spine density on adult hippocampal pyramidal neurons. *J Neurosci* (1990) 10:4035–9. doi:10.1523/JNEUROSCI.10-12-04035.1990
77. Woolley CS, McEwen BS. Estradiol mediates fluctuation in hippocampal synapse density during the estrous cycle in the adult rat. *J Neurosci* (1992) 12:2549–54. doi:10.1523/JNEUROSCI.12-07-02549.1992
78. Woolley CS, McEwen BS. Roles of estradiol and progesterone in regulation of hippocampal dendritic spine density during the estrous cycle in the rat. *J Comp Neurol* (1993) 336:293–306. doi:10.1002/cne.903360210
79. Kato A, Hojo Y, Higo S, Komatsuzaki Y, Murakami G, Yoshino H, et al. Female hippocampal estrogens have a significant correlation with cyclic fluctuation of hippocampal spines. *Front Neural Circuits* (2013) 7:149. doi:10.3389/fncir.2013.00149
80. Watanabe G, Taya K, Sasamoto S. Dynamics of ovarian inhibin secretion during the oestrous cycle of the rat. *J Endocrinol* (1990) 126:151–7. doi:10.1677/joe.0.1260151
81. Hojo Y, Okamoto M, Kato A, Higo S, Sakai F, Soya H, et al. Neurosteroid synthesis in adult female rat hippocampus, including androgens and allopregnanolone. *J Steroids Hormon Sci* (2014) S4:002. doi:10.4172/2157-7536.S4-002
82. Kimoto T, Ishii H, Higo S, Hojo Y, Kawato S. Semicomprehensive analysis of the postnatal age-related changes in the mRNA expression of sex steroidogenic enzymes and sex steroid receptors in the male rat hippocampus. *Endocrinology* (2010) 151:5795–806. doi:10.1210/en.2010-0581
83. Spencer JL, Waters EM, Milner TA, McEwen BS. Estrous cycle regulates activation of hippocampal Akt, LIM kinase, and neurotrophin receptors in C57BL/6 mice. *Neuroscience* (2008) 155:1106–19. doi:10.1016/j.neuroscience.2008.05.049
84. Znamensky V, Akama KT, McEwen BS, Milner TA. Estrogen levels regulate the subcellular distribution of phosphorylated Akt in hippocampal CA1 dendrites. *J Neurosci* (2003) 23:2340–7.
85. Balthazart J, Ball GF. Is brain estradiol a hormone or a neurotransmitter? *Trends Neurosci* (2006) 29:241–9. doi:10.1016/j.tins.2006.03.004
86. Balthazart J, Baillien M, Ball GF. Phosphorylation processes mediate rapid changes of brain aromatase activity. *J Steroid Biochem Mol Biol* (2001) 79:261–77. doi:10.1016/S0960-0760(01)00143-1
87. Balthazart J, Baillien M, Ball GF. Interactions between kinases and phosphatases in the rapid control of brain aromatase. *J Neuroendocrinol* (2005) 17:553–9. doi:10.1111/j.1365-2826.2005.01344.x
88. Fester L, Brandt N, Windhorst S, Prols F, Blaute C, Rune GM. Control of aromatase in hippocampal neurons. *J Steroid Biochem Mol Biol* (2016) 160:9–14. doi:10.1016/j.jsbmb.2015.10.009
89. Munetsuna E, Hojo Y, Hattori M, Ishii H, Kawato S, Ishida A, et al. Retinoic acid stimulates 17beta-estradiol and testosterone synthesis in rat hippocampal slice cultures. *Endocrinology* (2009) 150:4260–9. doi:10.1210/en.2008-1644
90. Fester L, Prange-Kiel J, Zhou L, Blittersdorf BV, Böhm J, Jarry H, et al. Estrogen-regulated synaptogenesis in the hippocampus: sexual dimorphism in vivo but not in vitro. *J Steroid Biochem Mol Biol* (2012) 131:24–9. doi:10.1016/j.jsbmb.2011.11.010
91. Prange-Kiel J, Schmutterer T, Fester L, Zhou L, Imholz P, Brandt N, et al. Endocrine regulation of estrogen synthesis in the hippocampus? *Prog Histochem Cytochem* (2013) 48:49–64. doi:10.1016/j.proghi.2013.07.002
92. Munetsuna E, Hattori M, Komatsu S, Sakimoto Y, Ishida A, Sakata S, et al. Social isolation stimulates hippocampal estradiol synthesis. *Biochem Biophys Res Commun* (2009) 379:480–4. doi:10.1016/j.bbrc.2008.12.076
93. Munetsuna E, Hattori M, Sakimoto Y, Ishida A, Sakata S, Hojo Y, et al. Environmental enrichment alters gene expression of steroidogenic enzymes in the rat hippocampus. *Gen Comp Endocrinol* (2011) 171:28–32. doi:10.1016/j.ygcen.2010.12.007
94. Okamoto M, Hojo Y, Inoue K, Matsui T, Kawato S, McEwen BS, et al. Mild exercise increases dihydrotestosterone in hippocampus providing evidence for androgenic mediation of neurogenesis. *Proc Natl Acad Sci U S A* (2012) 109:13100–5. doi:10.1073/pnas.1210023109
95. Gage FH. Mammalian neural stem cells. *Science* (2000) 287:1433–8. doi:10.1126/science.287.5457.1433
96. Galea LA, Wainwright SR, Roes MM, Duarte-Guterman P, Chow C, Hamson DK. Sex, hormones and neurogenesis in the hippocampus: hormonal modulation of neurogenesis and potential functional implications. *J Neuroendocrinol* (2013) 25:1039–61. doi:10.1111/jne.12070
97. Hamson DK, Wainwright SR, Taylor JR, Jones BA, Watson NV, Galea LA. Androgens increase survival of adult-born neurons in the dentate gyrus by an androgen receptor-dependent mechanism in male rats. *Endocrinology* (2013) 154:3294–304. doi:10.1210/en.2013-1129
98. Pawluski JL, Brummelte S, Barha CK, Crozier TM, Galea LA. Effects of steroid hormones on neurogenesis in the hippocampus of the adult female rodent during the estrous cycle, pregnancy, lactation and aging. *Front Neuroendocrinol* (2009) 30:343–57. doi:10.1016/j.yfrne.2009.03.007
99. Spritzer MD, Galea LA. Testosterone and dihydrotestosterone, but not estradiol, enhance survival of new hippocampal neurons in adult male rats. *Dev Neurobiol* (2007) 67:1321–33. doi:10.1002/dneu.20457
100. Marlatt MW, Potter MC, Lucassen PJ, van Praag H. Running throughout middle-age improves memory function, hippocampal neurogenesis, and BDNF levels in female C57BL/6J mice. *Dev Neurobiol* (2012) 72:943–52. doi:10.1002/dneu.22009
101. van Praag H, Christie BR, Sejnowski TJ, Gage FH. Running enhances neurogenesis, learning, and long-term potentiation in mice. *Proc Natl Acad Sci U S A* (1999) 96:13427–31. doi:10.1073/pnas.96.23.13427
102. Grassi S, Tozzi A, Costa C, Tantucci M, Colcelli E, Scarduzio M, et al. Neural 17beta-estradiol facilitates long-term potentiation in the hippocampal CA1 region. *Neuroscience* (2011) 192:67–73. doi:10.1016/j.neuroscience.2011.06.078
103. Tanaka M, Sokabe M. Continuous de novo synthesis of neurosteroids is required for normal synaptic transmission and plasticity in the dentate gyrus of the rat hippocampus. *Neuropharmacology* (2012) 62:2373–87. doi:10.1016/j.neuropharm.2012.02.007
104. Tanaka M, Sokabe M. Bidirectional modulatory effect of 17beta-estradiol on NMDA receptors via ERalpha and ERbeta in the dentate gyrus of juvenile male rats. *Neuropharmacology* (2013) 75:262–73. doi:10.1016/j.neuropharm.2013.07.029
105. Di Mauro M, Tozzi A, Calabresi P, Pettorossi VE, Grassi S. Neo-synthesis of estrogenic or androgenic neurosteroids determine whether long-term potentiation or depression is induced in hippocampus of male rat. *Front Cell Neurosci* (2015) 9:376. doi:10.3389/fncel.2015.00376
106. Hojo Y, Munetomo A, Mukai H, Ikeda M, Sato R, Hatanaka Y, et al. Estradiol rapidly modulates spinogenesis in hippocampal dentate gyrus: involvement of kinase networks. *Horm Behav* (2015) 74:149–56. doi:10.1016/j.yhbeh.2015.06.008
107. Tuscher JJ, Szinte JS, Starrett JR, Krentzel AA, Fortress AM, Remage-Healey L, et al. Inhibition of local estrogen synthesis in the hippocampus impairs hippocampal memory consolidation in ovariectomized female mice. *Horm Behav* (2016) 83:60–7. doi:10.1016/j.yhbeh.2016.05.001
108. Fan L, Zhao Z, Orr PT, Chambers CH, Lewis MC, Frick KM. Estradiol-induced object memory consolidation in middle-aged female mice requires dorsal hippocampal extracellular signal-regulated kinase and phosphatidylinositol 3-kinase activation. *J Neurosci* (2010) 30:4390–400. doi:10.1523/JNEUROSCI.4333-09.2010
109. Fernandez SM, Lewis MC, Pechenino AS, Harburger LL, Orr PT, Gresack JE, et al. Estradiol-induced enhancement of object memory consolidation involves hippocampal extracellular signal-regulated kinase activation and membrane-bound estrogen receptors. *J Neurosci* (2008) 28:8660–7. doi:10.1523/JNEUROSCI.1968-08.2008
110. Murakami G, Hojo Y, Ogiue-Ikeda M, Mukai H, Chambon P, Nakajima K, et al. Estrogen receptor KO mice study on rapid modulation of spines and long-term depression in the hippocampus. *Brain Res* (2015) 1621:133–46. doi:10.1016/j.brainres.2014.12.002

19

11β-HSD Types 1 and 2 in the Songbird Brain

Michelle A. Rensel[1,2], Jessica A. Ding[3], Devaleena S. Pradhan[2,3] and Barney A. Schlinger[2,3,4]*

[1] The Institute for Society and Genetics, University of California, Los Angeles, Los Angeles, CA, United States, [2] Laboratory of Neuroendocrinology, University of California, Los Angeles, Los Angeles, CA, United States, [3] Department of Integrative Biology and Physiology, University of California, Los Angeles, Los Angeles, CA, United States, [4] Department of Ecology and Evolutionary Biology, University of California, Los Angeles, Los Angeles, CA, United States

***Correspondence:**
Michelle A. Rensel
mrensel@ucla.edu

Glucocorticoid (GC) hormones act on the brain to regulate diverse functions, from behavior and homeostasis to the activity of the hypothalamic–pituitary–adrenal axis. Local regeneration and metabolism of GCs can occur in target tissues through the actions of the 11β-hydroxysteroid dehydrogenases [11 beta-hydroxysteroid dehydrogenase type 1 (11β-HSD1) and 11 beta-hydroxysteroid dehydrogenase type 2 (11β-HSD2), respectively] to regulate access to GC receptors. Songbirds have become especially important model organisms for studies of stress hormone action; however, there has been little focus on neural GC metabolism. Therefore, we tested the hypothesis that 11β-HSD1 and 11β-HSD2 are expressed in GC-sensitive regions of the songbird brain. Localization of 11β-HSD expression in these regions could provide precise temporal and spatial control over GC actions. We quantified GC sensitivity in zebra finch (*Taeniopygia guttata*) brain by measuring glucocorticoid receptor (GR) and mineralocorticoid receptor (MR) expression across six regions, followed by quantification of 11β-HSD1 and 11β-HSD2 expression. We detected GR, MR, and 11β-HSD2 mRNA expression throughout the adult brain. Whereas 11β-HSD1 expression was undetectable in the adult brain, we detected low levels of expression in the brain of developing finches. Across several adult brain regions, expression of 11β-HSD2 covaried with GR and MR, with the exception of the cerebellum and hippocampus. It is possible that receptors in these latter two regions require direct access to systemic GC levels. Overall, these results suggest that 11β-HSD2 expression protects the adult songbird brain by rapid metabolism of GCs in a context and region-specific manner.

Keywords: glucocorticoid, mineralocorticoid, 11 beta-hydroxysteroid dehydrogenase, stress response, songbird

INTRODUCTION

Glucocorticoid (GC) hormones regulate numerous biological processes, including crucial actions on the central nervous system such as feedback regulation of adrenal function, activation or suppression of cognitive and locomotor activity, and regulation of feeding behaviors (1). GC secretion is dynamic, varying according to time of day (2, 3), developmental and life history stage (4–7), as well as in response to acute and chronic stress (1). Following synthesis and secretion, primarily from the adrenals, GC effects are regulated by various mechanisms, including binding to circulating globulins that regulate access to tissues and local expression of catabolic and anabolic enzymes in target tissues (8). Ultimately, tissue genomic and cellular responses are guided by the degree to which GC receptors are expressed. Sensitivity to GC effects is mediated through the intracellular mineralocorticoid receptor (MR) and glucocorticoid receptor (GR); acute stress-induced effects are mediated by the lower-affinity GR, while the high-affinity MR mediates baseline and early stress-induced effects (1, 9). Membrane GR and MR, while less studied, are found in both birds and mammals where they likely mediate rapid, non-genomic effects of GCs (10–12).

The 11β hydroxysteroid dehydrogenase enzymes (11β-HSDs) mediate the interconversion of the GC corticosterone (birds, some rodents, and reptiles) or cortisol (other vertebrates; both hereafter referred to as CORT) to an inactive form, 11-dehydrocorticosterone (11-DHC) or cortisone, respectively. The enzyme 11 beta-hydroxysteroid dehydrogenase type 1 (11β-HSD1) catalyzes the conversion of 11-DHC or cortisone into CORT *in vivo* but is capable of catalyzing the reverse reaction *in vitro*; 11 beta-hydroxysteroid dehydrogenase type 2 (11β-HSD2) exclusively inactivates CORT by catalyzing its conversion into 11-DHC or cortisone (13). Dysregulation of these enzymes in peripheral tissues is implicated in mammalian models of hypertension, diabetes, obesity, and metabolic disorder (14). 11β-HSD2 plays a critical role in the mammalian kidney, where its expression preserves aldosterone access to MR, which binds both CORT and aldosterone with equal affinity (15).

In rodents, 11β-HSDs are expressed peripherally and in brain, although their localization and functional significance vary across developmental stages. For example, relatively little 11β-HSD1 is expressed in the early developing rodent brain (15, 16), whereas it is widely expressed in the adult brain and periphery. In the adult brain, this enzyme participates in hypothalamic–pituitary–adrenal (HPA) axis regulation (17, 18) and facilitates GC-induced memory impairments in aging animals (19). Conversely, 11β-HSD2 expression in the adult brain has a limited distribution associated with salt-based aldosterone sensitivity, while 11β-HSD2 is expressed abundantly in the fetal brain and placenta and is hypothesized to protect the fetal nervous system from excess GC exposure (15).

Evidence for 11β-HSD2 expression in the adult human brain is contradictory (20, 21), and it is possible that CORT is metabolized in the human brain *via* a unique hydroxysteroid dehydrogenase (22). Given the documented ill effects of stress and elevated GCs on adult neurogenesis and cognition (23), the presence of region-specific GC-inactivating and regenerating enzymatic machinery in the brain should be adaptive and expected.

Unlike the adult rodent brain, metabolism of CORT *via* 11β-HSD2 has been reported in hatchling and adult songbird brain using chicken-specific PCR primers (24) as well as species-specific primers (25). In the latter study, we confirmed expression of 11β-HSD2 in two regions of the adult zebra finch (*Taeniopygia guttata*) brain, the caudal nidopallium (cNp) and hippocampus (HP). In addition, expression covaried with free CORT sampled in these regions using *in vivo* microdialysis. Specifically, we found that CORT levels were higher in the region expressing lower levels of 11β-HSD2 (25) suggesting that 11β-HSD2 limits bioactive GC exposure in specific regions of the brain.

The cNp and HP both lie adjacent to the lateral ventricular zone (VZ), a region of the songbird brain in which adult neurogenesis is conspicuous and critical for seasonal growth of song control nuclei (26) and recruitment of hippocampal neurons (27). As previous work has established differential effects of GCs on neurogenesis (23), we predicted that both 11β-HSD1 and 11β-HSD2 expression in HP and cNp, as well as another adjacent region, the caudomedial nidopallium (NCM), should provide precise control over GCs within these sensitive proliferative zones. We therefore hypothesized that 11β-HSD2 and/or 11β-HSD1 expression regulates exposure of the adult songbird brain in regions with heightened expression of GC receptors.

We tested this hypothesis in adult male and female zebra finches, assessing expression in six brain regions. We included three brain regions, NCM, cNp, and HP because of their proximity to the VZ, the diencephalon (DIEN), because of its role in regulating HPA negative feedback, and the cerebellum and optic tectum as control regions. Previous studies have described expression profiles of GR and MR in songbirds (28–32). To the best of our knowledge, 11β-HSD1 expression has not been reported in songbirds, with little data on 11β-HSD2. To assess how metabolic enzymes might participate in controlling GC access to its receptors, we used quantitative PCR to simultaneously characterize expression of 11β-HSD1 and 11β-HSD2, as well as GR and MR, in adult brain. While we detected 11β-HSD2 in all brain regions, 11β-HSD1 expression was undetectable. To verify this result, which differs significantly from mammalian patterns of expression (15), we confirmed 11β-HSD1 expression in the brains of developing finches as well as two additional target tissues, the liver and kidney (33).

ANIMALS AND METHODS

Animals

This study was conducted at the University of California, Los Angeles. All procedures involving animals were approved by the Chancellor's Animal Research Committee. We utilized adult (>100 days of age) non-breeding zebra finches obtained from our captive colony. For one study, we utilized developing finches of variable ages (see below). Finches in our colony are kept in large open flight aviaries with up to 40 same-sex individuals residing in each enclosure. Breeding cages are comprised of four to five breeding pairs with access to breeding boxes filled with nesting material. Lights are maintained on a 14 h light/10 h dark cycle, and finches are supplied with *ad libitum* seed, water, cuttle bone, and grit at all times. Egg mix and nutritional supplements are provided at least once per week.

Dissections

Groups of four to five adult finches were captured together and transported in a darkened cage to a procedure room where each bird was then processed. Following rapid decapitation, the brain was removed and placed on a Petri dish situated in wet ice (see below). Upon dissection, the six brain regions of interest were immediately frozen on dry ice, transferred to tubes, and kept at −80°C until RNA extraction. The amount of time that passed from initial capture to sacrifice ranged from 1 to 87 min (mean time = 39 ± 6.5 min), and sacrifice time post-capture was included as a covariate in statistical analyses. Sampling times and ranges were highly similar between males and females (**Figure 1**). A total of 18 birds were sacrificed in this manner, over the course of four sessions in 2 days (one AM and one PM session/day—the order of sexes captured was counterbalanced across days). The same aviary was never entered more than once per day to reduce potential stress effects on gene expression.

Brain regions were dissected as follows: with the brain ventral side down, the whole cerebellum was removed. Next, we made two parasagittal cuts ~1 mm from the midline from the caudal to the rostral end, then removed 5 mm of the rostral portion of the brain. The HP was then carefully separated from the caudal portion and removed bilaterally [see Ref. (25)]. Using watchmaker's forceps, we next collected a roughly 1 mm^2 region of the underlying telencephalon (TEL) containing the caudomedial nidopallium (NCM) [see Ref. (34)]. A 1 mm^2 portion of cNp located lateral to the position of the HP cut was next made bilaterally [see Ref. (25)]. After removal of the remainder of the TEL, the optic tecta were easily separated. Finally, excess optic nerve and myelin was removed and discarded from the ventral DIEN. Liver and kidney were collected next and frozen.

To compare 11β-HSD1 expression across developmental stages, brain tissue was collected from four individuals per age group: 5–7 days post-hatch ("hatchlings"), 25 days post-hatch ("fledglings"), and 75 days post-hatch ("juveniles"). The entire TEL (including underlying DIEN) was collected from hatchlings due to their very small size, while only the caudal TEL was utilized from fledglings and juveniles. The HP was removed from the caudal TEL of these latter ages (for other studies). To enable a direct comparison of expression across ages, the remaining caudal TEL from four of the adults utilized in the main study above was processed in parallel with these developing finch samples.

RNA Extraction and cDNA Synthesis

RNA was extracted from frozen tissue samples using the Trizol method according to the manufacturer's guidelines (Ambion). All centrifugation steps were performed at 4°C. Briefly, tissue was homogenized in 1 ml cold Trizol for a maximum of 45 s, followed by centrifugation at 12,000 *g* for 10 min. The supernatant was decanted and incubated at room temperature for 5 min, and

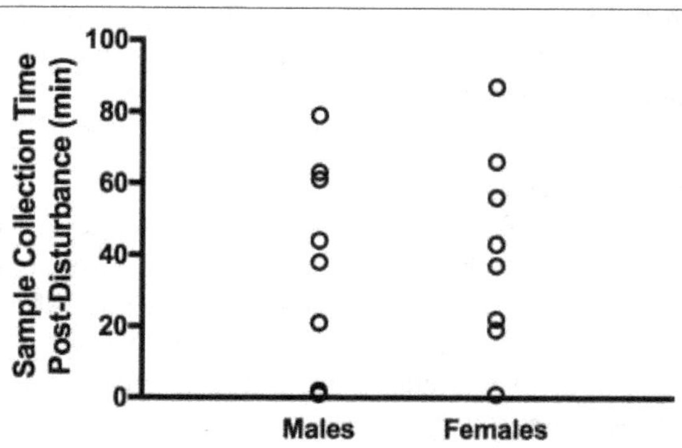

FIGURE 1 | Distribution of tissue collection times post-disturbance in adult male and female zebra finches. Males and females were sampled at similar times.

200 µl of chloroform was then added. Samples were vigorously shaken, incubated at room temp for 3 min and then centrifuged at 12,000 *g* for 15 min. After centrifugation, the aqueous layer was carefully removed and placed in a new tube. Next, 500 µl of isopropanol was added to each tube. For small tissues that produced tiny RNA pellets (HP, NCM, and cNp), we added 1 µl of 15 mg/ml glycoblue (Invitrogen) to improve visibility. Tubes were briefly vortexed, incubated at room temperature for 10 min, centrifuged at 12,000 *g* for 10 min, and the supernatant removed, leaving the RNA pellet in place. Finally, 1 ml of 75% ethanol (4°C) was added to the tube, and the tube was inverted to ensure that the pellet was free-floating. After centrifugation at 7,500 *g* for 5 min, the ethanol was carefully pipetted out of the tube, and residual ethanol was allowed to evaporate. The RNA pellet was then resuspended in 10–120 µl of sterile water based on pellet size, vortexed and then heated in a water bath at 58°C for 10 min. RNA quantity and integrity was then determined *via* nanodrop. Total RNA concentrations ranged from 100 to 600 ng/µl, and $A_{260/280}$ ratios were between 1.8 and 2.15.

To prepare cDNA from RNA samples, 600 ng RNA was reverse transcribed. Briefly, 0.5 µl of DNAse (Promega) and 1.1 µl of DNase buffer were added to each sample, then incubated at 37°C for 30 min and 65°C for 10 min. Next, 1.5 µl of oligoDT (Sigma) and 0.5 µl dNTPs (Bioline) were added, and tubes were incubated for 10 min at 65°C. Finally, a mix of reverse transcriptase (Superscript II, Invitrogen; 1 µl/sample), RT buffer (4 µl/sample), DTT (1 µl/sample), and RNAse inhibitor (RNAsin, Promega; 1 µl/sample) was added, followed by incubation at 42°C for 50 min and 70°C for 15 min. Samples were then frozen at −20°C until qPCR analysis.

Quantitative PCR

Mineralocorticoid receptor, 11β-HSD2, and 11β-HSD1 qPCR primers were designed based on the zebra finch genome using Primer3Plus and PrimerBlast (NCBI). GR primers were taken from Banerjee et al. (35). Concentrations were optimized for each primer pair and are listed along with primer sequences and amplicon lengths in **Table 1**. We used an Applied Biosystems 7300 Real-Time PCR system to quantify gene expression relative to glyceraldehyde-3-phosphate dehydrogenase (GAPDH) in samples using the SYBR Green method. Samples were run at a 1:10 dilution and in duplicate wells. Reaction volume was 25 µl, and cycling conditions were as follows: (1) 2 min at 50°C, (2) 10 min at 95°C, (3) 15 s at 95°C, (4) 1 min at 60°C, repeat steps 3 and 4 40 times, (5) 15 s at 95°C, (6) 1 min at 60°C, (7) 15 s at 95°C, and (8) 15 s at 60°C.

Standard curves were prepared for each gene and plate to confirm reaction efficiency (90–110%) and standard curve linearity (≥98%). For GR and MR, each plate contained a standard curve prepared from a mix of 1:1 cDNA representing all samples from the region represented on the plate. We included positive control tissue in the adult 11β-HSD2 standard curves, pooling all brain regions together with a small amount of kidney cDNA. The adult 11β-HSD1 standard curve was constructed from liver cDNA. All standard curves utilized a fourfold dilution with curves extending from 1:1 to 1:256 for GR, MR, and GAPDH, and standard curves ranging from 1:1 to 1:1,024 (11β-HSD1) or 1:4,096 (11β-HSD2).

TABLE 1 | Quantitative PCR primer details.

Gene name (accession #)	Primer sequence (5′–3′)	Amplicon length (bp)	[Primer] per reaction (μM)
Mineralocorticoid receptor (NM_001076690)	F: AAGAGTCGGCCAAACATCCTTGTTCT R: AAGAAACGGGTGGTCCTAAAATCCCAG	150	0.3
Glucocorticoid receptor (XM_002192952.3)	F: TGCAGTACTCCTGGATGTTCC R: GAGCATGTGTTTGCATTGTTC	155	0.3
11 Beta-hydroxysteroid dehydrogenase type 2 (XM_002187455.3)	F: AAAACAGGGACAACATGCGA R: CCCCTCTGTGATGCTGTTCA	189	0.6
11 Beta-hydroxysteroid dehydrogenase type 1 (XM_002196384.1[a])	F: CATCCATAGCGGGTAAAATTG R: CGCTCTCTGTGTTGATGTAGC	162	0.3
Glyceraldehyde-3-phosphate dehydrogenase (NM_001198610.1)	F: TGACCTGCCGTCTGGAAAA R: CCATCAGCAGCAGCCT	70	0.3

[a]*This transcript is "11 beta-dehydrogenase 1-like" in NCBI; Ensembl lists a nearly identical transcript as "HSD11B1." Therefore, we designed qPCR primers to cover a region of the transcript found in both versions.*

All sample values fell within the bounds of the standard curve for each gene and plate (except for 11β-HSD1; see below). Preliminary optimizations for 11β-HSD1 indicated low to no expression in adult brain; therefore, all samples within a given brain region and a given sex were pooled for the assay instead of running individual samples (n = 12 pooled samples from males and females in six regions).

In the absence of 11β-HSD1 expression in regions of the adult brain examined, we conducted further tests to verify the specificity and accuracy of our 11β-HSD1 primers. We first created individual pools of caudal and whole TEL (all ages), liver (all ages), and kidney (adults) and optimized the qPCR reaction. After confirming amplification in all three pools, we sequenced products and used NCBI Blast to confirm the specificity of the products. Because we successfully amplified 11β-HSD1 in the TEL pool, we next ran a single qPCR plate with TEL samples from all four ages (n = 4 per age). We constructed the standard curve for this plate from a pool of TEL, kidney, liver, and adrenal cDNA.

Specificity of amplification for GR, MR, 11β-HSD2, and 11β-HSD1 was established by (a) confirming the presence of a single peak on dissociation curves and (b) sequencing and subsequent BLAST analysis of qPCR products. Additional sequencing and gel electrophoresis were used to confirm expression of 11β-HSD1 in hatchling brain (see Results). No reverse transcriptase (no RT) controls were run for each gene to assess DNA contamination. We also confirmed that reaction mixes were not contaminated by running no-template controls on each plate.

Expression levels were calculated using the delta cycle threshold (CT) method, where expression = 1,000*power [2, $^{-(\mathrm{CT\ gene}\ -\ \mathrm{CT\ GAPDH})}$]. GAPDH was utilized as a reference gene for this calculation, as expression is relatively stable in the songbird brain (25, 36).

Statistics

Regional variation in MR, GR, and 11β-HSD2 relative expression was assessed using linear mixed models and general linear models where appropriate. For each gene, brain region, sex, the sex by brain region interaction, and sacrifice time post-disturbance were included as fixed effects, and bird ID (n = 17; one female was excluded from analyses due to aberrant GAPDH results) was included as a random factor to control for repeated sampling within individual birds. Initial analyses included the sex by sacrifice time interaction. In the absence of any sex-specific effects, this term was eliminated from the final models. The sample size in some brain regions was less than 17 due to technical error or depletion of sample (see figure legends for sample sizes). For GR and MR, there was no variance due to bird ID in the initial mixed model; therefore, general linear models were utilized (model results were identical with and without bird ID). If the interaction term was non-significant, it was removed and the model was re-run to obtain the final model. Significant effects of brain region or a significant interaction term were analyzed using LSD *post hoc* tests, with a significance value of $P < 0.05$. Liver and kidney expression levels in three to four samples were used as positive controls and were not statistically analyzed in comparison with brain.

We used linear regression to compare mean expression levels of 11β-HSD2 with those of MR and GR across regions. Using the same procedure, we tested whether regional patterns of GR expression predicted patterns of MR expression.

RESULTS

Regional Patterns of Gene Expression in Adult Brain

Mineralocorticoid receptor expression levels differed significantly between brain regions ($F_{5,89} = 26.2$; $P < 0.001$) with highest levels in HP, followed by NCM and cNp, and lowest levels in OT, CER, and DIEN (**Figure 2**). Levels did not differ between males and females ($F_{1,89} = 1.9$; $P = 0.171$) and were unrelated to time of sacrifice post-capture ($F_{1,89} = 0.8$; $P = 0.381$). There was no interaction between sex and region ($F_{5,84} = 0.7$; $P = 0.647$).

Glucocorticoid receptor expression levels also differed between brain regions ($F_{5,82} = 191.5$; $P < 0.001$) with highest levels in CER, followed by NCM and cNp, and lowest levels in DIEN, OT, and HP (**Figure 2**). A significant main effect of sex ($F_{1,82} = 11.4$; $P = 0.001$) was driven by the sex*region interaction term ($F_{5,82} = 6.6$, $P < 0.001$). Specifically, GR expression levels were elevated in the CER of females ($P < 0.001$), while there were no sex differences in any other brain regions (all $P > 0.2$). Time of sacrifice post-capture was unrelated to expression ($F_{1,82} = 0.1$; $P = 0.712$).

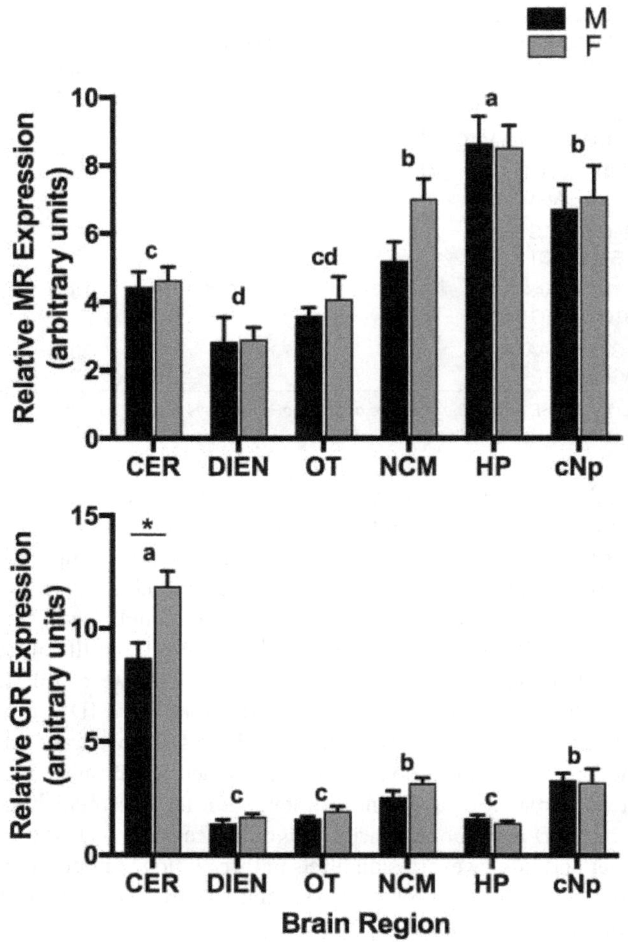

FIGURE 2 | Quantitative PCR results showing mineralocorticoid receptor (MR) (top panel) and glucocorticoid receptor (GR) (bottom panel) expression patterns (relative to glyceraldehyde-3-phosphate dehydrogenase) across six brain regions in adult male (M) and female (F) zebra finches. Letters above bars represent significant differences. *Indicates a significant difference between males and females in CER. Bars are means ± 1 SE. Sample sizes are as follows (*n* = MR/GR): CER, cerebellum (17/16); DIEN, diencephalon (17/16); OT, optic tectum (17/17); NCM, caudomedial nidopallium (16/16); HP, hippocampus (17/17); cNp, caudal nidopallium (13/13).

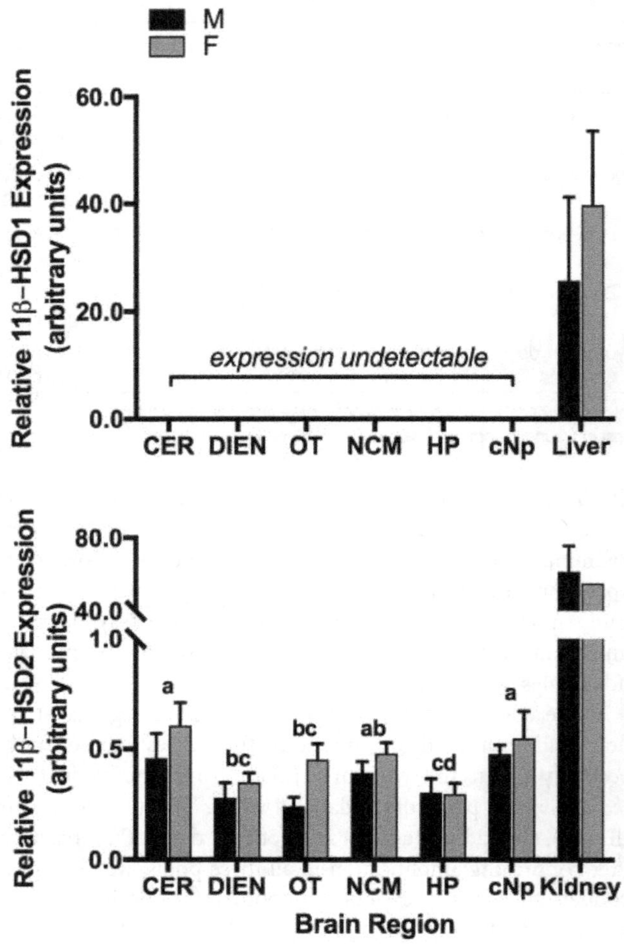

FIGURE 3 | Quantitative PCR results showing 11 beta-hydroxysteroid dehydrogenase type 1 (11β-HSD1) (top panel) and 11 beta-hydroxysteroid dehydrogenase type 2 (11β-HSD2) (bottom panel) expression patterns (relative to glyceraldehyde-3-phosphate dehydrogenase) across six brain regions in adult male (M) and female (F) zebra finches. Letters above bars represent significant differences. Positive control tissues are presented for comparison (11β-HSD1: liver; 11β-HSD2: kidney). Bars are means ± 1 SE. Sample sizes are as follows (*n* = 11β-HSD2): CER, cerebellum (17); DIEN, diencephalon (17); OT, optic tectum (17); NCM, caudomedial nidopallium (16); HP, hippocampus (17); cNp, caudal nidopallium (13).

Whereas expression levels were high in liver, we did not detect 11β-HSD1 expression in brain (**Figure 3**). Specifically, CT values were undetermined for all brain samples, indicating a lack of amplification within the 40-cycle qPCR program. The 11β-HSD1 primer concentrations (0.6 μM) were determined based on an optimization in liver, as previous validation attempts in brain with differing concentrations of primers and cDNA indicated low to no expression.

In contrast to 11β-HSD1, 11β-HSD2 was expressed in adult kidney and brain and differed significantly among brain regions ($F_{5,89} = 5.8$; $P < 0.001$). Levels were highest in CER, NCM, and cNp, followed by DIEN, OT, and HP (**Figure 3**). Expression levels did not vary between males and females ($F_{1,89} = 2.3$; $P = 0.136$) or according to time post-capture ($F_{1,89} = 0.2$; $P = 0.687$). There was no interaction between region and sex ($F_{5,84} = 0.8$; $P = 0.525$).

Coexpression Patterns across Brain Regions

Mean regional GR expression levels did not correlate with MR ($F_{1,4} = 0.1$; $P = 0.781$). If the two regions with exceptionally high MR and GR were removed, however (HP and CER), there was a strong and significant correlation between GR and MR in the remaining four regions ($F_{1,2} = 175.7$; $P = 0.006$; $R^2 = 0.99$; **Figure 4**). Similarly, regional 11β-HSD2 levels were not correlated with GR ($F_{1,4} = 5.6$; $P = 0.077$) or MR levels ($F_{1,4} = 0.02$; $P = 0.91$) when all regions were included in the analyses. However, exclusion of CER and HP resulted in a significant positive correlation between 11β-HSD2 and GR ($F_{1,2} = 126.1$; $P = 0.008$; $R^2 = 0.98$) and 11β-HSD2 and MR ($F_{1,2} = 64.5$; $P = 0.015$; $R^2 = 0.97$) among the remaining regions (**Figure 5**).

11β-HSD1 in Developing Zebra Finch Brain and Adult Kidney

After finding that 11β-HSD1 expression was absent in six brain regions of adults, but present in the liver (a major site of expression across taxa), we conducted an additional qPCR optimization to determine whether expression could be detected in a pool of TEL taken from hatchlings, fledglings, juveniles, and adults. We compared the CT value of this pool to those obtained from liver (all ages pooled) and kidney [an additional positive control tissue in rodents (33)]. Liver showed the highest signal, with CT values of ~24, followed by kidney (CTs ~27), followed by TEL (CTs ~30). Lower CT values indicate higher levels of expression in a sample. After sequencing, products from each of these pools correctly BLASTed to the 11β-HSD1 mRNA sequence in NCBI (see **Table 1** for details).

To further assess these findings in brain, we used qPCR to examine 11β-HSD1 expression in individual samples from all four age groups. Expression of 11β-HSD1 was detected in 2 of 3 hatchling whole TEL samples (the fourth hatchling sample was contaminated and omitted), 1 of 4 fledgling caudal TEL samples, 0 of 4 juvenile caudal TEL samples, and 0 of 4 adult caudal TEL samples. CT values for the two hatchlings were between 26 and 32, while all other amplification occurred at CT 35 or higher.

We further investigated the presence of 11β-HSD1 expression in these three brain samples by (1) running qPCR products on a gel and (2) sending samples for sequencing. Gel electrophoresis (5 μl product + 1 μl 6× loading dye; 2% gel) on the three brain samples with positive qPCR amplification revealed a single band at the expected size (~162 bp) for both hatchling samples and a faint band for the fledgling sample. Sequenced qPCR products from these three samples matched the 11β-HSD1 sequence in NCBI (using BLAST).

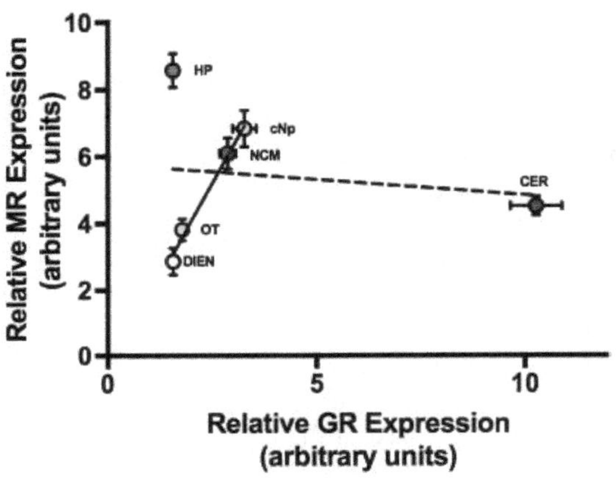

FIGURE 4 | The relationship between average (±1 SE) MR and GR expression levels across six brain regions. Dashed line = best fit line with all six brain regions included. Solid line = best fit line when CER and HP were excluded from the analysis. Abbreviations: CER, cerebellum; DIEN, diencephalon; OT, optic tectum; NCM, caudomedial nidopallium; HP, hippocampus; cNp, caudal nidopallium.

DISCUSSION

This study tested the hypothesis that the enzymes 11β-HSD1 and 11β-HSD2 are expressed in regions of the adult zebra finch brain with elevated sensitivity to GCs. Whereas widespread changes in GC exposure can be initiated by regulation of adrenal synthesis, secretion, and association with binding globulins, local regeneration and metabolism of GCs, respectively, may enable regions requiring precise GC regulation to control access to receptors on a fine scale (8). Our results in the finch vary significantly from expression patterns reported in rodents (15). In particular, we did not detect 11β-HSD1 expression in adult brain, though we confirmed expression of this enzyme in some hatchlings and fledglings. By contrast, 11β-HSD2 was expressed in all adult brain regions examined. In addition, in adult brains we observed distinct regional patterns of GR, MR, and 11β-HSD2 mRNA,

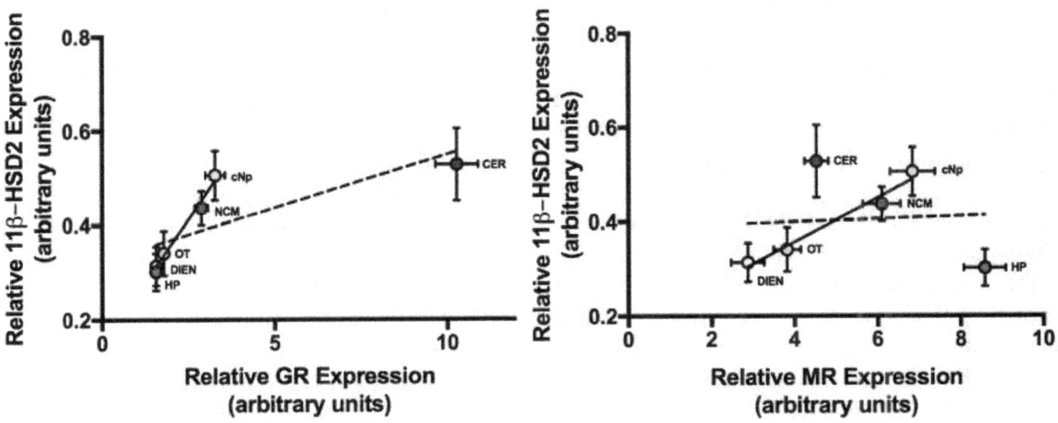

FIGURE 5 | The relationship between average (±1 SE) 11 beta-hydroxysteroid dehydrogenase type 2 (11β-HSD2) and GR (left panel) and average 11β-HSD2 and MR (right panel) expression levels across six brain regions. Dashed line = best fit line with all six brain regions included. Solid line = best fit line when CER and HP were excluded from the analysis. Abbreviations: CER, cerebellum; DIEN, diencephalon; OT, optic tectum; NCM, caudomedial nidopallium; HP, hippocampus; cNp, caudal nidopallium; MR, mineralocorticoid receptor; GR, glucocorticoid receptor.

with highest GR expression in CER and highest MR expression in HP. Regional 11β-HSD2 patterns were similar but not identical to GR and MR patterns. This suggests that 11β-HSD2 plays a role in regulating both baseline and stress-induced CORT access to receptors, but that the nature of this activity varies according to brain region and context.

Regional GR and MR Expression Patterns

Differential expression of GR and MR enables the brain to utilize GCs for a diversity of functions. For example, the paraventricular nucleus of the hypothalamus (PVN), which expresses abundant GR in mammals (37–40), is a key site for stress-induced negative feedback on the HPA axis (41). Similarly, the mammalian HP expresses abundant MR and GR (37, 39, 40) and provides feedback regulation of HPA axis activity (42). The nature of central GR and MR expression and function has been well characterized in mammals (40). In the avian brain, our results on the distribution and abundance of GC receptors align with the handful of other studies, showing elevated GR in CER (30, 31, 35, 43) and MR in the HP [(28, 29, 32, 43); but see Ref. (30, 35)]. We add to these studies the description of relatively low levels of both MR and GR in the songbird DIEN, and relatively high levels in NCM and cNp.

The expression of HP MR and, to a lesser extent, GR suggests that the avian HP plays a similar role in HPA axis regulation in birds and mammals. MR activation in the HP by baseline systemic CORT levels maintains basal activity of the HPA axis through inhibitory projections to the hypothalamus (44). In addition, relatively high GR expression in CER, which we report here, has been observed in the granule and Purkinje cell layers of adult mammals (37, 38) and the external granule cell layer of neonatal mammals (45). We also detected higher CER GR expression in females than males, with no differences elsewhere in brain. The functional significance of this heightened CER sensitivity in females remains unknown. Our results from DIEN differ somewhat from previous observations. For example, several studies show a lack of MR expression in the avian hypothalamus (28, 30, 32) and the mammalian PVN (40), whereas others provide evidence for expression (24, 35). We detected relatively low amounts of both GR and MR in zebra finch DIEN, which includes the hypothalamus. These discrepancies likely result from differential sensitivity of qPCR vs *in situ* hybridization procedures, or because our sampling of the hypothalamus included additional diencephalic regions excluded from other studies.

GR, MR, and 11β-HSD2 Coexpression

Coordinated GC regulation across the brain is necessary for management of the diverse central functions of CORT (44). It is therefore not surprising that we observed a positive correlation between average GR and MR expression levels across several regions, where those with elevated MR also expressed elevated GR. The same pattern was observed when correlating GR or MR expression with 11β-HSD2 expression: regions with elevated GR or MR expression exhibited the highest 11β-HSD2 mRNA levels. This relationship, however, was not identified in all regions, notably the two regions expressing the highest levels of GR (CER) and MR (HP). While 11β-HSD2 expression was relatively elevated in CER, the degree of elevation did not match that of GR expression. In addition, while HP MR was elevated, 11β-HSD2 expression in this region was among the lowest detected. Taken together, these results suggest that the CER and HP may depend on unmodified systemic levels of GCs to initiate appropriate responses on their respective receptors, while other regions may rely on co-regulation by 11β-HSD2, GR, and MR. Future studies should probe the activity and regulation of 11β-HSD2 particularly within the HP and CER, as these remain sites of elevated GC sensitivity.

The HP of adult finches in this study exhibited a greater degree of MR expression relative to GR than other regions examined, while 11β-HSD2 expression remained low. These results may reflect the critical role of HP MR in providing negative feedback on the HPA axis under basal conditions, as MR is virtually absent from the PVN and pituitary, where stress-induced, GR-mediated feedback predominates (46). While 11β-HSD2 preserves MR access for aldosterone in the kidney (47), HP MR is not an aldosterone target, and 11β-HSD2 expression is therefore unnecessary to enable this function. In addition, it is likely that enzymatic metabolism of GCs *via* 11β-HSD2 in HP would be detrimental, as MR binding in this region provides overarching control over the day-to-day activity of the HPA axis. It is therefore not surprising that 11β-HSD2 transcript levels were relatively low in HP.

In contrast to our finding of elevated MR in HP, GR expression was relatively elevated in the CER. Although this relationship has been observed previously in both birds and mammals, its significance is unclear. Very high GR expression relative to other regions has been observed in the neonatal rat cerebellum (48), and exogenous GC treatments can reduce cerebellar volume and initiate long-term cognitive impairments in children (49, 50). The role of GR in the adult CER is less clear, although stress and GC treatments have been shown to impair motor function in adult rats (51). Interestingly, some mood disorders associated with HPA axis dysregulation (52, 53) have been linked to cerebellar atrophy (54). We detected elevated 11β-HSD2 in adult zebra finch CER, although levels were not as high as expected given the correlation between GR and 11β-HSD2 across other brain regions. This suggests that CORT access to GR plays an important role in the avian CER.

High GR expression in the adult CER, which governs motor function, may be partially responsible for rapid, non-genomic changes in activity observed after acute CORT treatment in songbirds. A single dose of GCs administered non-invasively increased perch hopping activity in white-crowned sparrows within 15 min [*Zonotrichia leucophrys gambelii* (55, 56)]. GCs may affect HP-based cognition as well as motor behavior, leading to rapid changes in cache recovery behavior in chickadees within 5 min of administration [*Parus gambeli* (57)]. Rapid, non-genomic GC effects across vertebrate taxa are likely initiated by membrane GC receptor binding (11). A lower-affinity GC membrane receptor has been characterized in house sparrow [*Passer domesticus* (10)] and zebra finch brain (12). In addition, recent work on membrane GC receptors in mammals suggests that a single gene is responsible for both cytosolic and membrane receptors (11, 58). Therefore, it is possible that our characterization of GR and MR included membrane as well as intracellular GC receptor expression.

Although our study revealed expression patterns for several genes in the GC-signaling pathway, a full understanding of the interaction between GC-metabolizing enzymes and receptors requires assessing whether the molecules in these pathways are co-localized within individual neurons or glia. A higher resolution analysis might also be useful. In mammals, for example, 11β-HSD2 has been localized to the endoplasmic reticulum and the nucleus (59). Thus, cells expressing intracellular 11β-HSD2 might avoid effects of GC metabolism by expressing GR or MR receptors on the cell membrane. An investigation of the subcellular localization of 11β-HSD2 in songbird brain, along with a characterization of membrane GR and MR will provide a more conclusive picture of the nature of 11β-HSD2 expression and function in the songbird brain.

Functional Significance of 11β-HSD2 Expression in Brain

We observed 11β-HSD expression patterns that differ significantly from those in rodents. First, we found that 11β-HSD2 was expressed throughout the adult songbird brain, a finding that differs markedly from the adult rodent brain with its more limited distribution (15). This result builds on previous findings in our lab, in which 11β-HSD2 transcript, as well as dehydrogenase activity, was reported in hatchling and adult zebra finch brain (24, 25). Second, while we found robust expression of 11β-HSD1 in liver, expression was undetected in the adult zebra finch brain, though this enzyme is widely distributed in the brains of adult rodents (15). There are several possible explanations for this result. First, we did not attempt to quantify 11β-HSD1 expression in *all* brain regions of the adult zebra finch. Therefore, it is possible that other regions do express this enzyme. However, we noted an absence of 11β-HSD1 in the HP, a site of prominent expression in the rodent brain, which suggests a fundamental difference between birds and mammals. Another possibility is that differential splicing produces alternate transcripts in the zebra finch brain and liver. Future work will address this possibility by utilizing primers that target different regions of the gene. Finally, it is intriguing that we were able to detect 11β-HSD1 expression in the brains of very young finches. Such a result suggests that this enzyme could be developmentally down regulated. The role for this enzyme in developing brain is currently unknown, but future work should pinpoint the loci of expression in hatchlings and document more precisely its temporal patterns of expression.

Elevated expression of 11β-HSD2 in the developing rodent brain likely protects the growing brain from potential GC damage. This protection lasts through the first few weeks of neonatal life. This is clearly seen in the external granule cell layer of the cerebellum, where 11β-HSD2 reportedly protects neural progenitor cells from CORT-induced apoptosis, cerebellar atrophy, and developmental deficits (45, 60–62). These patterns in the developing mammal brain raise the question of whether 11β-HSD2 plays a similar role in the adult songbird brain, especially in the CER, cNp and NCM, regions where 11β-HSD2 transcript levels were highest. The HP, NCM and cNp are bordered by the VZ, where neurogenesis persists in adult songbirds (63). We found relatively high levels of GR, MR, and 11β-HSD2 expression in NCM and cNp, highlighting the potential importance of appropriate GC signaling in these areas. While adult neurogenesis in mammals is relatively restricted, it is conspicuous and widespread in songbirds and other taxa, including fish, reptiles, and amphibians (64, 65). GCs can impair hippocampal neurogenesis, depending on dose and context (23, 66–68). As 11β-HSD2 protects neurogenesis during mammalian fetal development (60, 69), it is plausible that the enzyme serves a similar function in adult songbirds, and potentially in fish, where 11β-HSD2 is also widely expressed in the adult brain (70).

The results of this study raise an important question: why are neural 11β-HSD1 and 2 expression patterns so different between rodents and songbirds? One possibility is that these taxa-specific patterns arose as a result of differences in HPA axis activity and regulation. For example, adult mice that are similar in body mass to songbirds have higher circulating baseline and stress-induced GCs, as well as higher brain GC levels when compared with zebra finches (71–73) (Rensel, unpublished data). Thus, one could speculate that mice would express higher levels of 11β-HSD2 to limit CORT exposure to the brain and potential damage to CORT-sensitive neural circuits. Obviously, this is not the case; instead, rodents display widespread expression of the GC-regenerating 11β-HSD1. A second possibility is that differences in neural GC metabolism could be accounted for by differences in MR or GR binding affinities in brain between rodents and songbirds. However, these receptors appear to be relatively conserved in their binding affinities in rodents and birds (10, 74). Interestingly, the mammalian and songbird GR respond quite similarly to GC agonists and antagonists, but some traditional MR agonists in mammals do not work well in songbirds (10), suggesting that there may be MR receptor differences which modify GC action on the receptor between species. Finally, this study and others suggest that neural MR is more widely expressed throughout the songbird brain than the rodent brain (10), providing support for the view that differential neural metabolism may exist to regulate GC action on MR instead of or in addition to GR. Thus, more work is needed to determine if GC actions on MR differ across taxa, possibly explaining differential 11β-HSD expression patterns.

Steroid hormone-binding globulins in the circulation also differ between birds and mammals. Mammals possess both corticosterone-binding globulin (CBG) and sex hormone-binding globulin (SHBG), the latter of which binds androgens and estrogens. By contrast, birds appear to lack SHBG, and instead some sex steroids also bind CBG [primarily androgens (75, 76)]. This difference may affect the amount of free CORT accessible to the brain, which in turn could necessitate neural GC regeneration or metabolism. For example, rodent CBG may bind a greater proportion of circulating GCs, necessitating 11β-HSD 1-based regeneration in brain, whereas free CORT may more easily reach the brain of the songbird because a greater portion of circulating GCs is unbound. However, while CBGs are thought to prevent access to target tissues (77), some studies suggest that CBGs are actually necessary for GC delivery to the brain, making any conclusions preliminary at this time (78). In the end, a vital difference between the brains of rodents and songbirds remains the widespread neuroplasticity that persists into adulthood in the songbird brain and which is present to a much smaller degree in rodents (8). Given the capacity for GCs to influence such plasticity, it seems likely that the expression of CORT metabolic enzymes in the adult avian brain is related to this inherent neuroplasticity.

Overall, our results highlight the complexity of GC signaling in the songbird brain. It is likely that 11β-HSD2 protects sensitive neural circuits from GC access to GR and MR, but the timing and localization of this activity undoubtedly depends on region and dose-specific effects. In addition, it is worthwhile to note that quantification of mRNA expression does not necessarily equate to presence of protein, as Medina et al. (79) documented a disparity between GR and MR mRNA and cytosolic protein in house sparrow brain. Rapid modulation of enzyme activity through post-translational modifications is also likely and may provide an additional layer of control over GC metabolism and action in the songbird brain [e.g., Ref. (80–82)]. Future studies will seek to elucidate the functional importance of 11β-HSD2 in those regions in which it is expressed.

ETHICS STATEMENT

This study was carried out in accordance with the recommendations of the UCLA Chancellor's Animal Research Committee. The protocol was approved by the Chancellor's Animal Research Committee.

AUTHOR CONTRIBUTIONS

MR and BS conceived and designed the study and wrote the manuscript. MR, JD, and DP conducted the experiments. MR analyzed the data. All the authors provided feedback on the manuscript.

ACKNOWLEDGMENTS

The authors thank Rice Zhang and the UCLA Division of Laboratory Animal Management for their excellent care of the finch colony. This work was supported by NIH R03 grant 5R03MH108921 awarded to MR and BS.

REFERENCES

1. Sapolsky R, Romero L, Munck A. How do glucocorticoids influence stress responses? Integrating permissive, suppressive, stimulatory, and preparative actions. *Endocr Rev* (2000) 21:55–89. doi:10.1210/edrv.21.1.0389
2. Breuner CW, Wingfield JC, Romero LM. Diel rhythms of basal and stress-induced corticosterone in a wild, seasonal vertebrate, Gambel's white-crowned sparrow. *J Exp Zool* (1999) 284:334–42. doi:10.1002/(SICI)1097-010X(19990801)284:3<334::AID-JEZ11>3.0.CO;2-#
3. Droste S, de Groote L, Atkinson H, Lightman SL, Reul JM, Linthorst AC. Corticosterone levels in the brain show a distinct ultradian rhythm but a delayed response to forced swim stress. *Endocrinology* (2008) 149:3244–53. doi:10.1210/en.2008-0103
4. Hau M, Ricklefs RE, Wikelski M, Lee KA, Brawn JD. Corticosterone, testosterone and life-history strategies of birds. *Proc Biol Sci* (2010) 277:3203–12. doi:10.1098/rspb.2010.0673
5. Rensel MA, Boughton RK, Schoech SJ. Development of the adrenal stress response in the Florida scrub-jay (*Aphelocoma coerulescens*). *Gen Comp Endocrinol* (2010) 165:255–61. doi:10.1016/j.ygcen.2009.07.002
6. Sapolsky RM, Meaney MJ. Maturation of the adrenocortical stress response: neuroendocrine control mechanisms and the stress hyporesponsive period. *Brain Res Rev* (1986) 11:65–76. doi:10.1016/0165-0173(86)90010-X
7. Wada H, Hahn TP, Breuner CW. Development of stress reactivity in white-crowned sparrow nestlings: total corticosterone response increases with age, while free corticosterone response remains low. *Gen Comp Endocrinol* (2007) 150:405–13. doi:10.1016/j.ygcen.2006.10.002
8. Rensel MA, Schlinger BA. Determinants and significance of corticosterone regulation in the songbird brain. *Gen Comp Endocrinol* (2016) 227:136–42. doi:10.1016/j.ygcen.2015.06.010
9. Romero LM. Physiological stress in ecology: lessons from biomedical research. *Trends Ecol Evol* (2004) 19:249–55. doi:10.1016/j.tree.2004.03.008
10. Breuner CW, Orchinik M. Pharmacological characterization of intracellular, membrane, and plasma binding sites for corticosterone in house sparrows. *Gen Comp Endocrinol* (2009) 163:214–24. doi:10.1016/j.ygcen.2009.01.027
11. Groeneweg FL, Karst H, de Kloet ER, Joëls M. Mineralocorticoid and glucocorticoid receptors at the neuronal membrane, regulators of nongenomic corticosteroid signalling. *Mol Cell Endocrinol* (2012) 350:299–309. doi:10.1016/j.mce.2011.06.020
12. Schmidt KL, Malisch JL, Breuner CW, Soma KK. Corticosterone and cortisol binding sites in plasma, immune organs and brain of developing zebra finches: intracellular and membrane-associated receptors. *Brain Behav Immun* (2010) 24:908–18. doi:10.1016/j.bbi.2010.02.008
13. Rajan V, Edwards CR, Seckl JR. 11 beta-Hydroxysteroid dehydrogenase in cultured hippocampal cells reactivates inert 11-dehydrocorticosterone, potentiating neurotoxicity. *J Neurosci* (1996) 16:65–70.
14. Draper N, Stewart PM. 11B-hydroxysteroid dehydrogenase and the pre-receptor regulation of corticosteroid hormone action. *J Endocrinol* (2005) 186:251–71. doi:10.1677/joe.1.06019
15. Wyrwoll CS, Holmes MC, Seckl JR. 11β-Hydroxysteroid dehydrogenases and the brain: from zero to hero, a decade of progress. *Front Neuroendocrinol* (2011) 32:265–86. doi:10.1016/j.yfrne.2010.12.001
16. Diaz R, Brown RW, Seckl JR. Distinct ontogeny of glucocorticoid and mineralocorticoid receptor and 11beta-hydroxysteroid dehydrogenase types I and II mRNAs in the fetal rat brain suggest a complex control of glucocorticoid actions. *J Neurosci* (1998) 18:2570–80.
17. Carter RN, Paterson JM, Tworowska U, Stenvers DJ, Mullins JJ, Seckl JR, et al. Hypothalamic-pituitary-adrenal axis abnormalities in response to deletion of 11β-HSD1 is strain-dependent. *J Neuroendocrinol* (2009) 21:879–87. doi:10.1111/j.1365-2826.2009.01899.x
18. Holmes MC, Seckl JR. The role of 11beta-hydroxysteroid dehydrogenases in the brain. *Mol Cell Endocrinol* (2006) 248:9–14. doi:10.1016/j.mce.2005.12.002
19. Yau JLW, Seckl JR. Local amplification of glucocorticoids in the aging brain and impaired spatial memory. *Front Aging Neurosci* (2012) 4:24. doi:10.3389/fnagi.2012.00024
20. Sandeep TC, Yau JLW, MacLullich AMJ, Noble J, Deary IJ, Walker BR, et al. 11B-hydroxysteroid dehydrogenase inhibition improves cognitive function in healthy elderly men and type 2 diabetics. *Proc Natl Acad Sci U S A* (2004) 101:6734–9. doi:10.1073/pnas.0306996101
21. Yu L, Romero DG, Gomez-Sanchez CE, Gomez-Sanchez EP. Steroidogenic enzyme gene expression in the human brain. *Mol Cell Endocrinol* (2002) 190:9–17. doi:10.1016/S0303-7207(02)00041-2
22. Huang C, Wan B, Gao B, Hexige S, Yu L. Isolation and characterization of novel human short-chain dehydrogenase/reductase SCDR10B which is highly expressed in the brain and acts as hydroxysteroid dehydrogenase. *Acta Biochim Pol* (2009) 56:279–89.
23. Schoenfeld T, Gould E. Stress, stress hormones, and adult neurogenesis. *Exp Neurol* (2012) 233:12–21. doi:10.1016/j.expneurol.2011.01.008.Stress
24. Katz A, Oyama RK, Feng N, Chen X, Schlinger BA. 11B-hydroxysteroid dehydrogenase type 2 in zebra finch brain and peripheral tissues. *Gen Comp Endocrinol* (2010) 166:600–5. doi:10.1016/j.ygcen.2010.01.016
25. Rensel MA, Comito D, Kosarussavadi S, Schlinger BA. Region-specific neural corticosterone patterns differ from plasma in a male songbird. *Endocrinology* (2014) 155:3572–81. doi:10.1210/en.2014-1231

26. Chen Z, Ye R, Goldman S. Testosterone modulation of angiogenesis and neurogenesis in the adult songbird brain. *Neuroscience* (2013) 239:139–48. doi:10.1016/j.biotechadv.2011.08.021.Secreted
27. Hall ZJ, Delaney S, Sherry DF. Inhibition of cell proliferation in black-capped chickadees suggests a role for neurogenesis in spatial learning. *Dev Neurobiol* (2014) 74:1002–10. doi:10.1002/dneu.22180
28. Dickens M, Romero LM, Cyr NE, Dunn IC, Meddle SL. Chronic stress alters glucocorticoid receptor and mineralocorticoid receptor mRNA expression in the European starling (*Sturnus vulgaris*) brain. *J Neuroendocrinol* (2009) 21:832–40. doi:10.1111/j.1365-2826.2009.01908.x
29. Krause JS, McGuigan MA, Bishop VR, Wingfield JC, Meddle SL. Decreases in mineralocorticoid but not glucocorticoid mRNA expression during the short Arctic breeding season in free-living Gambel's white-crowned sparrow (*Zonotrichia leucophrys gambelii*). *J Neuroendocrinol* (2015) 27:66–75. doi:10.1111/jne.12237
30. Senft RA, Meddle SL, Baugh AT. Distribution and abundance of glucocorticoid and mineralocorticoid receptors throughout the brain of the great tit (*Parus major*). *PLoS One* (2016) 11:e0148516. doi:10.1371/journal.pone.0148516
31. Shahbazi M, Schmidt M, Carruth LL. Distribution and subcellular localization of glucocorticoid receptor-immunoreactive neurons in the developing and adult male zebra finch brain. *Gen Comp Endocrinol* (2011) 174:354–61. doi:10.1016/j.ygcen.2011.09.017
32. Suzuki K, Matsunaga E, Kobayashi T, Okanoya K. Expression patterns of mineralocorticoid and glucocorticoid receptors in Bengalese finch (*Lonchura striata* var. *domestica*) brain suggest a relationship between stress hormones and song-system development. *Neuroscience* (2011) 194:72–83. doi:10.1016/j.neuroscience.2011.07.073
33. Roland BL, Krozowski ZS, Funder JW. Glucocorticoid receptor, mineralocorticoid receptors, 11β hydroxysteroid dehydrogenase-1 and -2 expression in rat brain and kidney: in situ studies. *Mol Cell Endocrinol* (1995) 111:R1–7. doi:10.1016/0303-7207(95)03559-P
34. Saldanha CJ, Clayton NS, Schlinger BA. Androgen metabolism in the juvenile oscine forebrain: a cross-species analysis at neural sites implicated in memory function. *J Neurobiol* (1999) 40:397–406. doi:10.1002/(SICI)1097-4695(19990905)40:3<397::AID-NEU11>3.0.CO;2-6
35. Banerjee SB, Arterbery AS, Fergus DJ, Adkins-Regan E. Deprivation of maternal care has long-lasting consequences for the hypothalamic-pituitary-adrenal axis of zebra finches. *Proc Biol Sci* (2012) 279:759–66. doi:10.1098/rspb.2011.1265
36. Zinzow-Kramer WM, Horton BM, Maney DL. Evaluation of reference genes for quantitative real-time PCR in the brain, pituitary, and gonads of songbirds. *Horm Behav* (2014) 66:267–75. doi:10.1016/j.yhbeh.2014.04.011
37. Meyer U, Kruhøffer M, Flugge G, Fuchs E. Cloning of glucocorticoid receptor and mineralocorticoid receptor cDNA and gene expression in the central nervous system of the tree shrew (*Tupaia belangeri*). *Mol Brain Res* (1998) 55:243–53. doi:10.1016/S0169-328X(98)00004-7
38. Morimoto M, Morita N, Ozawa H, Yokoyama K, Kawata M. Distribution of glucocorticoid receptor immunoreactivity and mRNA in the rat brain: an immunohistochemical and in situ hybridization study. *Neurosci Res* (1996) 26:235–69. doi:10.1016/S0168-0102(96)01105-4
39. Patel PD, Lopez JF, Lyons DM, Burke S, Wallace M, Schatzberg AF. Glucocorticoid and mineralocorticoid receptor mRNA expression in squirrel monkey brain. *J Psychiatr Res* (2000) 34:383–92. doi:10.1016/S0022-3956(00)00035-2
40. Pryce CR. Postnatal ontogeny of expression of the corticosteroid receptor genes in mammalian brains: inter-species and intra-species differences. *Brain Res Rev* (2008) 57:596–605. doi:10.1016/j.brainresrev.2007.08.005
41. Kretz O, Reichardt HM, Schütz G, Bock R. Corticotropin-releasing hormone expression is the major target for glucocorticoid feedback-control at the hypothalamic level. *Brain Res* (1999) 818:488–91. doi:10.1016/S0006-8993(98)01277-3
42. Feldman S, Weidenfeld J. Glucocorticoid receptor antagonists in the hippocampus modify the negative feedback following neural stimuli. *Brain Res* (1999) 821:33–7. doi:10.1016/S0006-8993(99)01054-9
43. Hodgson ZG, Meddle SL, Roberts ML, Buchanan KL, Evans MR, Metzdorf R, et al. Spatial ability is impaired and hippocampal mineralocorticoid receptor mRNA expression reduced in zebra finches (*Taeniopygia guttata*) selected for acute high corticosterone response to stress. *Proc Biol Sci* (2007) 274:239–45. doi:10.1098/rspb.2006.3704
44. De Kloet E, Vreugdenhil E, Oitzl M, Joels M. Brain corticosteroid receptor balance in health and disease. *Endocr Rev* (1998) 19:269–301. doi:10.1210/edrv.19.3.0331
45. Noguchi KK, Walls KC, Wozniak DF, Olney JW, Roth KA, Farber NB. Acute neonatal glucocorticoid exposure produces selective and rapid cerebellar neural progenitor cell apoptotic death. *Cell Death Differ* (2008) 15:1582–92. doi:10.1038/cdd.2008.97.Acute
46. Liposits Z, Uht RM, Harrison RW, Gibbs FP, Paull WK, Bohn MC. Ultrastructural localization of glucocorticoid receptor (GR) in hypothalamic paraventricular neurons synthesizing corticotropin releasing factor (CRF). *Histochemistry* (1987) 87:407–12. doi:10.1007/BF00496811
47. Rusvai E, Naray-Fejes-Toths A. A new isoform of 11 beta-hydroxysteroid dehydrogenase in aldosterone target cells. *J Biol Chem* (1993) 268:10717–20.
48. Pavlík A, Burešová M. The neonatal cerebellum: the highest level of glucocorticoid receptors in the brain. *Dev Brain Res* (1984) 12:13–20. doi:10.1016/0165-3806(84)90171-8
49. Allin M, Matsumoto H, Santhouse AM, Nosarti C, Alasady MH, Stewart AL, et al. Cognitive and motor function and the size of the cerebellum in adolescents born very pre-term. *Brain* (2001) 124:60–6. doi:10.1093/brain/124.1.60
50. Tam EWY, Chau V, Ferriero DM, Barkovich AJ, Poskitt KJ, Studholme C, et al. Preterm cerebellar growth impairment after postnatal exposure to glucocorticoids. *Sci Transl Med* (2011) 3:105ra105. doi:10.1126/scitranslmed.3002884.Preterm
51. Metz GA, Jadavji NM, Smith LK. Modulation of motor function by stress: a novel concept of the effects of stress and corticosterone on behavior. *Eur J Neurosci* (2005) 22:1190–200. doi:10.1111/j.1460-9568.2005.04285.x
52. Ozbolt L, Nemeroff C. HPA axis modulation in the treatment of mood disorders. In: Schoepf D, editor. *Psychiatric Disorders-New Frontiers in Affective Disorders*. InTech (2013). p. 21–40. doi:10.5772/51600
53. Watson S, Mackin P. HPA axis function in mood disorders. *Psychiatry* (2009) 8:97–101. doi:10.1016/j.mppsy.2008.11.006
54. Beyer JL, Krishnan KRR. Volumetric brain imaging findings in mood disorders. *Bipolar Disord* (2002) 4:89–104. doi:10.1034/j.1399-5618.2002.01157.x
55. Breuner CW, Greenberg AL, Wingfield JC. Noninvasive corticosterone treatment rapidly increases activity in Gambel's white-crowned sparrows (*Zonotrichia leucophrys gambelii*). *Gen Comp Endocrinol* (1998) 111:386–94. doi:10.1006/gcen.1998.7128
56. Breuner CW, Wingfield JC. Rapid behavioral response to corticosterone varies with photoperiod and dose. *Horm Behav* (2000) 37:23–30. doi:10.1006/hbeh.1999.1554
57. Saldanha CJ, Schlinger BA, Clayton NS. Rapid effects of corticosterone on cache recovery in mountain chickadees (*Parus gambeli*). *Horm Behav* (2000) 37:109–15. doi:10.1006/hbeh.2000.1571
58. Vernocchi S, Battello N, Schmitz S, Revets D, Billing AM, Turner JD, et al. Membrane glucocorticoid receptor activation induces proteomic changes aligning with classical glucocorticoid effects. *Mol Cell Proteomics* (2013) 12(7):1764–79. doi:10.1074/mcp.M112.022947
59. Farman N, Bocchi B. Mineralocorticoid selectivity: molecular and cellular aspects. *Kidney Int* (2000) 57:1364–9. doi:10.1046/j.1523-1755.2000.00976.x
60. Holmes MC, Sangra M, French KL, Whittle IR, Paterson J, Mullins JJ, et al. 11beta-Hydroxysteroid dehydrogenase type 2 protects the neonatal cerebellum from deleterious effects of glucocorticoids. *Neuroscience* (2006) 137:865–73. doi:10.1016/j.neuroscience.2005.09.037
61. Noguchi KK, Lau K, Smith DJ, Swiney BS, Farber NB. Glucocorticoid receptor stimulation and the regulation of neonatal cerebellar neural progenitor cell apoptosis. *Neurobiol Dis* (2011) 43:356–63. doi:10.1016/j.nbd.2011.04.004
62. Robson AC, Leckie CM, Seckl JR, Holmes MC. 11 Beta-hydroxysteroid dehydrogenase type 2 in the postnatal and adult rat brain. *Brain Res Mol Brain Res* (1998) 61:1–10. doi:10.1016/S0169-328X(98)00161-2
63. García-Verdugo JM, Ferrón S, Flames N, Collado L, Desfilis E, Font E. The proliferative ventricular zone in adult vertebrates: a comparative study using reptiles, birds, and mammals. *Brain Res Bull* (2002) 57:765–75. doi:10.1016/S0361-9230(01)00769-9
64. Chapouton P, Jagasia R, Bally-Cuif L. Adult neurogenesis in non-mammalian vertebrates. *Bioessays* (2007) 29:745–57. doi:10.1002/bies.20615
65. Nottebohm F. Neuronal replacement in adult brain. *Brain Res Bull* (2002) 57:737–49. doi:10.1016/S0361-9230(02)00750-5

66. Anacker C, Cattaneo A, Luoni A, Musaelyan K, Zunszain PA, Milanesi E, et al. Glucocorticoid-related molecular signaling pathways regulating hippocampal neurogenesis. *Neuropsychopharmacology* (2013) 38:872–83. doi:10.1038/npp.2012.253
67. Katz A, Mirzatoni A, Zhen Y, Schlinger BA. Sex differences in cell proliferation and glucocorticoid responsiveness in the zebra finch brain. *Eur J Neurosci* (2008) 28:99–106. doi:10.1111/j.1460-9568.2008.06303.x
68. Newman AEM, MacDougall-Shackleton SA, An YS, Kriengwatana B, Soma KK. Corticosterone and dehydroepiandrosterone have opposing effects on adult neuroplasticity in the avian song control system. *J Comp Neurol* (2010) 518:3662–78. doi:10.1002/cne.22395
69. Cottrell EC, Seckl JR, Holmes MC, Wyrwoll CS. Foetal and placental 11β-HSD2: a hub for developmental programming. *Acta Physiol* (2014) 210:288–95. doi:10.1111/apha.12187
70. Alderman SL, Vijayan MM. 11β-hydroxysteroid dehydrogenase type 2 in zebrafish brain: a functional role in hypothalamus-pituitary-interrenal axis regulation. *J Endocrinol* (2012) 215:393–402. doi:10.1530/JOE-12-0379
71. Little HJ, Croft AP, O'Callaghan MJ, Brooks SP, Wang G, Shaw SG. Selective increases in regional brain glucocorticoid: a novel effect of chronic alcohol. *Neuroscience* (2008) 156:1017–27. doi:10.1016/j.neuroscience.2008.08.029
72. Petersen HH, Andreassen TK, Breiderhoff T, Bräsen JH, Schulz H, Gross V, et al. Hyporesponsiveness to glucocorticoids in mice genetically deficient for the corticosteroid binding globulin. *Mol Cell Biol* (2006) 26:7236–45. doi:10.1128/MCB.00400-06
73. Tronche C, Piérard C, Coutan M, Chauveau F, Liscia P, Béracochéa D. Increased stress-induced intra-hippocampus corticosterone rise associated with memory impairments in middle-aged mice. *Neurobiol Learn Mem* (2010) 93:343–51. doi:10.1016/j.nlm.2009.11.009
74. Reul JMHM, de Kloet ER. Anatomical resolution of two types of corticosterone receptor sites in rat brain with in vitro radiography and computerized image analysis. *J Steroid Biochemistry* (1985) 24:269-72. doi:10.1016/0022-4731(86)90063-4
75. Deviche P, Breuner C, Orchinik M. Testosterone, corticosterone, and photoperiod interact to regulate plasma levels of binding globulin and free steroid hormone in dark-eyed juncos, *Junco hyemalis*. *Gen Comp Endocrinol* (2001) 122:67–77. doi:10.1006/gcen.2001.7613
76. Wingfield JC, Matt KS, Farner DS. Physiologic properties of steroid hormone-binding proteins in avian blood. *Gen Comp Endocrinol* (1984) 53:281–92. doi:10.1016/0016-6480(84)90254-5
77. Mendel CM. The free hormone hypothesis a physiologically based mathematical model. *Endocr Rev* (1989) 10:232–74. doi:10.1210/edrv-10-3-232
78. Minni AM, Dorey R, Pierard C, Dominguez G, Helbling JC, Foury A, et al. Critical role of plasma corticosteroid-binding-globulin during stress to promote glucocorticoid delivery to the brain: impact on memory retrieval. *Endocrinology* (2012) 153:4766–74. doi:10.1210/en.2012-1485
79. Medina CO, Lattin CR, McVey M, Romero LM. There is no correlation between glucocorticoid receptor mRNA expression and protein binding in the brains of house sparrows (*Passer domesticus*). *Gen Comp Endocrinol* (2013) 193:27–36. doi:10.1016/j.ygcen.2013.07.008
80. Comito D, Pradhan DS, Karleen BJ, Schlinger BA. Region-specific rapid regulation of aromatase activity in zebra finch brain. *J Neurochem* (2016) 136:1177–85. doi:10.1111/jnc.13513
81. Pradhan DS, Newman AEM, Wacker DW, Wingfield JC, Schlinger BA, Soma KK. Aggressive interactions rapidly increase androgen synthesis in the brain during the non-breeding season. *Horm Behav* (2010) 57:381–9. doi:10.1016/j.freeradbiomed.2008.10.025.The
82. Soma KK, Alday NA, Hau M, Schlinger BA. Dehydroepiandrosterone metabolism by 3B-hydroxysteroid dehydrogenase/5-4 isomerase in adult zebra finch brain: sex difference and rapid effect of stress. *Endocrinology* (2004) 145:1668–77. doi:10.1210/en.2003-0883

20

Stress and Corticosteroids Aggravate Morphological Changes in the Dentate Gyrus after Early-Life Experimental Febrile Seizures in Mice

Jolien S. van Campen[1,2], Ellen V. S. Hessel[1], Kirsten Bohmbach[1], Giorgio Rizzi[1], Paul J. Lucassen[3], Sada Lakshmi Turimella[1], Eduardo H. L. Umeoka[1,4], Gideon F. Meerhoff[3], Kees P. J. Braun[2], Pierre N. E. de Graan[1†] and Marian Joëls[1†]*

[1] Department of Translational Neuroscience, Brain Center Rudolf Magnus, University Medical Center Utrecht, Utrecht, Netherlands, [2] Department of Child Neurology, Brain Center Rudolf Magnus, University Medical Center Utrecht, Utrecht, Netherlands, [3] Swammerdam Institute for Life Sciences, Center for Neuroscience, University of Amsterdam, Amsterdam, Netherlands, [4] Neursocience and Behavioral Sciences Department, Ribeirão Preto School of Medicine, University of São Paulo, Ribeirão Preto, Brazil

***Correspondence:**
Jolien S. van Campen
j.s.vancampen@gmail.com

†These authors have share seniority.

Stress is the most frequently self-reported seizure precipitant in patients with epilepsy. Moreover, a relation between ear stress and epilepsy has been suggested. Although ear stress and stress hormones are known to influence seizure threshold in rodents, effects on the development of epilepsy (epileptogenesis) are still unclear. Therefore, we studied the consequences of ear corticosteroid exposure for epileptogenesis, under highly controlled conditions in an animal model. Experimental febrile seizures (eFS) were elicited in 10-day-old mice by warm-air induced hyperthermia, while a control group was exposed to a normothermic condition. In the following 2 weeks, mice received either seven corticosterone or vehicle injections or were left undisturbed. Specific measures indicative for epileptogenesis were examined at 25 days of age and compared with vehicle injected or untreated mice. We examined structural [neurogenesis, dendritic morphology, and mossy fiber sprouting (MFS)] and functional (glutamatergic postsynaptic currents and long-term potentiation) plasticity in the dentate gyrus (DG). We found that differences in DG morphology induced by eFS were aggravated by repetitive (mildly stressful) vehicle injections and corticosterone exposure. In the injected groups, eFS were associated with decreases in neurogenesis, and increases in cell proliferation, dendritic length, and spine density. No group differences were found in MFS. Despite these changes in DG morphology, no effects of eFS were found on functional plasticity. We conclude that corticosterone exposure during early epileptogenesis elicited by eFS aggravates morphological, but not functional, changes in the DG, which partly supports the hypothesis that ear stress stimulates epileptogenesis.

Keywords: stress, corticosteroids, epilepsy, epileptogenesis, febrile seizures, hyperthermia, early-life

---

Abbreviations: DG, dentate gyrus; eFS, experimental febrile seizures; HT, hyperthermia; NT, normothermia.

INTRODUCTION

Epilepsy is a common neurological disorder, especially in childhood where its prevalence is as high as 0.5–1.0% (1). An important factor influencing epilepsy and epileptic seizures is stress, which is the most frequently self-reported seizure precipitant in patients with epilepsy [reviewed in Ref. (2)]. The seizure precipitating effects of stress are also confirmed by prospective studies (3–7). Besides direct effects on seizure susceptibility, stress can also influence the risk of being diagnosed with epilepsy later in life (8–10). Thus, associations between stress and epilepsy exist on multiple levels. However, the mechanisms behind these relations are so far poorly understood.

Animal models can provide more insight into the exact mechanisms by which stress influences epilepsy. In various preclinical epilepsy models, stress has been shown to lower the threshold for the induction of epileptic seizures and to increase seizure severity (11–16). The effects of stress on epilepsy are largely attributed to neuronal exposure to stress hormones. Especially stress hormone exposure early in life can have profound effects on later brain morphology and function and predispose to the development of brain diseases [as reviewed in Ref. (17–21)]. Stress hormones have been shown to directly affect neuronal excitability [reviewed in Ref. (22, 23)]. Despite these effects of stress on seizures on the one hand, and on brain development on the other, effects of stress and stress hormones on the *development* of epilepsy (i.e., epileptogenesis) are currently unknown.

To improve insight into the impact of stress hormones on epileptogenesis, we studied the effects of corticosterone, an important stress hormone, during early-life epileptogenesis on neuronal morphology and functional plasticity in the rodent brain. Using a controlled design, we elicited experimental febrile seizures (eFS) in young mouse pups by warm-air induced hyperthermia (HT) and subsequently exposed them to repetitive (1) high concentrations of corticosterone, (2) vehicle injections (a control condition that is also a mild stressor), or (3) no injections. We next examined alterations in morphological and functional parameters in the dentate gyrus (DG), a hippocampal subarea that is affected by eFS (24–28) as well as stress hormones (29). To assess morphological changes, we investigated neurogenesis, cell proliferation, dendritic morphology, spine density, and mossy fiber sprouting (MFS). Functional plasticity was assessed measuring glutamatergic transmission and long-term potentiation (LTP) in the DG. We hypothesize that corticosterone aggravates the epileptogenic changes after eFS.

MATERIALS AND METHODS

Animals

Breeding pairs of C57BL6/J mice were obtained from The Jackson Laboratory (Bar Harbor, ME, USA) and subsequently bred in-house. Litters used in this experiment were derived from multiple breeding pairs ($n = 99$). On postnatal day (P) 1, litters were culled to four to six pups consisting of both males and females. The pups were not weaned during the experiment. Animals were kept in a controlled 12-h light–dark cycle (light on 7 a.m. to 7 p.m.) with a temperature of 22 ± 1°C. Food and water were available *ad libitum* (2111 RMH-TM diet; Hope Farms, Woerden, the Netherlands). All animals were housed in transparent Plexiglas cages (Macrolon type II) with sawdust bedding and paper tissues for nest building. Cages were cleaned at P7 and at P17/18 (in between injection days) by replacing half of the sawdust bedding. All experimental procedures were performed according to the institutional guidelines of the University Medical Center Utrecht and approved by the committee on ethical considerations in animal experiments of Utrecht University (DEC Utrecht, permit number 2012.I.03.047). All efforts were made to minimize suffering of the animals. Pups were assigned to multiple treatment groups per litter. A maximum of two pups per litter was used per treatment group per method of analysis to minimize litter effects on outcome measures. All animal experiments were performed within a period of 6 months and animals in all treatment groups were tested across the whole period to control for environmental or seasonal variation. For the purpose of this study, experiments were only performed on male animals.

Corticosterone Levels after Injection

To evaluate corticosterone levels after injection with corticosterone or vehicle, naïve P12 mice ($n = 4$–6 per time point per treatment group) were injected intraperitoneally with corticosterone (corticosterone-HBC complex 3 mg/kg dissolved in saline, total injection volume of 10 μl/g body weight) or vehicle (both obtained from Sigma-Aldrich, the Netherlands) between 8.30 and 9.00 a.m. Immediately before, or at 15, 30, 60, 120, 180, or 240 min after injection, mice were decapitated and trunk blood was collected. Between injection and decapitation, pups were returned to their home cage and left undisturbed. A separate group of non-injected mice was decapitated at the same time points to control for diurnal corticosterone variability.

Epileptogenesis

Epileptogenesis was induced using the HT-induced eFS model, a very subtle epilepsy model with close resemblance to the human situation in which children who experience complex febrile seizures are at increased risk to develop temporal lobe epilepsy later in life (30, 31). A unique aspect of this model is the relatively long-lasting latent phase of epileptogenesis, making it easier to study effects of additional risk factors prior to the actual onset of epilepsy, and irrespective of the damage and compensatory mechanisms induced by spontaneous seizures.

Prolonged eFS were induced in P10/11 mice by heated-air induced HT using a previously described paradigm in rats (32), which we adapted to mice ((33)). A temperature-sensitive transponder (IPTT-300 BioMedic Data Systems, Plexx BV, Elst, the Netherlands) was implanted subcutaneously on P9/10 in pups with a bodyweight between 5.0 and 6.5 g. One day after transponder implantation, body weight was determined and mice were placed in a preheated cylindrical chamber and exposed to a warm air stream of 41–48°C. To prevent skin burn and adverse effects on behavior, the temperature of the chamber floor was maintained at 39°C. Core body temperature was measured at least every 2.5 min period using a wireless temperature reader (WRS-6007; Plexx BV). To provoke prolonged seizures, air temperature was adjusted to maintain the core body temperature between 41.5 and 42°C. The presence of tonic–clonic convulsions was monitored by observation. These behavioral seizures correlate closely with electroencephalographic seizures, i.e., spike-wave discharges in the hippocampus, as shown by previous experiments in our lab (27, 34). After 30 min of HT (defined as core temperature ≥ 39°C) pups were rapidly cooled in a water bath at room temperature, gently dried with paper and returned to the dam. This procedure is known to induce epileptogenesis, as spontaneous (encephalographic) seizures are observed after a latent period of approximately 3 months in 35–68% of animals (26, 35, 36), and epileptiform interictal discharges in 88% (35). normothermia (NT) controls were treated as HT pups, except that the temperature of the air stream was kept at 30–32°C, resulting in a constant body temperature. All eFS experiments were performed between 10.00 a.m. and 3.00 p.m.

Injections and Decapitation

Animals were weighed at 2, 4, 6, 8, 10, 12, and 14 days after exposure to HT/NT and injected intraperitoneally with corticosterone or vehicle between 8.00 and 9.30 a.m., during the circadian trough. A separate group of animals was left undisturbed after HT/NT. One day (~24 h) after the last injection, mice were weighed and decapitated or perfused (see **Figure 1**). Decapitation was performed between 8.00 and 9.30 a.m.

Endocrinology

Trunk blood samples were collected immediately after decapitation at P25/26 from all animals subjected to HT/NT except those receiving perfusion fixation. Directly after decapitation, thymus and both adrenals were resected and weighed. Blood samples were centrifuged for 10 min at 4,000 rpm at 4°C. Plasma was stored at −80°C until assayed with an I^{125}-corticosterone radioimmunoassay for mice (MP Biomedicals, Inc., Aberdeen, UK) according to the manufacturer's instructions. All samples were processed in the same assay to exclude inter-assay variability.

Morphology and Functional Plasticity

All morphological and functional outcome parameters were examined in the DG. This hippocampal area was selected based on its functional and anatomical characteristics. First, the (epileptogenic) changes induced by eFS are located in the hippocampus, including the DG (24–28, 36, 37). Second, the DG has an important function in filtering excitation and seizure propagation to the other parts of the hippocampus (38, 39). Third, it is one of the few sites where neurogenesis continues in later life, a process that can be stimulated by seizures and has been implicated in epileptogenesis (40–44). Finally, the DG exhibits abundant receptors for corticosterone and therefore its morphology and function are largely influenced by early-life stress (29).

All following experimental procedures were performed by experimenters unaware of the treatment groups. Per outcome measure, tissue of animals belonging to different treatment groups was ordered in a semi-randomized way to control for environmental or experimenter effects on recording, staining and/or quantification over the total experimental period.

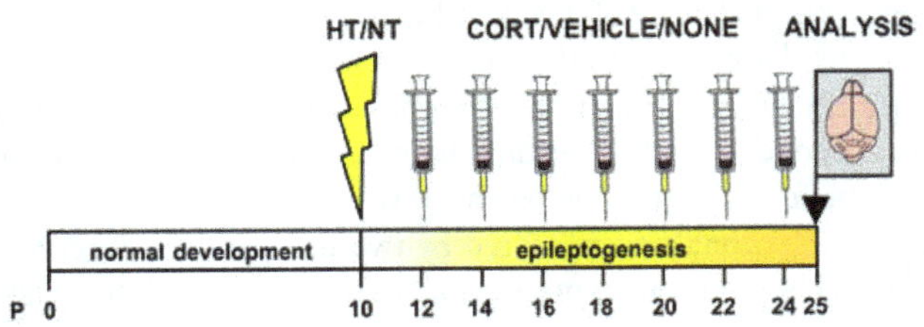

FIGURE 1 | Experimental design. Animals were exposed to hyperthermia (HT) or normothermia (NT) at postnatal day (P) 10 or 11 and subsequently received injections with corticosterone, vehicle or no injection every other day in the latent phase of epileptogenesis. Brains were dissected 24 h after the last injection, before the onset of spontaneous seizure activity.

Neurogenesis

Male mice (n = 6 per group) were decapitated between 9.00 and 10.30 a.m. Brains were dissected, post fixed at 4°C in 4% formaldehyde for 4 h, transferred to 30% sucrose for 24 h, frozen on powdered dry ice and stored at −80°C. Cryostat sections (20 μm) were cut in the coronal plane, collected in series of 15 on Superfrost slides and stored at −80°C until further use.

As a measure of neurogenesis, tissue was stained for Doublecortin (DCX), a marker for neuronal precursor cells and immature neurons, and Ki67, a marker for proliferating cells using modified protocols. Mounted sections were postfixed in acetone-methanol (1:1) at −20°C for 7.5 min, washed in 0.05 M Tris HCl 0.9% saline (TBS) pH 7.6 and heated in 0.01 M citrate buffer (pH 6.0) in a microwave oven for 10 min at 800 W followed by 5 min at 480 W and 5 min at 260 W. After a cool down period of 20 min, sections were washed in TBS. Endogenous peroxidase activity was blocked with 0.5% (for DCX) or 1.5% (for Ki67) H_2O_2 in TBS for 15 min. Sections were washed and, after incubation in 2% milk powder in TBS for 30 min, incubated with the primary antibody [DCX (polyclonal goat anti-DCX, SantaCruz; 1:800) or Ki67 (polyclonal rabbit anti-Ki67p, Novocastra, 1:5,000)], diluted in supermix (0.25% gelatine and 0.1% Triton in TBS) at room temperature for 1 h and then incubated overnight at 4°C. The next morning, sections were washed and incubated for 2 h with donkey antigoat biotinylated (for DCX, Jackson; 1:500) or goat antirabbit biotinylated (for Ki67, Vector; 1:200) secondary antibody diluted in supermix at room temperature. Sections were washed, incubated in avidin–biotin complex (ABC) (ABC Elite, Vector Laboratories; 1:800 in TBS) for 2 h (for DCX) or 1.5 h (for Ki67) at room temperature, washed again and incubated with biotinylated tyramide (1:500) in 0.01% H_2O_2 in TBS for 30 min. Sections were washed and incubated in ABC (1:800 in TBS) for 1.5 h at room temperature and washed in TBS. After washing in 0.05 M Tris HCl pH 7.6 (TB), chromogen development was performed with diaminobenzidine (DAB; 50 mg/100 ml Tris buffer, pH 7.6, 0.01% H_2O_2, 0.05% Nickel) for 40 min. Sections were washed in TB and stored overnight at 4°C. The next day, sections were washed in distilled water, counterstained with Hematoxylin and shortly rinsed in distilled water. After washing with running tap water, sections were dehydrated using a grading series of ethanol, cleared in xylene and coverslipped using Entallan.

DCX⁺ and Ki67⁺ cells in the granule cell layer and the subgranular zone of the DG were quantified unilaterally in every 15th section in a total of five sections per animal within Bregma range −1.46 to −2.80 (coronal) without a left/right preference within or between animals. DCX^+ cells were quantified stereologically using a StereoInvestigator system (Microbright field, USA) with a ×100 oil-immersion objective of a Zeiss Axiophot microscope and StereoInvestigator software, according to the optical fractionator method. The number of DCX^+ cells was estimated using a 25 μm × 25 μm counting frame, with a grid size of 70 μm × 80 μm. Section thickness was 10.5 μm. The estimated total of DCX^+ cells within the studied range was determined using the optical fractionator method and multiplied by two to correct for unilateral counting. The mean Gundersen coefficient of error of stereological quantification (m = 1) was 0.076 (range 0.06–0.10). $Ki67^+$ cells were counted manually using a light microscope (Olympus BH-2) with ×40 magnification and multiplied by the inverse of the sampling fraction and by two to correct for unilateral counting. The total estimated number of DCX^+ or $Ki67^+$ cells per animal was used for analysis.

Dendritic Morphology

Male mice (n = 6 per group) were decapitated between 9.00 and 10.30 a.m. Directly after decapitation, brains were dissected. Rapid Golgi staining (FD rapid-Golgi staining, Neurotechnologies) was performed according to the manufacturer's instructions with an impregnation time of 9 days. Vibratome sections (200 μm) were cut in the transversal plane (Leica VT 1000S; Leica Microsystems, Nussloch, Germany). Images were obtained using Zen 2011 (Carl Zeiss) in combination with an automated stage and focus control connected to the microscope. Golgi-impregnated dentate granule cells, fulfilling the following criteria, were randomly selected: (1) localization in the middle part (relative to the DG curvature and start of the CA3 region) of the suprapyramidal blade of the DG, within Bregma range −2.16 and −3.16 (transversal), (2) consistent and dark impregnation along the entire extent for all dendrites, and (3) relative isolation from neighboring impregnated neurons to avoid interference with analysis.

For morphological quantification, eight neurons from each animal in each treatment group were traced. Image stacks of 0.5 μm thickness were automatically acquired and combined. Neurons were traced using NeuroLucida software (MicroBrightField, Inc., Colchester, VT, USA) to obtain a 3D representation of each cell. Numerical analysis and graphical processing were performed with NeuroExplorer (MicroBrightField). Traced dendritic trees were evaluated by two investigators unaware of the treatment, on completeness of staining/tracing and on whether they belonged to a single cell, followed (if required) by a consensus meeting. Dendritic trees that were considered not completely stained/traced or belonging to multiple neurons were excluded from analysis [n = 50 (17%), 5–10 neurons per group, evenly distributed over the groups]. Spines were counted in two segments of ±20 μm per neuron, located on different dendrites. Segments were randomly chosen based on the following criteria: (1) localization at approximately 100 μm (80–120 μm) radial distance from the cell soma; (2) secondary or higher order dendritic branches; and (3) straight and remaining in a single focal-plane. Of each cell, dendritic properties were evaluated by analyzing the total dendritic length and maximum dendritic reach (radial distance), and the dendritic complexity index [(Σ branch tip orders + # branch tips) × (total dendritic length/total number of primary dendrites) (45)]. If dendritic length significantly differed between treatment groups, *post hoc* Sholl plots (46) were constructed by plotting the dendritic length as a function of radial distance from the soma center in 18 μm intervals. To normalize the distribution of the dendritic complexity index, neurons with a dendritic complexity index > 2 SD from the group mean were considered outliers and removed from the respective analysis [n = 12 (5%), 1–3 neurons per group, evenly distributed over the groups]. The remaining cells were subdivided into cells located in the inner-most part of the granule cell layer versus cells located in the middle or outer part of the granule cell layer (see Results). This subdivision was performed independently by two investigators blind to the treatment groups and compared afterward. In 96% of the cases the subdivision made by the two investigators was in agreement. In the remaining cases consensus was reached after in-depth investigation of the location.

Mossy Fiber Sprouting

Male mice (n = 6 per group) were killed between 9 and 12 a.m. under deep pentobarbital anesthesia (200 mg/kg body weight, i.p.) by transcardial perfusion with 0.1% sodium sulfide for 5 min, followed by 4% formaldehyde for 5 min (each in 0.01 phosphate-buffered saline, pH 7.4). Brains were removed from the skull, postfixed at 4°C in 4% formaldehyde/15% sucrose overnight, immersed at 4°C in 30% sucrose in phosphate-buffered saline until they sank and frozen on powered dry ice. Cryostat sections (30 μm) were cut in the coronal plane, mounted on superfrost slides in series of 15 and stored at −80°C until further use. Mossy fibers were stained with Timm histochemistry, according to Danscher (47). Staining was performed in two batches, each containing one slide of every animal to avoid staining-based variation between treatment groups. Sections were developed in the dark for 180 min in a freshly prepared 90/45/15/0.75 (volume/volume) solution of 50% arabic gum, 51% hydroquinone, 25.5% citric acid/23.5% sodium citrate, and 17% silver nitrate. After washing with running tap water, sections were dehydrated using a grading series of ethanol, cleared in xylene and coverslipped using malinol.

Mossy fiber staining in the hippocampal CA3 area and infrapyramidal blade of the DG (the main areas of possible MFS) was scored according to the scoring system described by Holmes et al. (48), ranging from 0 (no staining) to 5 (maximum staining). Eight sections of the septal hippocampus per animal (four sections for both staining batches), within Bregma range −1.46 to −2.80 (coronal), were scored by two independent observers, followed by a consensus meeting. Consensus scores of these eight sections were pooled per animal and the average was used for statistical analysis.

Slice Preparation for Electrophysiology

Male mice (n = 6–9 per group) were decapitated between 8.15 and 9.15 a.m., a few minutes after taking the animal out of its home cage. Only the first two mice of each litter were used for electrophysiological analysis to avoid confounding effects of a rise in plasma corticosterone due to acute stress. After rapid dissection, the brain was chilled in ice-cold, carbogenated (95% O_2:5% CO_2) artificial cerebrospinal fluid (aCSF) containing in mM: NaCl 120, KCl 3.5, $MgSO_4$ 5.0, NaH_2PO_4 1.25, $CaCl_2$ 0.2, $NaHCO_3$ 25.0, and D-glucose 10.0. After removing frontal lobes and cerebellum, 350 μm transversal hippocampal sections were prepared using a vibratome (Leica VT 1000S; Leica Microsystems, Nussloch, Germany). Both hemispheres were separated and all sections were incubated at room temperature in continuously carbogenated aCSF for at least 1 h.

Patch-Clamp Recording of Spontaneous Excitatory Postsynaptic Currents (sEPSCs)

Patching of DG neurons was performed using an upright microscope (Nicon Eclipse E600FN) with differential interference contrast and a water immersion objective (×40) to visually identify the cells. The sections were continuously perfused with carbogenated aCSF containing in mM NaCl 120, KCl 3.5, $MgSO_4$ 5.0, NaH_2PO_4 1.25, $CaCl_2$ 0.2, $NaHCO_3$ 25.0, and D-glucose 10 and 20 μM biccuculine to block γ-aminobutyric acid $(GABA)_A$-receptor mediated transmission (flow rate 2.0 ml/min, temperature 32°C, pH 7.4). Cell patching was performed as described by Pasricha et al. (49). Briefly, patch electrodes were pulled from a Sutter Instruments Micropipette puller and had a tip resistance of 4–6 MΩ when filled with the pipette (intracellular) solution containing in mM; Cs-methane sulfonate 120, CsCl 17.5, HEPES 10, BAPTA 5, MgATP 2, NaGTP 0.1, pH 7.3 (adjusted with CsOH). An Axopatch 200B amplifier (Axon Instruments, Foster City, CA, USA) was used for whole cell recordings, operating in the voltage-clamp mode. The patch-clamp amplifier was interfaced to a computer *via* a Digidata (type 1322A; Axon Instruments) analog-to-digital converter. Data acquisition was performed with Clampex, version 8.2 (Axon Instruments) at a sampling rate of 50 μs and a 5 kHz Bessel filter. The surface of the section was cleaned to have better vision of the cells in the deeper layers of DG. After establishing a gigaseal, the membrane patch was ruptured and the cell was clamped at a holding potential of −70 mV to allow measurement of currents mediated by the α-amino-3-hydroxy-5-methyl-4-isoxazolepropionic acid (AMPA) receptors, as at this potential, the *N*-methyl-D-aspartic acid or *N*-methyl-D-aspartate receptor is blocked by Mg^{2+}. sEPSCs were recorded for 5 min, starting 5–10 min after membrane rupture. After administration of tetrodotoxin (TTX, 0.5 μM, Bioconnect services) for 5 min to block voltage-gated Na channels and consequently also the development of action potentials, miniature EPSCs (mEPSCs) were measured for 5 min. Only one cell was recorded per slice and no more than two recordings were obtained per animal. Only recordings with an uncompensated series resistance of <2.5 times the pipette resistance, <20% variation during the recording period, and with frequencies <2 SD from the mean, were accepted for analysis. For each event, the area under the curve (AUC) and inter-event interval was analyzed using Clampfit version 9.2 (Axon Instruments). The median AUC and inter-event interval per cell were used for statistical analysis.

Field Potential Recordings

Sections were transferred to a submersion type recording chamber and continuously perfused with carbogenated aCSF containing in mM: NaCl 124, KCl 2.5, $MgSO_4$ 4.0, NaH_2PO_4 1.2, $CaCl_2$ 4.0, $NaHCO_3$ 26.0, D-glucose 10.0, and 20 μM bicuculline (flow rate 2 ml/min, temperature 32°C, pH 7.4). Field excitatory postsynaptic potentials (fEPSPs) were recorded in the DG, using glass microelectrodes filled with aCSF, positioned in the medial perforant pathway over the suprapyramidal blade of the DG, as confirmed by paired pulse stimulation elicited paired pulse inhibition. Minimum and maximum stimulation intensities were identified. After an incubation period of 20 min, an input–output response curve was generated by gradually increasing the stimulus intensity to define the stimulus intensity that generated the half-maximal response in peak-amplitude; this intensity was used for the remainder of the experiment. To measure paired pulse depression, paired pulses were delivered at an inter stimulus interval of 50, 100, and 200 ms. After 15–20 min of stable baseline recordings, sections were tetanized with 4 trains of 50 pulses of supramaximal intensity at 100 Hz (30 s inter train interval) to induce LTP. Field potentials were recorded for 1 h posttetanus at 30 s intervals. At the end of this period, the post-tetanic paired pulse depression and final input–output curve were determined. LTP was quantified by calculating the ratio between fEPSP slopes recorded post tetanization and pre tetanization. Data were acquired and analyzed with Signal 2.0 software (Cambridge Electronic Design, UK).

Statistical Analysis

The effect of eFS and injection type on outcome measures was analyzed with a general linear mixed model in a 2 × 3 design, examining the main effects of HT (HT versus NT) and injection type (corticosterone versus vehicle versus none), as well as their interaction. *A priori* we hypothesized that group differences would be caused by HT treatment or injection type. Therefore, not all possible group comparisons were included in statistical analysis. More specifically, in case of a significant main effect of injection type, *post hoc* tests were performed comparing injection types with Bonferroni correction for multiple comparison. Additionally, differences between HT and NT animals were analyzed per injection group with an independent samples *t*-test, Bonferroni corrected for multiple comparison. When data from multiple neurons per animal, or multiple segments per neuron, were analyzed, a linear mixed model was used, including the animal (for dendritic complexity and glutamatergic transmission) or neuron (for spine density) as subject variables. Effects of HT, injection type and their interaction on Sholl distribution were tested with a repeated measure general linear model. Correlation between parameters was assessed with Pearson correlation coefficient. Mean fEPSP slopes pre- and posttetanization were compared with a paired samples *t*-test.

Normality of residues was evaluated with Q–Q plots, variance of residues was evaluated with error plots. Differences were considered statistically significant at $p < 0.05$ (two-tailed) after correction for multiple comparison. Differences that were significant before, but not after correction for multiple comparison ($0.05 \leq p < 0.15$), were considered trends. Data were analyzed using SPSS 20.0 (SPSS, Inc., Chicago, IL, USA). Unless stated otherwise, data are presented as mean ± SEM.

RESULTS

Epileptic Seizures and Neuroendocrine Changes

Experimental seizures were elicited in all mice exposed to the HT protocol and the average seizure duration was 26.4 ± 2.0 min. Corticosterone injection resulted in a high peak concentration of corticosterone (1,043.3 ± 28.0 ng/ml at 15 min after injection) with a fast return to baseline in approximately 180 min, while vehicle injection elicited a much smaller (94.6 ± 8.2 ng/ml) and more short-termed increase in corticosterone levels (**Figure 2A**).

Weight increase between HT/NT treatment and decapitation, a 15 days interval, was significantly lower in HT animals compared to controls [main effect HT, $F_{(1,280)} = 10.73$, $p = 0.001$], but was not influenced by subsequent injections (**Figure 2B**). No group differences were observed in adrenal and thymus weights (data not shown). Although there were less than 2 min between successive decapitations of animals belonging to the same litter, later decapitation was associated with increased corticosterone levels (**Figure 2C**, left panel). While no group differences were observed in corticosterone levels in animals decapitated first of their litter (**Figure 2C**, middle panel), injection type did significantly influence corticosterone levels in animals decapitated as

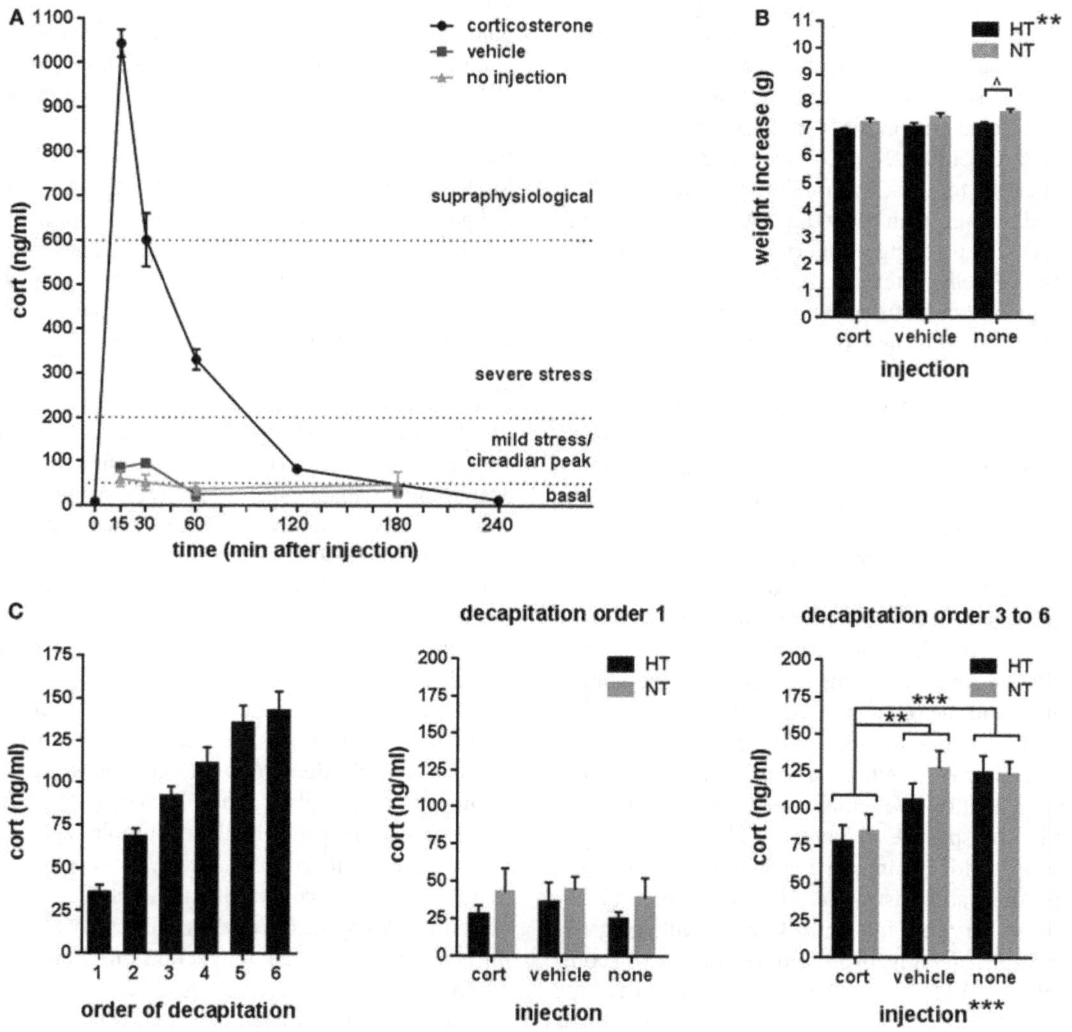

FIGURE 2 | Endocrinology. **(A)** Corticosterone (cort) levels at several time points after single intraperitoneal injection with corticosterone, vehicle, or no injection at 9.00 a.m. Reference corticosterone levels: basal < ±50 ng/ml, circadian peak or mild stress ±50–200 ng/ml, severe stress ±200–600 ng/ml, and supraphysiological > ±600 ng/ml (50–52). **(B)** Weight increase was significantly lower in hyperthermia (HT)- compared to normothermia (NT)-treated animals overall, while analyses per injection type only showed a trend difference in the not injected groups. **(C)** Corticosterone levels after decapitation increased with the order of decapitation within the litter (left panel). In animals decapitated as first of their litter (middle panel), corticosterone levels did not differ between treatment group, while in animals decapitated third to sixth of their litter (right panel), corticosterone levels differed between injection types—with significantly lower levels in the corticosterone injected animals—but not between HT- and NT-treated animals. Data represented as mean ± SEM. $^{***}p < 0.001$, $^{**}p < 0.01$, and $^{\wedge}p < 0.05$ before correction for multiple comparison (trend).

third to sixth of their litter [**Figure 2C**, right panel, main effect injection, $F_{(2,68)} = 8.7$, $p < 0.001$; corticosterone versus vehicle $p = 0.009$, corticosterone versus no injection $p < 0.001$, vehicle versus no injection $p = 0.36$], indicating that repetitive corticosterone injection indeed affected stress hormone regulation, which confirms successful manipulation.

Morphology

Neurogenesis

Neurogenesis significantly differed between HT and NT animals. HT was associated with a decrease in the number of immature DCX-positive neurons [main effect HT, $F_{(1,30)} = 6.21$, $p = 0.019$] (**Figure 3A**), and an increase in the number of proliferating cells in the DG [main effect HT, $F_{(1,30)} = 4.94$, $p = 0.034$] compared to NT (**Figure 3B**). Accordingly, the number of immature neurons and proliferating cells per animal were negatively correlated ($r = -0.55$, $p = 0.001$). Analyses per injection type revealed that the effects of HT on both DCX- and Ki67-staining were significant in the vehicle injected animals [$F_{(1,10)} = 12.16$, $p = 0.018$, respectively, $F_{(1,10)} = 15.89$, $p = 0.009$], while a similar effect was observed at trend level after corticosterone injection [$F_{(1,10)} = 5.71$, $p = 0.12$, respectively, $F_{(1,10)} = 6.88$, $p = 0.09$]. Non-injected HT and NT groups did not differ at all.

Dendritic Morphology

To assess the effects of eFS and injection type on dendritic morphology, we evaluated total dendritic length, dendritic reach, dendritic complexity and spine density. As dendritic complexity differed between dentate granule cells with a cell body located in the inner part of the granular cell layer, bordering the subgranular layer (referred to as "inner layer," $n = 15$–27 per group), versus the middle or outer part of the granule cell layer (referred to as "outer layer," $n = 11$–25 per group) (**Figure 4A**, A1), these cells were analyzed separately. In inner layer neurons, dendritic complexity index was increased in HT animals compared to NT controls [main effect HT, $F_{(1,111)} = 6.23$, $p = 0.014$], an effect that was only significant in animals receiving no subsequent injections [$F_{(1,7)} = 6.64$, $p = 0.04$] and was less pronounced after vehicle or corticosterone injection (**Figure 4A**, A2, left panel). Also the total dendritic length of inner layer neurons was increased in HT animals [main effect HT, $F_{(1,29)} = 4.47$, $p = 0.04$], an effect that aggravated with injection type, although analyses per injection type only revealed a difference in the corticosterone-injected group at trend level (**Figure 4A**, A2, right panel). No main nor interaction effects were observed on total dendritic reach. Sholl analyses per neuron revealed a main effect of HT [$F_{(1,120)} = 6.18$, $p = 0.01$] and radial distance from the soma [$F_{(3,358)} = 560.71$, $p < 0.001$] on dendrite length, as well as a

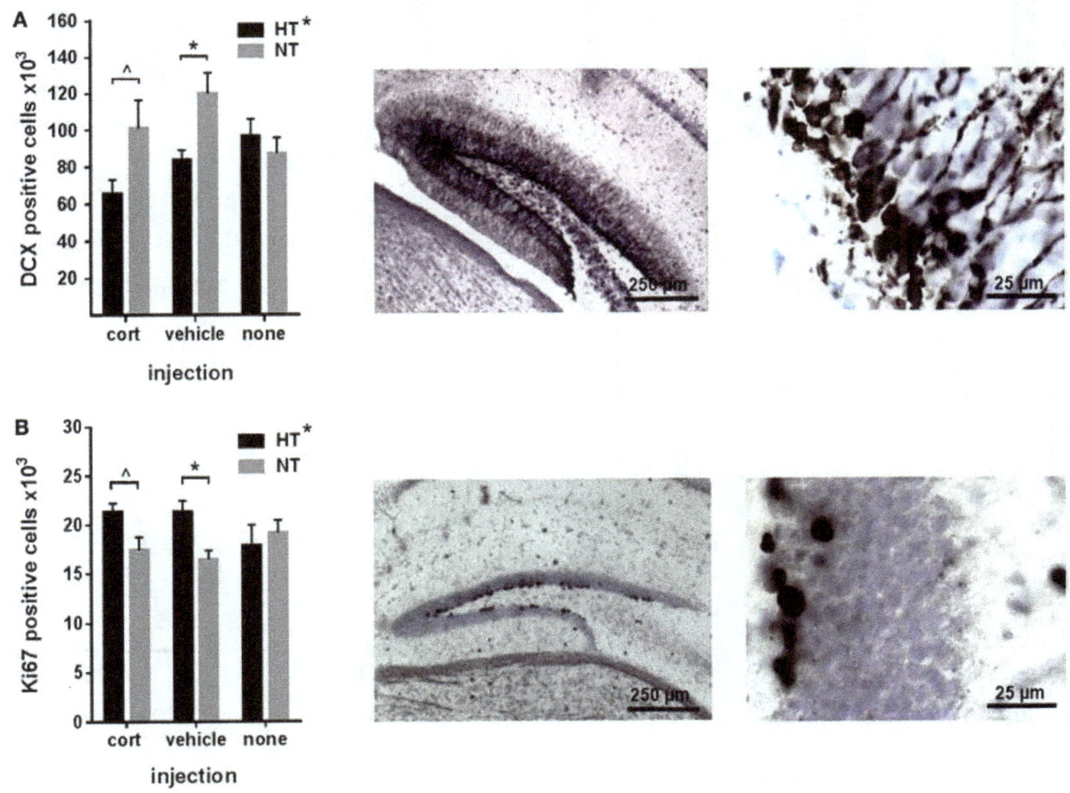

FIGURE 3 | Neurogenesis. **(A)** Left: the number of immature neurons in the dentate gyrus was decreased in male animals exposed to hyperthermia (HT) compared to normothermia (NT) after injection. Middle/right: representative example of DCX staining at lower and higher magnification. **(B)** Left: the number of proliferating cells in the dentate gyrus was increased in males exposed to HT. Middle/right: representative example of Ki67 staining at lower and higher magnification. Data represented as mean ± SEM. *$p < 0.05$ and ^$p < 0.05$ before correction for multiple comparison (trend).

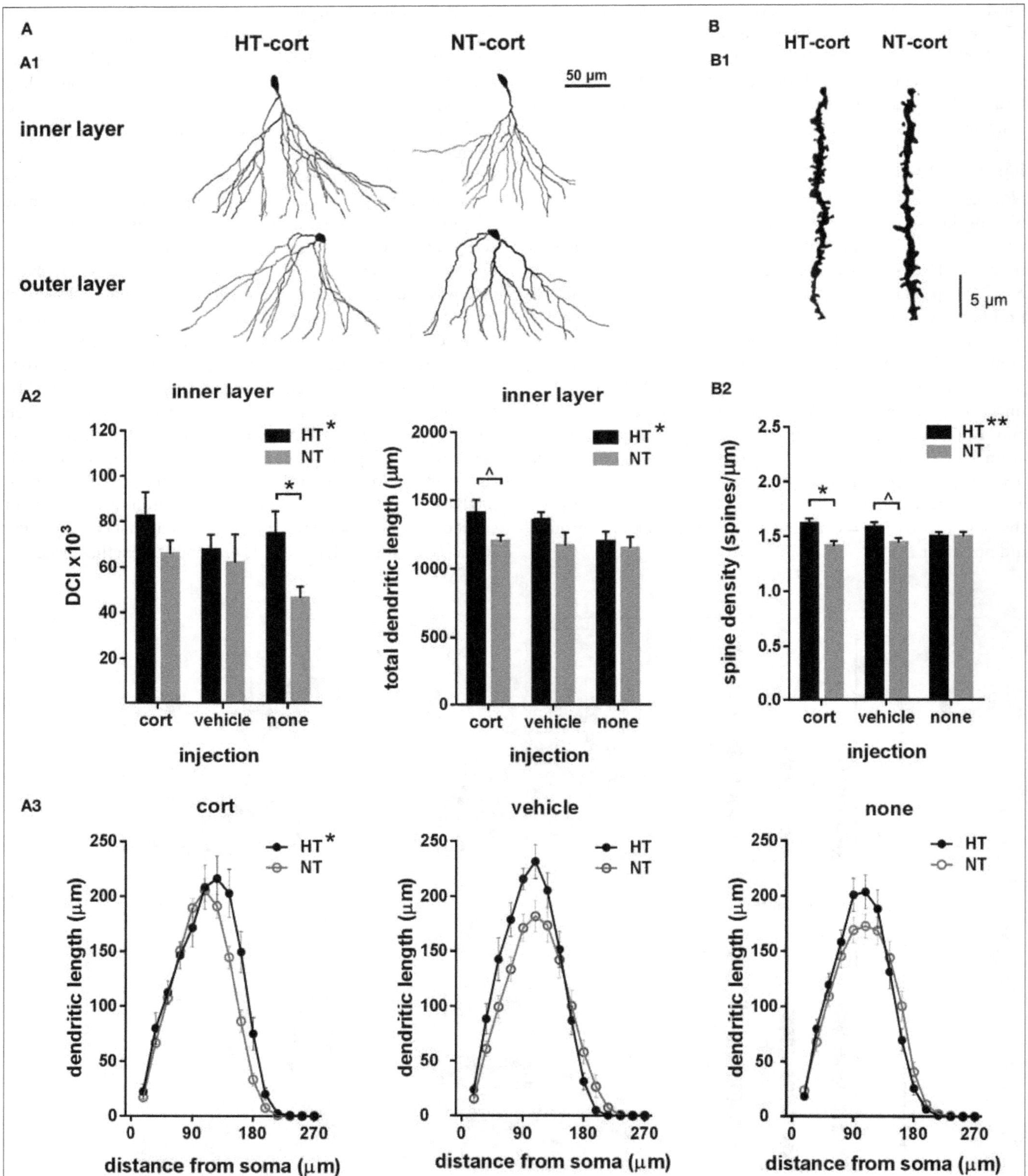

FIGURE 4 | Dendritic morphology. **(A)** Dendritic complexity. (A1) Dendritic complexity differed between dentate granule cells with a cell body located in the granular cell layer or inner part of the molecular layer (inner layer) versus the middle or outer part of the molecular cell layer (outer layer), representative examples of corticosterone (cort) injected animals after hyperthermia (HT) and normothermia (NT). (A2) Left: dendritic complexity index (DCI) in inner layer neurons was increased after HT compared to NT. Right: total dendritic length of inner layer neurons was increased after HT, an effect that increased with injection type. (A3) HT significantly influenced Sholl distribution. **(B)** Spine density. (B1) Representative example of HT-cort and NT-cort animal. (B2) Spine density was significantly higher in animals exposed to HT compared to NT, an effect that increased with injection type. Data represented as mean ± SEM. *$p < 0.05$ and ^$p < 0.05$ before correction for multiple comparison (trend).

HT × injection type × radial distance interaction [$F_{(6,358)} = 3.18$, $p = 0.005$] (**Figure 4A**, A3). In outer layer neurons, no main or interaction effects of HT or injection type were observed on dendritic complexity (data not shown).

Spine density was significantly higher in animals exposed to HT compared to NT [main effect HT, $F_{(1,165)} = 7.28, p = 0.008$]. This effect was significant after corticosterone injection [$F_{(1,58)} = 8.80$, $p = 0.01$], at trend level after vehicle injection [$F_{(1,55)} = 4.67$, $p = 0.11$], while it was not observed in animals receiving no injections [$F_{(1,52)} = 0.00, p = 1.00$] (**Figure 4B**, B1,B2).

Mossy Fiber Sprouting

Hippocampal MFS was assessed in the DG and the CA3 area of the hippocampus. As expected, intense Timm staining was observed in the hilus of the DG and in the stratum lucidum of the CA3 area, the main projection sites of mossy fibers. The amount of infrapyramidal Timm staining, characteristic for MFS, was very low in all treatment groups (mean MFS score DG 0.76 ± 0.09, CA3 1.07 ± 0.08, on a scale ranging from 0 to 5). HT or injection type did not significantly affect MFS score in both areas, although there was a trend towards an increased MFS score in the CA3 area after HT in animals receiving corticosterone injections [$F_{(1,10)} = 7.56, p = 0.06$, **Figure 5**].

Functional Plasticity

The eFS-induced changes in morphology and particularly the increased spine density may affect glutamatergic transmission in the DG, which could be reflected at the level of single cells as well as field potentials. To test this, we examined effects of HT and corticosterone injection on single cell spontaneous synaptic events (which are among other things determined by the number of synaptic contacts) and field excitatory potentials.

Single Cell Glutamatergic Transmission

Whole-cell voltage-clamp recordings of AMPA receptor mediated EPSCs in the DG were analyzed in 9–11 cells per treatment group. Input resistance and capacitance did not differ between groups (see **Table 1**). For both sEPSCs and mEPSCs, no HT × injection interaction or main effect of HT was observed. Interestingly, injection type did influence sEPSC and mEPSC properties (**Figures 6A,B**). A significant main effect of injection type existed on the interval between consecutive events for both sEPSC [main effect injection, $F_{(2,32)} = 3.48$, $p = 0.03$; corticosterone versus vehicle $p = 0.63$; corticosterone versus no injections $p = 0.06$, vehicle versus no injections $p = 0.01$] (**Figure 6A**, right panel) and mEPSC [main effect injection, $F_{(2,32)} = 3.95$, $p = 0.03$; corticosterone versus vehicle $p = 0.65$; corticosterone versus no injections $p = 0.07$, vehicle versus no injections $p = 0.01$] (**Figure 6B**, right panel), with a lower inter-event interval in the vehicle injection group compared to the non-injection group; a similar difference, although only at trend level, was observed for the corticosterone-injection versus non-injection groups. Also the AUC of the sEPSCs was influenced by injection type [$F_{(2,36)} = 4.39$, $p = 0.02$; corticosterone versus vehicle $p = 0.04$, vehicle versus no injections $p = 0.004$, corticosterone versus no injections not significant] with a smaller AUC after vehicle injection compared to the other groups (**Figure 6A**, middle panel), while the AUC of mEPSC did not significantly differ between groups (**Figure 6B**, middle panel).

Synaptic Plasticity

Changes in glutamatergic transmission at the single cell level may alter circuit properties and the ability to induce synaptic plasticity. This was tested with field potential recording and application of high-frequency stimulation. Treatment groups did not differ with respect to baseline slopes or stimulation intensity necessary to produce the half-maximal fEPSP, suggesting that HT and injection type did not influence baseline-evoked transmission (see **Table 1**). No significant differences were observed in paired pulse facilitation before and after high-frequency stimulation (**Figure 7A**). The input-output curve was increased after high frequency, and did not differ significantly between treatment groups (**Figure 7B**). A significant increase in fEPSP slope post tetanization (LTP) was elicited in 71% of all animals (38–88%

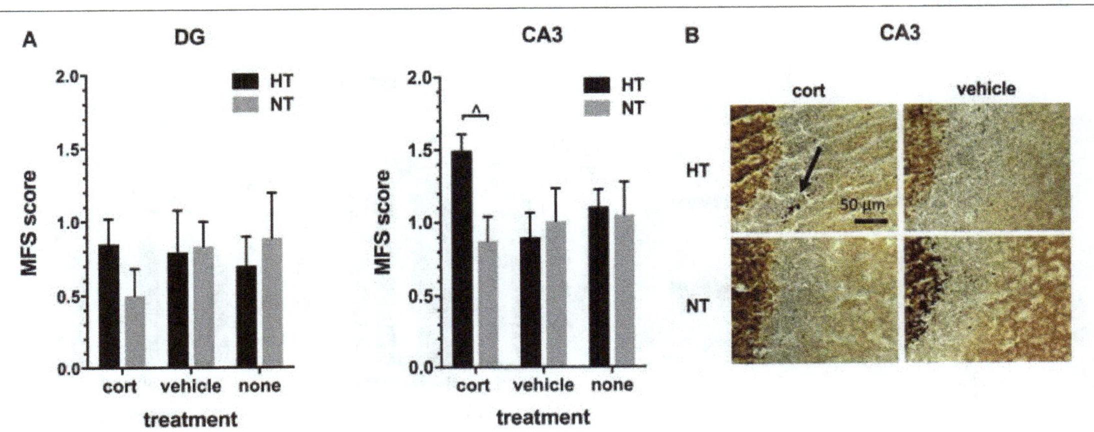

FIGURE 5 | Mossy fiber sprouting (MFS). **(A)** Left: the MFS score in dentate gyrus (DG) did not differ significantly between treatment groups. Right: in the CA3 area of the hippocampus only a trend was seen toward an increase in MFS score after hyperthermia (HT) in animals receiving corticosterone injections. **(B)** Representative example of MFS in the CA3 area in HT and normothermia (NT) animals with corticosterone versus vehicle injection. Arrow: MFS. Data represented as mean ± SEM. ^$p < 0.05$ before correction for multiple comparison (trend).

per group). Synaptic plasticity at half-maximal or maximal stimulation was not significantly influenced by the HT × injection interaction or by HT, but only by injection type [main effect injection, $F_{(2,38)} = 4.20$, $p = 0.02$; corticosterone versus vehicle $p = 0.02$, corticosterone versus no injections $p = 0.44$, vehicle versus no injections $p = 0.01$, other group comparisons not significant] (**Figure 7C**). At maximum stimulation intensities, no group differences were observed.

TABLE 1 | Baseline measurements of single cell glutamatergic transmission and synaptic plasticity.

Treatment group	Single cell transmission		Synaptic plasticity	
	Input resistance (mΩ)	Capacitance (pF)	Baseline slope (V/s)	Stimulation intensity (mA)
HT-cort	336 ± 49	9.8 ± 0.7	−0.13 ± 0.02	0.63 ± 0.05
NT-cort	338 ± 38	9.0 ± 0.8	−0.20 ± 0.02	0.71 ± 0.03
HT-vehicle	303 ± 33	9.0 ± 0.7	−0.19 ± 0.02	0.66 ± 0.02
NT-vehicle	320 ± 38	9.2 ± 0.7	−0.14 ± 0.03	0.77 ± 0.08
HT-none	285 ± 35	9.4 ± 0.8	−0.22 ± 0.02	0.80 ± 0.12
NT-none	302 ± 37	9.6 ± 1.1	−0.22 ± 0.04	0.84 ± 0.14

Baseline measurements of functional plasticity were not significantly influenced by the HT x injection type interaction, HT, or injection type. Data represented as mean ± SEM.

DISCUSSION

To increase understanding of the effects of stress and stress hormones on early-life epileptogenesis, we induced epileptogenesis in young mice using the HT-induced eFS model and subsequently exposed them to (1) corticosterone, (2) vehicle injection (a mild stressor), or (3) no injections, and evaluated morphological and functional parameters in the DG. In this latent phase of early epileptogenesis, few effects of eFS were observed in animals that were not subsequently injected. However, in mice that received repetitive corticosterone or vehicle injection (mild stress), eFS induced epileptogenesis was associated with changes in DG morphology, namely a lower number of immature cells, an increased cell proliferation and an increased dendritic length and spine density. These

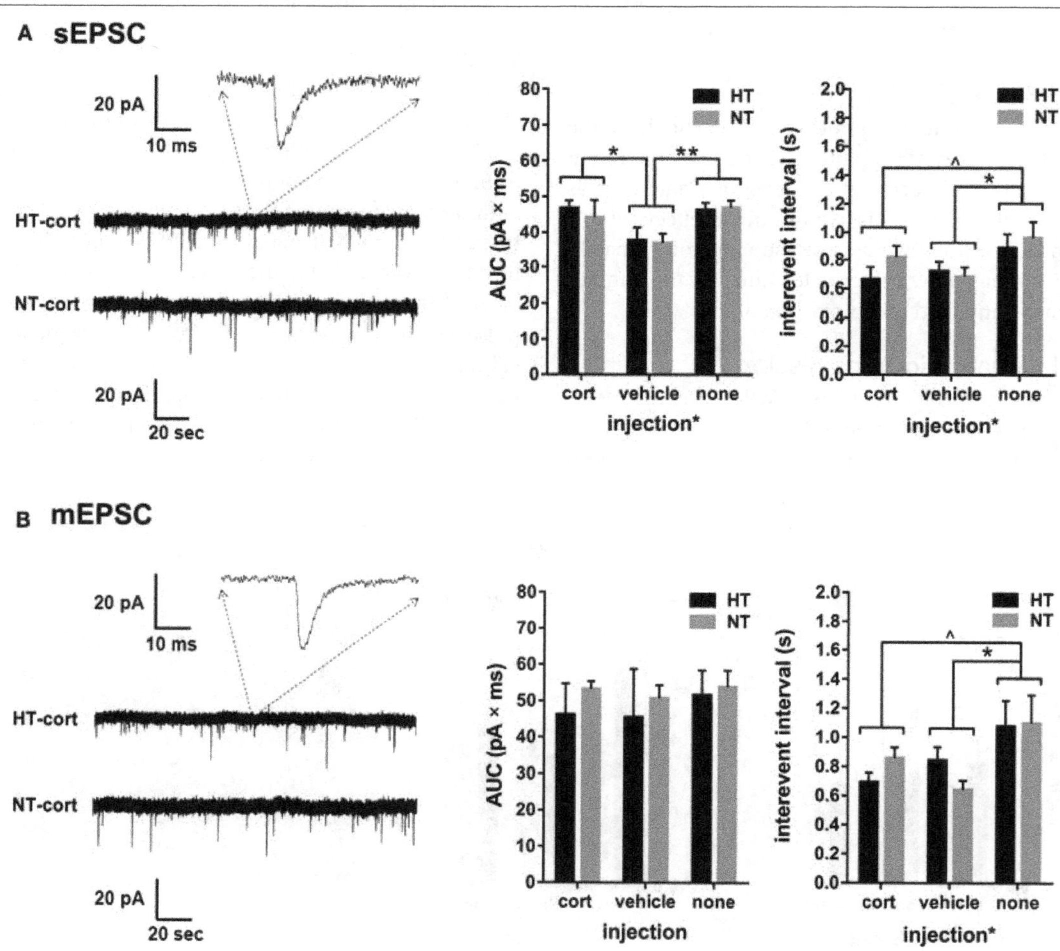

FIGURE 6 | Single cell glutamatergic transmission. **(A)** Left: example showing a spontaneous excitatory postsynaptic current (sEPSC) recording. Middle and right: a main effect of injection type, but not HT, is observed on sEPSC area under the curve (AUC) and interevent interval. **(B)** Left: example showing a miniature excitatory postsynaptic current (mEPSC) recording. Middle: no group differences are observed in mEPSC AUC. Right: a main effect of injection type, but not HT, is observed on mEPSC interevent interval. Data represented as mean ± SEM. **$p < 0.01$, *$p < 0.05$, and ^$p < 0.05$ before correction for multiple comparison (trend).

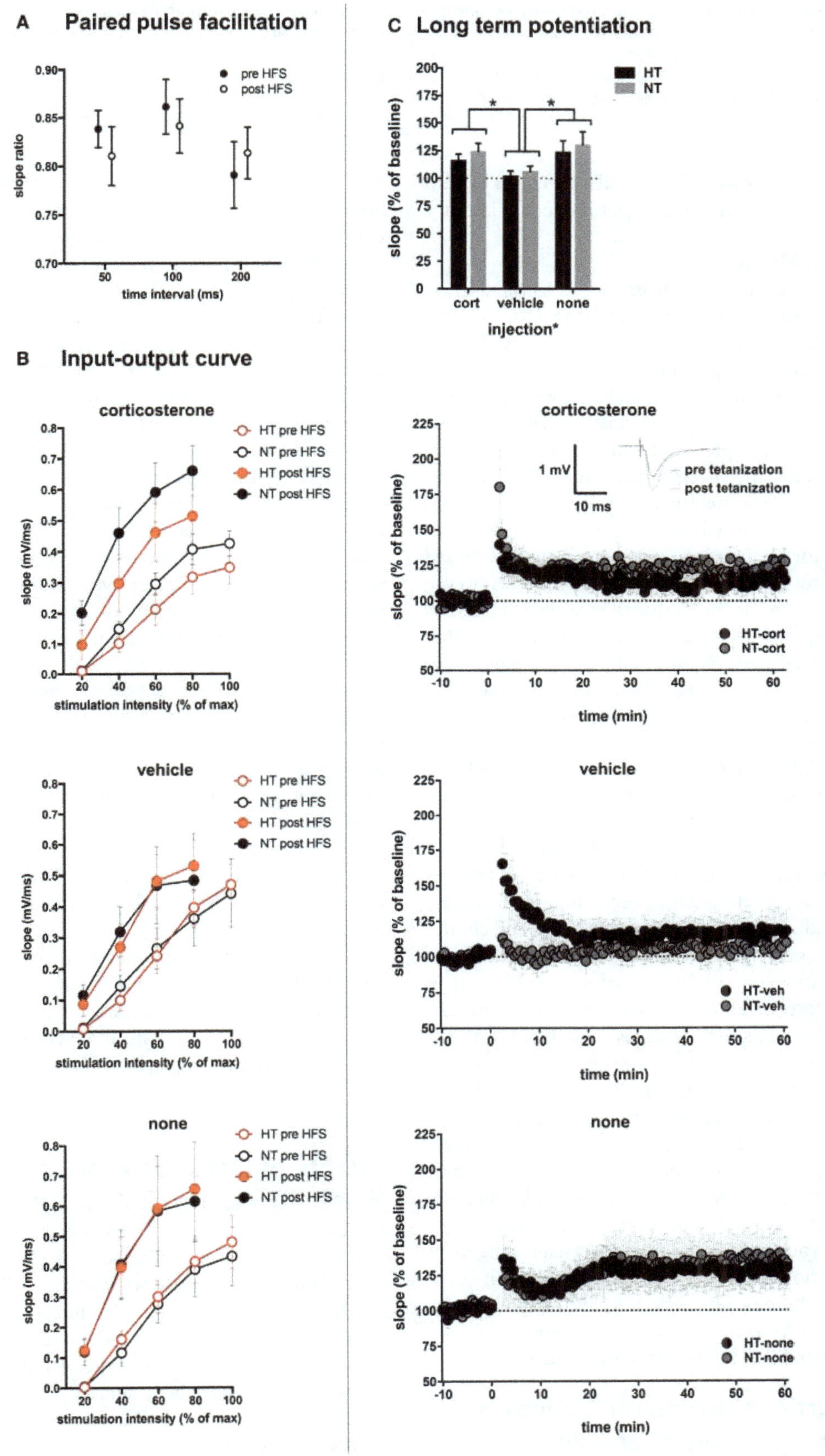

FIGURE 7 | Continued

FIGURE 7 | Synaptic plasticity. **(A)** Paired pulse facilitation before and after high-frequency stimulation (HFS). **(B)** The input–output curve is increased after HFS, but did not differ significantly between treatment groups. **(C)** Top: injection type, but not HT, influenced field-evoked postsynaptic potentials (fEPSP). Upper middle: LTP recordings of fEPSP in hyperthermia (HT) vs. normothermia (NT) animals after repetitive corticosterone injection (tetanization started at $t = 0$). Inset: example showing increased slope and amplitude of fEPSP after tetanization. Lower middle: fEPSP in HT vs. NT animals after repetitive vehicle injection. Bottom: fEPSP in HT vs. NT animals without subsequent injections. Data represented as mean ± SEM, $^{*}p < 0.05$.

morphological changes associated with epileptogenesis did not translate into differences in glutamatergic functional plasticity.

Experimental Model

The eFS model is a model of early-life prolonged febrile seizures with close resemblance to the human situation (30, 31). The relatively long-lasting latent phase of epileptogenesis in this model provides the unique opportunity to study epileptogenesis in the absence of spontaneous seizures and relatively apart from the damage and compensatory mechanisms that may arise due to recurrent electrographical or clinical seizure activity. However, non-epileptogenic effects of the initial eFS cannot be fully excluded. As we were interested in epileptogenic changes, outcome measures were assessed before the onset of spontaneous seizures. Based on earlier literature, a subset of animals exposed to eFS is expected not to develop epilepsy (26, 35, 36). However, the normal distribution of our outcome measures suggests a gradual distribution of epileptogenesis among animals. Further studies measuring long-term (seizure) outcome are required to determine whether the morphological and functional measures assessed are stable during the course of epileptogenesis, as well as their relevance for epilepsy outcome.

We hypothesized the mild epileptogenic changes in the latent phase after eFS to be aggravated by stress (hormone) exposure. As different stressors might differentially affect seizure-susceptibility [reviewed in Ref. (2, 23, 53)], we decided to use a clean design of injections with corticosterone—the end product of the stress response, exerting large effects on brain structure and function, including neuronal excitability (22)-, and control groups of mild injection stress and undisturbed animals. Stress paradigms in rodents are usually associated with a reduction in bodyweight and effects on adrenals and thymus. In our experiment, we did not observe such changes, possibly due to the mild nature of the injection stress. However, the reduced corticosterone levels in corticosterone-injected animals that were decapitated after prior handling of littermates, which can be considered an acute stressor, indicate that corticosterone injections *did* downregulate responsiveness of the hypothalamic–pituitary–adrenal axis. The effects of these supraphysiological doses of corticosterone were smaller than expected, which might relate to the young age of the animals, just after the stress hyporesponsive period. Also, the transient increases in corticosterone levels in the morning may not have interfered with the ultradian pulsatility of endogenous hormone levels (54), benefiting its comparability to real life stress exposure.

Effects of Corticosteroids on Structural Plasticity during Epileptogenesis

In animals that were *not* subsequently injected, HT only affected dendritic complexity, but none of the other outcome measures. The negative results during this early phase of epileptogenesis are in line with previous studies that also reported no differences in MFS (24, 27) or DG neurogenesis (24) around this age. Similarly, in non-injected mice we observed no effects of HT on DG spine density.

Differences between animals exposed to HT and NT only became manifest after repetitive corticosterone or vehicle injections. The increase of HT-associated changes after stress (hormone) exposure is in line with the vast amount of previous studies reporting stress exposure *before seizure induction* to increase seizure-susceptibility and seizure-severity [reviewed in Ref. (55)]. The effects of HT combined with corticosteroids or mild stress on proliferation are similar to those reported at a later stage of epileptogenesis after HT only (25, 26), suggesting that corticosterone and stress *accelerate* epileptogenesis-related structural plasticity. We observed an inverse relation between the number of proliferating cells and the amount of immature neurons, suggesting that the increased proliferation mainly occurs in non-neuronal (e.g., glial) cells, consistent with the gliosis prominent in many epilepsy models (56, 57).

Dendritic length, complexity and spine density are generally reported to decrease after seizures (58–63), which is considered a compensatory mechanism in response to the excess of excitatory input. Dendritic complexity was previously shown to be increased after eFS (28). The enhanced dendritic length and spine density that we found during the latent phase of early epileptogenesis in combination with corticosterone exposure and mild stress is therefore likely to be part of the epileptogenic process.

Clearly, the parameters that we investigated might not only be altered by epileptogenesis but also by corticosterone and stress themselves. This is shown for instance by the increased number of DCX^{+} cells in the vehicle injected compared to non-injected NT group, that is consistent with the literature (21, 64).

Effects of Corticosteroids on Functional Plasticity during Epileptogenesis

In non-injected animals, glutamatergic transmission and LTP were unaffected by HT. The latter is somewhat surprising, as around this age HT was shown to affect GABAergic transmission in DG (65) and both glutamateric and GABA-ergic transmission in CA1 (27, 66–69). Since we did not record GABAergic signals, we cannot exclude that in our model GABAergic transmission in the DG might have been altered.

In view of the increased dendritic length and spine density observed after HT when followed by corticosterone (and to a lesser degree vehicle) injection, the latent phase of early epileptogenesis may be accompanied by an expanded postsynaptic "potential" for synaptic transfer of signals. We tested whether this translated to the functional level; i.e., a higher spine density may result in increased mEPSC frequency and this, in turn, may enhance the ability to induce LTP (70). However, this appeared not to be the case. Rather than HT, the condition of mild stress related to vehicle injection resulted in a higher frequency of both sEPSCs and mEPSCs, and a smaller AUC of sEPSCs; the latter could explain the reduced ability to induce LTP in these groups. The discrepancy between structural changes in dendrites and spines versus sEPSC frequency is unexpected, but emphasizes that presynaptic changes, e.g., after mild injection stress, are important for the overall outcome in functional terms. Presynaptic effects of stress or corticosterone are indeed well documented (71, 72), also in the mouse DG (49), although these were never investigated with this particular paradigm and at this age. The data furthermore illustrate that the functional effect of mild injection stress cannot be extrapolated to effects of a high dose of corticosterone. This may relate to a bell-shaped dose-dependency for corticosterone, as indeed often observed (73, 74) or, importantly, the fact that mild (injection) stress causes the release of several stress-related hormones in addition to corticosterone.

Potential Implications for Epileptogenesis

The increase in morphological differences after HT when followed by corticosteroid and mild stress exposure suggests that stress (hormones) aggravates or accelerates epileptogenesis. Epileptogenesis, i.e., the neurobiological processes leading to epilepsy, is not limited to the time before the onset of spontaneous seizures, but continues during the course of epilepsy, contributing to the progression of the disease (75, 76). As none of the currently available anti-epileptic drugs can favorably modify the disease process, prevention or reduction of epileptogenesis remains one of the main challenges in the field of epilepsy (77–79) and could be beneficial for all patients, irrespective of the underlying pathology. Children with complex febrile seizures are of special interest, as they have a high risk to develop epilepsy—ranging from 21% after prolonged febrile seizures (80) to as much as 49% after prolonged seizures with focal semiology that reoccur within 24 h (81)—that is already identified at the very beginning of epileptogenesis, making them very suitable for early intervention. Large population-based studies, prospectively following children after complex febrile seizures and systematically documenting stress exposure, as well as epilepsy outcome, can provide more insight into the effects of stress on epileptogenesis in this human population.

In conclusion, our results suggest that stress and stress hormones modulate epileptogenesis, indicating that stress reduction strategies and possibly even medication targeting the stress system may have a potential role in reducing epileptogenesis. As studying epileptogenesis apart from seizure frequency is difficult, especially in humans, animal studies could provide valuable information on the effects of stress reduction on epileptogenesis, for example, by studying effects of an enriched environment during the latent phase of epileptogenesis on seizure outcome.

ETHICS STATEMENT

All experimental procedures were performed according to the institutional guidelines of the University Medical Center Utrecht and approved by the committee on ethical considerations in animal experiments of Utrecht University (DEC Utrecht, permit number 2012.I.03.047).

AUTHOR CONTRIBUTIONS

JC, KPJB, PG and MJ contributed conception and design of the study. JC, EH, KB, GR, ST, EU, and GM contributed to data acquisition. JC organized the database, performed the statistical analysis, and wrote the first draft of the manuscript. JC, KB, GR, PL, PG, and MJ contributed to data interpretation. All authors contributed to manuscript revision, read, and approved the submitted version.

ACKNOWLEDGMENTS

We acknowledge the expert help and technical assistance of H. Karst, R. A. Sarabdjitsingh, and B. Jongbloets. Moreover, we thank the practical assistance of B. Visser, V. Bonapersona, and T. Kliest in neuronal reconstructions for dendritic complexity or spine analyses, S. Vugts in optimizing neurogenesis stainings, M. Sep in Ki67 staining and quantification, and M. A. Pet in DCX quantification. This work was supported by a grant of the UMC Utrecht Alexandre Suerman Stipendium. This manuscript includes content that previously appeared in the first author's thesis (82).

REFERENCES

1. Shinnar S, Pellock JM. Update on the epidemiology and prognosis of pediatric epilepsy. *J Child Neurol* (2002) 17(Suppl 1):S4–17. doi:10.1177/08830738020170010201
2. van Campen JS, Jansen FE, de Graan PN, Braun KP, Joëls M. Early life stress in epilepsy: a seizure precipitant and risk factor for epileptogenesis. *Epilepsy Behav* (2013) 38:160–71. doi:10.1016/j.yebeh.2013.09.029
3. Feldman RG, Paul NL. Identity of emotional triggers in epilepsy. *J Nerv Ment Dis* (1976) 162:345–53. doi:10.1097/00005053-197605000-00005
4. Neufeld MY, Sadeh M, Cohn DF, Korczyn AD. Stress and epilepsy: the gulf war experience. *Seizure* (1994) 3:135–9. doi:10.1016/S1059-1311(05)80204-3
5. Swinkels WA, Engelsman M, Kasteleijn-Nolst Trenite DG, Baal MG, de Haan GJ, Oosting J. Influence of an evacuation in February 1995 in the Netherlands on the seizure frequency in patients with epilepsy: a controlled study. *Epilepsia* (1998) 39:1203–7. doi:10.1111/j.1528-1157.1998.tb01312.x
6. Bosnjak J, Vukovic-Bobic M, Mejaski-Bosnjak V. Effect of war on the occurrence of epileptic seizures in children. *Epilepsy Behav* (2002) 3:502–9. doi:10.1016/S1525-5050(02)00602-9
7. Klein P, van Passel L. Effect of stress related to the 9/11/2001 terror attack on seizures in patients with epilepsy. *Neurology* (2005) 64:1815–6. doi:10.1212/01.WNL.0000162026.52300.3C
8. Christensen J, Li J, Vestergaard M, Olsen J. Stress and epilepsy: a population-based cohort study of epilepsy in parents who lost a child. *Epilepsy Behav* (2007) 11:324–8. doi:10.1016/j.yebeh.2007.06.003

9. Shang NX, Zou LP, Zhao JB, Zhang F, Li H. Association between prenatal stress and infantile spasms: a case-control study in china. *Pediatr Neurol* (2010) 42:181–6. doi:10.1016/j.pediatrneurol.2009.09.003
10. Li J, Vestergaard M, Obel C, Precht DH, Christensen J, Lu M, et al. Prenatal stress and epilepsy in later life: a nationwide follow-up study in Denmark. *Epilepsy Res* (2008) 81:52–7. doi:10.1016/j.eplepsyres.2008.04.014
11. Huang LT, Holmes GL, Lai MC, Hung PL, Wang CL, Wang TJ, et al. Maternal deprivation stress exacerbates cognitive deficits in immature rats with recurrent seizures. *Epilepsia* (2002) 43:1141–8. doi:10.1046/j.1528-1157.2002.14602.x
12. Lai MC, Holmes GL, Lee KH, Yang SN, Wang CA, Wu CL, et al. Effect of neonatal isolation on outcome following neonatal seizures in rats – the role of corticosterone. *Epilepsy Res* (2006) 68:123–36. doi:10.1016/j.eplepsyres.2005.10.005
13. Lai MC, Lui CC, Yang SN, Wang JY, Huang LT. Epileptogenesis is increased in rats with neonatal isolation and early-life seizure and ameliorated by MK-801: a long-term MRI and histological study. *Pediatr Res* (2009) 66:441–7. doi:10.1203/PDR.0b013e3181b337d2
14. Salzberg M, Kumar G, Supit L, Jones NC, Morris MJ, Rees S, et al. Early postnatal stress confers enduring vulnerability to limbic epileptogenesis. *Epilepsia* (2007) 48:2079–85. doi:10.1111/j.1528-1167.2007.01246.x
15. Jones NC, Kumar G, O'Brien TJ, Morris MJ, Rees SM, Salzberg MR. Anxiolytic effects of rapid amygdala kindling, and the influence of early life experience in rats. *Behav Brain Res* (2009) 203:81–7. doi:10.1016/j.bbr.2009.04.023
16. Kumar G, Jones NC, Morris MJ, Rees S, O'Brien TJ, Salzberg MR. Early life stress enhancement of limbic epileptogenesis in adult rats: mechanistic insights. *PLoS One* (2011) 6:e24033. doi:10.1371/journal.pone.0024033
17. Lupien SJ, McEwen BS, Gunnar MR, Heim C. Effects of stress throughout the lifespan on the brain, behaviour and cognition. *Nat Rev Neurosci* (2009) 10:434–45. doi:10.1038/nrn2639
18. Lai MC, Huang LT. Effects of early life stress on neuroendocrine and neurobehavior: mechanisms and implications. *Pediatr Neonatol* (2011) 52:122–9. doi:10.1016/j.pedneo.2011.03.008
19. Lucassen PJ, Naninck EFG, Van Goudoever JB, Fitzsimons C, Joëls M, Korosi A. Perinatal programming of hippocampal structure and function; emerging roles of stress, neurogenesis, epigenetics and early nutrition. *Trends Neurosci* (2013) 36(11):621–31. doi:10.1016/j.tins.2013.08.002
20. Carr CP, Martins CM, Stingel AM, Lemgruber VB, Juruena MF. The role of early life stress in adult psychiatric disorders: a systematic review according to childhood trauma subtypes. *J Nerv Ment Dis* (2013) 201:1007–20. doi:10.1097/NMD.0000000000000049
21. Loi M, Koricka S, Lucassen PJ, Joëls M. Age- and sex-dependent effects of early life stress on hippocampal neurogenesis. *Front Endocrinol* (2014) 5:13. doi:10.3389/fendo.2014.00013
22. Joëls M. Stress, the hippocampus, and epilepsy. *Epilepsia* (2009) 50:586–97. doi:10.1111/j.1528-1167.2008.01902.x
23. Maguire J, Salpekar JA. Stress, seizures, and hypothalamic-pituitary-adrenal axis targets for the treatment of epilepsy. *Epilepsy Behav* (2013) 26:352–62. doi:10.1016/j.yebeh.2012.09.040
24. Bender RA, Soleymani SV, Brewster AL, Nguyen ST, Beck H, Mathern GW, et al. Enhanced expression of a specific hyperpolarization-activated cyclic nucleotide-gated cation channel (HCN) in surviving dentate gyrus granule cells of human and experimental epileptic hippocampus. *J Neurosci* (2003) 23:6826–36.
25. Lemmens EM, Lubbers T, Schijns OE, Beuls EA, Hoogland G. Gender differences in febrile seizure-induced proliferation and survival in the rat dentate gyrus. *Epilepsia* (2005) 46:1603–12. doi:10.1111/j.1528-1167.2005.00252.x
26. Kwak SE, Kim JE, Kim SC, Kwon OS, Choi SY, Kang TC. Hyperthermic seizure induces persistent alteration in excitability of the dentate gyrus in immature rats. *Brain Res* (2008) 1216:1–15. doi:10.1016/j.brainres.2008.04.026
27. Notenboom RG, Ramakers GM, Kamal A, Spruijt BM, de Graan PN. Long-lasting modulation of synaptic plasticity in rat hippocampus after early-life complex febrile seizures. *Eur J Neurosci* (2010) 32:749–58. doi:10.1111/j.1460-9568.2010.07321.x
28. Raijmakers M, Clynen E, Smisdom N, Nelissen S, Brône B, Rigo JM, et al. Experimental febrile seizures increase dendritic complexity of newborn dentate granule cells. *Epilepsia* (2016) 57:717–26. doi:10.1111/epi.13357
29. Joëls M. Role of corticosteroid hormones in the dentate gyrus. *Prog Brain Res* (2007) 163:355–70. doi:10.1016/S0079-6123(07)63021-0
30. Dubé CM, Brewster AL, Richichi C, Zha Q, Baram TZ. Fever, febrile seizures and epilepsy. *Trends Neurosci* (2007) 30:490–6. doi:10.1016/j.tins.2007.07.006
31. Dubé CM, Brewster AL, Baram TZ. Febrile seizures: mechanisms and relationship to epilepsy. *Brain Dev* (2009) 31:366–71. doi:10.1016/j.braindev.2008.11.010
32. Baram TZ, Gerth A, Schultz L. Febrile seizures: an appropriate-aged model suitable for long-term studies. *Brain Res Dev Brain Res* (1997) 98:265–70. doi:10.1016/S0165-3806(96)00190-3
33. van Gassen KL, Hessel EV, Ramakers GM, Notenboom RG, Wolterink-Donselaar IG, Brakkee JH, et al. Characterization of febrile seizures and febrile seizure susceptibility in mouse inbred strains. *Genes Brain Behav* (2008) 7:578–86. doi:10.1111/j.1601-183X.2008.00393.x
34. Hessel EV, van Gassen KL, Wolterink-Donselaar IG, Stienen PJ, Fernandes C, Brakkee JH, et al. Phenotyping mouse chromosome substitution strains reveal multiple QTLs for febrile seizure susceptibility. *Genes Brain Behav* (2009) 8:248–55. doi:10.1111/j.1601-183X.2008.00466.x
35. Dubé C, Richichi C, Bender RA, Chung G, Litt B, Baram TZ. Temporal lobe epilepsy after experimental prolonged febrile seizures: prospective analysis. *Brain* (2006) 129:911–22. doi:10.1093/brain/awl018
36. Koyama R, Tao K, Sasaki T, Ichikawa J, Miyamoto D, Muramatsu R, et al. GABAergic excitation after febrile seizures induces ectopic granule cells and adult epilepsy. *Nat Med* (2012) 18:1271–8. doi:10.1038/nm.2850
37. Tao K, Ichikawa J, Matsuki N, Ikegaya Y, Koyama R. Experimental febrile seizures induce age-dependent structural plasticity and improve memory in mice. *Neuroscience* (2016) 318:34–44. doi:10.1016/j.neuroscience.2016.01.011
38. Behr J, Lyson KJ, Mody I. Enhanced propagation of epileptiform activity through the kindled dentate gyrus. *J Neurophysiol* (1998) 79:1726–32. doi:10.1152/jn.1998.79.4.1726
39. Hsu D. The dentate gyrus as a filter or gate: a look back and a look ahead. *Prog Brain Res* (2007) 163:601–13. doi:10.1016/S0079-6123(07)63032-5
40. Cameron HA, McKay RD. Adult neurogenesis produces a large pool of new granule cells in the dentate gyrus. *J Comp Neurol* (2001) 435:406–17. doi:10.1002/cne.1040
41. Parent JM, Yu TW, Leibowitz RT, Geschwind DH, Sloviter RS, Lowenstein DH. Dentate granule cell neurogenesis is increased by seizures and contributes to aberrant network reorganization in the adult rat hippocampus. *J Neurosci* (1997) 17:3727–38.
42. Parent JM, Valentin VV, Lowenstein DH. Prolonged seizures increase proliferating neuroblasts in the adult rat subventricular zone-olfactory bulb pathway. *J Neurosci* (2002) 22:3174–88.
43. Bielefeld P, van Vliet EA, Gorter JA, Lucassen PJ, Fitzsimons CP. Different subsets of newborn granule cells: a possible role in epileptogenesis? *Eur J Neurosci* (2014) 39(1):1–11. doi:10.1111/ejn.12387
44. Danzer SC. Depression, stress, epilepsy and adult neurogenesis. *Exp Neurol* (2012) 233:22–32. doi:10.1016/j.expneurol.2011.05.023
45. Pillai AG, de Jong D, Kanatsou S, Krugers H, Knapman A, Heinzmann JM, et al. Dendritic morphology of hippocampal and amygdalar neurons in adolescent mice is resilient to genetic differences in stress reactivity. *PLoS One* (2012) 7:e38971. doi:10.1371/journal.pone.0038971
46. Sholl DA. Dendritic organization in the neurons of the visual and motor cortices of the cat. *J Anat* (1953) 87:387–406.
47. Danscher G. Histochemical demonstration of heavy metals. A revised version of the sulphide silver method suitable for both light and electronmicroscopy. *Histochemistry* (1981) 71:1–16. doi:10.1007/BF00592566
48. Holmes GL, Sarkisian M, Ben-Ari Y, Chevassus-Au-Louis N. Mossy fiber sprouting after recurrent seizures during early development in rats. *J Comp Neurol* (1999) 404:537–53. doi:10.1002/(SICI)1096-9861(19990222)404:4<537::AID-CNE9>3.0.CO;2-#

49. Pasricha N, Joëls M, Karst H. Rapid effects of corticosterone in the mouse dentate gyrus via a nongenomic pathway. *J Neuroendocrinol* (2011) 23:143–7. doi:10.1111/j.1365-2826.2010.02091.x
50. Barriga C, Martin MI, Tabla R, Ortega E, Rodriguez AB. Circadian rhythm of melatonin, corticosterone and phagocytosis: effect of stress. *J Pineal Res* (2001) 30:180–7. doi:10.1034/j.1600-079X.2001.300307.x
51. Malisch JL, Saltzman W, Gomes FR, Rezende EL, Jeske DR, Garland T Jr. Baseline and stress-induced plasma corticosterone concentrations of mice selectively bred for high voluntary wheel running. *Physiol Biochem Zool* (2007) 80:146–56. doi:10.1086/508828
52. Conboy L, Varea E, Castro JE, Sakouhi-Ouertatani H, Calandra T, Lashuel HA, et al. Macrophage migration inhibitory factor is critically involved in basal and fluoxetine-stimulated adult hippocampal cell proliferation and in anxiety, depression, and memory-related behaviors. *Mol Psychiatry* (2011) 16:533–47. doi:10.1038/mp.2010.15
53. Sawyer NT, Escayg A. Stress and epilepsy: multiple models, multiple outcomes. *J Clin Neurophysiol* (2010) 27:445–52. doi:10.1097/WNP.0b013e3181fe0573
54. Lightman SL, Wiles CC, Atkinson HC, Henley DE, Russell GM, Leendertz JA, et al. The significance of glucocorticoid pulsatiliy. *Eur J Pharmacol* (2008) 583:255–62. doi:10.1016/j.ejphar.2007.11.073
55. Jones NC, O'Brien TJ, Carmant L. Interaction between sex and early-life stress: influence on epileptogenesis and epilepsy comorbidities. *Neurobiol Dis* (2014) 72 (Pt B):233–41. doi:10.1016/j.nbd.2014.09.004
56. Represa A, Niguet J, Pollard H, Ben-Ari Y. Cell death, gliosis, and synaptic remodeling in the hippocampus of epileptic rats. *J Neurobiol* (1995) 26:413–25. doi:10.1002/neu.480260313
57. Aronica E, Ravizza T, Zurolo E, Vezzani A. Astrocyte immune responses in epilepsy. *Glia* (2012) 60:1258–68. doi:10.1002/glia.22312
58. Ward AA Jr, Thomas LB, Schmidt RP. Some properties of single epileptic neurones. *Arch Neurol* (1961) 5:301–13. doi:10.1001/archneur.1961.00450150074010
59. Belichenko P, Dahlstrom A, von Essen C, Lindstrom S, Nordborg C, Sourander P. Atypical pyramidal cells in epileptic human cortex: CFLS and 3-D reconstructions. *Neuroreport* (1992) 3:765–8. doi:10.1097/00001756-199209000-00011
60. Multani P, Myers RH, Blume HW, Schomer DL, Sotrel A. Neocortical dendritic pathology in human partial epilepsy: a quantitative Golgi study. *Epilepsia* (1994) 35:728–36. doi:10.1111/j.1528-1157.1994.tb02503.x
61. Nishimura A, Honda N, Sugioka N, Takada K, Shibata N. Evaluation of carbamazepine pharmacokinetic profiles in mice with kainic acid-induced acute seizures. *Biol Pharm Bull* (2008) 31:2302–8. doi:10.1248/bpb.31.2302
62. Gibbs S, Chattopadhyaya B, Desgent S, Awad PN, Clerk-Lamalice O, Levesque M, et al. Long-term consequences of a prolonged febrile seizure in a dual pathology model. *Neurobiol Dis* (2011) 43:312–21. doi:10.1016/j.nbd.2011.02.013
63. Singh SP, He X, McNamara JO, Danzer SC. Morphological changes among hippocampal dentate granule cells exposed to early kindling-epileptogenesis. *Hippocampus* (2013) 23:1309–20. doi:10.1002/hipo.22169
64. Oomen CA, Girardi CE, Cahyadi R, Verbeek EC, Krugers H, Joëls M, et al. Opposite effects of early maternal deprivation on neurogenesis in male versus female rats. *PLoS One* (2009) 4:e3675. doi:10.1371/journal.pone.0003675
65. Swijsen A, Brone B, Rigo JM, Hoogland G. Long-lasting enhancement of GABA(A) receptor expression in newborn dentate granule cells after early-life febrile seizures. *Dev Neurobiol* (2012) 72:1516–27. doi:10.1002/dneu.22016
66. Chen K, Baram TZ, Soltesz I. Febrile seizures in the developing brain result in persistent modification of neuronal excitability in limbic circuits. *Nat Med* (1999) 5:888–94. doi:10.1038/70932
67. Dubé C, Chen K, Eghbal-Ahmadi M, Brunson K, Soltesz I, Baram TZ. Prolonged febrile seizures in the immature rat model enhance hippocampal excitability long term. *Ann Neurol* (2000) 47:336–44. doi:10.1002/1531-8249(200003)47:3<336::AID-ANA9>3.0.CO;2-W
68. Kamal A, Notenboom RG, de Graan PN, Ramakers GM. Persistent changes in action potential broadening and the slow after hyperpolarization in rat CA1 pyramidal cells after febrile seizures. *Eur J Neurosci* (2006) 23:2230–4. doi:10.1111/j.1460-9568.2006.04732.x
69. Ouardouz M, Lema P, Awad PN, Di Cristo G, Carmant L. N-methyl-D-aspartate, hyperpolarization-activated cation current (Ih) and gamma-aminobutyric acid conductances govern the risk of epileptogenesis following febrile seizures in rat hippocampus. *Eur J Neurosci* (2010) 31:1252–60. doi:10.1111/j.1460-9568.2010.07159.x
70. Harms KJ, Dunaevsky A. Dendritic spine plasticity: looking beyond development. *Brain Res* (2007) 1184:65–71. doi:10.1016/j.brainres.2006.02.094
71. Karst H, Berger S, Turiault M, Tronche F, Schutz G, Joëls M. Mineralocorticoid receptors are indispensable for nongenomic modulation of hippocampal glutamate transmission by corticosterone. *Proc Natl Acad Sci U S A* (2005) 102:19204–7. doi:10.1073/pnas.0507572102
72. Karst H, Berger S, Erdmann G, Schutz G, Joëls M. Metaplasticity of amygdalar responses to the stress hormone corticosterone. *Proc Natl Acad Sci U S A* (2010) 107:14449–54. doi:10.1073/pnas.0914381107
73. Diamond DM, Bennett MC, Fleshner M, Rose GM. Inverted-U relationship between the level of peripheral corticosterone and the magnitude of hippocampal primed burst potentiation. *Hippocampus* (1992) 2:421–30. doi:10.1002/hipo.450020409
74. Joëls M. Corticosteroid effects in the brain: U-shape it. *Trends Pharmacol Sci* (2006) 27:244–50. doi:10.1016/j.tips.2006.03.007
75. Pitkanen A, Sutula TP. Is epilepsy a progressive disorder? Prospects for new therapeutic approaches in temporal-lobe epilepsy. *Lancet Neurol* (2002) 1:173–81. doi:10.1016/S1474-4422(02)00073-X
76. Williams PA, White AM, Clark S, Ferraro DJ, Swiercz W, Staley KJ, et al. Development of spontaneous recurrent seizures after kainate-induced status epilepticus. *J Neurosci* (2009) 29:2103–12. doi:10.1523/JNEUROSCI.0980-08.2009
77. Baulac M, Pitkanen A. Research priorities in epilepsy for the next decade – a representative view of the European scientific community. *Epilepsia* (2008) 50:571–8. doi:10.1111/j.1528-1167.2008.01811.x
78. Kelley MS, Jacobs MP, Lowenstein DH; NINDS Epilepsy Benchmark Stewards. The NINDS epilepsy research benchmarks. *Epilepsia* (2009) 50:579–82. doi:10.1111/j.1528-1167.2008.01813.x
79. Pitkanen A. Therapeutic approaches to epileptogenesis – hope on the horizon. *Epilepsia* (2010) 51(Suppl 3):2–17. doi:10.1111/j.1528-1167.2010.02602.x
80. Verity CM, Golding J. Risk of epilepsy after febrile convulsions: a national cohort study. *BMJ* (1991) 303:1373–6. doi:10.1136/bmj.303.6814.1373
81. Annegers JF, Hauser WA, Shirts SB, Kurland LT. Factors prognostic of unprovoked seizures after febrile convulsions. *N Engl J Med* (1987) 316:493–8. doi:10.1056/NEJM198702263160901
82. van Campen JS. *Stress and Childhood Epilepsy [Dissertation/PhD thesis]*. Utrecht: University of Utrecht (2015).

21

Identification of Transmembrane Protease Serine 2 and Forkhead Box A1 as the Potential Bisphenol A Responsive Genes in the Neonatal Male Rat Brain

Takayoshi Ubuka*, Shogo Moriya, Tomoko Soga and Ishwar Parhar

Jeffrey Cheah School of Medicine and Health Sciences, Brain Research Institute Monash Sunway, Monash University Malaysia, Bandar Sunway, Selangor, Malaysia

***Correspondence:**
Takayoshi Ubuka
takayoshi.ubuka@monash.edu

Perinatal exposure of Bisphenol A (BPA) to rodents modifies their behavior in later life. To understand how BPA modifies their neurodevelopmental process, we first searched for BPA responsive genes from androgen and estrogen receptor signaling target genes by polymerase chain reaction array in the neonatal male rat brain. We used a transgenic strain of Wistar rats carrying enhanced green fluorescent protein tagged to gonadotropin-inhibitory hormone (GnIH) promoter to investigate the possible interaction of BPA responsive genes and GnIH neurons. We found upregulation of transmembrane protease serine 2 (*Tmprss2*), an androgen receptor signaling target gene, and downregulation of Forkhead box A1 (*Foxa1*), an ER signaling target gene, in the medial amygdala of male rats that were subcutaneously administered with BPA from day 1 to 3. Tmprss2-immunoreactive (ir) cells were distributed in the olfactory bulb, cerebral cortex, hippocampus, amygdala, and hypothalamus in 3 days old but not in 1-month-old male rats. Density of Tmprss2-ir cells in the medial amygdala was increased by daily administration of BPA from day 1 to 3. Tmprss2 immunoreactivity was observed in 26.5% of GnIH neurons clustered from the ventral region of the ventromedial hypothalamic nucleus to the dorsal region of the arcuate nucleus of 3-day-old male rat hypothalamus. However, *Tmprss2* mRNA expression significantly decreased in the amygdala and hypothalamus of 1-month-old male rats. *Foxa1* mRNA expression was higher in the hypothalamus than the amygdala in 3 days old male rats. Intense Foxa1-ir cells were only found in the peduncular part of lateral hypothalamus of 3-day-old male rats. Density of Foxa1-ir cells in the hypothalamus was decreased by daily administration of BPA from day 1 to 3. *Foxa1* mRNA expression in the hypothalamus also significantly decreased at 1 month. These results suggest that BPA disturbs the neurodevelopmental process and behavior of rats later in their life by modifying *Tmprss2* and *Foxa1* expressions in the brain.

Keywords: transmembrane protease serine 2, forkhead box A1, androgen receptor, estrogen receptor, polymerase chain reaction array, gonadotropin-inhibitory hormone neurons

INTRODUCTION

Bisphenol A (BPA) is an organic synthetic compound widely used to make polycarbonate plastics and epoxy resins utilized in reusable food and drink containers and inner lining of cans and bottles (1). Hydrolysis of the ester-bond linking BPA can occur at high temperature, and BPA can be leached out into food and beverages. Fetuses or young animals during their developmental stages are thought to be susceptible to BPA exposure than adults (2). Therefore, detectable level of BPA in 88% of human cord blood samples (3) generated social concerns about the effect of BPA on the fetuses.

Dodds and Lawson were the first to show the estrogenic property of BPA (4). However, the estrogenic effect of BPA is 10,000 times less potent than estradiol-17β shown by uterine vascular permeability assay in ovariectomized mice (5). Similar level of agonistic activity of BPA to estrogen receptor (ER) was shown in yeast expressing human estrogen or androgen receptor (AR) (6). On the other hand, BPA is a potent ligand for the non-classic membrane bound G protein-coupled receptor for estrogen (GPR30) (7, 8). BPA did not have an agonistic activity but had an antagonistic activity to AR in the same yeast-based assay (6). Stronger antagonistic activity of BPA to human AR was shown in an African monkey kidney cell line (9). It is also known that BPA can disturb steroidogenesis by interfering the activity of steroidogenic enzymes, such as CYP450scc, 3βHSD, and CYP450arom (10). Perera et al. (11) examined the association between prenatal BPA exposure and child behavior. They found that high prenatal BPA exposure was associated with higher emotionally reactive and aggressive behavior syndromes in boys and lower anxious/depressed and aggressive behavior in girls (11). There are numerous studies showing the effect of perinatally administered BPA on social behavior of rodents. BPA exposure during pregnancy increased display of nose-to-nose contacts, play solicitations, and approaches in both sexes (12). Administration of BPA during pregnancy or lactation increased defensive behavior in male and sexual behavior in female rats (13). In the other study, BPA exposed males during gestation and lactation showed persistent deficits in sexual behavior in adulthood (14).

To find BPA responsive genes in the brain mediating its effect on social behavior, we first focused on amygdala, because amygdala is the integrative center for the processing of emotion, which is pivotal for social behavior. It is thought that deficits in the development of amygdala may cause autism, a neurodevelopmental disorder that is characterized by impaired social interaction (the amygdala theory of autism) (15). It is also known that these brain nuclei express ARs and ERs and abnormally enlarge in autism infants (16). We subcutaneously administered a reference dose of BPA (50 μg/kg BW/day) determined by United States Environmental Protection Agency (EPA, www.epa.gov/iris/subst/0356.htm) to neonatal male transgenic rats carrying enhanced green fluorescent protein tagged to gonadotropin-inhibitory hormone [EGFP-GnIH (17)] promoter from day 1 to 3 and differential expressions of AR and ER signaling target genes in the medial amygdala were analyzed by polymerase chain reaction (PCR) array. GnIH is a hypothalamic neuropeptide that decreases gonadotropin secretion directly acting on the pituitary or by decreasing the activity of gonadotropin-releasing hormone (GnRH) neurons (18, 19). Recent studies have shown that GnIH neurons also decrease motivated behavior (20, 21). We found upregulation of transmembrane protease serine 2 (*Tmprss2*) and downregulation of Forkhead box A1 (*Foxa1*) mRNAs in the amygdala by BPA exposure. We further studied the location of Tmprss2 and Foxa1 immunoreactive (ir) cells, effect of BPA on the density of Tmprss2 and Foxa1-ir cells and developmental changes in *Tmprss2* and *Foxa1* mRNA expressions in the male rat brain.

MATERIALS AND METHODS

Animals

EGFP-GnIH Wistar rats (17) were housed under a controlled 12 h light/dark cycle (light on at noon) and the temperature was maintained at 22°C in a specific pathogen free animal facility. All rats had free access to autoclaved food and water. The pups were counted after parturition, weighed, and remained with their biological mother. All procedures were approved by Monash University, Animal Ethics Committee (MARP/2016/037).

PCR Array

Bisphenol A at 50 μg/kg or vehicle (sesame oil) was subcutaneously injected to neonatal male rats after dawn daily from postnatal day 1 (P1) to P3. 2 h after the last injection the rats were deeply anesthetized by Zoletil/Ketamine/Xylazine (Z/K/X) at 13.5 mg/90 μl/kg and brains were collected and stored at −80°C. Medial amygdaloid tissue from both sides of the brain was dissected in a cryostat at −20°C by referring to a rat brain atlas (22). Medial amygdaloid tissues from two male siblings were combined in a tube for homogenization. Total medial amygdaloid tissue samples of six BPA treated rats from three different littermates and six vehicle treated rats from three different littermates were collected. Total RNA was extracted by using an RNA isolation kit (RNeasy mini kit; QIAGEN, Hilden, Germany) and reverse transcribed by using High-Capacity cDNA Reverse Transcription Kit (ThermoFisher SCIENTIFIC, Waltham, MA, USA). Differential gene expression was analyzed by PCR arrays, RT² Profiler™ PCR Array Rat AR Signaling Targets, and RT² Profiler™ PCR Array Rat ER Signaling Targets (QIAGEN). These PCR array kits analyze the expression levels of 84 AR signaling target genes (Table S1 in Supplementary Material) and 84 ER signaling target genes (Table S2 in Supplementary Material). Cbp/p300-interacting transactivator with Glu/Asp-rich carboxy-terminal domain 2 (Cited2, NM_053698), insulin-like growth factor binding protein 5 (Igfbp5, NM_012817), kallikrein B plasma 1 (Klkb1, NM_012725), and myelocytomatosis oncogene (Myc, NM_012603) were analyzed in both assays. Real-time PCR was performed using a StepOnePlus™ Real-Time PCR System (ThermoFisher SCIENTIFIC) with conditions of 95°C for 10 min, 40 cycles of 95°C for 15 s, and 60°C for 1 min, followed by a dissociation step according to the manufacturer's instruction. Expression levels of AR signaling target genes were normalized by the mean expression levels of housekeeping genes (HKGs), actin beta (Actb, NM_031144), Hypoxanthine

TABLE 1 | Effect of Bisphenol A (BPA) on androgen receptor (AR) and estrogen receptor (ER) signaling target gene expression in the medial amygdala of neonatal male rats.

AR signaling target genes			**ER signaling target genes**		
Gene symbol	**Fold changes**	***P* value**	**Gene symbol**	**Fold changes**	***P* value**
Abcc4	1.10	0.627	Adora1	1.09	0.735
Abhd2	1.12	0.508	Ahr	1.11	0.837
Acsl3	0.99	0.913	Akap1	1.23	0.424
Adamts1	0.91	0.751	Apbb1	1.11	0.665
Aldh1a3	0.89	0.646	Bcar1	1.13	0.634
Appbp2	0.99	0.944	Bcl2l1	1.08	0.634
Ar	0.95	0.434	Bdnf	1.07	0.810
Atad2	1.13	0.655	Bmp4	0.89	0.673
Camkk2	1.14	0.191	Bmp7	6.46	0.585
Cenpn	0.98	0.948	Brca1	0.62	0.0541
Cited2	1.11	0.696	C3	1.00	0.925
Ackr3	1.01	0.929	Cav1	1.06	0.719
Cyp2u1	1.00	0.897	Ccl12	0.87	0.916
Dhcr24	1.21	0.387	Ccnd1	0.98	0.944
Eaf2	0.56	0.0645	Cited2	1.26	0.526
Elk1	1.14	0.391	Ckb	0.97	0.853
Ell2	1.01	0.935	Ctgf	0.76	0.359
Ern1	1.21	0.392	Ctsd	1.06	0.899
Errfi1	1.16	0.564	Cyp19a1	1.01	0.975
Fam105a	0.99	0.832	Cyp1a1	–	–
Fkbp5	1.08	0.571	Ebag9	15.05	0.266
Fos	0.80	0.252	Efna5	1.27	0.257
Fzd5	0.99	0.795	Egr3	0.88	0.651
Gucy1a3	1.13	0.222	Erbb2	1.19	0.521
Herc3	1.01	0.974	Erbb3	1.52	0.992
Hpgd	1.17	0.482	Esr1	1.21	0.515
Igf1r	1.10	0.564	Esr2	0.86	0.606
Igfbp5	0.96	0.753	Fos	0.79	0.351
Irs2	1.08	0.733	Foxa1	0.32	0.0147*
Jun	1.08	0.639	Fst	0.97	0.814
Klk1c2	2.43	0.135	G6pd	1.11	0.599
Klk4	0.95	0.994	Gper1 G	1.06	0.791
Klkb1	–	–	Hsp90aa1	0.96	0.731
Krt8	1.06	0.931	Igf1	0.86	0.503
Lama1	0.90	0.304	Igfbp4	1.51	0.164
Lifr	0.90	0.545	Igfbp5	0.98	0.867
Lrig1	1.00	0.975	Irs1	1.12	0.629
Lrrfip2	1.03	0.854	Junb	0.99	0.790
Maf	1.09	0.692	Klkb1	–	–
Map7d1	1.01	0.926	L1cam	1.02	0.994
Mme	1.00	0.957	Lgals1	1.01	0.883
Mt2A	1.15	0.563	Lpl	1.02	0.890
Myc	1.23	0.286	Ltbp1	0.89	0.549
Ncapd3	1.00	0.990	Maff	0.71	0.473
Ndrg1	1.27	0.127	Med1	1.07	0.844
Nfkb1	1.05	0.866	Mmp9	2.81	0.357
Nfkb2	0.95	0.816	Mta1	1.06	0.678
Nfkbia	1.01	0.773	Myc	1.33	0.348
Nkx3-1	0.64	0.102	Nab2	1.28	0.685
Orm1	–	–	Ncoa2	1.01	0.979
Pak1ip1	1.11	0.0870	Ncoa3	1.01	0.969
Pgc	–	–	Ncor1	0.81	0.285
Pias1	1.10	0.789	Ncor2	0.98	0.888
Pik3r3	1.07	0.794	Nov	0.89	0.450
Pmepa1	1.14	0.489	Nr0b1	0.84	0.534
Ppap2a	0.92	0.341	Nr0b2	–	–
Rab4a	0.99	0.901	Nr2f6	1.07	0.787
Rel	0.80	0.131	Nr3c1	0.93	0.775
Rela	0.97	0.788	Nr5a2	1.33	0.703
Ripk4	1.01	0.888	Nrip1	1.21	0.467
Sgk1	1.18	0.369	Nrp1	1.39	0.285
Slc26a2	1.04	0.801	Pdzk1	1.02	0.987
Slc45a3	0.75	0.509	Pelp1	0.95	0.650
Sms	0.98	0.685	Pgr	0.71	0.397
Snai2	0.79	0.328	Phb2	1.16	0.178
Sord	0.97	0.896	Ptch1	1.14	0.725
Sp1	1.06	0.692	Ptgs2	1.43	0.504
Spdef	1.15	0.475	Rala	1.06	0.587
Srf	1.12	0.564	Rara	1.27	0.548
Steap4	0.61	0.302	S100a6	0.87	0.539
Stk39	0.93	0.560	Safb	1.05	0.831
Tbc1d8	1.01	0.876	Snai1	1.15	0.725
Tiparp	1.56	0.988	Socs3	1.04	0.885
Tmprss2	2.17	0.0449*	Spp1	0.74	0.650
Tpd52	1.03	0.862	Tff1	–	–
Trib1	1.09	0.715	Tgfa	0.99	0.993
Tsc22d1	1.03	0.370	Tgfb3	1.16	0.466
Tsc22d3	1.12	0.587	Thbs1	1.05	0.861
Vapa	0.99	0.942	Vdr	1.15	0.686
Vipr1	0.96	0.821	Vegfa	1.14	0.719
Wipi1	1.08	0.655	Wisp2	1.01	0.974
Zbtb10	1.10	0.305	Wnt4	0.99	0.997
Zbtb16	0.99	0.889	Wnt5a	1.04	0.804
Zfp189	1.02	0.925	Xbp1	1.07	0.808

Fold changes: ratio of the average of BPA group (n = 3, two siblings in one sample) to control group (n = 3, two siblings in one sample).
–, under detectable.
**P < 0.05 by Student's t-test.*

phosphoribosyltransferase 1 (Hprt1, NM_012583), lactate dehydrogenase A (Ldha, NM_017025), and ribosomal protein large P1 (Rplp1, NM_001007604) using the ΔΔCt method. Expression levels of ER signaling target genes were normalized by the mean expression levels of Hprt1 and Rplp1, which were selected from the HKGs by the software based on their consistent expression levels within all samples. Ct cut-off was set to 35 in both assays and treated as undetectable.

Real-Time PCR

Five P3 male brains and five P35 male brains were collected under deep anesthesia by Z/K/X at 13.5 mg/90 µl/kg and stored at −80°C. Amygdala, hypothalamus, and telencephalon excluding amygdala and hippocampus were collected in a cryostat at −20°C. Tissues were homogenized in TRIzol™ Reagent (ThermoFisher SCIENTIFIC) and total RNA was extracted by chloroform. Total RNA was reverse transcribed by using High-Capacity cDNA Reverse Transcription Kit (ThermoFisher SCIENTIFIC). Expression levels of *Rattus norvegicus* Tmprss2 mRNA (NM_130424.3) and Foxa1 mRNA (NM_012742.1) were measured using Rplp1 mRNA (NM_001007604.2) as a reference HKG. Real-time PCR was performed using SensiFAST SYBR Master Mix (BioLine Reagent, London, United Kingdom) and primers (Tmprss2 forward: 5′-CACCTGCCATCCACATACAG-3′, reverse: 5′-CCAGAACTTCCAAAGCAAGC-3′; Foxa1 forward:

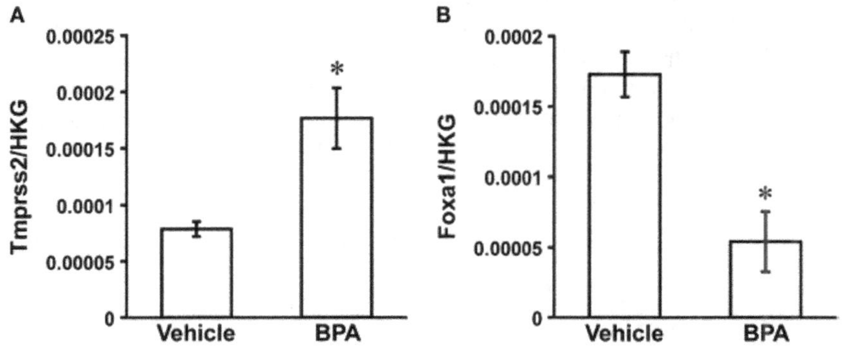

FIGURE 1 | Effect of Bisphenol A (BPA) administration on Tmprss2 and Foxa1 gene expression in the neonatal male rat medial amygdala. **(A)** Effect of BPA administration on the ratio of Tmprss2 gene expression level relative to housekeeping gene (HKG). Each column and the vertical line represent the mean ± SEM (n = 3 samples, both sides of medial amygdala of two male siblings in one sample). $^{*}P < 0.05$, vehicle vs. BPA by Student's t-test. **(B)** Effect of BPA administration on the ratio of Foxa1 gene expression level relative to HKG. Each column and the vertical line represent the mean ± SEM (n = 3 samples, both sides of medial amygdala of two male siblings in one sample). $^{*}P < 0.05$, vehicle vs. BPA by Student's t-test.

5′-GGAGGCCTACTCCTCTGTCC-3′, reverse: 5′-TTGGCGTA GGACATGTTGAA-3′; Rplp1 forward: 5′-GACGGTCACGGA GGATAAGA-3′,reverse:5′-GCAGATGAGGCTTCCAATGT-3′). Real-time PCR was performed using a StepOnePlus™ Real-Time PCR System (ThermoFisher SCIENTIFIC) with conditions of 95°C for 2 min, 40 cycles of 95°C for 5 s, and 60°C for 30 s, followed by a dissociation step. The levels of each mRNA were normalized to Rplp1 mRNA using the ΔΔCt method.

Immunohistochemistry and Fluorescent Microscopy

Immunohistochemistry was performed to investigate the location of Tmprss2 and Foxa1 protein in P3 male rat brains using rabbit monoclonal anti-TMPRSS2 antibody (EPR3861; abcam, Cambridge, United Kingdom) and anti-FOXA1 antibody (EPR10881: abcam). Briefly, five P3 male rats' brains were collected in 4% paraformaldehyde (PFA) under deep anesthetized by Z/K/X at 13.5 mg/90 µl/kg. After 5 days in 4% PFA at 4°C, brains were soaked in 30% sucrose in 0.1 M phosphate buffer at 4°C until they sank. Brains were kept at −80°C until sectioning at 20 µm thickness on a cryostat at −20°C. Sections were incubated in 0.3% H_2O_2 in 20% methanol in 0.01 M phosphate buffered saline (PBS; pH 7.0) for 20 min to suppress endogenous peroxidase activity. Sections were then washed three times in PBS and incubated overnight at 4°C in the primary antibody at concentrations of 1:300 for anti-TMPRSS2 antibody and 1:200 for anti-FOXA1 antibody in blocking solution (0.5% Triton X, 2% normal goat serum in PBS). The next day, three subsequent washes in PBS were followed by incubation in biotinylated goat anti-rabbit IgG at 1:500 in blocking solution for 40 min. After the sections were washed in PBS three times, they were then incubated for 45 min in avidin–biotin complex (Vectastain Elite Kit, Vector, Burlingame, CA, USA) in blocking solution. The resulting complex was visualized by 3,3-diaminobenzidine after the sections were washed three times in PBS and rinsed in 0.05 M Tris–HCl buffer (pH 7.5). Immunohistochemistry without the primary antibodies served as control. The location of the immunoreactivities was identified by Nissl staining of the adjacent sections.

Number of Tmprss2-ir cells in the medial amygdala was counted in three 100 µm grids and averaged for each P3 male rat that were subcutaneously injected with BPA at 50 µg/kg/day (n = 5) or vehicle (n = 4) from P1 to P3. Number of Foxa1-ir cells in the hypothalamus was counted in three 100 µm grids and averaged for each P3 male rat that were subcutaneously injected with BPA at 50 µg/kg/day (n = 4) or vehicle (n = 4) from P1 to P3.

Co-localization of Tmprss2 or Foxa1 immunoreactivity and GnIH-EGFP was studied using a fluorescent microscope with bright field function. The secondary antibody (biotinylated goat anti-rabbit IgG) for immunohistochemistry was used at 1:200 to investigate the co-localization of Tmprss2 or Foxa1 and GnIH-EGFP.

Statistics

Differential expression of AR and ER signaling target genes in the medial amygdala, number of Tmprss2-ir cells in the medial amygdala, and number of Foxa1-ir cells in the hypothalamus between BPA administered male rats and control rats were analyzed by Student's t-test. Differential expression of Tmprss2 and Foxa1 in the amygdala, hypothalamus, and telencephalon excluding amygdala and hippocampus in P3 and P35 male rat brains was analyzed by one-way ANOVA followed by Fisher's protected least significant difference test.

RESULTS

Effect of BPA on AR and ER Signaling Target Gene Expression in the Medial Amygdala of Neonatal Male Rats

Differential expression of AR and ER signaling target genes in the medial amygdala by BPA administration was analyzed in neonatal male rats. Klkb1 (NM_012725), orosomucoid 1 (Orm1, NM_053288), and progastricsin (pepsinogen C) (Pgc, NM_133284) were undetectable within the 84 AR signaling target genes, and cytochrome P450 family 1 subfamily a polypeptide 1 (Cyp1a1, NM_012540), Klkb1 (NM_012725), nuclear receptor subfamily 0 group B member 2 (Nr0b2, NM_057133) were undetectable within the 84 ER signaling target genes (**Table 1**). Genes analyzed in both assays (Cited2, Igfbp5, Klkb1, Myc) produced similar results in terms of detectability, fold changes by BPA treatment, and *P* values by Student's *t*-test (**Table 1**).

An AR signaling target gene, Tmprss2 (NM_130424) was the only gene that was significantly increased in the medial amygdala of neonatal male rats by BPA treatment (fold change 2.17, $P = 0.0449$; **Table 1**; **Figure 1A**). An ER signaling target gene, Foxa1 (NM_012742) was the only gene that decreased significantly in the medial amygdala of neonatal male rats by BPA treatment (fold change 0.32, $P = 0.0147$; **Table 1**; **Figure 1B**).

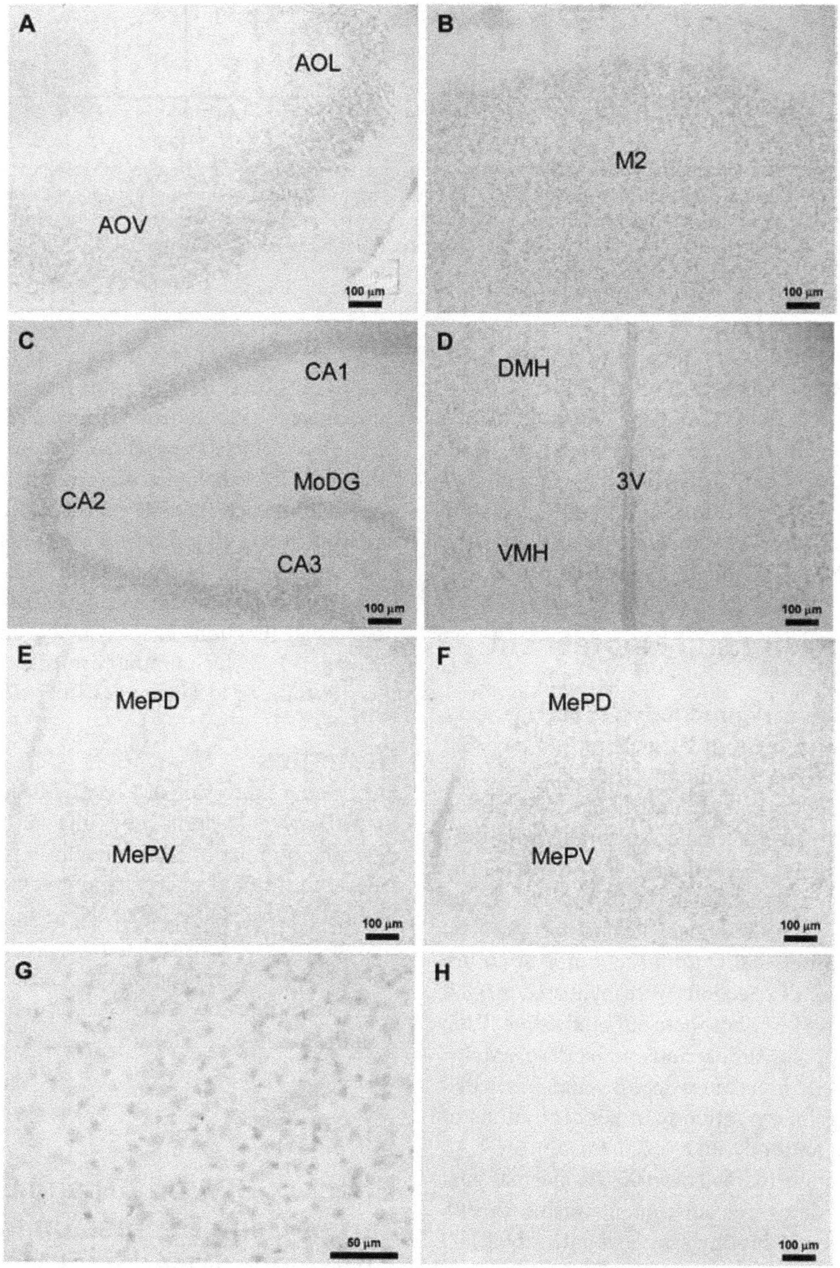

FIGURE 2 | Location of Tmprss2-immunoreactive cells in the neonatal male rat brain. **(A)** Tmprss2-immunoreactive (ir) cells in the olfactory bulb of Bisphenol A (BPA) treated P3 rat. AOL, anterior olfactory nucleus, lateral part. AOV, anterior olfactory nucleus, ventral part. **(B)** Tmprss2-ir cells in the secondary motor cortex (M2) of BPA treated P3 rat. **(C)** Tmprss2-ir cells in the hippocampus of BPA treated P3 rat. CA1, field CA1 of the hippocampus; CA2, field CA2 of the hippocampus; CA3, field CA3 of the hippocampus; MoDG, molecular layer of the dentate gyrus. **(D)** Tmprss2-ir cells in the hypothalamus of BPA treated P3 rat. DMH, dorsomedial hypothalamic area; VMH, ventromedial hypothalamic area; 3V, third ventricle. **(E)** Tmprss2-ir cells in the amygdala of vehicle treated P3 rat. MePD, medial amygdaloid nucleus, posterodorsal part; MePV, medial amygdaloid nucleus, posteroventral part. **(F)** Tmprss2-ir cells in the amygdala of BPA treated P3 rat. **(G)** Higher magnification of MePV of BPA treated P3 rat **(F)**. **(H)** Immunohistochemistry without the first antibody showed no immunoreactive cellular structure.

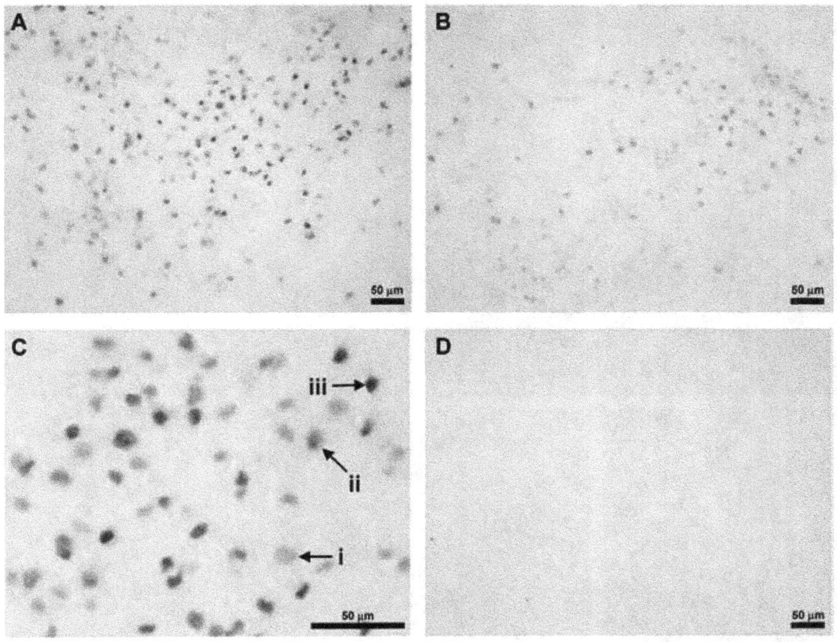

FIGURE 3 | Location of Foxa1-immunoreactive cells in the neonatal male rat brain. **(A)** Foxa1-ir cells in the peduncular part of lateral hypothalamus (PLH) of vehicle treated P3 rat. **(B)** Foxa1-ir cells in the PLH of Bisphenol A treated P3 rat. **(C)** Higher magnification of Foxa1-ir cells in the PLH of vehicle treated P3 rat **(A)**. (i) A cell showing even staining in the cytoplasm and the nucleus. (ii) A cell showing darker staining in the nucleus than the cytoplasm. (iii) A cell showing intense staining only in the nucleus. **(D)** Immunohistochemistry without the first antibody showed no immunoreactive cellular structure.

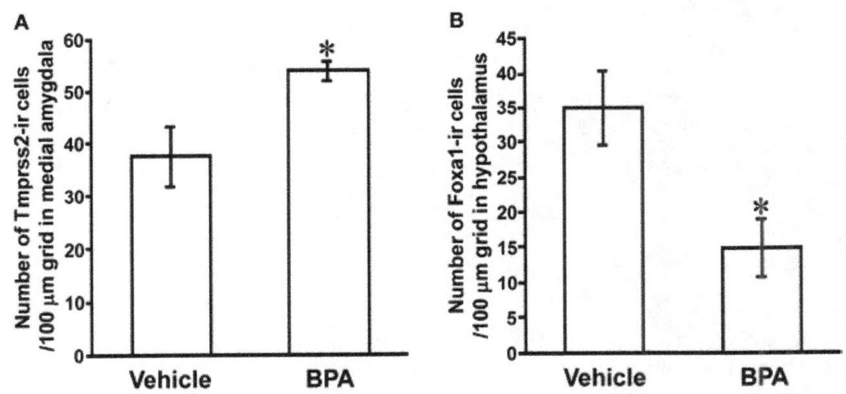

FIGURE 4 | Effect of Bisphenol A (BPA) administration on the number of Tmprss2-ir cells in the medial amygdala and Foxa1-ir cells in the hypothalamus of neonatal male rat. **(A)** Effect of BPA administration on the number of Tmprss2-ir cells in 100 µm grid in the medial amygdala. Each column and the vertical line represent the mean ± SEM. $^*P < 0.05$, vehicle ($n = 4$) vs. BPA ($n = 5$) by Student's *t*-test. **(B)** Effect of BPA administration on the number of Foxa1-ir cells in 100 µm grid in the hypothalamus. Each column and the vertical line represent the mean ± SEM. $^*P < 0.05$, vehicle ($n = 4$) vs. BPA ($n = 4$) by Student's *t*-test.

Distribution of Tmprss2 and Foxa1 Immunoreactive Cell Bodies in Neonatal Male Rat Brain

Location of Tmprss2 and Foxal-ir cell bodies in P3 male rat brains was analyzed by immunohistochemistry. Abundant Tmprss2-ir cell bodies were found in the olfactory bulb (**Figure 2A**), cerebral cortex (**Figure 2B**), hippocampus (**Figure 2C**), hypothalamus (**Figure 2D**), and amygdala (**Figures 2E–G**). Spindle-like Tmprss2-ir cell bodies of about 10 µm in diameter (**Figure 2G**) were consistently found in all brain areas. The weak blur staining of Tmprss2-ir cell bodies (**Figure 2G**) suggested that Tmprss2 exists in neuronal cellular membrane. Immunohistochemistry without the first antibody served as control (**Figure 2H**).

Foxal-ir cell bodies were only found in the peduncular part of lateral hypothalamus (PLH) (**Figures 3A–C**). Three kinds of staining were observed. The first type of staining was even through the cytoplasm and the nucleus, and the cellular diameter was about 10 µm (**Figure 3C**, i). The second type of staining was a weak staining in the cytoplasm and darker staining in the nucleus of about 7 µm in

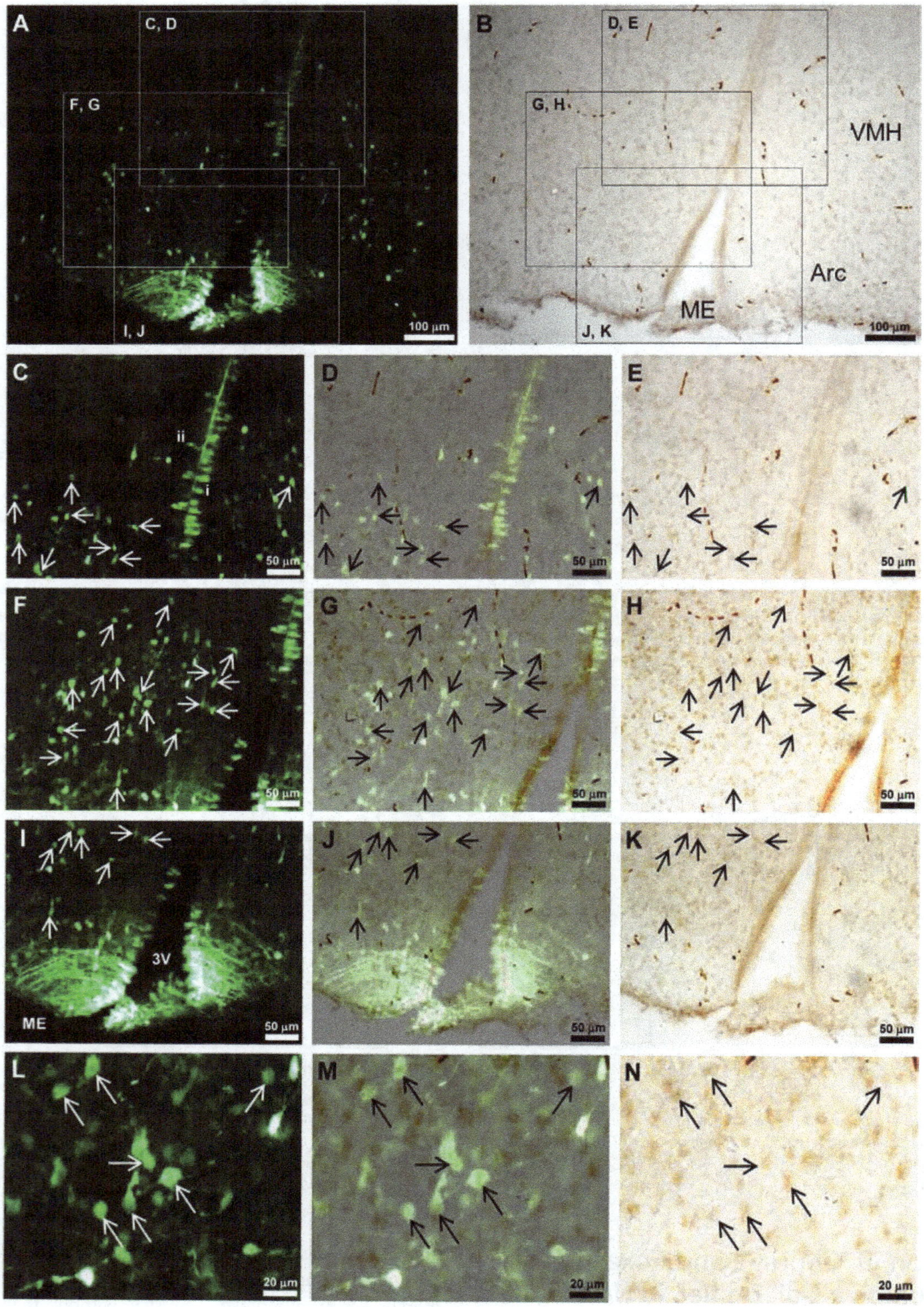

FIGURE 5 | Tmprss2-immunoreactive EGFP-GnIH neurons in the hypothalamus of neonatal male rat. **(A,B)** EGFP-GnIH neurons **(A)** and Tmprss2-immunoreactive (ir) cells **(B)** in the identical field and focus of hypothalamus. VMH, ventromedial hypothalamic area; Arc, arcuate hypothalamic nucleus; ME, median eminence. **(C–E)** Higher magnification of highlighted area in panel **(A,B)** with identical focus. Panel **(D)** is the merged image of **(C,E)**. Arrows show Tmprss2-ir EGFP-GnIH neurons. [**(C)** i] An example of ventricle contacting rod-like EGFP-GnIH cell. [**(C)** ii] An example of EGFP-GnIH cell projecting its process to the ventricle. **(F–H)** Higher magnification of highlighted area in panel **(A,B)** with identical focus. Panel **(G)** is the merged image of **(F,H)**. Arrows show Tmprss2-ir EGFP-GnIH neurons. **(I–K)** Higher magnification of highlighted area in panel **(A,B)** with identical focus. Panel **(J)** is the merged image of **(I,K)**. Arrows show Tmprss2-ir EGFP-GnIH neurons. 3V, third ventricle. **(L–N)** Higher magnification of the central area in panel **(F–H)** with identical focus. Arrows show Tmprss2-ir EGFP-GnIH neurons.

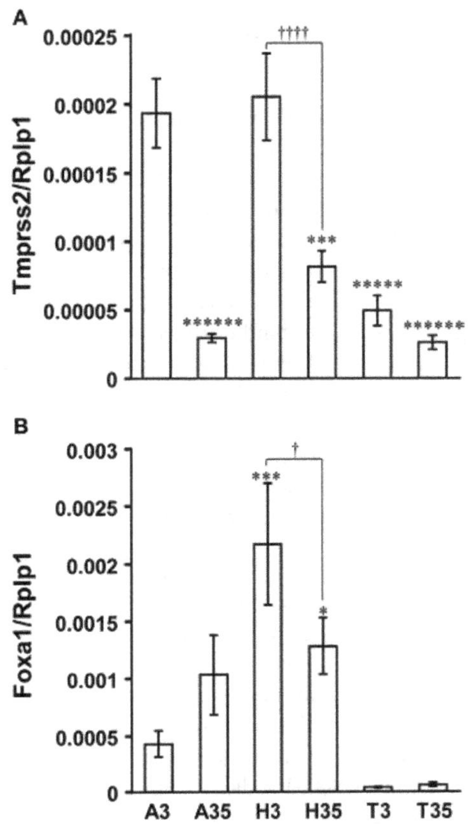

FIGURE 6 | Developmental changes in Tmprss2 and Foxa1 gene expression in the amygdala, hypothalamus, and telencephalon excluding amygdala and hippocampus of male rat. **(A)** The ratio of Tmprss2 gene expression level relative to a housekeeping gene, Rplp1. Each column and the vertical line represent the mean ± SEM (n = 5 samples, one sample from one rat). ******P < 0.000001; *****P < 0.00001, ***P < 0.001 vs. amygdala of P3 male rat (A3) by one-way ANOVA followed by Fisher's protected least significant difference (PLSD) test. ††††P < 0.0001, hypothalamus of P3 male rat (H3) vs. hypothalamus of P35 male rat (H35) by Student's t-test. A35, amygdala of P35 male rat; T3, telencephalon excluding amygdala and hippocampus of P3 male rat; T35, telencephalon excluding amygdala and hippocampus of P35 male rat. **(B)** The ratio of Foxa1 gene expression level relative to Rplp1. Each column and the vertical line represent the mean ± SEM (n = 5 samples, one sample from one rat). ***P < 0.001; *P < 0.05 vs. A3 by one-way ANOVA followed by Fisher's PLSD test. †P < 0.05, H3 vs. H35 by Student's t-test.

diameter (**Figure 3C**, ii). The third type of staining was an intense staining only in the nucleus (**Figure 3C**, iii). Immunohistochemistry without the first antibody served as control (**Figure 3D**).

Effect of BPA Administration on the Number of Tmprss2-ir Cells in the Medial Amygdala and Foxa1-ir Cells in the Hypothalamus

To investigate the effect of BPA on Tmprss2 and Foxal protein expressions, number of Tmprss2-ir cells and Foxal-ir cells were counted in the medial amygdala and hypothalamus, respectively, of P3 male rats that were daily administered with BPA or vehicle from P1 to P3. The number of Tmprss2-ir cells in the medial amygdala was significantly increased by BPA administration (P = 0.032; **Figures 2E,F** and **4A**). On the other hand, the number of Foxal-ir cells in the hypothalamus was significantly decreased by BPA administration (P = 0.042; **Figures 3A,B** and **4B**).

Co-Localization of Tmprss2 and EGFP-GnIH Cells in the Hypothalamus

Because Tmprss2 was highly expressed in the hypothalamus of P3 male rat (**Figure 2D**), where GnIH neuronal cell bodies are located, we investigated if some Tmprss2-ir cells are also EGFP-GnIH positive (17). Abundant EGFP-GnIH cells were observed from the ventral region of ventromedial hypothalamic nucleus (VMH) to the dorsal region of the arcuate nucleus (Arc) as well as along the third ventricle in P3 male rat hypothalamus (**Figures 5A,C,F,I,L**). The diameter of EGFP-GnIH cell bodies in the VMH and Arc was 6–11 μm and had typical GnIH neuronal structure with dendrite or axon-like processes (**Figures 5A,F,L**). 26.5 ± 6.8 (mean ± SD from four different brains) percent of EGFP-GnIH cells in the VMH and Arc were immunoreactive to Tmprss2 antibody (**Figures 5A–N**).

EGFP-GnIH cells along the third ventricle were different between the dorsal population (**Figure 5C**) and the ventral population in the median eminence (ME) (**Figure 5I**). The dorsal population of EGFP-GnIH cells along the third ventricle had two cell types. The first type had a rod-like structure with a diameter of 4–7 μm and they were directly attached to the ventricle (**Figure 5C,i**). The second type was round shape with a diameter of 4–7 μm situated in the sub-ventricular zone and had a protrusion to the ventricle (**Figure 5C,ii**). The ventral population of EGFP-GnIH cells in the ME had an oval shape with a minor axis of 4–7 μm directly contacted the ventricle and sent long processes to the external zone of the ME (**Figure 5I**). No clear cellular co-localization of Tmprss2 immunoreactivity was observed in EGFP-GnIH cells along the third ventricle either in the dorsal population (**Figures 5A–E**) or ventral population in the ME (**Figures 5I–K**).

Developmental Change in Tmprss2 and Foxa1 Gene Expression in the Amygdala, Hypothalamus, and Telencephalon in the Male Rat Brain

Tmprss2 was equally highly expressed in the amygdala and hypothalamus compared with the telencephalon excluding amygdala and hippocampus in P3 male rat brain (**Figure 6A**). However, Tmprss2 expression in the amygdala and hypothalamus decreased significantly in P35 male rat equivalent to Tmprss2 expression levels in the telencephalon (**Figure 6A**).

Foxal was expressed significantly higher in the hypothalamus compared with the amygdala of P3 male rats (**Figure 6B**). Although Foxal expression in the hypothalamus decreased significantly in P35, it was significantly higher than its expression level in the amygdala of P3 male rats (**Figure 6B**). Foxal expression in the telencephalon excluding amygdala and hippocampus was almost under detectable level (**Figure 6B**).

DISCUSSION

To understand how perinatal exposure of BPA can modify the neurodevelopmental process and behavior, we first searched for BPA responsive genes from AR and ER signaling target genes by PCR array in the neonatal male rat medial amygdala that were subcutaneously administered with a reference dose of BPA (50 μg/kg BW/day) determined by United States EPA. We found upregulation of *Tmprss2*, an AR signaling target gene, and down-regulation of *Foxa1*, an ER signaling target gene. Number of Tmprss2-ir cells in the medial amygdala was also increased and Foxa1-ir cells in the hypothalamus was also decreased in the hypothalamus by BPA administration to neonatal male rats.

Tmprss2 encodes a multimeric protein that is translated into an N-terminal short cytoplasmic domain, a transmembrane domain, extracellular low-density lipoprotein receptor A domain, a scavenger receptor cysteine-rich domain, and a serine protease domain at the C-terminal (23). In human tissue, *TMPRSS2* is highly expressed in the small intestine, followed by heart, lung, liver, and small amounts in thymus and prostate. *TMPRSS2* is very highly expressed in the fetal brain but its expression level in the adult brain is minimum (23). *TMPRSS2* was found to be induced by androgen exposure to prostate cancer cells by microarray containing 1,500 cDNAs (24). It was shown that TMPRSS2 mediates androgen-induced prostate cancer cell invasion, tumor growth, and metastasis by stimulating a proteolytic cascade (25).

There is no study investigating the function of Tmprss2 in the brain besides only one study showing its possibility to mediate cancer pain by acting on trigeminal neurons (26). Significant decrease of *Tmprss2* expression in the amygdala and hypothalamus at 1 month of age suggests that Tmprss2 is related to neurogenesis or neuronal differentiation. In humans, TMPRSS2 is highly expressed in the fetus brain but its expression decreases to undetectable level in the adult brain (23). Tmprss2-ir cells were consistently distributed in olfactory bulb, cerebral cortex, hippocampus, amygdala, and hypothalamus in 3 days old male rats. We attempted Tmprss2 immunohistochemistry in 1-month-old and adult rat brains but we could not observe positive staining possibly due to its low expression level. The site of Tmprss2 expression corresponds well with that of AR expression in the rat brain (27, 28), suggesting that Tmprss2 expression is regulated by androgen.

In 3-day-old male rat hypothalamus, Tmprss2 was expressed in 26.5% of EGFP-GnIH neurons in the hypothalamus. EGFP-GnIH neurons were clustered from the ventral region of VMH to the dorsal region of Arc at this age, which was similar to fetal rat brain (29), but unlike GnIH neuronal population in the dorsomedial hypothalamic area in the adult (17, 30, 31). Abundant EGFP-GnIH cells were also found along the third ventricle, but clear expression of Tmprss2 was not observed in this region. EGFP-GnIH cells along the third ventricle can be determined as tanicytes from their morphology. Recent lineage-tracing experiments have shown that tanicytes along the third ventricle are hypothalamic stem cells (32) and postnatally differentiate into neurons and astrocytes in the hypothalamus (33). These results suggest that Tmprs2 is involved in the construction of neural and glial cellular architecture as a transmembrane protease in neonatal rat brain. Previous study has found that daily subcutaneous injection of a reference dose of BPA (50 μg/kg BW/day) to female Wister rats whose GnRH neurons express EGFP from P0 to P3 decreases numbers of GnIH-ir cell bodies, fiber density, and contacts on GnRH neurons and advances puberty at 1 month of age (34).

FOXA1 belongs to the FOXA family of transcriptional regulators (FOXA1, FOXA2, and FOXA3) that play pivotal roles in mammalian development (35). FOXA proteins serve as pioneering factors in the early sequence of the transcriptional regulatory program. FOXA induces nucleosomal rearrangement that facilitates binding of other transcriptional regulators such as sex steroid hormone nuclear receptors (36). FOXA1 serves as a pioneering factor that is required for ERα to bind estrogen-response-element after estrogen stimulation (37). FOXA1 also facilitates AR/chromatin interactions at the regulatory loci near androgen responsive genes (38). It was shown that BPA promotes epithelial mesenchymal transition of ER-negative breast cancer cells through downregulation of FOXA1 by PI3K/Akt activation (39). It is possible that BPA also downregulates Foxa1 by activating PI3K/Akt in the brain.

Foxa1 was highly expressed in the hypothalamus of P3 male rat but significantly decreased in the 1-month-old rat brain, suggesting that Foxa1 is also involved in neuronal differentiation. It was shown that Foxa1 is one of the regulators of neuronal differentiation of midbrain dopamine cells (40). A recent study showed that ablation of Foxa1 causes impaired development of subthalamic nucleus in mice (41), a brain region that is next to PLH where intense Foxa1-ir cells were found in P3 male rats in this study. Foxa1 immunoreactivity in the nucleus of the cells in PLH where AR and ER are also expressed (27) suggests that Foxa1 is involved in transcriptional activities of AR and ER in PLH.

Finally, it was shown that BPA upregulates Tmprss2 and downregulates Foxa1 in the neonatal male rat brain. Location of Tmprss2 and Foxa1-ir cells as well as significant decrease in Tmprss2 and Foxa1 expression in 1-month-old male rat brain suggest that BPA disturbs the neurodevelopmental process and behavior by modifying the expression of Tmprss2 and Foxa1 in the brain.

ETHICS STATEMENT

All procedures were approved by Monash University, Animal Ethics Committee (MARP/2016/037).

AUTHOR CONTRIBUTIONS

TU conceived the project. TU, SM, and TS performed the experiments. TU wrote and IP edited the paper.

ACKNOWLEDGMENTS

We thank Dr. Satoshi Ogawa, Marshita Mohd Idris, Ng Kai We, Rachel Shalini Anthonysamy, Indah Maisarah binti Shani, and Vigneswaran Tambirajah for their technical assistances (Brain Research Institute Monash Sunway, Jeffrey Cheah School of Medicine and Health Sciences, Monash University Malaysia).

REFERENCES

1. Miyagawa S, Sato T, Iguchi T. Bisphenol A. In: Takei Y, Ando H, Tsutsui K, editors. *Handbook of Hormones*. Tokyo: Academic Press (2016). p. 577–8.
2. Gore AC, Martien KM, Gagnidze K, Pfaff D. Implications of prenatal steroid perturbations for neurodevelopment, behavior, and autism. *Endocr Rev* (2014) 35:961–91. doi:10.1210/er.2013-1122
3. Tan BL, Ali Mohd M. Analysis of selected pesticides and alkylphenols in human cord blood by gas chromatograph-mass spectrometer. *Talanta* (2003) 61:385–91. doi:10.1016/S0039-9140(03)00281-9
4. Dodds EC, Lawson W. Synthetic oestrogenic agents without the phenanthrene nucleus. *Nature* (1936) 137:996. doi:10.1038/137996a0
5. Milligan SR, Balasubramanian AV, Kalita JC. Relative potency of xenobiotic estrogens in an acute in vivo mammalian assay. *Environ Health Perspect* (1998) 106:23–6. doi:10.1289/ehp.9810623
6. Sohoni P, Sumpter JP. Several environmental oestrogens are also anti-androgens. *J Endocrinol* (1998) 158:327–39. doi:10.1677/joe.0.1580327
7. Dong S, Terasaka S, Kiyama R. Bisphenol A induces a rapid activation of Erk1/2 through GPR30 in human breast cancer cells. *Environ Pollut* (2011) 159:212–8. doi:10.1016/j.envpol.2010.09.004
8. Wang C, Zhang J, Li Q, Zhang T, Deng Z, Lian J, et al. Low concentration of BPA induces mice spermatocytes apoptosis via GPR30. *Oncotarget* (2017) 8:49005–15. doi:10.18632/oncotarget.16923
9. Xu LC, Sun H, Chen JF, Bian Q, Qian J, Song L, et al. Evaluation of androgen receptor transcriptional activities of bisphenol A, octylphenol and nonylphenol in vitro. *Toxicology* (2005) 216:197–203. doi:10.1016/j.tox.2005.08.006
10. Bloom MS, Mok-Lin E, Fujimoto VY. Bisphenol A and ovarian steroidogenesis. *Fertil Steril* (2016) 106:857–63. doi:10.1016/j.fertnstert.2016.08.021
11. Perera F, Vishnevetsky J, Herbstman JB, Calafat AM, Xiong W, Rauh V, et al. Prenatal bisphenol A exposure and child behavior in an inner-city cohort. *Environ Health Perspect* (2012) 120:1190–4. doi:10.1289/ehp.1104492
12. Wolstenholme JT, Taylor JA, Shetty SR, Edwards M, Connelly JJ, Rissman EF. Gestational exposure to low dose bisphenol A alters social behavior in juvenile mice. *PLoS One* (2011) 6:e25448. doi:10.1371/journal.pone.0025448
13. Farabollini F, Porrini S, Della Seta D, Bianchi F, Dessì-Fulgheri F. Effects of perinatal exposure to bisphenol A on sociosexual behavior of female and male rats. *Environ Health Perspect* (2002) 110(Suppl 3):409–14. doi:10.1289/ehp.02110s3409
14. Jones BA, Shimell JJ, Watson NV. Pre- and postnatal bisphenol A treatment results in persistent deficits in the sexual behavior of male rats, but not female rats, in adulthood. *Horm Behav* (2011) 59:246–51. doi:10.1016/j.yhbeh.2010.12.006
15. Baron-Cohen S, Ring HA, Bullmore ET, Wheelwright S, Ashwin C, Williams SC. The amygdala theory of autism. *Neurosci Biobehav Rev* (2000) 24:355–64. doi:10.1016/S0149-7634(00)00011-7
16. Nordahl CW, Scholz R, Yang X, Buonocore MH, Simon T, Rogers S, et al. Increased rate of amygdala growth in children aged 2 to 4 years with autism spectrum disorders: a longitudinal study. *Arch Gen Psychiatry* (2012) 69:53–61. doi:10.1001/archgenpsychiatry.2011.145
17. Soga T, Kitahashi T, Clarke IJ, Parhar IS. Gonadotropin-inhibitory hormone promoter-driven enhanced green fluorescent protein expression decreases during aging in female rats. *Endocrinology* (2014) 155:1944–55. doi:10.1210/en.2013-1786
18. Tsutsui K, Ubuka T. Gonadotropin-inhibitory hormone. In: Kastin A, editor. *Handbook of Biologically Active Peptides*. London: Academic Press (2013). p. 802–11.
19. Ubuka T, Son YL, Tsutsui K. Molecular, cellular, morphological, physiological and behavioral aspects of gonadotropin-inhibitory hormone. *Gen Comp Endocrinol* (2016) 227:27–50. doi:10.1016/j.ygcen.2015.09.009
20. Ubuka T, Mukai M, Wolfe J, Beverly R, Clegg S, Wang A, et al. RNA interference of gonadotropin-inhibitory hormone gene induces arousal in songbirds. *PLoS One* (2012) 7:e30202. doi:10.1371/journal.pone.0030202
21. Ubuka T, Haraguchi S, Tobari Y, Narihiro M, Ishikawa K, Hayashi T, et al. Hypothalamic inhibition of socio-sexual behaviour by increasing neuroestrogen synthesis. *Nat Commun* (2014) 5:3061. doi:10.1038/ncomms4061
22. Paxinos G, Watson C. *The Rat Brain in Stereotaxic Coordinates*. London: Academic Press (2007).
23. Paoloni-Giacobino A, Chen H, Peitsch MC, Rossier C, Antonarakis SE. Cloning of the TMPRSS2 gene, which encodes a novel serine protease with transmembrane, LDLRA, and SRCR domains and maps to 21q22.3. *Genomics* (1997) 44:309–20. doi:10.1006/geno.1997.4845
24. Lin B, Ferguson C, White JT, Wang S, Vessella R, True LD, et al. Prostate-localized and androgen-regulated expression of the membrane-bound serine protease TMPRSS2. *Cancer Res* (1999) 59:4180–4.
25. Ko CJ, Huang CC, Lin HY, Juan CP, Lan SW, Shyu HY, et al. Androgen-induced TMPRSS2 activates matriptase and promotes extracellular matrix degradation, prostate cancer cell invasion, tumor growth, and metastasis. *Cancer Res* (2015) 75:2949–60. doi:10.1158/0008-5472.CAN-14-3297
26. Lam DK, Dang D, Flynn AN, Hardt M, Schmidt BL. TMPRSS2, a novel membrane-anchored mediator in cancer pain. *Pain* (2015) 156:923–30. doi:10.1097/j.pain.0000000000000130
27. Simerly RB, Chang C, Muramatsu M, Swanson LW. Distribution of androgen and estrogen receptor mRNA-containing cells in the rat brain: an in situ hybridization study. *J Comp Neurol* (1990) 294:76–95. doi:10.1002/cne.902940107
28. Xiao L, Jordan CL. Sex differences, laterality, and hormonal regulation of androgen receptor immunoreactivity in rat hippocampus. *Horm Behav* (2002) 42:327–36. doi:10.1006/hbeh.2002.1822
29. Yano T, Iijima N, Hinuma S, Tanaka M, Ibata Y. Developmental expression of RFamide-related peptides in the rat central nervous system. *Brain Res Dev Brain Res* (2004) 152:109–20. doi:10.1016/j.devbrainres.2004.06.008
30. Hinuma S, Shintani Y, Fukusumi S, Iijima N, Matsumoto Y, Hosoya M, et al. New neuropeptides containing carboxy-terminal RFamide and their receptor in mammals. *Nat Cell Biol* (2000) 2:703–8. doi:10.1038/35036326
31. Ubuka T, Inoue K, Fukuda Y, Mizuno T, Ukena K, Kriegsfeld LJ, et al. Identification, expression, and physiological functions of Siberian hamster gonadotropin-inhibitory hormone. *Endocrinology* (2012) 153:373–85. doi:10.1210/en.2011-1110
32. Rizzoti K, Lovell-Badge R. Pivotal role of median eminence tanycytes for hypothalamic function and neurogenesis. *Mol Cell Endocrinol* (2017) 445:7–13. doi:10.1016/j.mce.2016.08.020
33. Haan N, Goodman T, Najdi-Samiei A, Stratford CM, Rice R, El Agha E, et al. Fgf10-expressing tanycytes add new neurons to the appetite/energy-balance regulating centers of the postnatal and adult hypothalamus. *J Neurosci* (2013) 33:6170–80. doi:10.1523/JNEUROSCI.2437-12.2013
34. Losa-Ward SM, Todd KL, McCaffrey KA, Tsutsui K, Patisaul HB. Disrupted organization of RFamide pathways in the hypothalamus is associated with advanced puberty in female rats neonatally exposed to bisphenol A. *Biol Reprod* (2012) 87:28. doi:10.1095/biolreprod.112.100826
35. Kaestner KH. The FoxA factors in organogenesis and differentiation. *Curr Opin Genet Dev* (2010) 20:527–32. doi:10.1016/j.gde.2010.06.005
36. Augello MA, Hickey TE, Knudsen KE. FOXA1: master of steroid receptor function in cancer. *EMBO J* (2011) 30:3885–94. doi:10.1038/emboj.2011.340
37. Carroll JS, Liu XS, Brodsky AS, Li W, Meyer CA, Szary AJ, et al. Chromosome-wide mapping of estrogen receptor binding reveals long-range regulation requiring the forkhead protein FoxA1. *Cell* (2005) 122:33–43. doi:10.1016/j.cell.2005.05.008
38. Wang Q, Li W, Zhang Y, Yuan X, Xu K, Yu J, et al. Androgen receptor regulates a distinct transcription program in androgen-independent prostate cancer. *Cell* (2009) 138:245–56. doi:10.1016/j.cell.2009.04.056
39. Zhang XL, Wang HS, Liu N, Ge LC. Bisphenol A stimulates the epithelial mesenchymal transition of estrogen negative breast cancer cells via FOXA1 signals. *Arch Biochem Biophys* (2015) 585:10–6. doi:10.1016/j.abb.2015.09.006
40. Metzakopian E, Bouhali K, Alvarez-Saavedra M, Whitsett JA, Picketts DJ, Ang SL. Genome-wide characterisation of Foxa1 binding sites reveals several mechanisms for regulating neuronal differentiation in midbrain dopamine cells. *Development* (2015) 142:1315–24. doi:10.1242/dev.115808
41. Gasser E, Johannssen HC, Rülicke T, Zeilhofer HU, Stoffel M. Foxa1 is essential for development and functional integrity of the subthalamic nucleus. *Sci Rep* (2016) 6:38611. doi:10.1038/srep38611

Permissions

All chapters in this book were first published by Frontiers; hereby published with permission under the Creative Commons Attribution License or equivalent. Every chapter published in this book has been scrutinized by our experts. Their significance has been extensively debated. The topics covered herein carry significant findings which will fuel the growth of the discipline. They may even be implemented as practical applications or may be referred to as a beginning point for another development.

The contributors of this book come from diverse backgrounds, making this book a truly international effort. This book will bring forth new frontiers with its revolutionizing research information and detailed analysis of the nascent developments around the world.

We would like to thank all the contributing authors for lending their expertise to make the book truly unique. They have played a crucial role in the development of this book. Without their invaluable contributions this book wouldn't have been possible. They have made vital efforts to compile up to date information on the varied aspects of this subject to make this book a valuable addition to the collection of many professionals and students.

This book was conceptualized with the vision of imparting up-to-date information and advanced data in this field. To ensure the same, a matchless editorial board was set up. Every individual on the board went through rigorous rounds of assessment to prove their worth. After which they invested a large part of their time researching and compiling the most relevant data for our readers.

The editorial board has been involved in producing this book since its inception. They have spent rigorous hours researching and exploring the diverse topics which have resulted in the successful publishing of this book. They have passed on their knowledge of decades through this book. To expedite this challenging task, the publisher supported the team at every step. A small team of assistant editors was also appointed to further simplify the editing procedure and attain best results for the readers.

Apart from the editorial board, the designing team has also invested a significant amount of their time in understanding the subject and creating the most relevant covers. They scrutinized every image to scout for the most suitable representation of the subject and create an appropriate cover for the book.

The publishing team has been an ardent support to the editorial, designing and production team. Their endless efforts to recruit the best for this project, has resulted in the accomplishment of this book. They are a veteran in the field of academics and their pool of knowledge is as vast as their experience in printing. Their expertise and guidance has proved useful at every step. Their uncompromising quality standards have made this book an exceptional effort. Their encouragement from time to time has been an inspiration for everyone.

The publisher and the editorial board hope that this book will prove to be a valuable piece of knowledge for researchers, students, practitioners and scholars across the globe.

List of Contributors

Jun Zhang and Ping Xu
Department of Neurology, Affiliated Hospital of Zunyi Medical University, Guizhou, China

Xiaowei Qiu, Dongxu Li, Changyin Yu and Zucai Xu
Department of Neurology, Affiliated Hospital of Zunyi Medical University, Guizhou, China
Key Laboratory of Brain Science, Zunyi Medical University, Guizhou, China

Haiqing Zhang, Yixue Gu and Zheng Xiao
Department of Neurology, The First Affiliated Hospital of Chongqing Medical University, Chongqing, China

Jing Wang
Department of Preventive Health Care, Affiliated Hospital of Zunyi Medical University, Guizhou, China

Zhigang Jiang and Yuanzhong Zhou
School of Public Health, Zunyi Medical University, Guizhou, China

Zhanhui Feng
Department of Neurology, Affiliated Hospital of Guizhou Medical University, Guizhou, China

Min Zhong
Department of Neurology, Children's Hospital of Chongqing Medical University, Chongqing, China

Liang He and Yangmei Chen
Department of Neurology, The Second Affiliated Hospital of Chongqing Medical University, Chongqing, China

Wei Li
Department of Neurology, Daping Hospital & Research Institute of Surgery, The Army Military Medical University, Chongqing, China

Yuanyuan Huang
Department of Neurology, Southwest Hospital, The Third Military Medical University (Army Medical University), Chongqing, China

Jing Liu
Department of Neurology, Chongqing Three Gorges Central Hospital, Chongqing, China

Tracy A. Larson
Department of Biology, University of Virginia, Charlottesville, VA, United States

John C. Wingfield
Department of Neurobiology Physiology and Behavior, University of California, Davis, Davis, CA, United States

Douglas W. Wacker
Division of Biological Sciences, School of STEM, University of Washington Bothell, Bothell, WA, United States

George E. Bentley
Department of Integrative Biology, Helen Wills Neuroscience Institute, University of California, Berkeley, Berkeley, CA, United States

Kazuyoshi Tsutsui
Department of Biology, Waseda University, Shinjuku, Japan

Raffaele Nuzzi, Simona Scalabrin and Alice Becco
Eye Clinic, Department of Surgical Sciences, University of Turin, Turin, Italy

Giancarlo Panzica
Laboratory of Neuroendocrinology, Department of Neuroscience Rita Levi-Montalcini, University of Torino, Torino, Italy
Neuroscience Institute Cavalieri-Ottolenghi (NICO), Orbassano, Italy

David M. Dorris
Department of Biological Sciences, North Carolina State University, Raleigh, NC, United States

Jinyan Cao
Department of Biological Sciences, North Carolina State University, Raleigh, NC, United States
W.M. Keck Center for Behavioral Biology, North Carolina State University, Raleigh, NC, United States

Jaime A. Willett
Department of Biological Sciences, North Carolina State University, Raleigh, NC, United States
W.M. Keck Center for Behavioral Biology, North Carolina State University, Raleigh, NC, United States
Graduate Program in Physiology, North Carolina State University, Raleigh, NC, United States

Fengzhen Li
Department of Neurology, First Affiliated Hospital of Xinxiang Medical University, Weihui, China

John Meitzen
Department of Biological Sciences, North Carolina State University, Raleigh, NC, United States
W.M. Keck Center for Behavioral Biology, North Carolina State University, Raleigh, NC, United States
Center for Human Health and the Environment, North Carolina State University, Raleigh, NC, United States
Comparative Medicine Institute, North Carolina State University, Raleigh, NC, United States

Dillon F. Da Fonte, Lei Xing and Vance L. Trudeau
Department of Biology, University of Ottawa, Ottawa, ON, Canada

Chris J. Martyniuk
Department of Physiological Sciences, College of Veterinary Medicine, UF Genetics Institute, University of Florida, Gainesville, FL, United States

Etienne-Emile Baulieu
INSERM UMR 1195, Université Paris-Saclay, Hôpital Le Kremlin Bicêtre, Val de Marne, France

Jie Li
Department of Neurology, First Affiliated Hospital of Xinxiang Medical University, Weihui, China
Xinxiang Medical University, Xinxiang, China

Jianzhao Zhang, Taoyun Ji, Yanan Jiang, Huan Cheng, Wenqiang Ma, Ting Lei, Yao Zhang, Yiwen Jin, Cuijie Wei, Ye Wu, Xingzhi Chang, Xinhua Bao, Yuehua Zhang, Hui Xiong and Yuwu Jiang
Division of Pediatric Neurology, Pediatrics Department, Peking University First Hospital, Beijing, China

Qian Chen, Ping Zheng, Xinna Ji, Shuo Feng and Jian Yang
Department of Pediatric Neurology, Children's Hospital Affiliated to the Capital Institute of Pediatrics, Beijing, China

Haitao Ren
Department of Neurology, Peking Union Medical College Hospital, Chinese Academy of Medical Science, Beijing, China

Daniel J. Tobiansky and Stan B. Floresco
Department of Psychology, University of British Columbia, Vancouver, BC, Canada
Djavad Mowafaghian Centre for Brain Health, University of British Columbia, Vancouver, BC, Canada

Kathryn G. Wallin-Miller
Neuroscience Graduate Program, University of Southern California, Los Angeles, CA, United States

Ruth I. Wood
Department of Integrative Anatomical Sciences, Keck School of Medicine of the University of Southern California, Los Angeles, CA, United States

Kiran K. Soma
Department of Psychology, University of British Columbia, Vancouver, BC, Canada
Djavad Mowafaghian Centre for Brain Health, University of British Columbia, Vancouver, BC, Canada
Department of Zoology, University of British Columbia, Vancouver, BC, Canada

Min Zhang, Wenhui Li, Shuizhen Zhou, Yuanfeng Zhou, Lifei Yu, Ji Wang, Yi Wang and Linmei Zhang
Department of Neurology, Children's Hospital of Fudan University, Shanghai, China

Haowei Yang
Department of Radiology, Children's Hospital of Fudan University, Shanghai, China

Carlton P. Frost, Roxanne M. Hoks and Heather C. Abercrombie
Department of Psychiatry, University of Wisconsin-Madison, Madison, WI, United States

Rasmus M. Birn
Department of Psychiatry, University of Wisconsin-Madison, Madison, WI, United States
Department of Medical Physics, University of Wisconsin-Madison, Madison, WI, United States

M. Elizabeth Meyerand
Department of Medical Physics, University of Wisconsin-Madison, Madison, WI, United States
Department of Biomedical Engineering, University of Wisconsin-Madison, Madison, WI, United States

Erin C. Walsh
Department of Psychiatry, University of North Carolina at Chapel Hill, Chapel Hill, NC, United States

Shanshan Zhang and Ge Tan
Department of Neurology, The First Affiliated Hospital of Chongqing Medical University, Chongqing, China

Dongli Yuan
The Institute of Medical Information, Chongqing Medical University, Chongqing, China

Yuting Jiang, Xin Tian, Yixue Gu and Feng Li
Chongqing Key Laboratory of Neurology, Department of Neurology, the First Affiliated Hospital of Chongqing Medical University, Chongqing, China

Yasushi Hojo
Department of Biochemistry, Faculty of Medicine, Saitama Medical University, Moroyama, Saitama, Japan

Xuefeng Wang
Chongqing Key Laboratory of Neurology, Department of Neurology, the First Affiliated Hospital of Chongqing Medical University, Chongqing, China
Center of Epilepsy, Beijing Institute for Brain Disorders, Beijing, China

Giovanna Ponti
Department of Veterinary Sciences, University of Turin, Grugliasco, Turin, Italy
Neuroscience Institute Cavalieri Ottolenghi (NICO), Orbassano, Turin, Italy

Alice Farinetti, Marilena Marraudino, GianCarlo Panzica and Stefano Gotti
Neuroscience Institute Cavalieri Ottolenghi (NICO), Orbassano, Turin, Italy
Department of Neuroscience "Rita Levi-Montalcini", University of Turin, Turin, Italy

Kathleen M. Munley, Nikki M. Rendon and Gregory E. Demas
Program in Neuroscience, Department of Biology, Center for the Integrative Study of Animal Behavior, Indiana University, Bloomington, IN, United States

Suguru Kawato
Department of Biophysics and Life Sciences, Graduate School of Arts and Sciences, The University of Tokyo, Tokyo, Japan
Department of Urology, Graduate School of Medicine, Juntendo University, Tokyo, Japan
Department of Cognitive Neuroscience, Faculty of Pharma-Science, Teikyo University, Tokyo, Japan

Michelle A. Rensel
The Institute for Society and Genetics, University of California, Los Angeles, Los Angeles, CA, United States
Laboratory of Neuroendocrinology, University of California, Los Angeles, Los Angeles, CA, United States

Jessica A. Ding
Department of Integrative Biology and Physiology, University of California, Los Angeles, Los Angeles, CA, United States

Devaleena S. Pradhan
Laboratory of Neuroendocrinology, University of California, Los Angeles, Los Angeles, CA, United States
Department of Integrative Biology and Physiology, University of California, Los Angeles, Los Angeles, CA, United States

Barney A. Schlinger
Laboratory of Neuroendocrinology, University of California, Los Angeles, Los Angeles, CA, United States
Department of Integrative Biology and Physiology, University of California, Los Angeles, Los Angeles, CA, United States
Department of Ecology and Evolutionary Biology, University of California, Los Angeles, Los Angeles, CA, United States

Ellen V. S. Hessel, Kirsten Bohmbach, Giorgio Rizzi, Sada Lakshmi Turimella, Pierre N. E. de Graan and Marian Joëls
Department of Translational Neuroscience, Brain Center Rudolf Magnus, University Medical Center Utrecht, Utrecht, Netherlands

Kees P. J. Braun
Department of Child Neurology, Brain Center Rudolf Magnus, University Medical Center Utrecht, Utrecht, Netherlands

Jolien S. van Campen
Department of Translational Neuroscience, Brain Center Rudolf Magnus, University Medical Center Utrecht, Utrecht, Netherlands
Department of Child Neurology, Brain Center Rudolf Magnus, University Medical Center Utrecht, Utrecht, Netherlands

Paul J. Lucassen and Gideon F. Meerhoff
Swammerdam Institute for Life Sciences, Center for Neuroscience, University of Amsterdam, Amsterdam, Netherlands

Eduardo H. L. Umeoka
Department of Translational Neuroscience, Brain Center Rudolf Magnus, University Medical Center Utrecht, Utrecht, Netherlands
Neursocience and Behavioral Sciences Department, Ribeirão Preto School of Medicine, University of São Paulo, Ribeirão Preto, Brazil

Takayoshi Ubuka, Shogo Moriya, Tomoko Soga and Ishwar Parhar
Jeffrey Cheah School of Medicine and Health Sciences, Brain Research Institute Monash Sunway, Monash University Malaysia, Bandar Sunway, Selangor, Malaysia

Index

www.ingramcontent.com/pod-product-compliance
Lightning Source LLC
LaVergne TN
LVHW082151200926
848484LV00008B/2142